Brief Contents

An Introduction to Community Health

Brief   ion

James F. Mc   PhD, MPH,
Profe   n State-He
Professor   s, Ball Sta

        t R. Pin
Professor Emeritus, Ball State University

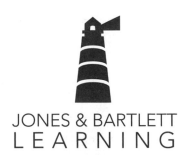

JONES & BARTLETT
LEARNING

World Headquarters
Jones & Bartlett Learning
5 Wall Street
Burlington, MA 01803
978-443-5000
info@jblearning.com
www.jblearning.com

Jones & Bartlett Learning books and products are available through most bookstores and online booksellers. To contact Jones & Bartlett Learning directly, call 800-832-0034, fax 978-443-8000, or visit our website, www.jblearning.com.

Substantial discounts on bulk quantities of Jones & Bartlett Learning publications are available to corporations, professional associations, and other qualified organizations. For details and specific discount information, contact the special sales department at Jones & Bartlett Learning via the above contact information or send an email to specialsales@jblearning.com.

Production Credits
Publisher: William Brottmiller
Executive Editor: Cathy L. Esperti
Editorial Assistant: Agnes Burt
Associate Director of Production: Julie Champagne Bolduc
Production Editor: Jessica Steele Newfell
Senior Marketing Manager: Andrea DeFronzo
VP, Manufacturing and Inventory Control: Therese Connell

Composition: Cenveo Publisher Services
Cover Design: Scott Moden
Director of Photo Research and Permissions: Amy Wrynn
Cover Image: © Denis Cristo/ShutterStock, Inc.
Printing and Binding: Edwards Brothers Malloy
Cover Printing: Edwards Brothers Malloy

To order this product, use ISBN: 978-1-284-02689-4

Library of Congress Cataloging-in-Publication Data
McKenzie, James F., 1948–
  An introduction to community health / by James F. McKenzie and Robert R. Pinger. — Brief ed.
     p. ; cm.
  Abridgement of: An introduction to community health / James F. McKenzie, Robert R. Pinger, Jerome E. Kotecki. 7th ed. c2012.
  Includes bibliographical references and index.
  ISBN 978-1-4496-5150-3 — ISBN 1-4496-5150-X
  I. Pinger, R. R. II. Title.
  [DNLM: 1. Community Health Services—United States. 2. Delivery of Health Care—United States. 3. Environmental Health—United States. 4. Public Health Practice—United States. WA 546 AA1]

  362.1—dc23

                                 2012048915

6048

Printed in the United States of America
17 16 15 14 13   10 9 8 7 6 5 4 3 2 1

Contents

CHAPTER 8   Community Health and Minorities 183

Miguel A. Pérez, PhD, MCHES

CHAPTER 9   Community Mental Health 205

David V. Perkins, PhD

CHAPTER 10   Alcohol, Tobacco, and Other Drugs:
A Community Concern 227

Robert R. Pinger, PhD

CHAPTER 11   Healthcare Delivery
in the United States............................. 253

James F. McKenzie, PhD, MPH, MCHES

Preface

An Introduction to Community Health, Brief Edition (hereafter referred to as the *Brief Edition*) was written in response to requests from adopters of *An Introduction to Community Health* for an abbreviated version. The *Brief Edition* retains many of the features found in the full version—chapter objectives, up-to-date content, marginal definitions of key terms, chapter summaries, review questions, activities, Web activities, and references—but it achieves its brevity through a more concise writing style, a reduction of the historical framework, a reduction in the number and size of tables and figures, the transfer of selected features to the companion website, and the combining of chapters. We believe that students will find the *Brief Edition* easy to read, understand, and use. If they read the chapters carefully and make an honest effort to answer the review questions and complete the activities, we are confident that students will gain a good understanding of the realm of community health. The following is a summary of the key features and pedagogical elements of the *Brief Edition.*

Content

Although essential content has been retained, some examples have been excluded, and explanations of how we have arrived at the current state of affairs have been reduced. For example, the current status of HIV/AIDS in the community may be stated without detailed reference to its past status. Many figures, tables, boxes, and photos have been retained, but others have been shortened or deleted. Also retained are examples of our national health goals and objectives drawn from *Healthy People 2020*. To enhance and facilitate learning, the chapters are organized into three units: Foundations of Community Health, The Nation's Health and Healthcare Delivery, and Environmental Health and Safety.

Chapter Objectives, Review Questions, and Activities

Chapter objectives identify key content and will help students focus on the major points in each chapter. Review questions and activities at the end of each chapter help students achieve the learning objectives and skills that should be mastered through chapter readings.

Key Terms

Boldfaced key terms are defined in the margin when they first appear and again in the glossary at the end of this text. In addition, some words in the text have been italicized for emphasis and are often key terms defined in another chapter.

Chapter Summaries

At the end of each chapter, students will find several bulleted points that review the major concepts contained within the chapter.

Community Health on the Web

The Internet contains a wealth of information about community and public health. The Web activities are presented to encourage students to further explore the chapter's content by visiting relevant websites. These activities recap three concepts or issues from the text in each chapter. The starting point for these activities is the Navigate Companion Website (go.jblearning.com/McKenzieBrief).

Once students are connected to the Navigate Companion Website, they will be provided with activity instructions for further exploration. Animated flashcards, an interactive glossary, and crossword puzzles are also available online. When more up-to-date information becomes available at an assigned website, we are able to immediately edit the exercise to reflect this most recent material.

The Web activities bring to life the content and theory presented in the text, thus furnishing students with a real-world context for understanding community health concepts and issues. The intent of including Web activities with this text is to inspire the students, in real time, to authentically assess and critically think about what they have just read by asking them thought-provoking questions related to the assigned website. By integrating the Web into this text, we have created a dynamic learning environment that is as up-to-date as today's newspaper.

Accompanying Ancillaries

The *Brief Edition* is accompanied by a suite of updated instructor resources, including PowerPoint Lecture Outlines, a Test Bank, and an Instructor's Manual. These products are available to adopters of this text. For more information about these ancillary products, please contact your sales representative at Jones & Bartlett Learning.

Acknowledgments

A project of this nature could not be completed without the assistance and understanding of a number of individuals. First, we would like to thank those individuals who have brought their expertise to the writing team: Sara A. Baker, MSW, Senior Instructor, Penn State–Hershey, Department of Public Health Sciences, provided revisions for Chapter 5 (Maternal, Infant, and Child Health); Denise M. Seabert, PhD, MCHES, Associate Professor, Department of Physiology and Health Science, Ball State University, completed revisions for Chapter 6 (Adolescents, Young Adults, and Adults); Charity Bishop, MS, CHES, Instructor, Department of Physiology and Health Science, Ball State University, was responsible for the revisions to Chapter 7 (Elders); Miguel A. Pérez, PhD, MCHES, Professor and Chair, Department of Public Health, Fresno State University, revised Chapter 8 (Community Health and Minorities); David V. Perkins, PhD, Professor, Department of Psychological Sciences, Ball State University, completed the revisions for Chapter 9 (Community Mental Health); and Farah Kauffman, MPH, Instructor, Department of Public Health Sciences, Penn State–Hershey, created the book's ancillary materials. Their expertise is both welcomed and appreciated.

We would also like to thank all of the employees at Jones & Bartlett Learning whose hard work, support, guidance, and confidence in us have been most helpful in creating this and all previous editions of this text. Specifically, we would like to thank: Cathy Esperti, Executive Editor; Julie Bolduc, Associate Director of Production; Agnes Burt, Editorial Assistant; Amy Wrynn, Director of Permissions and Photo Research; and Andrea DeFronzo, Senior Marketing Manager.

Finally, we would like to thank our families for their love, support, encouragement, and tolerance of all of the time that writing takes away from time together.

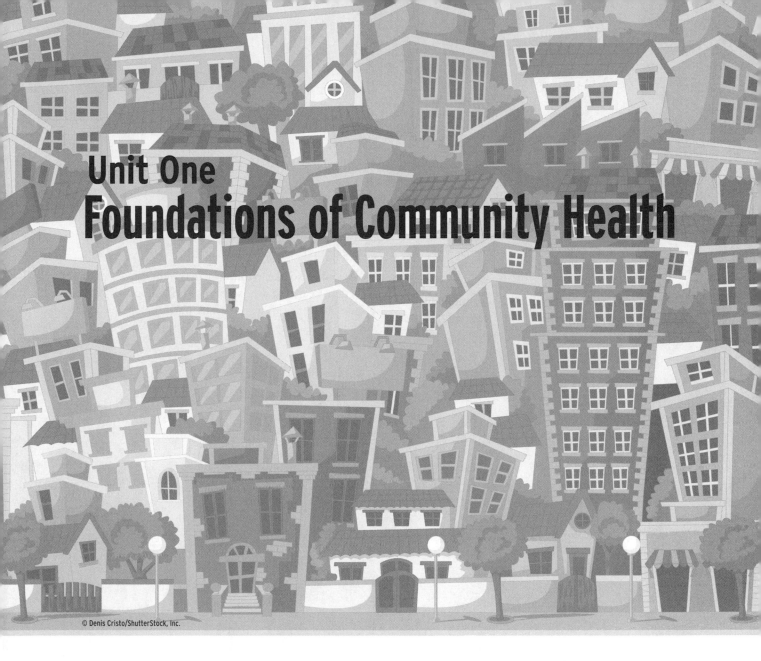

Unit One
Foundations of Community Health

© Denis Cristo/ShutterStock, Inc.

Chapter 1

Understanding Community Health and the Organizations That Help Shape It

James F. McKenzie, PhD, MPH, MCHES

Chapter Objectives

1. Define the terms *health*, *community*, *community health*, *population health*, *public health*, *public health system*, and *global health*, and explain the difference between personal and community health activities.

2. Briefly describe the five major determinants of health.

3. List and discuss the factors that influence a community's health.

4. Briefly relate the history of community/public health.

5. Provide a brief overview of the current health status of Americans.

6. Describe the major community health problems facing the United States today.

7. Describe the major community health problems facing the world today.

8. Describe the purpose of the *Healthy People 2020* goals and objectives.

9. Explain the need for organizing to improve community health.

10. Explain what a governmental health organization is and give an example of one at each of the following levels—international, national, state, and local.

11. Explain the role the World Health Organization (WHO) plays in community health.

12. Briefly describe the structure and function of the U.S. Department of Health and Human Services (HHS).

13. State the three core functions of public health.

14. List the 10 essential public health services.

15. Explain the relationship between a state and local health department.

16. Explain what is meant by the term *coordinated school health program*.

17. Define the term *quasi-governmental* and explain why some health organizations are classified under this term.

18. List the four primary activities of most voluntary health organizations.

19 Explain the purpose of a professional health organization/association.

20 Explain how philanthropic foundations contribute to community health.

21 Discuss the role that service, social, and religious organizations play in community health.

22 Identify the major reason why corporations are involved in community health and describe some corporate activities that contribute to community health.

Introduction

In looking back over the last 100-plus years, it is easy to point to the tremendous progress that was made in the health and life expectancy of those in the United States (see **Box 1.1**) and of many people of the world. Infant mortality dropped, many of the infectious diseases were brought under control, and better family planning became available. However, there is still room for improvement! Individual health behaviors, such as the use of tobacco, poor diet, and physical inactivity, have given rise to an unacceptable number of cases of illness and death from noninfectious diseases

---

Box 1.1   Ten Great Public Health Achievements—United States, 1900-1999 and 2001-2010

As the twentieth century came to a close, the overall health status and life expectancy in the United States were at all-time highs. Between 1900 and 2000, U.S. residents' life expectancy at birth increased by 62% to a high in 2000 of 76.8 years[2]; most of the increase is attributed to advances in public health.[3] There were many public health achievements that can be linked to this gain in life expectancy. The Centers for Disease Control and Prevention (CDC), the U.S. government agency charged with protecting the public health of the nation, singled out the "Ten Great Public Health Achievements" in the United States between 1900 and 1999. Here is the list:[4]

1. Vaccination
2. Motor vehicle safety
3. Safer workplaces
4. Control of infectious diseases
5. Decline of deaths from coronary heart disease and stroke
6. Safer and healthier foods
7. Healthier mothers and babies
8. Family planning
9. Fluoridation of drinking water
10. Recognition of tobacco use as a health hazard

At the conclusion of 2010, public health scientists at the CDC were asked to nominate noteworthy public health achievements that occurred in the United States between 2001 and 2010. Following, in no specific order, are the ones selected from the nominations[5]:

- *Vaccine-preventable deaths:* Over the 10-year period there was a substantial decline in cases, hospitalizations, deaths, and healthcare costs associated with vaccine-preventable diseases.

- *Prevention and control of infectious diseases:* Improvements in public health infrastructure along with innovative and targeted prevention efforts yielded significant progress in controlling infectious diseases (e.g., tuberculosis cases).

- *Tobacco control:* Tobacco still remains the single largest preventable cause of death and disease in the United States, but the adult smoking prevalence dropped to 19.3% in 2010,[6] and approximately half of the states have comprehensive smoke-free laws.

- *Maternal and infant health:* During the 10-year period there were significant reductions in the number of infants born with neural tube defects and an expansion of screening of newborns for metabolic and other heritable disorders.

- *Motor vehicle safety:* There were significant reductions in motor vehicle deaths and injuries, as well as pedestrian and bicyclist deaths. All were attributed to safer vehicles, safer roads, and safer road use.

- *Cardiovascular disease prevention:* Death rates for both stroke and coronary heart disease continue to trend down. Most can be attributed to reduction in the prevalence of risk factors, and improved treatments, medications, and quality of care.

- *Occupational safety:* Much progress was made in improving working conditions and reducing the risk for workplace-associated injuries over the 10 years.

- *Cancer prevention:* A number of death rates due to various cancers dropped during the 10 years; much of the progress can be attributed to the implementation of evidence-based screening recommendations.

- *Childhood lead poisoning prevention:* There was a steep decline in the percentage of children ages 1-5 years with blood levels > 10 µg/dL. Much of the progress can be traced to the 23 states in 2010 that had comprehensive lead poisoning prevention laws.

- *Public health preparedness and response.* Following the terrorist attacks of 2001 in the United States, great effort was made to both expand and improve the capacity of the public health system to respond to public health threats.

Source: Modified from Centers for Disease Control and Prevention (1999). "Ten Great Public Health Achievements—United States, 1900–1999." *Morbidity and Mortality Weekly Report,* 48(12): 241–243; and U.S. Department of Health and Human Services, Centers for Disease Control and Prevention (2011). "Ten Great Public Health Achievements—United States, 2001–2010." *Morbidity and Mortality Weekly Report,* 60(19): 619–623. Available at http://www.cdc.gov/mmwr/preview/mmwrhtml/mm6019a5.htm?s_cid=mm6019a5_w.

such as cancer, diabetes, and heart disease. New and emerging infectious diseases, such as the 2009 H1N1 flu and those caused by drug-resistant pathogens, are stretching resources available to control them. And events stemming from natural disasters such as floods and hurricanes, and humanmade disasters such as the Gulf oil spill and terrorism around the world have caused us to refocus our priorities. All of these events have severely disrupted Americans' sense of security[1] and sense of safety in the environment. In addition, many of these events revealed the vulnerability of the United States' ability to respond to such circumstances and highlighted the need for improvement in emergency response preparedness and the infrastructure of the public health system.

Even with all that has happened in recent years in the United States and around the world, the achievement of good health remains a worldwide goal in the twenty-first century. Governments, private organizations, and individuals throughout the world are working to improve health. Although individual actions to improve one's own personal health certainly contribute to the overall health of the community, organized community actions are often necessary when health problems exceed the resources of any one individual. When such actions are not taken, the health of the entire community is at risk.

This chapter introduces the concepts and principles of community health, explains how community health differs from personal health, provides a brief history of community health, identifies some health problems facing Americans, provides an outlook for the twenty-first century, and examines the organizations that help shape community health.

Understanding Community Health

Definitions

The word *health* means different things to different people. Similarly, there are other words that can be defined in various ways. Some basic terms we will use in this text are defined in the following paragraphs.

Health

The word *health* is derived from *hal*, which means "hale, sound, whole." When it comes to the health of people, the word *health* has been defined in a number of different ways. The most widely quoted definition of health was the one created by the World Health Organization (WHO) in 1946. That definition states that "health is a state of complete physical, mental, and social well-being and not merely the absence of disease and infirmity."[7] Further, the WHO has indicated that "health is a resource for everyday life, not the object of living, and is a positive concept emphasizing social and personal resources as well as physical capabilities."[7] Others have stated that health cannot be defined as a state because it is ever-changing. Therefore, we have chosen to define **health** as a *dynamic* state or condition of the human organism that is multidimensional in nature (i.e., physical, emotional, social, intellectual, spiritual, and occupational), a resource for living, and results from a person's interactions with and adaptations to his or her environment. Therefore, it can exist in varying degrees and is specific to each individual and his or her situation. "For example, a person can be healthy while dying, or a person who is a quadriplegic can be healthy in the sense that his or her mental and social well-being are high and physical health is as good as it can be."[8]

A person's health status is dynamic in part because of the many different factors that determine one's health. It is widely accepted that health status is determined by the interaction of five domains: genetic makeup, social circumstances (e.g., education, income, poverty, crime, and social cohesion), environmental conditions (e.g., toxic and microbial agents, and structural hazards), behavioral choices (e.g., diet, physical activity, substance use and abuse), and the availability of quality medical care.[9]

> Ultimately, the health fate of each of us is determined by factors acting not mostly in isolation but by our experience where domains interconnect. Whether a gene is expressed can be determined by environmental exposures or behavioral patterns. The nature and consequences of behavioral choices are affected by social circumstances. Our genetic predispositions affect the health care we need, and our social circumstances affect the health care we receive.[10]

Community

Traditionally, a community has been thought of as a geographic area with specific boundaries—for example, a neighborhood, city, county, or state. However, in the context of community health, a **community** is "a collective body of individuals identified by common characteristics such as geography, interests, experiences, concerns, or values."[11] Today we can even talk about a cyber community.[12]

Examples of communities include the people of the city of Columbus

community a collective body of individuals identified by common characteristics

health a dynamic state or condition of the human organism that is multidimensional in nature, a resource for living, and results from a person's interactions with and adaptations to his or her environment; therefore, it can exist in varying degrees and is specific to each individual and his or her situation (geography), the Asian community (race), seniors (age), the homeless (specific problem), those on welfare (particular outcome), or those who are members of a social network (cyber). A community may be as small as the group of people who live on a residence hall floor at a university or as large as all of the individuals who make up a nation.

Public, Community, Population, and Global Health

Prior to defining the four terms *public health*, *community health*, *population health*, and *global health*, it is important to note that often the terms are used interchangeably by both laypeople and professionals who work in the various health fields. When the terms are used interchangeably, most people are referring to the collective health of those in society and the actions or activities taken to obtain and maintain that health. The definitions provided here for the four terms more precisely define the group of people in question and the origin of the actions or activities.

Of the four terms, *public health* is the most inclusive. The Institute of Medicine (IOM) defined **public health** in 1988 as "what we as a society do collectively to assure the conditions in which people can be healthy."[13] The **public health system**, which has been defined as "activities undertaken within the formal structure of government and the associated efforts of private and voluntary organizations and individuals,"[13] is the organizational mechanism for providing such conditions.

Community health refers to the health status of a defined group of people and the actions and conditions to promote, protect, and preserve their health. For example, the health status of the people of Muncie, Indiana, and the private and public actions taken to promote, protect, and preserve the health of these people would constitute community health.

The term *population health* is similar to *community health*. The primary

difference between these two terms is the degree of organization or identity of the people. **Population health** refers to the health status of people who are not organized and have no identity as a group or locality and the actions and conditions to promote, protect, and preserve their health. Men younger than 50, adolescents, prisoners, and white-collar workers are all examples of populations.[14]

A term that has been used increasingly in recent years is *global health*. **Global health** describes "health problems, issues, and concerns that transcend national boundaries, may be influenced by circumstances or experiences in other countries, and are best addressed by cooperative actions and solutions."[15] Therefore, an issue such as a flu pandemic can be viewed as a global health issue. Much of the rise in concern about global health problems comes from the speed of international travel and how easy it is for people who may be infected with a disease to cross borders into another country.

Personal Health Activities Versus Community Health Activities

To further clarify the definitions presented in this chapter, it is important to distinguish between the terms *personal health activities* and *community health activities*.

Personal health activities are individual actions and decision making that affect the health of an individual or his or her immediate family members or friends. These activities may be preventive or curative in nature but seldom directly affect the behavior of others. Choosing to eat wisely, to regularly wear a safety belt, and to visit the physician are all examples of personal health activities.

Community health activities are activities that are aimed at protecting or improving the health of a population or community. Maintenance of accurate birth and death records, protection of the food and water supply, and participating in fund drives for voluntary health organizations such as the American Lung Association are examples of community health activities. Within this text you are introduced to the many community health activities and to the organizations that are responsible for carrying them out.

Factors That Affect the Health of a Community

There are many factors that affect the health of a community. As a result, the health status of each community is different. These factors may be physical, social, and/or cultural. They

community health the health status of a defined group of people and the actions and conditions to promote, protect, and preserve their health

global health describes health problems, issues, and concerns that transcend national boundaries, may be influenced by circumstances or experiences in other countries, and are best addressed by cooperative actions and solutions

population health the health status of people who are not organized and have no identity as a group or locality and the actions and conditions to promote, protect, and preserve their health

public health actions that society takes collectively to ensure that the conditions in which people can be healthy can occur

public health system the organizational mechanism of those activities undertaken within the formal structure of government and the associated efforts of private and voluntary organizations and individuals also include the ability of the community to organize and work together as a whole as well as the individual behaviors of those in the community (see Figure 1.1).

Physical Factors

Physical factors include the influences of geography, the environment, community size, and industrial development.

Geography

A community's health problems can be directly influenced by its altitude, latitude, and climate. In tropical countries where warm, humid temperatures and rain prevail throughout the year, parasitic and infectious diseases are a leading community health problem (see Figure 1.2). In many tropical countries, survival from these diseases is made more difficult because poor soil conditions result in inadequate food production and malnutrition. In temperate climates with fewer parasitic and infectious diseases and a more than adequate food supply, obesity and heart disease are important community health problems.

Environment

The quality of our environment is directly related to the quality of our stewardship of it. Many experts believe that if we continue to allow uncontrolled population growth and continue to deplete nonrenewable natural resources, succeeding generations will inhabit communities that are less desirable than ours.

Community Size

The larger the community, the greater its range of health problems and the greater its number of health resources. For example, larger communities have more health professionals and better health facilities than smaller communities. These resources are often needed because communicable diseases can spread more quickly and environmental

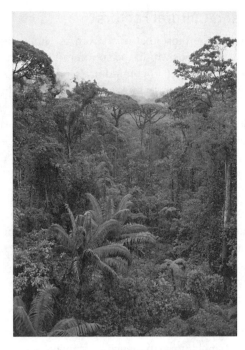

Figure 1.2 In tropical countries, parasitic and infectious diseases are leading community health problems.
© Rubberball Productions/Getty Images

problems are often more severe in densely populated areas. For example, the amount of trash generated by the approximately 8.2 million people in New York City is many times greater than that generated by the entire state of Wyoming, with its population of about 568,158.

It is important to note that a community's size can have both a positive and a negative impact on that community's health. The ability of a community to effectively plan, organize, and utilize its resources can determine whether its size can be used to its advantage.

Industrial Development

Industrial development, like size, can have either positive or negative effects on the health status of a community. Industrial development provides a community with added resources for community health programs, but it may bring with it environmental pollution and occupational injuries and illnesses. Communities that experience rapid industrial development must eventually regulate (e.g., laws and ordinances) the way in which industries (1) obtain raw materials, (2) discharge by-products, (3) dispose of wastes, (4) treat and protect their employees, and (5) clean up environmental accidents.

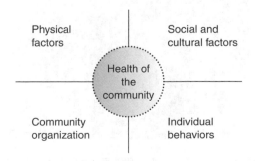

Figure 1.1 Factors that affect the health of a community.

Social and Cultural Factors

Social factors are those that arise from the interaction of individuals or groups within the community. For example, people who live in urban communities, where life is fast-paced, experience higher rates of stress-related illnesses than those who live in rural communities, where life is more leisurely. On the other hand, those in rural areas may not have access to the same quality or selection of health care (i.e., hospitals or medical specialists) that is available to those who live in urban communities.

Cultural factors arise from guidelines (both explicit and implicit) that individuals "inherit" from being a part of a particular society. Some of the factors that contribute to culture are discussed in the following sections.

Beliefs, Traditions, and Prejudices

The beliefs, traditions, and prejudices of community members can affect the health of the community. The beliefs of those in a community about such specific health behaviors as exercise and smoking can influence policy makers on whether they will spend money on bike trails and work toward no-smoking ordinances. The traditions of specific ethnic groups can influence the types of food, restaurants, retail outlets, and services available in a community. Prejudices of one specific ethnic or racial group against another can result in acts of violence and crime. Racial and ethnic disparities will continue to put certain groups at greater risk.

The Economy

Both national and local economies can affect the health of a community through reductions in health and social services. An economic downturn means lower tax revenues (fewer tax dollars) and fewer contributions to charitable groups. Such actions will result in fewer dollars being available for programs such as welfare, the Supplemental Nutrition Assistance Program (formerly know as Food Stamp Program), community health care, and other community services. This occurs because revenue shortfalls cause agencies to experience budget cuts. With less money, these agencies often must alter their eligibility guidelines, thereby restricting aid to only the neediest individuals. Many people who had been eligible for assistance before the economic downturn become ineligible.

Employers usually find it increasingly difficult to provide health benefits for their employees as their income drops. The unemployed and underemployed face poverty and deteriorating health. Thus, the cumulative effect of an economic downturn significantly affects the health of the community.

Politics

Those who happen to be in political office can improve or jeopardize the health of their community by the decisions (i.e., laws and ordinances) they make. In the most general terms, the argument is over greater or lesser governmental participation in health issues. For example, there has been a long-standing discussion in the United States on the extent to which the government should involve itself in health care. Historically, Democrats have been in favor of such action whereas Republicans have been against it.

Religion

A number of religions have taken a position on health care and health behaviors. For example, some religious communities limit the type of medical treatment their members may receive. Some do not permit immunizations; others do not permit their members to be treated by physicians. Still others prohibit certain foods. For example, Kosher dietary regulations permit Jews to eat the meat only of animals that chew cud and have cloven hooves and the flesh only of fish that have both gills and scales; others, like the Native American Church of the Morning Star, use peyote, a hallucinogen, as a sacrament.

Some religious communities actively address moral and ethical issues such as abortion, premarital intercourse, and homosexuality. Other religions teach health-promoting codes of living to their members (see **Figure 1.3**).

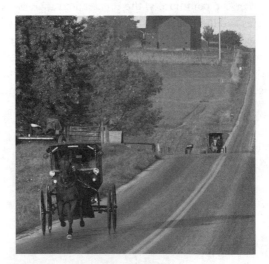

Figure 1.3 Religion can affect a community's health either positively or negatively.
© Weldon Schloneger/ShutterStock, Inc.

Social Norms

The influence of social norms can be positive or negative and can change over time. Cigarette smoking is a good example. During the 1940s, 1950s, and 1960s, it was socially acceptable to smoke in most settings. As a matter of fact, in 1960, 53% of American men and 32% of American women smoked. Thus, in 1960 it was socially acceptable to be a smoker, especially if you were male. Now, early in the twenty-first century, those percentages have dropped to 21.5% for men and 17.3% for women, and in most public places it has become socially unacceptable to smoke.[6] The lawsuits against tobacco companies by both the state attorneys general and private citizens provide further evidence that smoking has fallen from social acceptability. Because of this change in the social norm, there is less secondhand smoke in many public places, and in turn the health of the community has improved.

Unlike smoking, alcohol consumption represents a continuing negative social norm in the United States, especially on college campuses. The normal expectation seems to be that drinking is fun. Despite the fact that most college students are too young to drink legally, approximately 66% of college students drink.[16] It seems fairly obvious that the American alcoholic-beverage industry has influenced our social norms.

Socioeconomic Status

Differences in individual- and community-level socioeconomic status, whether defined by education, employment, or income, have independent effects on health.[17] "In the United States today, the health of poor people is threatened by the adverse environmental conditions of the inner cities, such as lead paint and air pollution, crime, and violence. Poor people also have poorer nutrition, less access to medical care, and more psychological stress."[1]

Community Organizing

The way in which a community is able to organize its resources directly influences its ability to intervene and solve problems, including health problems. **Community organizing** is "the process by which community groups are helped to identify common problems or change targets, mobilize resources, and develop and implement strategies to reach their collective goals."[18] If a community can organize its resources effectively into a unified force, it "is likely to produce benefits in the form of increased effectiveness and productivity by reducing duplication of efforts and avoiding the imposition of solutions that are not congruent with the

local culture and needs."[19] For example, many communities in the United States have faced community-wide drug problems. Some have been able to organize their resources to reduce or resolve these problems, whereas others have not.

Individual Behavior

The behavior of the individual community members contributes to the health of the entire community. For example, if each individual consciously recycles his or her trash each week, community recycling will be successful. Likewise, the more individuals who become immunized against a specific disease, the slower the disease will spread and fewer people will be exposed. This concept is known as **herd immunity**.

A Brief History of Community and Public Health

The history of community and public health is almost as long as the history of civilization. This brief summary (see also **Box 1.2**) provides an account of some of the accomplishments and failures in community and public health. It is hoped that knowledge of the past will enable us to better prepare for future challenges to our community's health. Although the history of community and public health can be traced back to the earliest civilizations on earth, we begin our discussion in the late eighteenth century.

The Eighteenth Century

The eighteenth century was characterized by industrial growth. Despite the beginnings of recognition of the nature of disease, living conditions were hardly conducive to good health. Cities were overcrowded, and water supplies were inadequate and often unsanitary. Streets were usually unpaved, filthy, and heaped with trash and garbage. Many homes had unsanitary dirt floors.

Workplaces were unsafe and unhealthy. A substantial portion of the workforce was made up of the poor, which included children, who were forced to work long hours as indentured servants. Many of these jobs were unsafe or involved working in unhealthy environments, such as textile factories and coal mines.

community organizing the process by which community groups are helped to identify common problems or change targets, mobilize resources, and develop and implement strategies to reach their collective goals

herd immunity the resistance of a population to the spread of an infectious agent based on the immunity of a high proportion of individuals

---

Box 1.2   Timeline and Highlights of Community and Public Health from 1700 to 2000

A. Eighteenth Century (1700s)
1. Period characterized by industrial growth; workplaces were unsafe and unhealthy
2. 1790: first U.S. census
3. 1793: yellow fever epidemic in Philadelphia
4. 1796: Dr. Edward Jenner successfully demonstrated smallpox vaccination
5. 1798: Marine Hospital Service (forerunner to U.S. Public Health Service) was formed
6. By 1799: several of America's largest cities, including Boston, Philadelphia, New York, and Baltimore, had municipal boards of health

B. First Half of Nineteenth Century (1800–1848)
1. U.S. government's approach to health was laissez faire
2. 1813: first visiting nurse in United States

C. Second Half of Nineteenth Century (1848–1900)
1. 1849, 1854: London cholera epidemics
2. 1850: Modern era of public health begins
3. 1850: Shattuck's report
4. 1854: Snow had pump handle removed from Broad Street pump
5. 1863: Pasteur proposed germ theory
6. 1872: American Public Health Association founded
7. 1875–1900: Bacteriological period of public health
8. 1876: Koch established relationship between a particular microbe and a particular disease
9. 1900: Reed announced that yellow fever was transmitted by mosquitos
10. 1900: Life expectancy in the United States was 47 years

D. Twentieth Century
1. Health Resources Development Period (1900–1960)
   a. The Reform Phase (1900–1920)
      - 1902: First national-level voluntary health agency created: National Association for the Study and Prevention of Tuberculosis
      - 1906: Sinclair's *The Jungle* published
      - 1910: First International Congress on Occupational Diseases
      - 1910: 45% of U.S. population lived in cities

- 1911: First local health department established
- 1917: United States ranked fourteenth of 16 in maternal death rate
- 1918: Birth of school health instruction
- 1918: First school of public health established in United States

2. 1920s
   a. 1922: Wood created first professional preparation program for health education specialists
   b. 1930: Life expectancy in the United States was 59.7 years
3. The Great Depression and WWII
   a. 1933: New Deal; included unsuccessful attempt at national healthcare program
   b. 1935: Social Security Act passed
   c. 1937: National Cancer Institute formed
4. Postwar Years
   a. 1946: National Hospital Survey and Construction (Hill-Burton) Act passed
   b. 1952: Development of polio vaccine
   c. 1955: Eisenhower's heart attack

E. Period of Social Engineering (1960–1973)
1. 1965: Medicare and Medicaid bills passed

F. Period of Health Promotion (1974–present)
1. 1974: Nixon's unsuccessful attempt at national healthcare program
2. 1974: *A New Perspective on the Health of Canadians* published
3. 1976: Health Information and Health Promotion Act passed
4. 1979: *Healthy People* published
5. 1980: *Promoting Health/Preventing Disease: Objectives of the Nation* published
6. 1990: *Healthy People 2000* published
7. 1997: Clinton's unsuccessful attempt at a national healthcare program
8. 2000: *Healthy People 2010* published
9. 2010: Affordable Health Care Act (ACA) passed
10. 2010: *Healthy People 2020* published

One medical advance made at the end of the eighteenth century deserves mention because of its significance for public health. In 1796, Dr. Edward Jenner successfully demonstrated the process of vaccination as a protection against smallpox. He did this by inoculating a boy with material from a cowpox (*Vaccinia*) pustule. When challenged later with material from a smallpox (*Variola*) pustule, the boy remained healthy.

Dr. Jenner's discovery remains as one of the great discoveries of all time for both medicine and for public health. Prior to his discovery, millions died or were severely disfigured by smallpox (see **Figure 1.4**). The only known prevention had been "variolation," inoculation with smallpox material itself. This was a risky procedure because people sometimes became quite ill with smallpox. Nonetheless, during the American Revolution, General George Washington ordered the Army of the American Colonies "variolated." He did this so that he could be sure an epidemic of smallpox would not wipe out his colonial forces.[20]

Following the American Revolution, George Washington ordered the first U.S. census for the purpose of the

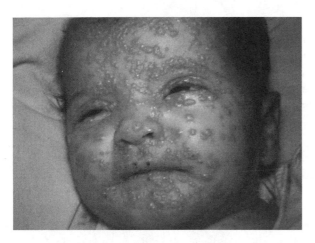

Figure 1.4 Prior to the elimination of smallpox, millions died or were severely disfigured by the disease.
Courtesy of Dr. John Noble, Jr./CDC

apportionment of representation in the House of Representatives. The census, first taken in 1790, is still conducted every 10 years and serves as an invaluable source of information for community health planning.

As the eighteenth century came to a close, a young United States faced numerous disease problems, including continuing outbreaks of smallpox, cholera, typhoid fever, and yellow fever. Yellow fever outbreaks usually occurred in port cities such as Charleston, Baltimore, New York, and New Orleans, where ships arrived to dock from tropical America. The greatest single epidemic of yellow fever in the United States occurred in Philadelphia in 1793, where there were an estimated 23,000 cases, including 4,044 deaths in a population estimated at only 37,000.[21]

In response to these continuing epidemics and the need to address other mounting health problems, such as sanitation and protection of the water supply, several governmental health agencies were created. In 1798, the Marine Hospital Service (forerunner to the U.S. Public Health Service) was formed to deal with disease that was occurring onboard water vessels. By 1799, several of the United States' largest cities, including Boston, Philadelphia, New York, and Baltimore, also had founded municipal boards of health.

The Nineteenth Century

During the first half of the nineteenth century, few remarkable advancements in public health occurred. Living conditions in Europe and England remained unsanitary, and industrialization led to an even greater concentration of the population within cities. However, better agricultural methods led to improved nutrition for many.

During this period, the United States experienced westward expansion, characterized by a spirit of pioneering, self-sufficiency, and rugged individualism. The federal government's approach to health problems was characterized by the French term *laissez faire*, meaning noninterference. There were also few health regulations or health departments in rural areas. Health quackery thrived; this was truly a period when "buyer beware" was good advice.

Epidemics continued in major cities in both Europe and the United States. In 1854, another cholera epidemic struck London. Dr. John Snow studied the epidemic and hypothesized that the disease was being caused by the drinking water from the Broad Street pump. He obtained permission to remove the pump handle, and the epidemic was abated (see Figure 1.5). Snow's action was remarkable because it predated the discovery that microorganisms can cause disease. The predominant theory of contagious disease at the time was the "miasmas theory." According to this theory, vapors, or miasmas, were the source of many diseases. The miasmas theory remained popular throughout much of the nineteenth century.

In the United States in 1850, Lemuel Shattuck drew up a health report for the Commonwealth of Massachusetts that

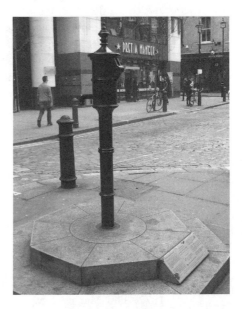

Figure 1.5 In London, England, in 1854, John Snow helped interrupt a cholera epidemic by having the handle removed from this pump, located on Broad Street.

outlined the public health needs for the state. It included recommendations for the establishment of boards of health, the collection of vital statistics, the implementation of sanitary measures, and research on diseases. Shattuck also recommended health education and controlling exposure to alcohol, smoke, adulterated food, and nostrums (quack medicines).[22] Although some of his recommendations took years to implement (the Massachusetts Board of Health was not founded until 1869), the significance of Shattuck's report is such that 1850 is a key date in U.S. public health; it marks the beginning of the **modern era of public health**.

Real progress in the understanding of the causes of many communicable diseases occurred during the last third of the nineteenth century. One of the obstacles to progress was the theory of spontaneous generation, the idea that living organisms could arise from inorganic or nonliving matter. Akin to this idea was the thought that one type of contagious microbe could change into another type of organism. In 1862, Louis Pasteur of France proposed his germ theory of disease. Throughout the 1860s and 1870s, he and others carried out experiments and made observations that supported this theory. Pasteur is generally given credit for providing the death blow to the theory of spontaneous generation.

It was the German scientist Robert Koch who developed the criteria and procedures necessary to establish that a particular microbe, and no other, causes a particular disease. His first demonstration, with the anthrax bacillus, was in 1876. Between 1877 and the end of the century, the identity of numerous bacterial disease agents was established, including those that caused gonorrhea, typhoid fever, leprosy, tuberculosis, cholera, diphtheria, tetanus, pneumonia, plague, and dysentery. This period (1875–1900) has come to be known as the **bacteriological period of public health**.

bacteriological period of public health the period of 1875-1900, during which the causes of many bacterial diseases were discovered

health resources development period the years 1900-1960, a time of great growth in healthcare facilities and providers

modern era of public health the era of public health that began in 1850 and continues today

Although most scientific discoveries in the late nineteenth century were made in Europe, there were significant public health achievements occurring in the United States as well. The first law prohibiting the adulteration of milk was passed in 1856, the first sanitary survey was carried out in New York City in 1864, and the American Public Health Association was founded in 1872. The Marine Hospital Service gained new powers of inspection and investigation under the Port Quarantine Act of 1878.[22] In 1890,

the pasteurization of milk was introduced, and in 1891 meat inspection began. It was also during this time that nurses were first hired by industries (in 1895) and schools (in 1899). Also in 1895, septic tanks were introduced for sewage treatment. In 1900, Major Walter Reed of the U.S. Army announced that yellow fever was transmitted by mosquitoes.

The Twentieth Century

As the twentieth century began, the leading causes of death were still communicable diseases—influenza, pneumonia, tuberculosis, and infections of the gastrointestinal tract. Other communicable diseases, such as typhoid fever, malaria, and diphtheria, also killed many people.

There were other health problems as well. Thousands of children were afflicted with conditions characterized by noninfectious diarrhea or by bone deformity. Although the symptoms of pellagra and rickets were known and described, the causes of these ailments remained a mystery at the turn of the century. Discovery that these conditions resulted from vitamin deficiencies was slow because some scientists were searching for bacterial causes.

Vitamin deficiency diseases and one of their contributing conditions, poor dental health, were extremely common in the slum districts of both European and U.S. cities. The unavailability of adequate prenatal and postnatal care meant that deaths associated with pregnancy and childbirth were also high.

Health Resources Development Period (1900-1960)

Much growth and development took place during the 60-year period from 1900 to 1960. Because of the growth of healthcare facilities and providers, this period of time is referred to as the **health resources development period**. This period can be further divided into the reform phase (1900–1920), the 1920s, the Great Depression and World War II, and the postwar years.

The Reform Phase (1900-1920)

By the beginning of the twentieth century, there was a growing concern about the many social problems in the United States. The remarkable discoveries in microbiology made in the previous years had not dramatically improved the health of the average citizen. By 1910, the urban population had grown to 45% of the total population (up from 19% in 1860). Much of the growth was the result of immigrants who came to the United States for the jobs created by new industries

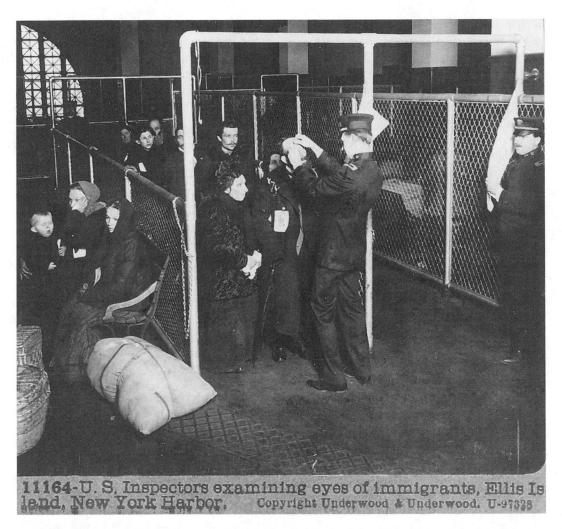

11164-U. S. Inspectors examining eyes of immigrants, Ellis Is
land, New York Harbor.   Copyright Underwood & Underwood. U-97328

Figure 1.6 Ellis Island immigration between 1860 and 1910 resulted in dramatic increases in urban population in the United States.
Courtesy of Library of Congress, Prints & Photographs Division, [reproduction number LC-USZ62-7386]

(see **Figure 1.6**). Northern cities wcre also swelling from the northward migration of black Americans from the southern states. Many of these workers had to accept poorly paying jobs involving hard labor and low wages. There was also a deepening chasm between the upper and lower classes, and social critics began to clamor for reform.

The years 1900 to 1920 have been called the **reform phase of public health**. The plight of the immigrants working in the meat packing industry was graphically depicted by Upton Sinclair in his book *The Jungle*. Sinclair's goal was to draw attention to unsafe working conditions. What he achieved was greater governmental regulation of the food industry through the passage of the Pure Food and Drugs Act of 1906.

The reform movement was broad, involving both social and moral as well as health issues. Edward T. Devine noted in 1909 that "Ill health is perhaps the most constant of the attendants of poverty."[23] The reform movement finally took hold when it became evident to the majority that neither the discoveries of the causes of many communicable diseases nor the continuing advancement of industrial production could overcome continuing disease and poverty. Even by 1917, the United States ranked fourteenth of 16 "progressive" nations in maternal death rate.[23]

Although the relationship between occupation and disease had been

> **reform phase of public health** the years 1900–1920, characterized by social movements to improve health conditions in cities and in the workplace

pointed out 200 years earlier in Europe, occupational health in the United States in 1900 was an unknown quantity. Then in 1910 the first International Congress on Occupational Diseases was held in Chicago.[24] That same year, the state of New York passed a tentative Workman's Compensation Act, and over the next 10 years most other states passed similar laws. Also in 1910, the U.S. Bureau of Mines was created and the first clinic for occupational diseases was established in New York at Cornell Medical College.[23] By 1910, the movement for healthier conditions in the workplace was well established.

This period also saw the birth of the first national-level volunteer health agencies. The first of these agencies was the National Association for the Study and Prevention of Tuberculosis, which was formed in 1902. It arose from the first local voluntary health agency, the Pennsylvania Society for the Prevention of Tuberculosis, organized in 1892.[25] That same year, the Rockefeller Foundation was established in New York. This philanthropic foundation has funded a great many public health projects, including work on hookworm and pellagra, and the development of a vaccine against yellow fever.

Another movement that began about this time was that of public health nursing. The first school nursing program was begun in New York City in 1902. In 1918, the first School of Public Health was established at Johns Hopkins University in Baltimore. Also in 1918 was the birth of school health instruction as we know it today.

These advances were matched with similar advances by governmental bodies. The Marine Hospital Service was renamed the Public Health and Marine Hospital Service in 1902 in keeping with its growing responsibilities. In 1912, it became the U.S. Public Health Service.[22]

By 1900, 38 states had state health departments. The rest followed during the first decades of the twentieth century. The first two local (county) health departments were established in 1911, one in Guilford County, North Carolina, and the other in Yakima County, Washington.

The 1920s

In comparison with the preceding period, the 1920s represented a decade of slow growth in public health, except for a few health projects funded by foundations. Prohibition resulted in a decline in the number of alcoholics and alcohol-related deaths. Although the number of county health departments had risen to 467 by 1929, 77% of the rural population still lived in areas with no health services.[25] However, it was during this period in 1922 that the first professional preparation program for health education specialists was begun at Columbia University by Thomas D. Wood, MD, whom many consider the father of health education.

The Great Depression and World War II

Until the Great Depression (1929–1935), individuals and families in need of social and medical services were dependent on friends and relatives, private charities, voluntary agencies, community chests, and churches. By 1933, after 3 years of economic depression, it became evident that private resources could never meet the needs of all the people who needed assistance. The drop in tax revenues during the Depression also reduced health department budgets and caused a virtual halt in the formation of new local health departments.[25]

Beginning in 1933, President Franklin D. Roosevelt created numerous agencies and programs for public works as part of his New Deal. Much of the money was used for public health, including the control of malaria, the building of hospitals and laboratories, and the construction of municipal water and sewer systems.

The Social Security Act of 1935 marked the beginning of the government's major involvement in social issues, including health. This act provided substantial support for state health departments and their programs, such as maternal and child health and sanitary facilities. As progress against the communicable diseases became visible, some turned their attention toward other health problems, such as cancer. The National Cancer Institute was formed in 1937.

The United States' involvement in World War II resulted in severe restrictions on resources available for public health programs. Immediately following the conclusion of the war, however, many of the medical discoveries made during wartime made their way into civilian medical practice. Two examples are the antibiotic penicillin, used for treating pneumonia, rheumatic fever, syphilis, and strep throat, and the insecticide DDT, used for killing insects that transmit diseases.

During World War II, the Communicable Disease Center was established in Atlanta, Georgia. Now called the Centers for Disease Control and Prevention (CDC), it has become the premier epidemiological center in the world.

The Postwar Years

Following the end of World War II, there was still concern about medical care and the adequacy of the facilities in which that care could be administered. In 1946, Congress passed the National Hospital Survey and Construction Act (the Hill-Burton Act). The goal of the legislation was to improve the distribution of medical care and to enhance the quality of hospitals. From 1946 through the 1960s, hospital construction occurred at a rapid rate with relatively little thought given to planning. Likewise, attempts to set national health priorities or to establish a national health agenda were virtually nonexistent.

The two major health events in the 1950s were the development of a vaccine to prevent polio and President Eisenhower's heart attack. The latter event helped the United States to focus on its number 1 killer, heart disease. When the president's physician suggested exercise, some Americans heeded his advice and began to exercise on a regular basis.

Period of Social Engineering (1960-1973)

The 1960s marked the beginning of a period when the federal government once again became active in health matters. The primary reason for this involvement was the growing realization that many Americans were still not reaping any of the benefits of 60 years of medical advances. These Americans, most of whom were poor or elderly, either lived in underserved areas or simply could not afford to purchase medical services.

In 1965, Congress passed the Medicare and Medicaid bills (amendments to the Social Security Act of 1935). **Medicare** assists in the payment of medical bills for older adults and certain people with disabilities, and **Medicaid** assists in the payment of medical bills for the poor. These pieces of legislation helped provide medical care for millions and also improved standards in healthcare facilities. Unfortunately, the influx of federal dollars accelerated the rate of increase in the cost of health care for everyone. As a result, the 1970s, 1980s, and 1990s saw repeated attempts and failures to bring the growing costs of health care under control.

Period of Health Promotion (1974-Present)

By the mid-1970s, it had become apparent that the greatest potential for saving lives and reducing healthcare costs in the United States was to be achieved through means other than health care.

> Most scholars, policymakers, and practitioners in health promotion would pick 1974 as the turning point that marks the beginning of health promotion as a significant component of national health policy in the twentieth

century. That year Canada published its landmark policy statement, *A New Perspective on the Health of Canadians*.[26] In the United States, Congress [in 1976] passed PL 94-317, the Health Information and Health Promotion Act, which created the Office of Health Information and Health Promotion, later renamed the Office of Disease Prevention and Health Promotion.[27]

In the late 1970s, the CDC conducted a study that examined premature deaths in the United States in 1977. That study revealed that approximately 48% of all premature deaths could be traced to one's lifestyle or health behavior—choices that people make. Lifestyles characterized by a lack of exercise, unhealthy diets, smoking, uncontrolled hypertension, and the inability to control stress were found to be contributing factors to premature mortality.[28] This led the way for the U.S. government's publication *Healthy People: The Surgeon General's Report on Health Promotion and Disease Prevention*,[29] which provided Americans with the prescription for reducing their health risks and increasing their chances for good health.

Healthy People was then followed by the release of the first set of health goals and objectives for the nation, called *Promoting Health/Preventing Disease: Objectives for the Nation*.[30] *Healthy People 2020* is the fourth edition of these goals and objectives. Since their inception, these *Healthy People* documents have defined the nation's health agenda and guided its health policy.

All four editions of the *Healthy People* documents have included several overarching goals and many supporting objectives for the nation's health. The goals provide a general focus and direction, and the objectives are used to measure progress within a specified period of time. Formal reviews (i.e., measured progress) of these objectives are conducted both at midcourse (i.e., halfway through the 10-year period) and again at the end of 10 years. The midcourse review provides an opportunity to update the document based on the events of the first half of the decade for which the objectives are written.

Healthy People 2020 was released in December 2010, and includes a vision statement, a mission statement, four overarching goals (see **Table 1.1**), and almost 600 objectives spread over 42 different topic areas (see **Table 1.2**). On the Healthy People.gov website, each topic has its own page. At a minimum, each page contains a concise goal statement, a brief overview of the topic that provides the background and context for

Medicaid government health insurance for the poor
Medicare government health insurance for older adults and those with certain disabilities

Table 1.1 *Healthy People 2020* Vision, Mission, and Goals

Vision
A society in which all people live long, healthy lives.
Mission
Healthy People 2020 strives to:
• Identify nationwide health improvement priorities
• Increase public awareness and understanding of the determinants of health, disease, and disability and the opportunities for progress
• Provide measurable objectives and goals that are applicable at the national, state, and local levels
• Engage multiple sectors to take actions to strengthen policies and improve practices that are driven by the best available evidence and knowledge
• Identify critical research, evaluation, and data collection needs
Overarching Goals
• Attain high-quality, longer lives free of preventable disease, disability, injury, and premature death
• Achieve health equity, eliminate disparities, and improve the health of all groups
• Create social and physical environments that promote good health for all
• Promote quality of life, healthy development, and healthy behaviors across all life stages

Source: U.S. Department of Health and Human Services (2010). "About Healthy People." Available at http://www.healthypeople.gov/2020/about/default.aspx.

Table 1.2 *Healthy People 2020* Topic Areas

1. Access to Health Services
2. Adolescent Health
3. Arthritis, Osteoporosis, and Chronic Back Conditions
4. Blood Disorders and Blood Safety
5. Cancer
6. Chronic Kidney Disease
7. Dementias, Including Alzheimer's Disease
8. Diabetes
9. Disability and Health
10. Early and Middle Childhood
11. Educational and Community-Based Programs
12. Environmental Health
13. Family Planning
14. Food Safety
15. Genomics
16. Global Health
17. Health Communication and Health Information Technology
18. Healthcare-Associated Infections
19. Health-Related Quality of Life and Well-Being
20. Hearing and Other Sensory or Communication Disorders
21. Heart Disease and Stroke
22. HIV
23. Immunization and Infectious Diseases
24. Injury and Violence Prevention
25. Lesbian, Gay, Bisexual, and Transgender Health
26. Maternal, Infant, and Child Health
27. Medical Product Safety
28. Mental Health and Mental Disorders
29. Nutrition and Weight Status
30. Occupational Safety and Health
31. Older Adults
32. Oral Health
33. Physical Activity
34. Preparedness
35. Public Health Infrastructure
36. Respiratory Diseases
37. Sexually Transmitted Diseases
38. Sleep Health
39. Social Determinants of Health
40. Substance Abuse
41. Tobacco Use
42. Vision

Source: U.S. Department of Health and Human Services (2010). "Topics & Objectives Index—Healthy People." Available at http://www.healthypeople.gov/2020/topicsobjectives2020/default.aspx.

the topic, a statement about the importance of the topic backed up by appropriate evidence, and references.

The developers of *Healthy People 2020* think that the best way to implement the national objectives is with the framework referred to as MAP-IT (see **Figure 1.7**). MAP-IT stands for Mobilize, Assess, Plan, Implement, and Track. The Mobilize step of MAP-IT deals with bringing interested parties together within communities to deal with health issues. The second step, Assess, is used to find out who is affected by the health problem and examine what resources are available to deal with it. In the Plan step, goals and objectives are created and an intervention is planned that has the best chance of dealing with the health problem. The Implement step deals with putting the intervention into action. The final step, Track, deals with evaluating the impact of the intervention on the health problem.[31]

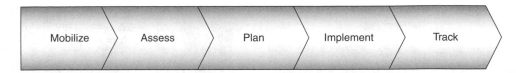

Figure 1.7 The action model to achieve *Healthy People* goals.

U.S. Department of Health and Human Services (2012). "Implementing Healthy People 2020." Available at http://www.healthypeople.gov/2020/implementing/default.aspx.

Community Health in the United States in the Early 2000s

Early in the new millennium, it is widely agreed that although decisions about health are an individual's responsibility to a significant degree, society has an obligation to provide an environment in which the achievement of good health is possible and encouraged. Furthermore, many recognize that certain segments of our population whose disease and death rates exceed those of the general population may require additional resources, including education, to achieve good health.

The American people face a number of serious public health problems. In the paragraphs that follow, we provide a brief overview of some of the problems that will make up a significant portion of the community health agenda in the United States for the years ahead.

Healthcare Delivery

In March 2010, significant changes were made to the U.S. healthcare system when President Barack Obama signed the Affordable Care Act (ACA) into law. Although the law has many components, the primary focus is to increase the number of Americans with health insurance. The ACA does this, but by providing health insurance to an additional 32 million Americans, the costs will also go up, which will continue to make U.S. health care the most expensive in the world. By 2013, health expenditures were projected to be almost $3 trillion and consume 17.6% of the gross domestic product (GDP); by 2020 they were expected to reach $4.6 trillion and 19.8% of the GDP.[32] The United States spends more per capita annually on health care (estimated at $9,348 in 2013)[32] than any other nation. The cost of health care is an issue that still needs to be addressed.

Environmental Problems

Millions of Americans live in communities where the air is unsafe to breathe, the water is unsafe to drink, or solid waste is disposed of improperly. With a few minor exceptions, the rate at which we pollute our environment continues to increase. Many Americans still believe that our natural resources are unlimited and that their individual contributions to the overall pollution are insignificant. In actuality, we must improve on our efforts in resource preservation and energy conservation if our children are to enjoy an environment as clean as ours. These environmental problems are compounded by the fact that the world population continues to grow; it now consists of more than 7 billion people and is expected to reach 8 billion by the year 2026.[33]

Lifestyle Diseases

The leading causes of death in the United States today are not the communicable diseases that were so feared 100 years ago, but chronic illnesses resulting from unwise lifestyle choices. The prevalence of obesity and diseases like diabetes is increasing. The four leading causes of death today are heart disease, cancer, chronic lower respiratory diseases, and stroke.[34] Although it is true that everyone has to die from some cause sometime, too many Americans die prematurely because of their unhealthy lifestyles (i.e., lack of exercise, poor diet, use of tobacco and drugs, and alcohol abuse). In the twenty-first century, behavior patterns continue to "represent the single most prominent domain of influence over health prospects in the United States"[10] (see Table 1.3).

Communicable Diseases

Although communicable (infectious) diseases no longer constitute the leading causes of death in the United States, they remain a concern for several reasons. First, they are the primary reason for days missed at school or at work. The success in reducing the life-threatening nature of these diseases has made many Americans complacent about obtaining vaccinations or taking other precautions against contracting these diseases. With the exception of smallpox, none of these diseases has been eradicated, although several should have been, such as measles.

Second, as new communicable diseases continue to appear, old ones such as tuberculosis reemerge, sometimes in drug-resistant forms, demonstrating that communicable diseases still represent a serious community health problem in the United States. Legionnaires' disease, toxic shock syndrome,

Table 1.3 Comparison of Most Common Causes of Death and Actual Causes of Death

Most Common Causes of Death, United States, 2010	Actual Causes of Death, United States, 2000
1. Diseases of the heart	1. Tobacco
2. Malignant neoplasms (cancers)	2. Poor diet and physical inactivity
3. Chronic lower respiratory diseases	3. Alcohol consumption
4. Cerebrovascular diseases (stroke)	4. Microbial agents
5. Unintentional injuries (accidents)	5. Toxic agents
6. Alzheimer's disease	6. Motor vehicles
7. Diabetes mellitus	7. Firearms
8. Nephritis, nephrotic syndrome, and nephrosis	8. Sexual behavior
9. Influenza and pneumonia	9. Illicit drug use
10. Intentional self-harm (suicide)	

Source: Data from Murphy, S. L., J. Q. Xu, and K. D. Kochanek (2012). "Deaths: Preliminary Data for 2010." *National Vital Statistics Reports,* 60(4). Available at http://www.cdc.gov/nchs/products/nvsr.htm. Mokdad, A. H., J. S. Marks, D. F. Stroup, and J. L. Gerberding (2004). "Actual Causes of Death in the United States, 2000." *Journal of the American Medical Association,* 291(10): 1238–1245; and Mokdad, A. H., J. S. Marks, D. F. Stroup, and J. L. Gerberding (2005). "Correction: Actual Causes of Death in the United States, 2000." *Journal of the American Medical Association,* 293(3): 293–294.

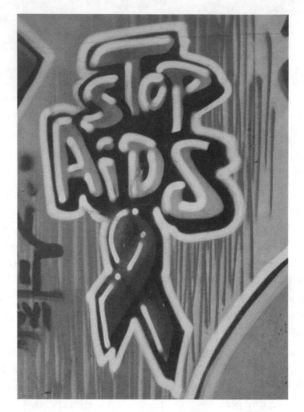

Figure 1.8 AIDS is one of the most feared communicable diseases today.
© coka/ShutterStock, Inc.

Lyme disease, acquired immune deficiency syndrome (AIDS), and severe acute respiratory syndrome (SARS) are diseases that were unknown only 40 years ago. The first cases of AIDS were reported in June 1981.[35] Since then an estimated 1.7 million people in the United States have been infected with human immunodeficiency virus (HIV)[36] (see **Figure 1.8**). The total number of cases continues to grow, with close to 50,000 new cases being diagnosed each year.[36] Also, diseases that were once found only in animals are now crossing over to human populations and causing much concern and action. Included in this group of diseases are avian flu, *Escherichia coli* O157:H7, hantavirus, mad cow disease, and SARS.[1]

Third, and maybe the most disturbing, is the use of communicable diseases for bioterrorism. **Bioterrorism** involves "the threatened or intentional release of biological agents (virus, bacteria, or their toxins) for the purpose of influencing the conduct of government

bioterrorism the threatened or intentional release of biological agents for the purpose of influencing the conduct of government or intimidating or coercing a civilian population to further political or social objectives

or intimidating or coercing a civilian population to further political or social objectives. These agents can be released by way of the air (as aerosols), food, water or insects."[37] Concern in the United States over bioterrorism was heightened after 9/11 and the subsequent intentional distribution of *Bacillus anthracis* spores through the U.S. postal system (the anthrax mailings).

Alcohol and Other Drug Abuse

"Abuse of legal and illegal drugs has become a national problem that costs this country thousands of lives and billions of dollars each year. Alcohol and other drugs are often associated with unintentional injuries, domestic violence, and violent crimes."[38] Federal, state, and local governments as well as private agencies attempt to address the supply and demand problems associated with the abuse of alcohol and other drugs, but a significant challenge remains for the United States.

Health Disparities

It has long been "recognized that some individuals are healthier than others and that some live longer than others do, and that often these differences are closely associated with social characteristics such as race, ethnicity, gender, location, and socioeconomic status."[39] These gaps between groups have been referred to as health disparities. **Health disparities** have been defined as the difference in health among different populations. Health disparities are a problem in the United States in that many minority groups' health status, on many different measures, is not as good as that of the white population. Efforts have been put forth to eliminate the disparities, as evidenced by one of the *Healthy People 2020* overarching goals to "achieve health equity, eliminate disparities, and improve the health for all groups." Many experts think these differences have been caused by two health inequities—lack of access to health care, and/or when health care is received the quality has not been as good for those in minority groups. Whatever the reason, health disparities continue to be a problem and much more needs to be done.

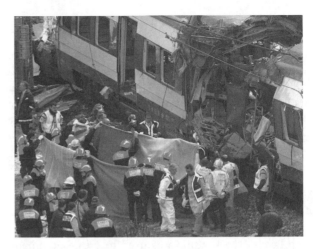

Figure 1.9 Terrorism has become a concern throughout the world.
© Reuters/Kai Pfaffenbach/Landov

Disasters

Disasters can be classified into two primary categories— natural (or conventional) and humanmade (or technological disasters).[1] Whereas natural disasters are the result of the combination of the forces of nature (e.g., hurricane, flood, blizzard, tornado, earthquake, landslide) and human activities, humanmade disasters result from either unintentional (e.g., spill of a toxic substance into the environment) or intentional (e.g., bioterrorism) human activities, often associated with the use or misuse of technology. Both types of disasters have the potential to cause injury, death, disease, and damage to property on a large scale.[1] In recent years, the United States has felt the large-scale impact of both types of disasters via the Gulf oil spill; Hurricanes Katrina, Rita, and Sandy; and the severe flooding in the middle of the country. All of these events showed us that the preparation for such disasters was not adequate and that each type of disaster required different resources and a different response.

Even though the causes of the two categories of disasters are different, preparedness for them has many common elements. A major difference in preparedness for the two categories of disasters is the specific other steps needed to deal with the peculiarity of the humanmade disasters. An example of this would be the need for decontamination following exposure to a biological agent.

Even given the devastating consequences of natural disasters each year, it has been the intentional humanmade disasters—specifically terrorism—that have occupied much of our attention in recent years (see **Figure 1.9**). Mention was made earlier of the use of a communicable disease as part of terrorism; however, a number of agents could be used as part of terrorism. Since the anthrax mailings, community and public health professionals have focused on the possibility that future terrorism could include chemical, biological, and/or radiological/nuclear (CBRN) agents, resulting in mass numbers of casualties. Such concern led to an evaluation of community and public health emergency preparedness and response. "Determining the level of state and local health departments' emergency preparedness and response capacities is crucial because public health officials are among those, along with firefighters, emergency medical personnel, and local law enforcement personnel, who serve on 'rapid response' teams when large-scale emergency situations arise."[40] Results of that evaluation showed that the public health infrastructure was not where it should be to handle large-scale emergencies, as well as a number of more common public health concerns.

Based on the results of several different evaluations that exposed many weaknesses in emergency preparedness in general and in the public health infrastructure more specifically, investment in public health preparedness has increased since September 11, 2001. Those federal departments that have been responsible for most of the effort have been the Departments of Homeland Security (DHS) and Health and Human Services (HHS). The DHS has the responsibility of protecting the United States, whereas the HHS has taken the leadership for public health and medical preparedness.

health disparities the difference in health among different populations

Public health preparedness has been defined as "the ability of the public health system, community, and individuals to prevent, protect against, quickly respond to, and recover from health emergencies, particularly those in which scale, timing, or unpredictability threatens to overwhelm routine capabilities."[41] **Medical preparedness** has been defined as "the ability of the health care system to prevent, protect against, quickly respond to, and recover from health emergencies, particularly those whose scale, timing, or unpredictability threatens to overwhelm routine capabilities."[41]

After 9/11, the federal government, through a variety of funding sources and programs, worked to strengthen homeland security, emergency preparedness, and response at all levels. The funding was used to create or enhance the various components needed in disaster situations (i.e., communication, coordination, and the workforce). The funding also was used to bring much of the public health system up-to-date (i.e., laboratories, personnel, and surveillance) after many years of neglect. However, in part because of the downturn in the economy, there has been a decrease in public health preparedness funding the past few years,[42] which has started to erode a decade's worth of progress.[43]

Although the United States is better prepared than prior to 9/11, much still needs to be done. In December 2011, the Trust for America's Health (TFAH), a nonprofit, nonpartisan organization, and the Robert Wood Johnson Foundation released their ninth report on the state of public health preparedness in the United States.[43] Although previous years' reports contained preparedness scores for all 50 states and the District of Columbia, much of the ninth report focuses on the impact of budget cuts that are putting preparedness programs and capabilities at risk for major cuts or elimination.

Overall, the report concludes that while it is impossible to be prepared for every potential threat, it is possible and essential to maintain a basic, core level of preparedness and response capabilities. Being prepared means the country must have enough resources and vigilance to prevent what we can and respond when we have to. In an era of scarce resources, it is more important than ever to think

medical preparedness the ability of the healthcare system to prevent, protect against, quickly respond to, and recover from health emergencies, particularly those whose scale, timing, or unpredictability threatens to overwhelm routine capabilities

public health preparedness the ability of the public health system, community, and individuals to prevent, protect against, quickly respond to, and recover from health emergencies, particularly those in which scale, timing, or unpredictability threatens to overwhelm routine capabilities

strategically to ensure Americans are not left unnecessarily vulnerable.[43]

Community Health in the World in the Early 2000s

Like the United States, much progress has been made in the health of people throughout the world in recent years. Life expectancy has increased by between 6 and 7 years globally in the last 30 years, due primarily to (1) social and economic development, (2) the wider provision of safe water and sanitation facilities, and (3) the expansion of national health services.[44] And, like in the United States, a number of public health achievements took place in the first 10 years of the twenty-first century (see Box 1.3). However, all do not share in this increased life expectancy and better health.

> There are widening health inequities between and within countries, between rich and poor, between men and women, and between different ethnic groups. More than a billion of the world's poorest people are not benefiting from the major advances in health care and several countries, particularly in sub-Saharan Africa, have seen a decline in life expectancy due in part to the HIV/AIDS epidemic.[44]

In the following paragraphs we identify some of the community health issues that the peoples of the world will be facing in the years ahead.

Communicable Diseases

Even though information presented in Box 1.3 suggests that there have been a number of achievements with regard to communicable diseases throughout the world between 2001 and 2010, the burden of communicable diseases worldwide is still great. It is most vivid when looking at mortality. The leading causes of death in the world do not look much different than the leading causes of death in the United States. In fact, heart disease and cerebrovascular disease are the number one and two killers worldwide. However, when the leading causes of death are broken down by the wealth of the countries, big differences appear. Four of the 10 leading causes of death in low- and middle-income countries are infectious diseases (i.e., lower respiratory infections, diarrheal disease, HIV/AIDS, and tuberculosis), whereas 9 of the 10 leading causes are noncommunicable diseases in high-income countries. Similar trends appear when the age of those who die are compared with the wealth of the countries. In low-income countries less than one in five of all people reach the age of 70, and more than a third of all deaths are among children under the age of 15. In middle-income countries, nearly half of all people live to

---

Box 1.3   Ten Great Public Health Achievements Worldwide 2001–2010

At the conclusion of 2010, experts in global public health were asked to nominate noteworthy public health achievements that occurred outside of the United States during 2001-2010. From them, 10 were selected. Following, in no specific order, are the ones selected from the nominations[45]:

- *Reductions in child mortality:* Currently, an estimated 8.1 million children die each year before reaching their fifth birthday, a decrease of approximately 2 million between 2001 and 2010. Almost all childhood deaths (~99%) occur in low-income and middle-income countries, with 49% occurring in sub-Saharan Africa and 33% in southern Asia.

- *Vaccine-preventable deaths:* Over the 10-year period, an estimated 2.5 million deaths were prevented each year among children less than 5 years of age through the use of measles, polio, and diphtheria-tetanus-pertussis vaccines.

- *Access to safe water and sanitation:* Diarrhea, most of which is related to inadequate water, sanitation, and hygiene (WASH), kills 1.5 million children under 5 years of age annually. The proportion of the world's population with access to improved drinking water sources increased from 83% to 87% (covering an additional 800 million persons), and the proportion with access to improved sanitation increased from 58% to 61% (covering an additional 570 million persons).

- *Malaria prevention and control:* Malaria is the fifth leading cause of death from infectious disease worldwide and the second leading cause in Africa. Increased coverage with insecticide-treated bednets, indoor residual spraying, rapid diagnosis and prompt treatment with artemisinin combination therapy, and intermittent preventive treatment during pregnancy resulted in a 21% decrease in estimated global malaria deaths between 2000 and 2009.

- *Prevention and control of HIV/AIDS:* The HIV epidemic continues to be a global health challenge, with 33.3 million people living with HIV at the end of 2009.[46] However, a number of public health interventions, including provider-initiated HIV testing and counseling, prevention of mother-to-child HIV transmission, expanded availability and use of condoms and sterile injection equipment, improved blood safety, and antiretroviral

therapy (ART), have helped to reduce the number of new infections.

- *Tuberculosis (TB) control.* Due in large part to the World Health Organization's (WHO's) directly observed therapy, short-course (DOTS) strategy for TB control, focusing on finding and successfully treating TB cases with standardized regimens and rigorous treatment and program monitoring, during the decade case detection and treatment success rates each have risen nearly 20%, with incidence and prevalence declining in every region.

- *Control of neglected tropical diseases:* Neglected tropical diseases affect approximately 1 billion persons worldwide. Three of these diseases have been targeted for elimination or eradication: dracunculiasis (Guinea worm disease), onchocerciasis (river blindness), and lymphatic filariasis. Those programs targeting dracunculiasis and onchocerciasis in the Americas are on the verge of success, and the lymphatic filariasis programs are making progress.

- *Tobacco control:* In 2010, 5.4 million premature deaths were attributable to tobacco use.[47] However, during the decade, 168 countries adopted the WHO's first global health treaty aimed at tobacco, 163 countries tracked tobacco use via surveys, and the total global population covered by smoke-free laws increased.

- *Increased awareness and response for improving global road safety:* Approximately 1.3 million persons die on the world's roads each year (3,000 every day), and this number is projected to double by 2030. Although the number of road deaths did not slow down during the past 10 years, a significant global effort was made to create a plan to reduce the forecasted growth in road fatalities.

- *Improved preparedness and response to global health threats:* During the 10-year period of time, the public health community has improved preparedness for and detection of pandemic threats and is now responding more effectively than before. This is due in part to modernization of the international legal framework, better disease surveillance techniques, better public health networking, and better global disease detection systems.

Source: Modified from U.S. Department of Health and Human Services, Centers for Disease Control and Prevention (2011). "Ten Great Public Health Achievements –Worldwide, 2001–2010." *Morbidity and Mortality Weekly Report,* 60(24): 814–818. Available at http://www.cdc.gov/mmwr/preview/mmwrhtml/mm6024a4.htm?s_cid=mm6024a4_w.

---

the age of 70, and in high-income countries more than two-thirds of all people live beyond the age of 70.[48]

Poor Sanitation and Unsafe Drinking Water

A significant portion of the deaths caused by communicable diseases can be traced to poor sanitation and unsafe drinking water. Those most impacted by these conditions are the poorest of the poor. Over a third of the world's population (~2.6 million people) still does not have access to a flush toilet or other forms of improved sanitation.[49] Although the percentage is not as large as those without a flush toilet,

about 13% of the world's population does not have access to clean drinking water. Both urbanites and rural dwellers are impacted, but the conditions are much worse for those in rural areas. "In sub-Saharan Africa, an urban dweller is 1.8 times more likely to use an improved drinking water source than a person living in a rural area."[49]

Hunger

The distribution of food worldwide is far from equal. Despite some gains on the issue of poverty, the proportion of people going hungry in the developing regions of the world has plateaued at 16% after being around 20% in 1990.[48] Some of the hardest hit in these regions are the children. In some regions nearly one-fourth of the children under the age of 5 are underweight. Their lack of weight is due to a combination of factors including "lack of quality food, suboptimal feeding practices, repeated attacks of infectious diseases and pervasive undernutrition."[49]

Organizations That Help Shape Community Health

As noted earlier in the chapter, the history of community health dates to antiquity. For much of that history, community health issues were addressed only on an emergency basis. For example, if a community faced a drought or an epidemic, a town meeting would be called to deal with the problem. It has been only in the last 100 years or so that communities have taken explicit actions to deal aggressively with health issues on a continual basis.

Today's communities differ from those of the past in several important ways. Although individuals are better educated, more mobile, and more independent than in the past, communities are less autonomous and are more dependent on state and federal funding for support. Contemporary communities are too large and complex to respond effectively to sudden health emergencies or to make long-term improvements in public health without community organization and careful planning. Better community organizing and careful long-term planning are essential to ensure that a community makes the best use of its resources for health, both in times of emergency and over the long run.

governmental health agencies health agencies that are part of the governmental structure (federal, state, or local) and that are funded primarily by tax dollars

top-down funding a method of funding in which funds are transmitted from federal or state government to the local level

World Health Organization (WHO) the most widely recognized international governmental health organization

The ability of today's communities to respond effectively to their own problems is hindered by the following characteristics: (1) highly developed and centralized resources in our national institutions and organizations; (2) continuing concentration of wealth and population in the largest metropolitan areas; (3) rapid movement of information, resources, and people made possible by advanced communication and transportation technologies that eliminate the need for local offices where resources were once housed; (4) the globalization of health; (5) limited horizontal relationships between/among organizations;

and (6) a system of **top-down funding** (money that comes from either the federal or state government to the local level) for many community programs.[50]

In the following sections we discuss organizations that help to shape a community's ability to respond effectively to health-related issues by protecting and promoting the health of the community and its members. These community organizations can be classified as governmental, quasi-governmental, or nongovernmental, based on their sources of funding, responsibilities, and organizational structure.

Governmental Health Agencies

Governmental health agencies are part of the governmental structure. They are funded primarily by tax dollars and managed by government officials. Each governmental health agency is designated as having authority over some geographic area. Such agencies exist at the four governmental levels—international, national, state, and local.

International Health Agencies

The most widely recognized international governmental health organization today is the **World Health Organization (WHO)** (see **Figure 1.10**). Its headquarters is located in Geneva, Switzerland, and there are six regional offices around the world. The names, acronyms, and cities and countries of location for WHO regional offices are as follows: Africa (AFRO), Brazzaville, Congo; Americas (PAHO), Washington, D.C., United States; Eastern Mediterranean (EMRO), Cairo, Egypt; Europe (EURO), Copenhagen, Denmark; Southeast Asia (SEARO), New Delhi, India; and Western Pacific (WPRO), Manila, Philippines.[50]

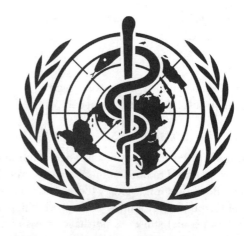

Figure 1.10 The emblem of the World Health Organization.
© PR Newswire/AP Photos

Although the WHO is now the largest international health organization, it is not the oldest. Among the organizations (listed with their founding dates) that predate the WHO are the following:

- International D'Hygiene Publique (1907), which was absorbed by the WHO.
- The Health Organization of the League of Nations (1919), which was dissolved when the WHO was created.
- The United Nations Relief and Rehabilitation Administration (1943), which was dissolved in 1946. Its work is carried out today by the Office of the United Nations High Commissioner for Refugees (UNHCR) (1950).
- The United Nations Children's Fund (UNICEF) (1946), which was formerly known as the United Nations International Children's Emergency Fund.
- The Pan American Health Organization (PAHO) (1902), which is still an independent organization but is integrated with WHO in a regional office.

Because the WHO is the largest and most visible international health agency, it is discussed at greater length in the following sections.

History of the World Health Organization

Planning for the WHO began when a charter of the United Nations was adopted at an international meeting in 1945. Contained in the charter was an article calling for the establishment of a health agency with wide powers. In 1946, at the International Health Conference, representatives from all of the countries in the United Nations succeeded in creating and ratifying the constitution of the WHO. However, it was not until April 7, 1948, that the constitution went into force and the organization officially began its work. In recognition of this beginning, April 7 is commemorated each year as World Health Day.[50]

Organization of the World Health Organization

Membership in the WHO is open to any nation that has ratified the WHO constitution and receives a majority vote of the World Health Assembly. In 2012, 194 countries were members. The **World Health Assembly** is composed of delegates from the member nations. This assembly, which meets in general sessions annually and in special sessions when necessary, has the primary tasks of approving the WHO program and the budget for the following biennium and deciding major policy questions.[50]

The WHO is administered by a staff that includes a director-general, deputy director-general, and nine assistant directors-general. Great care is taken to ensure political balance in staffing WHO positions, particularly at the higher levels of administration.

Purpose and Work of the World Health Organization

The primary objective of the WHO, as stated in its constitution, is the attainment by all peoples of the highest possible level of health.[50] To achieve this objective, the WHO has six core functions:

1. Providing leadership on matters critical to health and engaging in partnerships where joint action is needed;
2. Shaping the research agenda and stimulating the generation, translation and dissemination of valuable knowledge;
3. Setting norms and standards, and promoting and monitoring their implementation;
4. Articulating ethical and evidence-based policy options;
5. Providing technical support, catalysing [sic] change, and building sustainable institutional capacity;
6. Monitoring the health situation and assessing health trends.

The work of the WHO is financed by its member nations, each of which is assessed according to its ability to pay; the wealthiest countries contribute the greatest portion of the total budget.

Although the WHO has sponsored and continues to sponsor many worthwhile programs, an especially noteworthy one was the work of the WHO in helping to eradicate smallpox. In 1967, smallpox was active in 31 countries. During that year, 10 million to 15 million people contracted the disease, and of those, approximately 2 million died and many millions of others were permanently disfigured or blinded. The last known case of smallpox was diagnosed on October 26, 1977, in Somalia.[50] In 1979, the World Health Assembly declared the global eradication of this disease. Using the smallpox mortality figures from 1967, it can be estimated that more than 40 million lives have been saved since the eradication.

The current work of the WHO is guided by two documents—the 11th General Programme of Work[43] and the United Nations Millennium Declaration, which was adopted at the Millennium Summit in 2003.[51] Much of what is included in the 11th General Programme of Work is summarized in Box 1.4 (the WHO Agenda). The Millennium Declaration set out

World Health Assembly a body of delegates of the member nations of the WHO

Box 1.4   The WHO Agenda

1. *Promoting development.* During the past decade, health has achieved unprecedented prominence as a key driver of socioeconomic progress, and more resources than ever are being invested in health. Yet poverty continues to contribute to poor health, and poor health anchors large populations in poverty. Health development is directed by the ethical principle of equity: Access to life-saving or health-promoting interventions should not be denied for unfair reasons, including those with economic or social roots. Commitment to this principle ensures that WHO activities aimed at health development give priority to health outcomes in poor, disadvantaged, or vulnerable groups. Attainment of the health-related Millennium Development Goals, preventing and treating chronic diseases and addressing the neglected tropical diseases, are the cornerstones of the health and development agenda.

2. *Fostering health security.* Shared vulnerability to health security threats demands collective action. One of the greatest threats to international health security arises from outbreaks of emerging and epidemic-prone diseases. Such outbreaks are occurring in increasing numbers, fueled by such factors as rapid urbanization, environmental mismanagement, the way food is produced and traded, and the way antibiotics are used and misused. The world's ability to defend itself collectively against outbreaks has been strengthened since June 2007, when the revised International Health Regulations came into force.

3. *Strengthening health systems.* For health improvement to operate as a poverty-reduction strategy, health services must reach poor and underserved populations. Health systems in many parts of the world are unable to do so, making the strengthening of health systems a high priority for WHO. Areas being addressed include the provision of adequate numbers of appropriately trained staff, sufficient financing, suitable systems for collecting vital statistics, and access to appropriate technology including essential drugs.

4. *Harnessing research, information, and evidence.* Evidence provides the foundation for setting priorities, defining strategies, and measuring results. WHO generates authoritative health information, in consultation with leading experts, to set norms and standards, articulate evidence-based policy options, and monitor the evolving global heath situation.

5. *Enhancing partnerships.* WHO carries out its work with the support and collaboration of many partners, including UN agencies and other international organizations, donors, civil society, and the private sector. WHO uses the strategic power of evidence to encourage partners implementing programs within countries to align their activities with best technical guidelines and practices, as well as with the priorities established by countries.

6. *Improving performance.* WHO participates in ongoing reforms aimed at improving its efficiency and effectiveness, both at the international level and within countries. WHO aims to ensure that its strongest asset–its staff–works in an environment that is motivating and rewarding. WHO plans its budget and activities through results-based management, with clear expected results to measure performance at country, regional and international levels.

Source: Reprinted with permission of World Health Organization (2012). "The WHO Agenda." Available at http://www.who.int/about/agenda/en/index.html.

---

principles and values in seven areas (peace, security, and disarmament; development and poverty eradication; protecting our common environment; human rights, democracy, and good governance; protecting the vulnerable; meeting special needs of Africa; and strengthening the United Nations) that should govern international relations in the twenty-first century.[52] Following the summit, the Road Map was prepared, which established goals and targets to be reached by 2015 in each of the seven areas.[53] The resulting eight goals in the area of development and poverty eradication are now referred to as the Millennium Development Goals (MDGs). More specifically, the MDGs are aimed at reducing poverty and hunger, and tackling ill health, gender inequality, lack of education, lack of access to clean water, and environmental degradation (see Table 1.4).

As can be seen from this description, the MDGs are not exclusively aimed at health, but there are interactive processes between health and economic development that create a crucial link; that is, better health is "a prerequisite and major contributor to economic growth and social cohesion. Conversely, improvement in people's access to health technology is a good indicator of the success of other development processes."[54] As such, "three of the eight goals, eight of the 18 targets required to achieve them, and 18 of the 48 indicators of progress are health-related"[54] (see Table 1.4).

To date, progress has been made to achieve the MDGs by the target date of 2015; however, this progress has been relatively slow. Strategies for achieving large-scale and rapid progress toward meeting the MDGs involve strong government leadership and policies and strategies that meet the needs of the poor, combined with sufficient funding and technical support from the international community.[55] Much work lies ahead, by all people of the world, to improve the health of those most in need.

National Health Agencies

Each national government has a department or agency that has the primary responsibility for the protection of the health and welfare of its citizens. These national health agencies meet their responsibilities through the

Table 1.4 Health-Related Millennium Development Goals, Targets, and Indicators

Goal: 1. Eradicate Extreme Poverty and Hunger

Target: 2.	Halve, between 1990 and 2015, the proportion of people who suffer from hunger
Indicator:	**4.** Prevalence of underweight children under 5 years of age
	5. Proportion of population below minimum level of dietary energy consumption[a]

Goal: 4. Reduce Child Mortality

Target: 5.	Reduce by two-thirds, between 1990 and 2015, the under-5 mortality rate
Indicator:	**13.** Under-5 mortality rate
	14. Infant mortality rate
	15. Proportion of 1-year-old children immunized against measles

Goal: 5. Improve Maternal Health

Target: 6.	Reduce by three-quarters, between 1990 and 2015, the maternal mortality ratio
Indicator:	**16.** Maternal mortality ratio
	17. Proportion of births attended by skilled health personnel

Goal: 6. Combat HIV/AIDS, Malaria, and Other Diseases

Target: 7.	Have halted by 2015 and begun to reverse the spread of HIV/AIDS
Indicator:	**18.** HIV prevalence among young people aged 15 to 24 years[b]
	19. Condom use rate of the contraceptive prevalence rate
	20. Number of children orphaned by HIV/AIDS
Target: 8.	Have halted by 2015 and begun to reverse the incidence of malaria and other major diseases
Indicator:	**21.** Prevalence and death rates associated with malaria
	22. Proportion of population in malaria-risk areas using effective malaria prevention and treatment measures
	23. Prevalence and death rates associated with tuberculosis
	24. Proportion of tuberculosis cases detected and cured under Directly Observed Treatment, Short-course (DOTS)

Goal: 7. Ensure Environmental Sustainability

Target: 9.	Integrate the principles of sustainable development into country policies and programmes and reverse the loss of environmental resources
Indicator:	**29.** Proportion of population using solid fuel
Target: 10.	Halve by 2015 the proportion of people without sustainable access to safe drinking water
Indicator:	**30.** Proportion of population with sustainable access to an improved water source, urban and rural
Target: 11.	By 2020 to have achieved a significant improvement in the lives of at least 100 million slum dwellers
Indicator:	**31.** Proportion of urban population with access to improved sanitation

Goal: 8. Develop a Global Partnership for Development

Target: 17.	In cooperation with pharmaceutical companies, provide access to affordable essential drugs in developing countries
Indicator:	**46.** Proportion of population with access to affordable essential drugs on a sustainable basis

[a]Health-related indicator reported by the Food and Agriculture Organization only.
[b]Indicators from the MDG list reformulated by WHO and United Nations General Assembly Special Session on HIV/AIDS.
Source: World Health Organization (2003). *World Health Report 2003: Shaping the Future.* Geneva, Switzerland: Author, 28. Used with permission of the World Health Organization.

development of health policies, the enforcement of health regulations, the provision of health services and programs, the funding of research, and the support of their respective state and local health agencies.

In the United States, the primary national health agency is the Department of Health and Human Services (HHS). HHS "is the United States government's principal agency for protecting the health of all Americans and providing essential human services, especially for those who are least able to help themselves."[56] It is important to note, however, that other federal agencies also contribute to the betterment of our nation's health. For example, the Department of Agriculture inspects meat and dairy products and coordinates the Women, Infants, and Children (WIC) food assistance program; the Environmental Protection Agency (EPA) regulates hazardous wastes; the Department of Labor houses the Occupational Safety and Health Administration (OSHA), which is concerned with safety and health in the workplace; the Department of Commerce, which includes the Bureau of the Census, collects much of the national data that drive our nation's health programs; and the Department of Homeland Security (DHS) deals with all aspects of terrorism within the United States. A detailed description of the Department of Health and Human Services follows.

Department of Health and Human Services

The HHS is headed by the Secretary of Health and Human Services, who is appointed by the president and is a member of his or her cabinet. The Department of Health and Human Services was formed in 1980 (during the administration of President Jimmy Carter), when the Department of Health, Education, and Welfare (HEW) was divided into two new departments, HHS and the Department of Education. HHS is the department most involved with the nation's human concerns. In one way or another it touches the lives of more Americans than any other federal agency. It is literally a department of people serving people, from newborn infants to persons requiring health services to our most elderly citizens. With an annual budget in excess of $909 billion (representing about 24% of the federal budget), HHS is the largest department in the federal government, and it spends approximately $170 billion more per year than the Department of Defense.[57]

Since its formation, HHS has undergone several reorganizations. Some of the more recent changes have been the addition of the Center for Faith-Based and Community Initiatives and an Assistant Secretary for Public Health Emergency Preparedness. Currently, the HHS is organized into 11 operating agencies (see Figure 1.11) whose heads report directly to the Secretary. In addition, the HHS has 10 regional offices, which serve as representatives of the Secretary of HHS in direct, official dealings with state and local governmental organizations. Eight of the 11 operating divisions of the HHS (AHRQ, CDC, ATSDR, FDA, HRSA, IHS, NIH, and SAMSHA—see their descriptions in the following list), along with the Office of Global Health Affairs (OGHA), the Office of the Assistant Secretary for Health (ASH), and the Office of the Assistant Secretary for Preparedness and Response (ASPR), now constitute the Public Health Service (PHS). Another three operating divisions (CMS, ACF, and ACL) comprise the human services operating divisions.

Superfund legislation
legislation enacted to deal with the cleanup of hazardous substances in the environment

- *Administration for Children and Families (ACF):* The ACF is composed of a number of smaller agencies and is responsible for federal programs that promote the economic and social well-being of families, children, individuals, and communities. One of the better-known programs originating from this division is Head Start, which promotes the school readiness of children from birth to 5 years of age from low-income families by enhancing their cognitive, social, and emotional development. Other programs are aimed at family assistance, refugee resettlement, and child support enforcement.
- *Administration on Community Living (ACL):* The ACL is the newest operating division, formed in 2012. It combines the former Administration on Aging, the Office on Disability, and the Administration on Developmental Disabilities into a single agency. The goal of this new division is to increase access to community supports and full participation, while focusing attention and resources on the unique needs of older Americans and people with disabilities.
- *Agency for Healthcare Research and Quality (AHRQ):* The mission of AHRQ "is to improve the quality, safety, efficiency, and effectiveness of health care for all Americans."[58] AHRQ sponsors research that provides evidence-based information on healthcare outcomes; quality; and cost, use, and access. The information helps healthcare decision makers—patients and clinicians, health system leaders, and policy makers—make more informed decisions and improve the quality of healthcare services.
- *Agency for Toxic Substances and Disease Registry (ATSDR):* This agency was created by the **Superfund legislation** (Comprehensive Environmental Response, Compensation, and Liability Act) in 1980. This legislation was enacted to deal with the cleanup of hazardous substances in the environment. ATSDR's mission is to "serve the public through responsive public health actions to promote healthy and safe environments and prevent harmful exposures."[59] To carry out its mission and to serve the needs of the U.S. public, ATSDR evaluates information on hazardous substances released into the environment in order to assess the impact on public health; conducts and sponsors studies and other research related to hazardous substances and adverse human health effects; establishes and maintains registries of human exposure (for long-term follow-up) and complete listings of areas closed to the public or otherwise restricted in use due to contamination; summarizes and makes data available on the effects of hazardous substances; and provides consultations

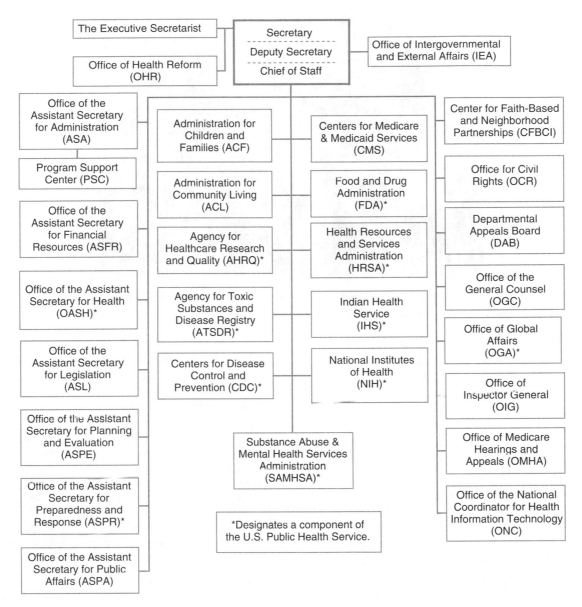

Figure 1.11 Organizational chart for the U.S. Department of Health and Human Services (HHS).

Reproduced from U.S. Department of Health and Human Services (2010). "U.S. Department of Health and Human Services Organizational Chart." Available at http://www.hhs.gov/about/orgchart.html.

and training to ensure adequate response to public health emergencies.

- *Centers for Disease Control and Prevention (CDC):* The CDC, located in Atlanta, Georgia (see **Figure 1.12**), "is the primary Federal agency for conducting and supporting public health activities in the United States."[60] Its mission "is to collaborate to create the expertise, information, and tools that people and communities need to protect their health—through health promotion, prevention

of disease, injury and disability, and preparedness for new health threats."[61] The CDC is composed of the Office of the Director, the National Institute for Occupational Safety and Health, the Center for Global Health, and five offices: Public Health Preparedness and Response; State, Tribal, Local, and Territorial Support; Surveillance, Epidemiology and Laboratory Services; Noncommunicable Diseases, Injury and Environmental Health; and Infectious Diseases.[60] Within its offices are the many "national centers"

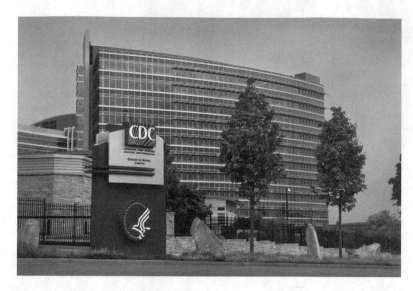

Figure 1.12 The Centers for Disease Control and Prevention (CDC) in Atlanta, Georgia, is one of the major operating divisions of the Department of Health and Human Services (HHS).
Courtesy of James Gathany/CDC

(e.g., National Center for Health Statistics and National Center for Injury Prevention and Control); thus the term *Centers* in CDC. Further, the CDC "employs more than 15,000 employees in more than 50 countries and in 168 occupational categories."[60] Once known solely for its work to control communicable diseases, the CDC now also maintains records, analyzes disease trends, and publishes epidemiological reports on all types of diseases, including those that result from lifestyle, occupational, and environmental causes. Beyond its own specific responsibilities, the CDC also supports state and local health departments and cooperates with similar national health agencies from other WHO member nations.

- *Centers for Medicare and Medicaid Services (CMS):* The CMS is responsible for overseeing the Medicare program (health care for the elderly and the disabled), the federal portion of the Medicaid program (health care for low-income individuals), and the related quality assurance activities. Both Medicare and Medicaid were created in 1965 to ensure that the special groups covered by these programs would not be deprived of health care because of cost. In 2010, more than 92 million Americans were covered by these programs.[62] In 1997, the Children's Health Insurance Program (CHIP) also became the responsibility of the CMS.
- *Food and Drug Administration (FDA):* The FDA touches the lives of virtually every American every day. The FDA is responsible for:

- Protecting the public health by assuring that foods are safe, wholesome, sanitary and properly labeled; human and veterinary drugs, and vaccines and other biological products and medical devices intended for human use are safe and effective
- Protecting the public from electronic product radiation
- Assuring cosmetics and dietary supplements are safe and properly labeled
- Regulating tobacco products
- Advancing the public health by helping to speed product innovations
- Helping the public get the accurate science-based information they need to use medicines, devices, and foods to improve their health[63]

Much of this work revolves around regulatory activities and the setting of health and safety standards as spelled out in the Federal Food, Drug, and Cosmetic Act and other related laws. However, because of the complex nature of its standards and the agency's limited resources, enforcement of many FDA regulations is left to other federal agencies and to state and local agencies. For example, the Department of Agriculture is responsible for the inspection of many foods, such as meat and dairy products. Restaurants, supermarkets, and other food outlets are inspected by state and local public health agencies.

- *Health Resources and Services Administration (HRSA):* HRSA "is the primary federal agency for improving access to health care services for people who are underinsured, isolated, or medically vulnerable."[64] The cited mission of HRSA is "to improve health and achieve health equity through access to quality services, a skilled health workforce and innovative programs."[64] HRSA maintains the National Health Service Corps and helps build the healthcare workforce through training and education programs. The agency "administers a variety of programs to improve the health of mothers and children and serves people living with HIV/AIDS through the Ryan White CARE Act programs." HRSA is also responsible for overseeing the nation's organ, bone marrow, and cord blood donations.[64]

- *Indian Health Service (IHS):* The IHS "is responsible for providing federal health services to American Indians and Alaska Natives."[65] Currently, it "provides a comprehensive health service delivery system for approximately 1.9 million American Indians and Alaska Natives who belong to 564 federally recognized tribes in 35 states."[65]

  - The provision of health services to members of federally recognized tribes grew out of the special government-to-government relationship between the federal government and Indian tribes. This relationship, established in 1787, is based on Article I, Section 8 of the Constitution, and has been given form and substance by numerous treaties, laws, Supreme Court decisions, and Executive Orders. The IHS is the principal federal health care provider and health advocate for Indian people and its goal is to raise their health status to the highest possible level.[65]

- *National Institutes of Health (NIH):* Begun as a one-room Laboratory of Hygiene in 1887, the NIH is the nation's medical research agency and today is one of the world's foremost medical research centers. NIH is made up of 21 institutes (e.g., National Cancer Institute [NCI], National Human Genome Research Institute [NHGRI]) and six centers (e.g., Center for Information Technology [CIT], National Center for Complementary and Alternative Medicine [NCCAM]). The mission of the NIH "is to seek fundamental knowledge about the nature and behavior of living systems and the application of that knowledge to enhance health, lengthen life, and reduce the burdens of illness and disability."[66] Although a significant amount of research is carried out by NIH scientists at NIH laboratories in Bethesda, Maryland, and elsewhere, a much larger portion of this research is conducted by scientists at public and private universities and other research institutions. These scientists receive NIH funding for their research proposals through a competitive, peer-reviewed grant application process. Through this process of proposal review by qualified scientists, NIH seeks to ensure that federal research monies are spent on the best-conceived research projects.

- *Substance Abuse and Mental Health Services Administration (SAMHSA):* SAMHSA is the primary federal agency responsible for ensuring that up-to-date information and state-of-the-art practice are effectively used for the prevention and treatment of addictive and mental disorders. SAMHSA's "mission is to reduce the impact of substance abuse and mental illness on American's communities."[67] Within SAMHSA, there are four centers—the Center for Substance Abuse Treatment (CSAT), the Center for Substance Abuse Prevention (CSAP), the Center for Mental Health Services (CMHS), and the Center for Behavioral Health Statistics and Quality (CBHSQ). Each of these centers has its own mission that contributes to the overall mission of SAMHSA.

State Health Agencies

All 50 states have their own state health departments (see Figure 1.13). Although the names of these departments may vary from state to state (e.g., Ohio Department of Health, Indiana State Department of Health), their purposes remain the same: to promote, protect, and maintain the health and welfare of their citizens. These purposes are represented in the **core functions of public health**, which are assessment of information on the health of the community, comprehensive public health policy development, and assurance that public health services are provided to the community.[68] These core functions have been defined further with the following 10 essential public health services[69] (see Figure 1.14):

1. Monitor health status to identify community health problems.
2. Diagnose and investigate health problems and health hazards in the community.
3. Inform, educate, and empower people about health issues.
4. Mobilize community partnerships to identify and solve health problems.
5. Develop policies and plans that support individual and community health efforts.
6. Enforce laws and regulations that protect health and ensure safety.
7. Link people to needed personal health services and assure the provision of health care when otherwise unavailable.

core functions of public health assessment, policy development, and assurance

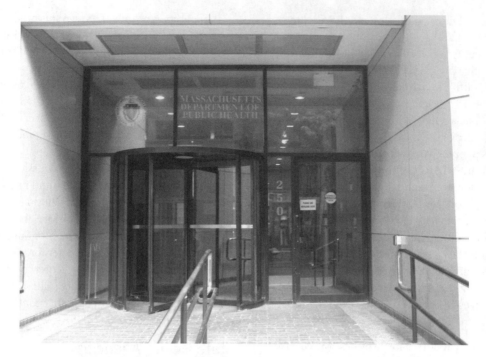

Figure 1.13 Each of the 50 states has its own health department.

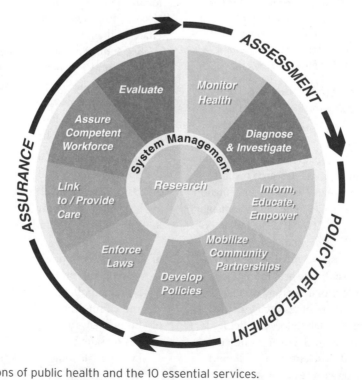

Figure 1.14 Core functions of public health and the 10 essential services.
Public Health Functions Steering Committee, Members (July 1995). "Public Health in America." Available at http://web.health.gov/phfunctions/public.htm.

8. Ensure a competent public health and personal healthcare workforce.
9. Evaluate effectiveness, accessibility, and quality of personal- and population-based health services.
10. Research for new insights and innovative solutions to health problems.

The head of the state health department is usually a medical doctor, appointed by the governor, who may carry the title of director, commissioner, or secretary. However, because of the political nature of the appointment, this individual may or may not have extensive experience in community or public health. Unfortunately, political influence sometimes reaches below the level of commissioner to the assistant commissioners and division chiefs; it is the commissioner, assistant commissioners, and division chiefs who set policy and provide direction for the state health department. Middle- and lower-level employees are usually hired through a merit system and may or may not be able to influence health department policy. Although not always, these employees, who carry out the routine work of the state health department, are professionally trained health specialists such as microbiologists, engineers, sanitarians, epidemiologists, nurses, and health education specialists.

Most state health departments are organized into divisions or bureaus that provide certain standard services. Typical divisions include Administration, Communicable Disease Prevention and Control, Chronic Disease Prevention and Control, Vital and Health Statistics, Environmental Health, Health Education or Promotion, Health Services, Maternal and Child Health, Mental Health, Occupational and Industrial Health, Dental Health, Laboratory Services, Public Health Nursing, Veterinary Public Health, and most recently, a division of Public Health Preparedness to deal with bioterrorism issues.

In promoting, protecting, and maintaining the health and welfare of their citizens, state health departments play many different roles. They can establish and promulgate health regulations that have the force and effect of law throughout the state. The state health departments also provide an essential link between federal and local (city and county) public health agencies. As such, they serve as conduits for federal funds aimed at local health problems. Federal funds come to the states as block grants. Funds earmarked for particular health projects are distributed to local health departments by their respective state health departments in accordance with previously agreed upon priorities. State health departments may also link local needs with federal expertise. For example, epidemiologists from the CDC are sometimes made available to investigate local disease outbreaks at the request of the state health department. State health departments usually must approve appointments of local health officers and can also remove any local health officers who neglect their duties.

The resources and expertise of the state health department are also at the disposal of local health departments. One particular area where the state health departments can be helpful is laboratory services; many modern diagnostic tests are simply too expensive for local health departments. Another area is environmental health. Water and air pollution problems usually extend beyond local jurisdictions, and their detection and measurement often require equipment too expensive for local governments to afford. This equipment and expertise are often provided by the state health department.

Local Health Departments

Local-level governmental health organizations, referred to as local health departments (LHDs), are usually the responsibility of the city or county governments. In large metropolitan areas, community health needs are usually best served by a city health department. In smaller cities with populations of up to 75,000, people often come under the jurisdiction of a county health department. In some rural counties where most of the population is concentrated in a single city, an LHD may have jurisdiction over both city and county residents. In sparsely populated rural areas, it is not uncommon to find more than one county served by a single health department. In 2010, there were approximately 2,700 LHDs; of that number, 75% were located in nonmetropolitan areas and 25% were in metropolitan areas.[70]

It is through LHDs that health services are provided to the people of the community. A great many of these services are mandated by state laws, which also set standards for health and safety. Examples of mandated local health services include the inspection of restaurants, public buildings, and public transportation systems; the detection and reporting of certain diseases; and the collection of vital statistics such as births and deaths. Other programs such as safety belt programs and immunization clinics may be locally planned and implemented. In this regard, local health jurisdictions are permitted (unless preemptive legislation is in place) to enact ordinances that are stricter than those of the state, but these jurisdictions cannot enact codes that fall below state standards. It is at this level of governmental health agencies that sanitarians implement the environmental health programs, nurses and physicians offer the clinical services, and health education specialists present health education and promotion programs.

Organization of Local Health Departments

Each LHD is headed by a health officer/administrator/commissioner. In most states, there are laws that prescribe who can hold such a position. Those often noted are physicians, dentists, veterinarians, or individuals with a master's or doctoral degree in public health. If the health officer is not a physician, then a physician is usually hired on a consulting basis to advise as needed. Usually this health officer is appointed by a board of health, the members of which are themselves appointed by officials in the city or county government or, in some situations, elected by the general public. The health officer and administrative assistants may recommend which programs will be offered by the LHDs. However, they may need final approval from a board of health. Although it is desirable that those serving on the local board of health have some knowledge of community health programs, most states have no such requirement. Often, politics plays a role in deciding the makeup of the local board of health.

The local health officer, like the state health commissioner, has far-reaching powers, including the power to arrest someone who refuses to undergo treatment for a communicable disease (tuberculosis, for example) and who thereby continues to spread disease in the community. The local health officer has the power to close a restaurant on the spot if it has serious health law violations or to impound a shipment of food if it is contaminated. Because many local health departments cannot afford to employ a full-time physician, the health officer is usually hired on a part-time basis. In such cases, the day-to-day activities of the LHD are carried out by an administrator trained in public health. The administrator is also hired by the board of health based on qualifications and the recommendation of the health officer.

Local sources provide the greatest percentage of LHD revenues (26%), followed by state funds (21%) and federal pass-through funds (14%).[70] A limited number of LHD services are provided on a fee-for-service basis. For example, there is usually a fee charged for birth and death certificates issued by the LHD. Also, in some communities, minimal fees are charged to offset the cost of providing immunizations, lab work, or inspections. Seldom do these fees cover the actual cost of the services provided. Therefore, income from service fees usually makes up a very small portion

sliding scale the scale used to determine the fee for services based on ability to pay

of any LHD budget. It also is not unusual to find that many LHDs use a **sliding scale** to determine the fee for a service.

Coordinated School Health Programs

Few people think of public schools as governmental health agencies. Consider, however, that schools are funded by tax dollars, are under the supervision of an elected school board, and include as a part of their mission the improvement of the health of those in the school community. Because school attendance is required throughout the United States, the potential for school health programs to make a significant contribution to community health is enormous. In fact, Allensworth and Kolbe have stated that schools "could do more perhaps than any other single agency in society to help young people, and the adults they will become, to live healthier, longer, more satisfying, and more productive lives."[71] Yet coordinated school health programs have faced a number of barriers, including: (1) insufficient local administrative commitment, (2) inadequately prepared teachers, (3) too few school days to teach health in the school year, (4) inadequate funding, (5) the lack of credibility of health education as an academic subject, (6) insufficient community/parental support, and (7) concern for the teaching of controversial topics (e.g., sex education).[72] If communities were willing to work to overcome these barriers, the contribution of coordinated school health programs to community health could be almost unlimited.

A coordinated school health program is defined as follows:

an organized set of policies, procedures, and activities designed to protect, promote, and improve the health and well-being of students and staff, thus improving a student's ability to learn. It includes but is not limited to comprehensive school health education; school health services; a healthy school environment; school counseling; psychological and social services; physical education; school nutrition services; family and community involvement in school health; and school-site health promotion for staff.[11]

Although all components of the coordinated school health program are important, there are three essential components: health education, a healthy school environment, and health services. Health instruction should be based on a well-conceived, carefully planned curriculum that has an appropriate scope (coverage of topics) and logical sequencing. Instructional units should include cognitive (knowledge), affective (attitudes), and psychomotor (behavioral) components. The healthy school environment should provide a learning environment that is both physically and mentally safe and healthy. Finally, each school's health program should provide the essential health services, from emergency care through health appraisals, to ensure that students will be healthy learners.

Quasi-governmental Health Organizations

Quasi-governmental health organizations—organizations that have some official health responsibilities but operate, in part, like voluntary health organizations—make important contributions to community health. Although they derive some of their funding and legitimacy from governments, and carry out tasks that may be normally thought of as government work, they operate independently of government supervision. In some cases, they also receive financial support from private sources. Examples of quasi-governmental agencies are the American Red Cross (ARC), the National Science Foundation, and the National Academy of Sciences.

The American Red Cross

The ARC, founded in 1881 by Clara Barton (see **Figure 1.15**), is a prime example of an organization that has quasi-governmental status. Although it has certain "official" responsibilities placed on it by the federal government, it is funded by voluntary contributions. "Official" duties of the ARC include: (1) providing relief to victims of natural disasters such as floods, tornadoes, hurricanes, and fires (Disaster

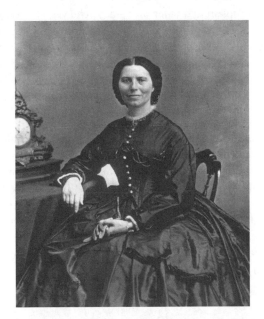

Figure 1.15 The American Red Cross was founded by Clara Barton in 1881.
© National Library of Medicine

Services) and (2) serving as the liaison between members of the active armed forces and their families during emergencies (Services to the Armed Forces and Veterans). In this latter capacity, the ARC can assist active-duty members of the armed services in contacting their families in case of an emergency, or vice versa.

In addition to these "official" duties, the ARC also engages in many nongovernmental services. These include blood drives, safety services (including water safety, first aid, cardiopulmonary resuscitation [CPR], and HIV/AIDS instruction), nursing and health services, youth services, community volunteer services, and international services.

The ARC was granted a charter by Congress in 1900, and the ARC and the federal government have had a special relationship ever since. The president of the United States is the honorary chairman of the ARC. The U.S. Attorney General and Secretary of the Treasury are honorary counselor and treasurer, respectively.

The Red Cross idea was not begun in the United States. It was begun in 1863 by five Swiss men in Geneva, Switzerland, who were concerned with the treatment provided to the wounded during times of war. The group, which was called the International Committee for the Relief to the Wounded, was led by Henry Dunant. With the assistance of the Swiss government, the International Committee brought together delegates from 16 nations in 1864 to the Geneva Convention for the Amelioration of the Condition of the Wounded in Armies in the Field (now known as the first Geneva Convention) to sign the Geneva Treaty.

The efforts of Henry Dunant and the rest of the International Committee led to the eventual establishment of the International Committee of the Red Cross (ICRC). The ICRC, which still has its headquarters in Geneva and is still governed by the Swiss, continues to work today during times of disaster and international conflict. It is the organization that visits prisoners of war to ensure they are being treated humanely.[73,74]

Today, the international movement of the Red Cross comprises the Geneva-based ICRC, the International Federation of Red Cross and Red Crescent Societies (the red crescent emblem is used in Moslem countries), and the over 180 National Red Cross and Red Crescent Societies.[73] There are a number of other countries that believe in the principles of the Red Cross Movement, but have not officially joined because the emblems used by the movement are offensive.

quasi-governmental health organizations organizations that have some responsibilities assigned by the government but operate more like voluntary agencies

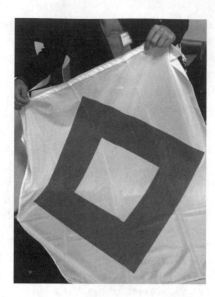

Figure 1.16 The red crystal: an additional emblem of the ICRC.

© Keystone/Laurent Gillieron/AP Photos

Thus, the ICRC has created a third emblem that meets all the criteria for use as a protective device and at the same time is free of any national, political, or religious connotations. The design is composed of a red frame in the shape of a square on the edge of a white background. The name chosen for this distinctive emblem was "red crystal," to signify purity (see **Figure 1.16**).[74]

Nongovernmental Health Agencies

Nongovernmental health agencies (sometimes referred to as NGOs) are funded by private donations or, in some cases, by membership dues. There are thousands of these organizations that all have one thing in common: They arose because there was an unmet need. For the most part, the agencies operate free from governmental interference as long as they meet Internal Revenue Service guidelines with regard to their specific tax status. In the following sections, we discuss the following types of nongovernmental health agencies—voluntary, professional, philanthropic, service, social, religious, and corporate.

Voluntary Health Agencies

Voluntary health agencies are an American creation. Each of these agencies was created by one or more concerned citizens who felt that a specific health need was not being met by existing governmental agencies. New voluntary agencies continue to be born each year. Examples of recent additions to the perhaps 100,000 agencies already in existence are the Alzheimer's Association and the First Candle (formerly SIDS Alliance). A discussion of the commonalities of voluntary health agencies follows.

Organization of Voluntary Health Agencies

Most voluntary agencies exist at three levels—national, state, and local. At the national level, policies that guide the agency are formulated. A significant portion of the money raised locally is forwarded to the national office, where it is allocated according to the agency's budget. Much of the money is designated for research. By funding research, the agencies hope to discover the cause of and cure for a particular disease or health problem. There have been some major successes. The March of Dimes, for example, helped to eliminate polio as a major disease problem in the United States through its funding of immunization research.

There is not always a consensus of opinion about budget decisions made at the national level; some believe that less should be spent for research and more for treating those afflicted with the disease. Another common internal disagreement concerns how much of the funds raised at the local level should be sent to the national headquarters instead of being retained for local use. Those outside the agency sometimes complain that when an agency achieves success, as the March of Dimes did in its fight against polio, it should dissolve. This does not usually occur; instead, successful agencies often find a new health concern. The March of Dimes now fights birth defects, and when tuberculosis was under control, the Tuberculosis Society changed its name to the American Lung Association to fight all lung diseases.

The state-level offices of voluntary agencies are analogous to the state departments of health in the way that they link the national headquarters with local offices. The primary work at this level is to coordinate local efforts and to ensure that policies developed at the national headquarters are carried out. The state-level office may also provide training services for employees and volunteers of local-level offices and are usually available as consultants and problem solvers. In recent years, some voluntary agencies have been merging several state offices into one to help reduce overhead expenses.

The local-level office of each voluntary agency is usually managed by a paid staff worker who has been hired either by the state-level office or by a local board of directors.

> **voluntary health agencies** nonprofit organizations created by concerned citizens to deal with a health need not met by governmental health agencies

Members of the local board of directors usually serve in that capacity on a voluntary basis. Working under the manager of each agency are local volunteers, who are the backbone of voluntary agencies. This is where most of the money is raised, most of the education takes place, and most of the service is rendered. Volunteers are of two types, professional and lay. Professional volunteers have had training in a medical profession, whereas lay volunteers have had no medical training. The paid employees help facilitate the work of the volunteers with expertise, training, and other resources.

Purpose of Voluntary Health Agencies

Voluntary agencies share four basic objectives: (1) to raise money to fund their programs, with the majority of the money going to fund research; (2) to provide education both to professionals and to the public; (3) to provide service to those individuals and families that are afflicted with the disease or health problem; and (4) to advocate for beneficial policies, laws, and regulations that affect the work of the agency and in turn the people they are trying to help.

Fundraising is a primary activity of many voluntary agencies. Whereas in the past this was accomplished primarily by door-to-door solicitations, today mass mailing, telephone, and social media solicitations are more common. In addition, most agencies sponsor special events such as golf outings, dances, walk-a-thons, dinners, or other special events (see **Figure 1.17**). In addition, some of these agencies have become United Way agencies and receive some funds derived from the annual United Way campaign, which conducts fundraising efforts at worksites. The three largest voluntary agencies in the United States today (in terms of dollars raised) are the American Cancer Society, the American Heart Association, and the American Lung Association.

Over the years, the number of voluntary agencies formed to help meet special health needs has continually increased. Because of the growth in the number of new agencies, several consumer "watchdog" groups have taken a closer look into the practices of the agencies. A major concern of these consumer groups has been the amount of money that the voluntary agencies spend on the cause (e.g., cancer, heart disease, AIDS) and how much they spend on fundraising and overhead (e.g., salaries, office furniture, leasing of office space). Well-run agencies will spend less than 15% of what they raise on fundraising. Some of the not-so-well-run agencies spend as much as 80% to 90% on fundraising. All consumers should ask agencies how they spend their money prior to contributing.

Professional Health Organizations/ Associations

Professional health organizations and associations are made up of health professionals who have completed specialized education and training programs and have met the standards of registration, certification, and/or licensure for

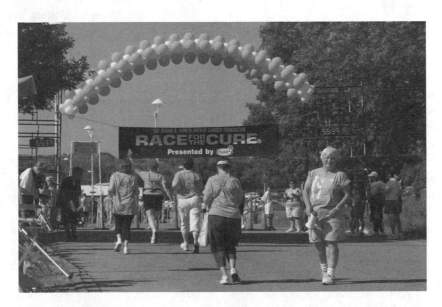

Figure 1.17 Most voluntary health agencies hold special events to raise money for their causes.
© Suzanne Tucker/ShutterStock, Inc.

their respective fields. Their mission is to promote high standards of professional practice for their specific profession, thereby improving the health of society by improving the people in the profession. Professional organizations are funded primarily by membership dues. Examples of such organizations are the American Medical Association, American Dental Association, American Nursing Association, American Public Health Association, and the Society for Public Health Education.

Although each professional organization is unique, most provide similar services to their members. These services include the certification of continuing-education programs for professional renewal, the hosting of annual conventions where members share research results and interact with colleagues, and the publication of professional journals and other reports. Some examples of journals published by professional health associations are the *Journal of the American Medical Association* and the *American Journal of Public Health*.

Like voluntary health agencies, another important activity of some professional organizations is advocating on issues important to their membership. The American Medical Association, for example, has a powerful lobby nationally and in some state legislatures. Its purpose is to affect legislation in such a way as to benefit its membership and its profession. Many professional health organizations provide the opportunity for benefits, including group insurance and discount travel rates. There are hundreds of professional health organizations in the United States, and it would be difficult to describe them all here.

Philanthropic Foundations

Philanthropic foundations have made and continue to make significant contributions to community health in the United States and throughout the world. These foundations support community health by funding programs and research on the prevention, control, and treatment of many diseases. Foundation directors, sometimes in consultation with a review committee, determine the types of programs that will be funded. Some foundations fund an array of health projects, whereas others have a much narrower scope of interests. Some foundations, such as the Bill and Melinda Gates Foundation, fund international health projects, whereas others restrict their funding to domestic projects. The geographical scope of domestic foundations can be national, state, or local. Local foundations may restrict their funding to projects that benefit only local citizens.

> **philanthropic foundation** an endowed institution that donates money for the good of humankind

The activities of these foundations differ from those of the voluntary health agencies in two important ways. First, foundations have money to give away, and therefore no effort is spent on fundraising. Second, foundations can afford to fund long-term or innovative research projects, which might be too risky or expensive for voluntary or even government-funded agencies. The development of a vaccine for yellow fever by a scientist funded by the Rockefeller Foundation is an example of one such long-range project.

Some of the larger foundations, in addition to the Bill and Melinda Gates Foundation, that have made significant commitments to community health are the Commonwealth Fund, which has contributed to community health in rural communities, improved hospital facilities, and tried to strengthen mental health services; the Robert Wood Johnson Foundation, which has worked to improve access to medical and dental care throughout the United States and lessen the impact of tobacco on health; the Henry J. Kaiser Family Foundation, which has supported the development of health maintenance organizations (HMOs) and community health promotion; and the W. K. Kellogg Foundation, which has funded many diverse health programs that address human issues and provide a practical solution.

Service, Social, and Religious Organizations

Service, social, and religious organizations have also played a part in community health over the years (see **Figure 1.18**). Examples of service and social groups involved in community health are the Jaycees, Kiwanis Club, Fraternal Order of Police, Moose, Shriners, and American Legion. Members of these groups enjoy social interactions with

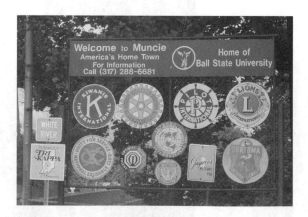

Figure 1.18 Community service groups contribute needed resources for the improvement of the health of the community.

people of similar interests in addition to fulfilling the groups' primary reason for existence—service to others in their communities. Although health may not be the specific focus of their mission, several of these groups make important contributions in that direction by raising money and funding health-related programs. Sometimes, their contributions are substantial. Examples of such programs include the Shriners' children's hospitals and burn centers, and the Lions' contributions to guide dog programs and other services for those who are visually impaired, such as the provision of eyeglasses for school-aged children unable to afford them.

The contributions of religious groups to community health have also been substantial. Such groups also have been effective avenues for promoting health programs because (1) they have had a history of volunteerism and preexisting reinforcement contingencies for volunteerism, (2) they can influence entire families, and (3) they have accessible meeting-room facilities.[75] One way in which these groups contribute is through donations of money for missions for the less fortunate. Examples of religious organizations that solicit donations from their members include the Protestants' One Great Hour of Sharing, the Catholics' Relief Fund, and the United Jewish Appeal. Other types of involvement in community health by religious groups include (1) the donation of space for voluntary health programs such as blood donations, Alcoholics Anonymous, and other support groups; (2) the sponsorship of food banks and shelters for the hungry, poor, and homeless; (3) the sharing of the doctrine of good personal health behavior; and (4) allowing community health professionals to deliver their programs through the congregations. This latter contribution has been especially useful in black American communities because of the importance of churches in the culture of this group of people.

In addition, it should be noted that some religious groups have hindered the work of community health workers. Almost every community in the country can provide an example in which a religious organization has protested the offering of a school district's sex education program, picketed a public health clinic for providing reproductive information or services to women, or spoken out against homosexuality.

Corporate Involvement in Community Health

From the way it treats the environment by its use of natural resources and the discharge of wastes, to the safety of the work environment, to the products and services it produces and provides, to the provision of healthcare benefits for its employees, corporate America is very much involved in community health. Although each of these aspects of community health is important to the overall health of a community, because of the concern for the "bottom line" in corporate America, it is the provision of healthcare benefits that often receives the most attention. In fact, many corporations today find that their single largest annual expenditure behind salaries and wages is for employee healthcare benefits. Consider, for example, the cost of manufacturing a new car. The cost of health benefits for those who build the car now exceeds the cost of the raw materials for the car itself.

In an effort to keep a healthy workforce and reduce the amount paid for healthcare benefits, many companies support health-related programs both at and away from the worksite. Worksite programs aimed at trimming employee medical bills have been expanded beyond the traditional safety awareness programs and first aid services to include such programs as substance abuse counseling, nutrition education, smoking cessation, stress management, physical fitness, and disease management. Many companies also are implementing health promotion policies and enforcing state and local laws that prohibit (or severely restrict) smoking on company grounds or that mandate the use of safety belts at all times in all company-owned vehicles.

Chapter Summary

- A number of key terms are associated with the study of community health, including *health*, *community*, *community health*, *population health*, *public health*, *public health system*, and *global health*.

- The four factors that affect the health of a community are physical (e.g., community size), social and cultural (e.g., religion), community organization, and individual behaviors (e.g., exercise and diet).

- It is important to be familiar with and understand the history of community health to be able to deal with present and future community health issues.
- The eighteenth century was characterized by industrial growth. Science was being used more in medicine, and it was during this century that the first vaccine was discovered.
- The nineteenth century ushered in the modern era of public health. The germ theory was introduced during this time, and the last fourth of the century is known as the bacteriological period of public health.
- The twentieth century can be divided into several periods. The health resources development period (1900–1960) was a time when many public and private resources were used to improve health. The period of social engineering (1960–1973) saw the U.S. government's involvement in health insurance through Medicare and Medicaid. The health promotion period began in 1974 and continues today.
- Great concern still exists for health care, the environment, diseases caused by an impoverished lifestyle, the spread of communicable diseases (such as AIDS, Legionnaires' disease, toxic shock syndrome, and Lyme disease), the harm caused by alcohol and other drug abuse, and terrorism.
- Contemporary society is too complex to respond effectively to community health problems on either an emergency or a long-term basis. This fact necessitates organizations and planning for health in our communities.
- The different types of organizations that contribute to the promotion, protection, and maintenance of health in a community can be classified into three groups according to their sources of funding and organizational structure—governmental, quasi-governmental, and nongovernmental.
- Governmental health agencies exist at the local, state, federal, and international levels and are funded primarily by tax dollars.
- The World Health Organization (WHO) is the largest and most visible governmental health agency on the international level.
- The Department of Health and Human Services (HHS) is the U.S. government's principal agency for the protection of the health of all Americans and for providing essential human services, especially for those who are least able to help themselves.
- The core functions of public health include the assessment of information on the health of the community, comprehensive public health policy development, and assurance that public health services are provided to the community.
- Quasi-governmental agencies, such as the American Red Cross, share attributes with both governmental and nongovernmental agencies.
- Nongovernmental organizations include voluntary and professional associations; philanthropic foundations; and service, social, and religious groups.
- Corporate America has also become more involved in community health, both at the worksite and within the community.

Review Questions

1. How did the WHO define health in 1946? How has that definition been modified?
2. What is public health?
3. What are the differences among community health, population health, and global health?
4. What are the five major domains that determine a person's health?
5. What is the difference between personal health activities and community health activities?
6. Define the term *community*.
7. What are four major factors that affect the health of a community? Provide an example of each.
8. What are some of the major events of community health that occurred in the eighteenth and nineteenth centuries?
9. Provide a brief explanation of the origins from which the following twentieth-century periods get their names:
   a. Health resources development period
   b. Period of social engineering
   c. Period of health promotion

10. What are the major community health problems facing the United States in the twenty-first century?

11. What are some of the major community health problems facing other parts of the world in the twenty-first century?

12. What characteristics of modern society necessitate planning and organization for community health?

13. What is a governmental health agency?

14. What is the World Health Organization (WHO), and what does it do?

15. What federal department in the United States is the government's principal agency for protecting the health of all Americans and for providing essential human services, especially to those who are least able to help themselves? What major services does this department provide?

16. What are the three core functions of public health?

17. What are the 10 essential public health services?

18. How do state and local health departments interface?

19. What is meant by the term *coordinated school health program*? What are the major components of it?

20. What is meant by the term *quasi-governmental agency*? Name one such agency.

21. Describe the characteristics of a nongovernmental health agency.

22. How do philanthropic foundations contribute to community health? List three well-known foundations.

23. How do service, social, and religious groups contribute to the health of the community?

24. Why has corporate America become involved in community health?

Activities

1. Write your own definition for *health*.

2. Select a community health problem that exists in your hometown; then, using the factors that affect the health of a community noted in this chapter, analyze and discuss in a two-page paper at least three factors that contribute to the problem in your hometown.

3. Review a copy of *Healthy People 2020* on the Web. Then, set up a time to talk with an administrator in your hometown health department. Find out which of the objectives the health department has been working on as priorities. Summarize in a paper what the objectives are, what the health department is doing about them, and what it hopes to accomplish by the year 2020.

4. Call a local voluntary health organization in your community and ask if you could volunteer to work 10 to 15 hours during this academic term. Then, volunteer those hours and keep a journal of your experience.

5. Carefully review your community newspaper each day for an entire week. Keep track of all articles or advertisements that make reference to local health organizations. Summarize your findings in a one-page paper. (If you do not subscribe to your local paper, copies are available in libraries, or on the Web.)

Community Health on the Web

The Internet contains a wealth of information about community and public health. Increase your knowledge of some of the topics presented in this chapter by accessing the Jones & Bartlett Learning website at **go.jblearning.com/McKenzieBrief** and follow the links to complete the following Web activities.

- Department of Homeland Security
- Department of Health and Human Services
- *Healthy People 2020*
- Global Health
- World Health Organization

References

1. Schneider, M.-J. (2011). *Introduction to Public Health*, 3rd ed. Burlington, MA: Jones & Bartlett Learning.
2. National Center for Health Statistics (2011). *Health, United States, 2010: With Special Feature on Death and Dying.* Hyattsville, MD: CDC, National Center for Health Statistics. Available at http://www.cdc.gov/nchs/hus.htm.
3. Bunker, J. P., H. S. Frazier, and F. Mosteller (1994). "Improving Health: Measuring Effects of Medical Care." *Milbank Quarterly*, 72: 225-258.
4. Centers for Disease Control and Prevention (1999). "Ten Great Public Health Achievements–United States, 1900-1999." *Morbidity and Mortality Weekly Report*, 48(12): 241-243.
5. U.S. Department of Health and Human Services, Centers for Disease Control and Prevention (2011). "Ten Great Public Health Achievements–United States, 2001-2010." *Morbidity and Mortality Weekly Report*, 60(19): 619-623. Available at http://www.cdc.gov/mmwr/preview/mmwrhtml/mm6019a5.htm?s_cid=mm6019a5_w.
6. U.S. Department of Health and Human Services, Centers for Disease Control and Prevention (2011). "Vital Signs: Current Cigarette Smoking Among Adults Aged ≥18 Years–United States, 2005-2010." *Morbidity and Mortality Weekly Report*, 60(35): 1207-1212. Available at http://www.cdc.gov/mmwr/preview/mmwrhtml/mm6035a5.htm?s_cid=%20mm6035a5.htm_w.
7. World Health Organization (2010). *Glossary of Globalization, Trade, and Health Terms.* Geneva, Switzerland: Author. Available at http://www.who.int/trade/glossary/en/.
8. Hancock, T., and M. Minkler (2005). "Community Health Assessment or Healthy Community Assessment." In M. Minkler, ed., *Community Organizing and Community Building for Health*, 2nd ed. New Brunswick, NJ: Rutgers University Press, 138-157.
9. McGinnis, J. M. (2001). "United States." In C. E. Koop, ed., *Critical Issues in Global Health*. San Francisco: Jossey-Bass, 80-90.
10. McGinnis, J. M., P. Williams-Russo, and J. R. Knickman (2002). "The Case for More Active Policy Attention to Health Promotion." *Health Affairs*, 21(2): 78-93.
11. Joint Committee on Health Education and Promotion Terminology (2012). *Report of the 2011 Joint Committee on Health Education and Promotion Terminology.* Reston, VA: American Association of Health Education.
12. Minkler, M., N. Wallerstein, and N. Wilson (2008). "Improving Health Through Community Organizing and Community Building." In K. Glanz, B. K. Rimer, and K. Viswanath, eds., *Health Behavior and Health Education Practice: Theory, Research, and Practice*, 4th ed. San Francisco: Jossey-Bass, 287-312.
13. Institute of Medicine (1988). *The Future of Public Health.* Washington, DC: National Academies Press.
14. Green, L. W., and J. F. McKenzie (2002). "Community and Population Health." In L. Breslow, ed., *Encyclopedia of Public Health*. New York: Macmillan Reference USA, 247-255.
15. Institute of Medicine (1997). *America's Vital Interest in Global Health: Protecting Our People, Enhancing Our Economy, and Advancing Our International Interests.* Washington, DC: National Academy Press. Available at http://books.nap.edu/openbook.php?record_id=5717&page=R1.
16. American College Health Association (2012). *American College Health Association–National College Health Assessment II (ACHA-NCHA II) Spring 2011: Reference Group Executive Summary.* Available at http://www.achancha.org/reports_ACHA-NCHAII.html.
17. Shi, L., and D. A. Singh (2013). *Essentials of the US Health Care System*, 3rd ed. Burlington, MA: Jones & Bartlett Learning.
18. Minkler, M., and N. Wallerstein (2012). "Improving Health through Community Organizing and Community Building: Perspectives from Health Education and Social Work." In M. Minkler, ed., *Community Organizing and Community Building for Health and Welfare*, 3rd ed. New Brunswick, NJ: Rutgers University Press, 37-58.
19. Institute of Medicine (2003). *The Future of the Public's Health in the 21st Century.* Washington, DC: National Academies Press.
20. Rosen, G. (1958). *A History of Public Health.* New York: MD Publications.
21. Woodruff, A. W. (1977). "Benjamin Rush, His Work on Yellow Fever and His British Connections." *American Journal of Tropical Medicine and Hygiene*, 26(5): 1055-1059.
22. Pickett, G., and J. J. Hanlon (1990). *Public Health: Administration and Practice*, 9th ed. St. Louis, MO: Times Mirror/Mosby.
23. Rosen, G. (1975). *Preventive Medicine in the United States, 1900-1975.* New York: Science History Publications.
24. Smillie, W. G. (1955). *Public Health: Its Promise for the Future.* New York: Macmillan.
25. Duffy, J. (1990). *The Sanitarians: A History of American Public Health.* Chicago: University of Illinois Press.
26. Lalonde, M. (1974). *A New Perspective on the Health of Canadians: A Working Document.* Ottawa, Canada: Minister of Health.
27. Green, L. W. (1999). "Health Education's Contributions to the Twentieth Century: A Glimpse through Health Promotion's Rearview Mirror." In J. E. Fielding, L. B. Lave, and B. Starfield, eds., *Annual Review of Public Health*. Palo Alto, CA: Annual Reviews, 67-88.
28. U.S. Department of Health and Human Services, Public Health Service (1980). *Ten Leading Causes of Death in the United States, 1977.* Washington, DC: U.S. Government Printing Office.
29. U.S. Department of Health, Education, and Welfare (1979). *Healthy People: The Surgeon General's Report on Health Promotion and Disease Prevention* (DHEW pub. no. 79-55071). Washington, DC: U.S. Government Printing Office.
30. U.S. Department of Health and Human Services (1980). *Promoting Health/Preventing Disease: Objectives for the Nation.* Washington, DC: U.S. Government Printing Office.
31. U.S. Department of Health and Human Services (2012). *Implementing Healthy People 2020.* Available at http://www.healthypeople.gov/2020/implementing/default.aspx.
32. U.S. Department of Health and Human Services, Centers for Medicare and Medicaid Services (2010). *National Health Expenditure Data.* Available at http://www.cms.gov

/Research-Statistics-Data-and-Systems/Statistics-Trends-and-Reports/NationalHealthExpendData/index.html.

33. U.S. Census Bureau (2012). *World Population 1950-2050*. Available at http://www.census.gov/population/international /data/worldpop/table_population.php.

34. Murphy, S. L., J. Q. Xu, and K. D. Kochanek (2012). "Deaths: Preliminary Data for 2010." *National Vital Statistics Reports*, 60(4).

35. Centers for Disease Control (1981). "Pneumocystis Pneumonia–Los Angeles." *Morbidity and Mortality Weekly Report*, 30: 250-252.

36. The Henry J. Kaiser Family Foundation (2012). "Fact Sheet: The HIV/AIDS Epidemic in the United States." Available at http://www.kff.org/hivaids/3029.cfm.

37. Turnock, B. J. (2012). *Public Health: What It Is and How It Works*, 5th ed. Burlington, MA: Jones & Bartlett Learning.

38. Pinger, R. R., W. A. Payne, D. B. Hahn, and E. J. Hahn (1998). *Drugs: Issues for Today*, 3rd ed. Boston: WCB McGraw-Hill.

39. King, N. (2009). "Health Inequalities and Health Inequities." In E. E. Morrison, ed., *Health Care Ethics: Critical Issues for the 21st Century*. Sudbury, MA: Jones and Bartlett, 339-354.

40. Institute of Medicine (2003). *The Future of the Public's Health in the 21st Century*. Washington, DC: National Academies Press.

41. Centers for Disease Control and Prevention (2012). *Emergency Preparedness and Response: What CDC Is Doing*. Available at http://www.bt.cdc.gov/cdc/.

42. Katz, R. (2013). *Essentials of Public Health Preparedness*. Burlington, MA: Jones & Bartlett Learning.

43. Trust for America's Health and the Robert Wood Johnson Foundation (2011). *Ready or Not? 2011: Protecting the Public's Health from Disease, Disasters, and Bioterrorism*. Available at http://healthyamericans.org/report/92/.

44. World Health Organization (2006). *Engaging for Health: Eleventh General Programme of Work 2006-2015*. Available at http://www.euro.who.int/en/who-we-are/technical-programmes-in-the-european-region/engaging-for-health-eleventh-general-programme-of-work-2006-2015,-a-global-health-agenda.

45. U.S. Department of Health and Human Services, Centers for Disease Control and Prevention (2011). "Ten Great Public Health Achievements–Worldwide, 2001-2010." *Morbidity and Mortality Weekly Report*, 60(24): 814-818. Available at http://www.cdc.gov/mmwr/preview/mmwrhtml/mm6024a4.htm?s_cid=mm6024a4_w.

46. Joint United Nations Programme on HIV/AIDS (UNAIDS) (2010). *Global Report: UNAIDS Report on the Global AIDS Epidemic 2010*. Geneva, Switzerland: UNAIDS. Available at http://www.unaids.org/globalreport/global_report.htm.

47. World Health Organization (2011). *WHO Report on the Global Tobacco Epidemic, 2008: The MPOWER Package*. Geneva, Switzerland: Author. Available at http://www.who.int/tobacco /mpower/2008/en/index.html.

48. World Health Organization (2012). *The Top 10 Causes of Death*. Geneva, Switzerland: Author. Available at http://www.who.int /mediacentre/factsheets/fs310/en/index.html.

49. United Nations (2011). *The Millennium Development Goals Report 2011*. New York: Author. Available at http://mdgs .un.org/unsd/mdg/News.aspx?ArticleId=59.

50. Green, L. W. (1990). "The Revival of Community and the Public Obligation of Academic Health Centers." In R. E. Bulger and S. J. Reiser, eds., *Integrity in Institutions: Humane Environments for Teaching, Inquiry and Health*. Iowa City: University of Iowa Press, 163-180.

51. World Health Organization (2012). "World Health Organization." Available at http://www.who.int/about/en/.

52. United Nations (2000). *United Nations Millennium Declaration*. New York: Author.

53. United Nations (2002). *Road Map Towards the Implementation of the United Nations Millennium Declaration*. New York: Author.

54. World Health Organization (2003). *World Health Report 2003: Shaping the Future*. Geneva, Switzerland: Author.

55. United Nations (2007). *The Millennium Development Goals Report*. New York: Author.

56. U.S. Department of Health and Human Services (2012). "United States Department of Health and Human Services." Available at http://www.hhs.gov/about/whatwedo.html.

57. U.S. Census Bureau (2012). "Federal Budget." *The 2012 Statistical Abstract: The National Data Book*. Available at http://www.census.gov/compendia/statab/.

58. Agency for Healthcare Research and Quality (2012). "AHRQ at a Glance." Available at http://ahrq.hhs.gov/about/ataglance .htm.

59. Agency for Toxic Substances and Disease Registry (2009). "Vision, Mission, Goals, & Core Values." Available at http://www.atsdr.cdc.gov/about/mission_vision_goals.html.

60. Centers for Disease Control and Prevention (2012). "Fact Sheet: The Centers for Disease Control and Prevention." Available at http://www.cdc.gov/about/resources/facts.htm.

61. Centers for Disease Control and Prevention (2012). "CDC Organization." Available at http://www.cdc.gov/about /organization/cio.htm.

62. National Center for Health Statistics. (2011). "Health, United States, 2012: With Special Feature on Socioeconomic Status and Health." Hyattsville, MD: Author.

63. U.S. Food and Drug Administration (2010). "About the FDA: What Does the FDA Do?" Available at http://www.fda.gov /AboutFDA/Transparency/Basics/ucm194877.htm.

64. Health Resources and Services Administration (2012). "About HRSA." Available at http://www.hrsa.gov/about /index.html.

65. Indian Health Service (2012). "Indian Health Service Introduction." Available at http://www.ihs.gov/index. cfm?module=ihsIntro.

66. National Institutes for Health (2011). "About NIH: Mission." Available at http://www.nih.gov/about/mission.htm.

67. Substance Abuse and Mental Health Services Administration (2012). "About the Agency (SAMHSA)." Available at http://www.samhsa.gov/about/#org.

68. National Academy of Sciences, Institute of Medicine (1988). *The Future of Public Health*. Washington, DC: National Academy Press.

69. Office of Disease Prevention and Health Promotion (2008). "Public Health in America." Available at http://web.health.gov /phfunctions/public.htm.

70. National Association of County and City Health Officials (2011). *2010 National Profile of Local Health Departments*. Washington, DC: Author.

71. Allensworth, D. D., and L. J. Kolbe (1987). "The Comprehensive School Health Program: Exploring an Expanded Concept." *Journal of School Health,* 57(10): 409–412.

72. Butler, S. C. (1993). "Chief State School Officers Rank Barriers to Implementing Comprehensive School Health Education." *Journal of School Health,* 63(3): 130–132.

73. American Red Cross (2012). "Red Cross History." Available at http://www.redcross.org.

74. International Committee of the Red Cross (2002). "History of the ICRC." Available at http://www.icrc.org.

75. Lasater, T. M., B. L. Wells, R. A. Carleton, and J. P. Elder (1986). "The Role of Churches in Disease Prevention Research Studies." *Public Health Report,* 101(2): 123–131.

Chapter 2

Epidemiology: The Study, Prevention, and Control of Diseases, Injuries, and Other Health Conditions in the Community

Robert R. Pinger, PhD

Chapter Objectives

1. Define the terms *epidemic*, *epidemiology*, and *epidemiologist*, and explain their importance in community health.

2. List some past and current epidemic diseases.

3. Explain the importance of rates in epidemiology.

4. Define incidence and prevalence rates and provide examples of each.

5. Discuss the reasons for and importance of disease reporting to a community's health and outline the disease reporting process.

6. Define the following terms: *life expectancy*, *years of potential life lost (YPLL)*, *disability-adjusted life years (DALYs)*, and *health-adjusted life expectancy (HALE)*.

7. Identify sources of standardized data used by epidemiologists, community health workers, and health officials and list the types of data available from each source.

8. Explain the purpose behind each of the types of epidemiological studies.

9. Describe three approaches community leaders might use to prioritize the importance of diseases and health-related conditions in a community.

10. Define primary, secondary, and tertiary prevention of diseases.

11. Use the chain of infection model to explain how a specific communicable disease is transmitted among members in a community.

⑫ Describe the multicausation disease model and explain how it helps to conceptualize the development of a noncommunicable disease such as heart disease.

⑬ Explain the purpose and importance of health screenings in a community and provide an example.

⑭ Provide examples of the application of primary, secondary, and tertiary prevention approaches for controlling at least one communicable and one noncommunicable disease.

Introduction

Epidemiology is "the study of the distribution and determinants of health-related states or events in specified populations, and the application of this study to control health problems."[1] The goal of epidemiology is to limit disease, injury, and death in a community by intervening to prevent or limit outbreaks or epidemics of disease and injury. This is accomplished by (1) describing disease outbreaks, and (2) designing studies to analyze them. Epidemiologic methods are also used to evaluate new approaches to prevention, control, and treatment. Through these practices, epidemiologists contribute to our knowledge of how diseases begin and spread through populations, and how they can be prevented, controlled, and treated.

When an unusually high number of cases of a disease occur in a population, the disease is said to have become **epidemic**. Diseases that have a constant presence in a given population but do not occur at unexpectedly high levels are called **endemic diseases**. To determine whether a disease is epidemic or endemic in a population, one must specify the disease and the population. For example, whereas malaria can occur in 25% of the population in parts of equatorial Africa and still be considered endemic, one or two unexplained cases in a community in the United States would be considered an epidemic. Some recent examples of epidemics in the United States are presented in Table 2.1.

An **epidemiologist** is "an investigator who studies the occurrence of disease or other health-related conditions or events in defined populations."[1] Some epidemics begin as outbreaks of disease in animals, known as epizootics, and then spread to human populations. Examples include bubonic plague, which first affects rodents, and West Nile fever virus, which first affects birds. Occasionally, an epidemic will spread over a wide area, perhaps even across an entire continent or around the world. Such a widespread epidemic is termed a **pandemic**. In the influenza pandemic of 1918, for example, an estimated 50 million people died around the world.[2] The global economy and increasingly rapid international travel mean that more and more epidemics are likely to become pandemics. Acquired immune deficiency syndrome (AIDS) is another example of a pandemic disease. During 2000, an estimated 1.8 million people died of AIDS worldwide, and about 33.3 million people were living with HIV (human immunodeficiency virus).[3]

endemic disease
a disease that occurs regularly in a population as a matter of course

epidemic an unexpectedly large number of cases of an illness, specific health-related behavior, or other health-related event in a particular population

epidemiologist
one who practices epidemiology

epidemiology
the study of the distribution and determinants of health-related states or events in specified populations

pandemic an outbreak of disease over a wide geographical area such as a continent

Table 2.1 Recent Epidemics in the United States

Disease	Cases in Previous Years	Epidemic Period	Number of Cases
HIV/AIDS	Unknown (before 1975)	Currently	1,200,000[4]
Lyme disease	Unknown (before 1975)	2009	29,959[5]
West Nile virus	Unknown (before 1999)	2011	690[6]
Influenza A	2,585-10,609	2009-2010	66,589[7]
Overdose drug deaths from opioid analgesics	2,700 (in 1999)	2008	9,100[8]

Source: Data from Centers for Disease Control and Prevention.

The practice of epidemiology began with the study of infectious diseases such as yellow fever, cholera, and plague. In the nineteenth century, large cities such as London often experienced recurring epidemics, especially of waterborne diseases like cholera. In 1854 Dr. John Snow and others, following an exhaustive investigation, were able to extinguish a cholera epidemic in London by insisting that the handle be removed from the Broad Street water pump (the contaminated water source).[9] This is one of the earliest examples of applied epidemiology.

From this early use for the investigation and control of a communicable disease outbreak, epidemiology has developed into a sophisticated applied science. Epidemiological methods are now used to evaluate everything from the effectiveness of vaccines to the possible causes of occupational illnesses and motor-vehicle deaths.

Community health workers use epidemiology to establish the needs or conditions required for a particular health program or to justify a request for funding. Likewise, epidemiological methods are used to evaluate the effectiveness of programs already in existence and to plan to meet anticipated needs for personnel, equipment, or facilities.

The Importance of Rates

Epidemiologists are concerned with numbers and rates. Of prime importance is the number of health-related events, the number of **cases** (people who are sick), and, of course, the number of deaths. Numbers alone, however, do not provide an adequate description of the extent of the disease in a community. Epidemiologists must also know the total number in the susceptible population so that rates can be calculated. A **rate** is the number of events (births, cases of disease, or deaths) in a given population over a given period or at a given point in time. Three general categories of rates are **natality (birth) rates**, **morbidity (sickness) rates**, and **mortality or fatality (death) rates**.

Why are rates important? Why not simply enumerate the sick or dead? The answer is that rates enable one to compare the injury, disease, or death experiences of one population to those of another population. The two populations might differ in location, time, or human composition (age, sex, race). For example, by using rates it is possible to determine that the number of gonorrhea cases per capita was higher in South Carolina than in California in 2008, or that the number of gonorrhea cases per capita fell to its lowest rate in 10 years in the United States in 2008.

The following is an example of the importance of rates for the transportation industry. The example compares transportation deaths associated with travel by autos and airplanes. In this hypothetical situation, consider that for a given time period, 1,000 people died in auto crashes whereas 50 people died in airplane crashes. Without calculating rates, one might assume that auto travel is 20 times more dangerous than air travel. However, if you knew the population exposed (100,000 people for auto travel versus 1,000 people for air travel), you could calculate fatality rates, the number of deaths divided by the population, for each mode of travel.[10] (See Table 2.2.) These rates have greater meaning than the numbers of deaths because they are based on the **population at risk**, those who are susceptible to disease or death from a particular cause. In this case, the fatality rates are 1/100 for autos and 5/100 for airplanes, thus indicating that in this hypothetical example air travel is five times more dangerous than auto travel.

Incidence, Prevalence, and Attack Rates

Three important types of morbidity rates are incidence rates, prevalence

> **cases** people afflicted with a disease
> **morbidity (sickness) rate** the rate of illness in a population
> **mortality (fatality) rate** the number of deaths in a population divided by the total population
> **natality (birth) rate** the number of live births divided by the total population
> **population at risk** those in the population who are susceptible to a particular disease or condition
> **rate** the number of events that occur in a given population in a given period of time

Table 2.2   Hypothetical Number of Deaths and Death Rates for Two Modes of Travel

	Source of Fatalities	
	Auto	Airplane
Number of fatalities per year	1,000	50
Number exposed to risk	100,000	1,000
Rate of fatality	0.01 (1/100)	0.05 (5/100)

Source: Mausner, J. S., and S. Kramer (1985). *Mausner and Bahn Epidemiology—An Introductory Text,* 2nd ed. Philadelphia, PA: W. B. Saunders, p. 5.

rates, and attack rates. An **incidence rate** is defined as the number of new health-related events or cases of a disease in a population exposed to that risk in a given time period—the number of new cases of influenza in a community over a week's time, for example. Those who became ill with influenza during the previous week and remain ill during the week in question are not counted in an incidence rate. Incidence rates are important in the study of **acute diseases**—diseases in which the peak severity of symptoms occurs and subsides within days or weeks. These diseases usually move quickly through a population. Examples of acute diseases are the common cold, influenza, chickenpox, measles, and mumps.

Prevalence rates are calculated by dividing all current cases of a disease (old and new) by the total population. Prevalence rates are useful for the study of **chronic diseases**—diseases that usually last 3 months or longer. In these cases, it is more important to know how many people are currently suffering from a chronic disease—such as arthritis, heart disease, cancer, or diabetes—than it is to know when they became afflicted. Furthermore, with many chronic diseases, it is difficult or impossible to determine the date of onset of disease. Because a preponderance of health services and facilities are used for the treatment of persons with chronic diseases and conditions, prevalence rates are more useful than incidence rates for

the planning of public health programs, personnel needs, and facilities.

An **attack rate** is a special incidence rate calculated for a particular population for a single disease outbreak and expressed as a percentage. For example, suppose a number of people who traveled on the same airline flight developed a similar illness, and epidemiologists suspected that the cause of this illness was associated with the flight itself. An attack rate could be calculated for the passengers on that flight to express the percentage who became ill. Furthermore, attack rates could be calculated for various subpopulations, such as those seated at various locations in the plane, those who selected specific entrees from the menu, those of particular age groups, or those who boarded the flight at specific stops. Differences in attack rates for different subpopulations might indicate to the epidemiologists the source or cause of the illness.

Crude and Age-Adjusted Rates

Incidence and prevalence rates can be expressed in two forms—crude and specific. **Crude rates** are those in which the denominator includes the total population. The most important of these are the crude birth rate and the crude death rate. The **crude birth rate (CBR)** is the number of live births in a given year, divided by the midyear population. The **crude death rate (CDR)** is the total number of deaths in a given year from all causes, divided by the midyear population (see **Table 2.3**). Crude rates are relatively easy to obtain and are useful when comparing similar populations, but they can be misleading when populations differ by age structure or by some other attribute. For example, CBRs are normally higher in younger populations, which have a higher proportion of people of reproductive age, than in populations with more elderly people. Conversely, CDRs are normally higher in older populations. For these reasons, it is inappropriate to use crude rates to compare the risk of death in populations with different age structures, such as those of Florida and Alaska. To show what the level of mortality would be if the age composition of different populations were the same,

acute disease a disease that lasts 3 months or less

attack rate an incidence rate calculated for a particular population for a single disease outbreak and expressed as a percentage

chronic disease a disease or health condition that lasts longer than 3 months

crude birth rate (CBR) the number of live births per 1,000 in a population in a given period of time

crude death rate (CDR) the number of deaths (from all causes) per 1,000 in a population in a given period of time

crude rate a rate in which the denominator includes the total population

incidence rate the number of new health-related events or cases of a disease in a population exposed to that risk during a particular period of time, divided by the total number in that same population

prevalence rate the number of new and old cases of a disease in a population in a given period of time, divided by the total number in that population

Table 2.3 Crude Rates

Name of Rate	Definition of Rate	Multiplier
Crude birth rate =	$\dfrac{\text{Number of live births}}{\text{Estimated midyear population}}$ ×	1,000
Crude death rate =	$\dfrac{\text{Number of deaths (all causes)}}{\text{Estimated midyear population}}$ ×	100,000

Table 2.4 Crude and Age-Adjusted Mortality Rates for Alaska and Florida, 2010

State	Number of Deaths	Crude Death Rate*	Age-Adjusted Death Rate*
Alaska	3,727	524.8	771.3
Florida	173,763	924.2	701.0

*Deaths per 100,000 population.
Source: Data from Murphy, S. L., J. Q. Xu, and K. D. Kochanek (2012). "Deaths: Preliminary Data for 2010." *National Vital Statistics Reports*, 60(4). Hyattsville, MD: National Center for Health Statistics. Available at http://www.cdc.gov /nchs/data/nvsr/nvsr60/nvsr60_04.pdf.

epidemiologists use **age-adjusted rates**. For example, because of its larger senior population, in 2010 Florida had a higher crude death rate (924.2 per 100,000) compared with Alaska's (524.8 per 100,000), where the population is younger. However, when these death rates are adjusted for differences in the age structures of the populations of these two states, one can see that the death rate in Florida (701.0 per 100,000) compares favorably with the death rate in Alaska (771.3 per 100,000). See Table 2.4.[11] Methods for calculating age-adjusted rates can be found in standard epidemiology textbooks.

Specific Rates

Specific rates measure morbidity and mortality for particular populations or for particular diseases. One could, for example, calculate the age-specific mortality rate for a population of 35- to 44-year-olds by dividing the number of deaths in that age group by the midyear population of 35- to 44-year-olds. Similarly, one could calculate race- and sex-specific mortality rates.

A very important specific rate is the **cause-specific mortality rate (CSMR)**, which measures the death rate for a specific disease. This rate can be calculated by dividing the number of deaths due to a particular disease by the total population. One could also calculate an age-specific, cause-specific mortality rate. Because fewer people can be expected to die from each cause than to die from all causes, CSMRs are usually reported per 100,000 population. Table 2.5 lists some important rates used in epidemiology, defines them, and gives an example of each.

Two other important measures of disease are the **case fatality rate (CFR)** and the **proportionate mortality ratio (PMR)**. The CFR is simply the percentage of cases that result in death. It is a measure of the severity of a disease and is directly related to the virulence of the disease agent. It is calculated by dividing the number

age-adjusted rate a rate used to make comparisons of relative risks across groups and over time when groups differ in age structure
case fatality rate (CFR) the percentage of cases of a particular disease that result in death
cause-specific mortality rate (CSMR) the death rate due to a particular disease
proportionate mortality ratio (PMR) the percentage of overall mortality in a population that is attributable to a particular cause
specific rate a rate that measures morbidity or mortality for a particular population or disease

Table 2.5 Important Rates in Epidemiology

Rate	Definition	Multiplier	Examples (U.S. 2010)[12,13]
Crude birth rate =	$\frac{\text{Number of live births}}{\text{Estimated midyear population}}$	× 1,000	13.0/1,000
Crude death rate =	$\frac{\text{Number of deaths (all causes)}}{\text{Estimated midyear population}}$	× 100,000	798.7/100,000
Age-specific death rate =	$\frac{\text{Number of deaths, 15–24 years}}{\text{Estimated midyear population, 15–24 years}}$	× 100,000	67.6/100,000
Infant mortality rate =	$\frac{\text{Number of deaths under 1 year of age}}{\text{Number of live births}}$	× 1,000	6.14/1,000
Neonatal mortality rate =	$\frac{\text{Number of deaths under 28 days of age}}{\text{Number of live births}}$	× 1,000	4.04/1,000
Cause-specific death rate =	$\frac{\text{Number of deaths (diabetes mellitus)}}{\text{Estimated midyear population}}$	× 100,000	22.3/100,000
Age-specific, cause-specific death rate =	$\frac{\text{Number of deaths, 15–24 years (motor vehicles)}}{\text{Estimated midyear population}}$	× 100,000	16.5/100,000

of deaths from a particular disease in a specified period of time by the number of cases of that same disease in the same time period. The resulting fraction is multiplied by 100 and is reported as a percentage. For example, if there were 200 cases of a severe illness and 10 of them resulted in death, the CFR would be 10 ÷ 200 × 100 = 5%.

The PMR describes the relationship between the number of deaths from a specific cause and the total number of deaths attributable to all causes. It is calculated by dividing the number of deaths attributed to a particular disease by the total number of deaths from all causes in the same population during the same period of time. This rate is also reported as a percentage. For example, in the United States, there were 595,444 deaths due to diseases of the heart in 2010, and 2,465,936 total deaths reported that same year.[11] Thus, the PMR for diseases of the heart can be calculated as follows: 595,444 ÷ 2,465,936 = 24%. In other words, in the United States, heart disease was responsible for nearly one in four deaths in 2010.

Reporting of Births, Deaths, and Diseases

Births, deaths, and specific diseases are reported to, and recorded by, local, state, and federal health agencies. Births must be recorded so each of the jurisdictions has a record of the arrival of a new person. Similarly, deaths must be recorded so that jurisdictions have a record of the date and time of each person's death. These data, along with marriage, divorce, and adoption records, are known as vital records or **vital statistics** and are maintained permanently by the appropriate local government. Local agencies send copies of these records to their respective state departments of health, where they are collated and forwarded to the National Center for Health Statistics at the Centers for Disease Control and Prevention (CDC).

Notifiable (reportable) diseases are infectious diseases that can become epidemic and for which the CDC requests reports from each state and territorial health department. Each state and territorial government has the legal power to require physicians, clinics, and hospitals to report all births and deaths as well as notifiable diseases to their local health departments. Local health departments are required by their respective state health departments to summarize all records of births, deaths, and notifiable diseases and to report them. State health departments summarize these reports and relay them to the CDC through the **National Electronic Telecommunications System (NETS)**. The reporting scheme for notifiable disease is shown in **Figure 2.1**.

The CDC summarizes state and territorial data and publishes them in *Morbidity and Mortality Weekly Reports* (*MMWRs*), which are available to the public electronically at the CDC website, www.cdc.gov/mmwr. Paper copies can usually be found in the government documents areas of certain larger libraries.

Unfortunately, the information reported is not always as good as it should be. One study estimated that local health

National Electronic Telecommunications System (NETS) the electronic reporting system used by state health departments and the CDC.

notifiable (reportable) diseases infectious diseases for which health officials request or require reporting for public health reasons

vital statistics statistical summaries of records of major life events such as births, deaths, marriages, divorces, and infant deaths

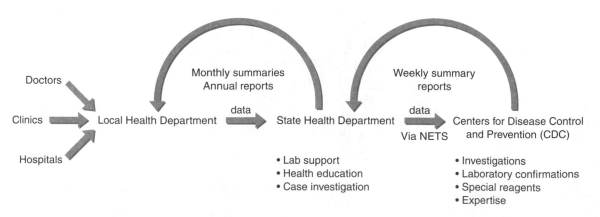

Figure 2.1 Scheme for the reporting of notifiable diseases.

departments may receive notification of only 35% of the cases of some communicable diseases. Doctors' offices and clinics may be understaffed or simply too busy to keep up with reporting, or may not be familiar with the reporting requirement. In other cases, patients recover—with or without treatment—before a diagnosis is confirmed. Also, changes in local and state government administration or other key personnel often interfere with the timely reporting of disease data. The accuracy of disease reporting also depends on the virulence of the disease agent. Rabies cases, for example, are almost 100% reported, whereas German measles cases may be only 80% to 90% reported. Therefore, morbidity data—although useful for reflecting disease trends—cannot always be considered to be precise counts of the actual number of cases of diseases.

Standardized Measurements of the Health Status of Populations

Mortality statistics are the single most reliable indicator of a population's health status. Although they provide an incomplete description of a population's health, mortality

statistics underlie other important measurements; two of these are life expectancy and years of potential life lost. Finally, there are measurements of ill health that, although less precise than mortality, can nonetheless be meaningful. Two of these measurements are disability-adjusted life years and health-adjusted life expectancy.

Mortality Statistics

In 2010, 2,465,936 deaths were registered in the United States, resulting in a crude mortality rate of 798.7 per 100,000. The age-adjusted death rate, which eliminates the effects of the aging population, was 746.2 deaths per 100,000 U.S. standard population, a record low.[11] Age-adjusted death rates show what the level of mortality would be if no changes occurred in the age makeup of the population from year to year. Thus, they are a better indicator than are unadjusted (crude) death rates for examining changes in the risk of death over a period of time when the age distribution of the population is changing. Deaths and age-adjusted death rates for the 15 leading causes of death for the entire population in the United States in 2010 are presented in **Table 2.6**.[11]

Naturally, morbidity and mortality rates vary greatly depending on age, sex, race, and ethnicity. For example,

Table 2.6 Deaths and Death Rates for 2010 and Age-Adjusted Rates

Rank[a]	Cause of Death (based on the International Classification of Diseases, Tenth Revision, 2nd ed., 2004)	Number	Death Rate	Age-Adjusted Death Rate 2010	2009[b]	Percent Change
...	All causes	2,465,932	798.7	746.2	749.6	-0.5
1	Diseases of heart (I00-I09, I11, I13, I20-I51)	595,444	192.9	178.5	182.8	-2.4
2	Malignant neoplasms (C00-C97)	573,855	185.9	172.5	173.5	-0.6
3	Chronic lower respiratory diseases (J40-J47)	137,789	44.6	42.1	42.7	-1.4
4	Cerebrovascular diseases (I60-I69)	129,180	41.8	39.0	39.6	-1.5
5	Accidents (unintentional injuries) (V01-X59, Y85-Y86)[c]	118,043	38.2	37.1	37.5	-1.1
6	Alzheimer's disease (G30)	83,308	27.0	25.0	24.2	3.3
7	Diabetes mellitus (E10-E14)	68,905	22.3	20.8	21.0	-1.0
8	Nephritis, nephrotic syndrome, and nephrosis (N00-N07, N17-N19, N25-N27)	50,472	16.3	15.3	15.1	1.3
9	Influenza and pneumonia (J09-J18)[d]	50,003	16.2	15.1	16.5	-8.5
10	Intentional self-harm (suicide) (X60-X84, Y87.0)[3]	37,793	12.2	11.9	11.8	0.8

(continues)

Table 2.6 Deaths and Death Rates for 2010 and Age-Adjusted Rates (*Continued*)

Rank[a]	Cause of Death (based on the *International Classification of Diseases, Tenth Revision,* 2nd ed., 2004)	Number	Death Rate	Age-Adjusted Death Rate 2010	2009[b]	Percent Change
11	Septicemia (A40-A41)	34,843	11.3	10.6	11.0	-3.6
12	Chronic liver disease and cirrhosis (K70, K73-K74)	31,802	10.3	9.4	9.1	3.3
13	Essential hypertension and hypertensive renal disease (I10, I12, I15)	26,577	8.6	7.9	7.8	1.3
14	Parkinson's disease (G20-G21)	21,963	7.1	6.8	6.5	4.6
15	Pneumonitis due to solids and liquids (J69)	17,001	5.5	5.1	4.9	4.1
...	All other causes (residual)	488,954	158.5	...	...	...

... Category not applicable.
[a]Based on number of deaths.
[b]Rates are revised and may differ from rates previously published.
[c]For unintentional injuries and suicides, preliminary and final data may differ significantly because of the truncated nature of the preliminary file.
[d]Expanded ICD-10 code J09 (Influenza due to certain identified influenza virus) was added to the category in 2009.
Notes: Data based on a continuous file of records received from the states. Rates are per 100,000 population. Rates are based on populations enumerated in the 2010 U.S. census as of April 1 for 2010 and estimated as of July 1 for 2009. Age-adjusted rates per 100,000 U.S. standard population are based on the year 2000 standard. Figures for 2010 are based on weighted data rounded to the nearest individual, so categories may not add to totals. Data are subject to sampling and random variation.
Source: Reproduced from Murphy, S. L., J. Q. Xu, and K. D. Kochanek (2012). "Deaths: Preliminary Data for 2010." *National Vital Statistics Reports*, 60(4). Hyattsville, MD: National Center for Health Statistics. 2010. Available at: http://www.cdc.gov/nchs/data/nvsr/nvsr60/nvsr60_04.pdf.

whereas heart disease is the leading cause of death for the overall population and particularly for adults 65 years of age or older, cancer is the leading cause of death for the 45- to 64-year-old age group, and unintentional injuries are the leading cause of death for all age groups between 1 and 44 years.

A study of the mortality statistics from the beginning of the twentieth century through the beginning of the twenty-first century reveals a shift in the leading causes of death. When the twentieth century began, communicable diseases such as pneumonia, tuberculosis, and gastrointestinal infections were the leading causes of death.[13] As a result of progress in public health practice and in biomedical research, heart disease, cancer, chronic lower respiratory disease, stroke, and unintentional injuries (accidents and adverse effects) accounted for about 65% of all deaths in 2010 (see Table 2.7).

Communicable diseases remain frequent causes of deaths in certain age groups. For example, pneumonia and influenza still kill many older adults in this country each year. Also, HIV/AIDS, listed as the eighth overall leading cause of death for Americans as recently as 1996, kills more males than females. Thus, it is important to remember that viewing the leading causes of death for the entire population does not provide a clear picture of the health for any one segment of the population.

Life Expectancy

Life expectancy is defined as the average number of years a person from a specific cohort is projected to live from a given point in time. Whereas life insurance companies are interested in life expectancy at every age, health statisticians are usually concerned with life expectancy at birth, at the age of 65 years, and, more recently, at age 75. It must be remembered that life expectancy is an average for an entire cohort (usually of a single birth year) and is not necessarily a useful prediction for any one individual. Moreover, it certainly cannot describe the quality of one's life. However, the ever-increasing life expectancy for Americans suggests

life expectancy
the average number of years a person from a specific cohort is projected to live from a given point in time

Table 2.7 Leading Causes of Death in the United States: 1900, 1940, 2010

1900	
1.	Pneumonia, influenza
2.	Tuberculosis
3.	Diarrhea
4.	Diseases of the heart
5.	Cerebrovascular diseases (stroke)
6.	Nephritis
7.	Unintentional injuries (accidents)
8.	Malignant neoplasms (cancers)
9.	Senility
10.	Diphtheria
1940	
1.	Diseases of the heart
2.	Malignant neoplasms (cancers)
3.	Cerebrovascular diseases (stroke)
4.	Nephritis
5.	Pneumonia, influenza
6.	Unintentional injuries (non-motor vehicle)
7.	Tuberculosis
8.	Diabetes mellitus
9.	Unintentional injuries (motor vehicle)
10.	Premature birth
2010	
1.	Diseases of the heart
2.	Malignant neoplasms (cancers)
3.	Chronic lower respiratory diseases
4.	Cerebrovascular diseases (stroke)
5.	Unintentional injuries (all)
6.	Alzheimer's disease
7.	Diabetes mellitus
8.	Nephritis (kidney diseases)
9.	Influenza and pneumonia
10.	Intentional self-harm (suicide)

Source: Data from Murphy, S. L., J. Q. Xu, and K. D. Kochanek (2012). "Deaths: Preliminary Data for 2010." *National Vital Statistics Reports*, 60(4). Hyattsville, MD: National Center for Health Statistics. Available at http://www.cdc.gov /nchs/data/nvsr/nvsr60/nvsr60_04.pdf; and Centers for Disease Control and Prevention, National Center for Health Statistics (1998). "Leading Causes of Death, 1900–1998." Available at http://www.cdc.gov/nchs/data/dvs /lead1900_98.pdf.

that, as a country, we have managed to control some of those factors that contribute to early deaths.

Table 2.8 provides a summary of life expectancy figures for the United States population at birth, at age 65, and at age 75 years from 1900 to 2008. The data presented indicate that the overall life expectancy has increased more than 30 years since 1900. Life expectancies at birth for both sexes increased from 47.3 years in 1900 to 78.1 years in 2008, when the life expectancy for newborn girls was 80.6 years and newborn boys was 75.6 years.[14] Although life expectancy has risen dramatically for Americans, it remains well below that of Japan, where life expectancies for newborn girls and boys are 86 and 79 years, respectively.[15]

Years of Potential Life Lost

Whereas standard mortality statistics, such as leading causes of death, provide one measure of the importance of various diseases, **years of potential life lost (YPLL)** provides another, different measure. YPLL is calculated by subtracting a person's age at death from his or her life expectancy. Such calculations are impossible because each person may have a different life expectancy at any given time. For this reason, 75 years is now used in these calculations. Thus, for a person who dies at age 59, the YPLL-75 is 16.

YPLL weights deaths such that the death of a very young person counts more than the death of a very old person. **Table 2.9** provides a summary of the age-adjusted YPLL before 75 (YPLL-75) for the 10 leading causes of death in the United States for 1990 and 2007.[13] In examining this table, note that the number of YPLL-75 per 100,000 population was higher for malignant neoplasms (cancer) than for heart disease. Also, YPLL resulting from unintentional injuries was the second highest. This is because unintentional injuries and malignant neoplasms (cancer) often kill people when they are young. These differences can also be seen in the two pie charts shown in **Figure 2.2**. Also, notice that the YPLL-75 per 100,000 population declined for most of the leading causes of death between 1990 and 2007. An important exception is for diabetes mellitus, a disease that is becoming epidemic in the United States.

YPLL from specific causes varies depending on the gender and race of the subpopulation under consideration. For example, the YPLL-75 per

> **years of potential life lost (YPLL)** the number of years lost when death occurs before the age of 65 or 75

Table 2.8 Life Expectancy at Birth, at 65 Years of Age, and at 75 Years of Age According to Sex: In the United States, During the Selected Years 1900–2008

	At Birth Year			At 65 Years			At 75 Years		
	Both Sexes	Male	Female	Both Sexes	Male	Female	Both Sexes	Male	Female
1900	47.3	46.3	48.3	11.9	11.5	12.2	*	*	*
1950	68.2	65.6	71.1	13.9	12.8	15.0	*	*	*
1960	69.7	66.6	73.1	14.3	12.8	15.8	*	*	*
1970	70.8	67.1	74.7	15.2	13.1	17.0	*	*	*
1980	73.7	70.7	77.4	16.4	14.1	18.3	10.4	8.8	11.5
1990	75.4	71.8	78.8	17.2	15.1	18.9	10.9	9.4	12.0
2000	76.8	74.1	79.3	17.6	16.0	19.0	11.0	9.8	11.8
2008	78.1	75.6	80.6	18.8	17.3	20.0	11.8	10.7	12.6

*Data not available.
Source: Modified from National Center for Health Statistics (2010). *Health, United States, 2009 with Special Feature on Medical Technology.* DHHS pub. no. 2010-1232. Hyattsville, MD: Author. Available at http://www.cdc.gov/nchs/hus.htm; and Murphy, S. L., J. Q. Xu, and K. D. Kochanek (2012). "Deaths: Preliminary Data for 2010." *National Vital Statistics Reports,* 60(4). Hyattsville, MD: National Center for Health Statistics. Available at http://www.cdc.gov/nchs/data/nvsr/nvsr60/nvsr60_04.pdf.

Table 2.9 Age-Adjusted Years of Potential Life Lost Before 75 (YPLL-75) for the 10 Leading Causes of Death, United States, 1990 and 2007

Cause	YPLL per 100,000 Population	
	1990	2007
Diseases of the heart	1,617.7	1,042.4
Malignant neoplasms (cancer)	2,003.8	1,461.4
Cerebrovascular diseases (stroke)	259.6	184.5
Chronic lower respiratory diseases	187.4	172.1
Unintentional injuries	1,162.1	1,159.5
Influenza and pneumonia	141.5	71.6
Diabetes mellitus	155.9	170.1
Human immunodeficiency virus infection (HIV/AIDS)	383.8	115.2
Suicide	393.1	357.5
Homicide and legal intervention	417.4	278.3

Source: Modified from National Center for Health Statistics (2011). *Health, United States, 2010: With Special Feature on Death and Dying.* Hyattsville, MD: Author. Available at http://www.cdc.gov/nchs/data/hus/hus10.pdf.

---

disability-adjusted life years (DALYs) a measure for the burden of disease that takes into account premature death and loss of healthy life resulting from disability

100,000 population resulting from unintentional injuries is nearly three times as high for men as it is for women. The YPLL-75 per 100,000 for diseases of the heart for blacks is nearly twice that for whites, and for homicide, it is nearly six times greater.[15]

Disability-Adjusted Life Years

Mortality does not entirely express the burden of disease. For example, chronic depression and paralysis caused by polio are responsible for great loss of healthy life but are not reflected in mortality tables. Because of this, the World Health Organization (WHO) and the World Bank have developed a measure called the **disability-adjusted life years (DALYs)**.[16]

Deaths by Cause, United States, 2007

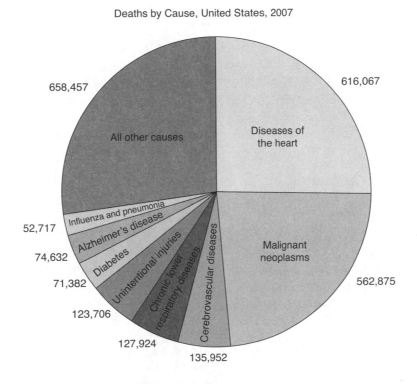

YPLL Before Age 75 for Selected Causes of Death, 2007

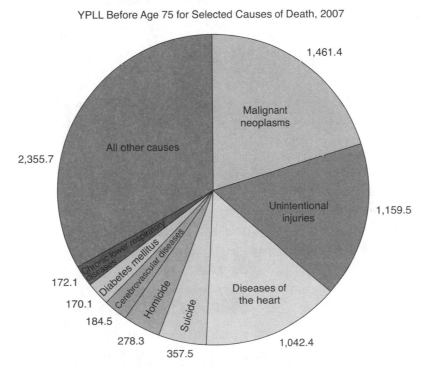

Figure 2.2 Deaths by cause in the United States, 2007, and the years of potential life lost before age 75 (YPLL-75) per 100,000 population for selected causes of death within the United States, 2007.

Data from National Center for Health Statistics (2011). *Health, United States, 2010: With Special Feature on Death and Dying.* Hyattsville, MD: Author. Available at http://www.cdc.gov/nchs/data/hus/2010/fig24.pdf.

One DALY is one lost year of healthy life. Total DALYs for a given condition for a particular population can be calculated by estimating the total YPLL and the total years of life lived with disability, and then summing these totals. As an example, the DALYs incurred through firearm injuries in the United States could be calculated by adding the total YPLL incurred from fatal firearm injuries to the total years of life lived with disabilities by survivors of firearm injuries.

Health-Adjusted Life Expectancy

Health-adjusted life expectancy (HALE), sometimes referred to as healthy life expectancy, is the number of years of healthy life expected, on average, in a given population or region of the world. The HALE indicator used by the WHO is similar to the disability-adjusted life expectancy (DALE) first reported in the original Global Burden of Disease study.[16] The methods used to calculate HALE are beyond the scope of this text, but have been described elsewhere.[17] Worldwide, HALE at birth in 2001 was 57.4 years, 7.5 years lower than overall life expectancy at birth. As with life expectancy, HALE in sub-Saharan Africa is very low—less than 40 years for males, compared with about 70 years for females in high-income countries (**Figure 2.3**).[18]

> **health-adjusted life expectancy (HALE)** the number of years of healthy life expected, on average, in a given population
>
> **U.S. Census** the enumeration of the population of the United States that is conducted every 10 years

Sources of Standardized Data

Because demographic and epidemiological data are used to plan community health programs and services, students should be aware of the sources of these standardized data. National data for use in community health work are available from the following sources: the U.S. Census Bureau (www.census.gov), several of the centers located within the Centers for Disease Control and Prevention (www.CDC.gov), and some of the larger voluntary health organizations, including the American Cancer Society (www.cancer.org), the American Heart Association (www.americanheart.org), and the American Lung Association (www.lungusa.org). International statistics can be found at the World Health Organization (www.who.int). Each of these sources of national data has a specific value and usefulness to those in the public health field. Students interested in studying local health problems can obtain data from state and local health departments, hospitals, volunteer agencies, and disease registries. The study and analysis of these data provide a basis for planning appropriate health programs and facilities in your communities.

The U.S. Census Bureau

Two useful publications by the U.S. Census Bureau are the U.S. Census reports and the *Statistical Abstract of the United States*. The **U.S. Census**, taken every 10 years since 1790, is an enumeration of the population living in the United

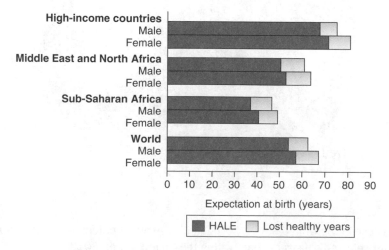

Figure 2.3 Life expectancy, health-adjusted life expectancy (HALE), and lost healthy years by region and sex, 2001.

States. The current census, taken in 2010, is much more complex than the original one. Data are gathered about income, employment, family size, education, dwelling type, and many other social indicators (see **Figure 2.4**). Census data are used by epidemiologists and public health statisticians to calculate disease and death rates and for health program planning. The **Statistical Abstract of the United States**, published annually, is the standard summary of statistics on the social, political, and economic organization of the United States. Information is divided into sections under headings such as Population, Vital Statistics, Health and Nutrition, Education, Law Enforcement, Courts and Prisons, and many more. It is also available at www.census.gov/compendia/statab/.

The Centers for Disease Control and Prevention

The single best source for health statistics in the United States is the Centers for Disease Control and Prevention (CDC).

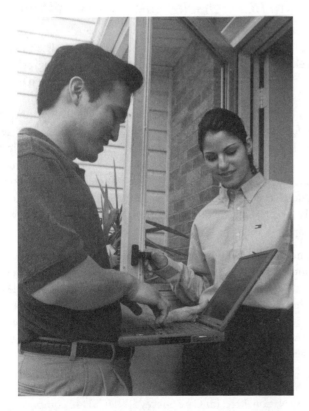

Figure 2.4 A census worker collects data used to calculate disease rates.

Photographed by Lloyd Wolf for the U.S. Census Bureau, Public Information Office (PIO).

Morbidity and Mortality Weekly Report

Reported cases of specified notifiable diseases, discussed earlier, are reported weekly in the *Morbidity and Mortality Weekly Report (MMWR)*, which lists morbidity and mortality data by state and region of the country. The report is prepared by the CDC based on reports from state health departments. Each weekly issue also contains several reports of outbreaks of disease, environmental hazards, unusual cases, or other public health problems. The *MMWR* and its annual summary reports are available at www.cdc.gov/mmwr.

Monthly Vital Statistics Report

The National Center for Health Statistics (NCHS), located in Hyattsville, Maryland, publishes national vital statistics in its *Monthly Vital Statistics Report*. Vital statistics, as described previously, are records of major life events (live births, deaths, marriages, divorces, and infant deaths). These monthly data are then summarized by sex, age, race and ethnicity, state, and other factors and published in annual reports. The statistics in these annual reports are used by public health officials and cited in this text. These data are available at www.cdc.gov/nchs/.

National Health Surveys

Another source of standardized data available from the NCHS are the National Health Surveys. These surveys are designed to ascertain the amount, distribution, and effects of illness and disability in the United States. The National Health Surveys comprise three types of surveys: (1) health interviews of people; (2) clinical tests, measurements, and physical examinations of people; and (3) surveys of places where people receive medical care, such as hospitals, clinics, and doctors' offices. The following paragraphs describe these surveys. More information about these surveys and results is available at the NCHS website.

National Health Interview Survey

In the National Health Interview Survey (NHIS), people are asked numerous questions about their health. One of the questions asks respondents to describe their health status using one of five categories—excellent, very good, good, fair, or poor. Fewer than 1 in 10 of the respondents in 2010 described their health status as either fair or poor, whereas nearly 7 in 10 Americans believe they are in very good or excellent health. College graduates (39%)

> **Statistical Abstract of the United States** the standard summary of statistics on the social, political, and economic organization of the United States

were about two times as likely as persons who had not graduated from high school (16%) to be in excellent health. Also, persons with family incomes of $100,000 or more were almost twice as likely as those with incomes of less than $35,000 to be in excellent health (49% vs. 26%).[19]

It is important to remember that these data were generated by self-reported responses to NHIS questions and not by actual examinations objectively generated in a clinic. As such, respondents may overreport good health habits or underreport bad ones. Such reporting is often dependent on the respondent's perceived social stigma or support for a response and the degree to which people's responses are confidential or anonymous. Furthermore, people have widely divergent views on what constitutes poor or good health. For example, many sedentary, cigarette-smoking, high-stress people see themselves as being in good health, whereas "health nuts" feel their health is deteriorating when they miss a day of exercise. In general, the young assess their health better than the old do, males better than females, whites better than blacks, and those with large family incomes better than those with smaller ones.

National Health and Nutrition Examination Survey

Another of the National Health Surveys is the National Health and Nutrition Examination Survey (NHANES). The purpose of the NHANES is to assess the health and nutritional status of the general U.S. population. Using mobile examination centers, doctors and other medical practitioners collect health data on representative Americans by conducting direct physical examinations, clinical and laboratory testing, and related procedures. Each year, the survey examines a nationally representative sample of about 5,000 persons, located in 15 counties across the country using mobile examination centers.

These examinations provide the most authoritative source of standardized clinical, physical, and physiological data on our population. Included in the data are the prevalence of specific conditions and diseases and data on blood pressure, serum cholesterol, body measurements, nutritional status and deficiencies, and exposure to environmental toxins.

Results of NHANES benefit people in the United States in important ways. Facts about the distribution of health problems and risk factors in the population give researchers important clues to the causes of disease. Information collected from the current survey is compared with information collected in previous surveys, allowing health planners

to detect the changes in various health problems and risk factors over time. By identifying the healthcare needs of the population, government agencies and private sector organizations can establish policies and plan research, education, and health promotion programs that help improve present health status and prevent future health problems.[20]

Behavioral Risk Factor Surveillance System

"The Behavioral Risk Factor Surveillance System (BRFSS) is a state-based system of health surveys that collects information on health risk behaviors, preventive health practices, and health care access primarily related to chronic disease and injury."[21] This survey seeks to ascertain the prevalence of such high-risk behaviors as cigarette smoking, excessive alcohol consumption, and physical inactivity, and the lack of preventive health care such as screening for cancer. BRFSS data are used by the states to identify emerging health problems, establish and track health objectives, and develop and evaluate public health policies and programs. Survey results are published as part of *MMWR*'s CDC Surveillance Summaries and are available online.

Youth Risk Behavior Surveillance System

The national Youth Risk Behavior Surveillance System (YRBSS) monitors six categories of priority health-risk behaviors among youth and young adults, including behaviors that contribute to unintentional injuries and violence; tobacco use; alcohol and other drug use; sexual behaviors that contribute to unintended pregnancy and sexually transmitted infections (STIs), including human immunodeficiency virus (HIV) infection; unhealthy dietary behaviors; and physical inactivity. In addition, the national YRBSS monitors the prevalence of obesity and asthma. The national YRBSS is conducted every 2 years during the spring semester and provides data representative of ninth- through twelfth-grade students in public and private schools in the United States.[22]

The YRBSS includes a national school-based survey conducted by the CDC, and state and local school-based surveys conducted by state and local education and health agencies. The YRBSS is conducted by the Division of Adolescent and School Health in the CDC's National Center for Chronic Disease Prevention and Health Promotion (www.cdc.gov /healthyyouth/yrbs/).

National Health Care Surveys

The National Health Care Surveys (NHCS) are composed of nine different national surveys that gather information on the nation's healthcare system. Two of the best-known healthcare surveys are the National Hospital Discharge Survey (NHDS) and the National Hospital Ambulatory Medical Care Survey (NHAMCS). The NHDS provides data on the characteristics of patients discharged from nonfederal, short-stay hospitals. These data can be used to examine a variety of important public health issues such as hospitalization rates for selected inpatient surgical procedures, infectious diseases, injuries, substance abuse, and other health problems. It can also be used to estimate costs for public health problems. The NHAMCS gathers and disseminates information about the health care provided by hospital outpatient departments and emergency departments. Summaries of the results of these surveys are published by the National Center for Health Statistics and are available at www.cdc.gov/nchs/dhcs.htm.

Epidemiological Studies

When disease and/or death occurs in unexpected or unacceptable numbers, epidemiologists may carry out investigations. These investigations may be descriptive or analytic (observational or experimental/interventional), depending on the objectives of the specific study.

Descriptive Studies

Descriptive studies seek to describe the extent of disease in regard to person, time, and place. These studies are designed to answer the questions who, when, and where. To answer the first question, epidemiologists first take a "head count" to determine how many cases of a disease have occurred. At this time, they also try to determine who is ill—children, older adults, men, women, or both. The data they gather should permit them to develop a summary of cases by age, sex, race, marital status, occupation, and employer.

To answer the second question (when), epidemiologists must determine the time of the onset of illness for each case. The resulting data can be used to prepare an **epidemic curve**, a graphic display of the cases of disease by the time or date of the onset of their symptoms. Three types of epidemic curves are commonly used in descriptive studies—secular, seasonal, and single epidemic curves. The secular display of a disease shows the distribution of cases over many years (e.g., cases of chickenpox for the period 1993 to 2009; see **Figure 2.5**). Secular graphs illustrate the long-term trend of a disease. A graph of the case data by season or month is usually prepared to show cyclical changes in the number of cases of a disease. For example, in North America, cases of arthropodborne viral infections peak in the late summer months following the amplification of the virus during

descriptive study an epidemiological study that describes an epidemic with respect to person, place, and time

epidemic curve a graphic display of the cases of disease according to the time or date of onset of symptoms

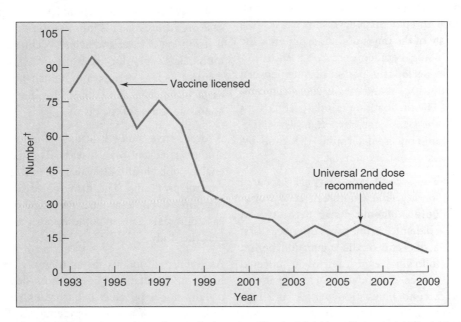

Figure 2.5 Varicella (chickenpox), number of reported cases—Illinois, Michigan, Texas, and West Virginia, 1992–2009.
Reproduced from Centers for Disease Control and Prevention (2011). "Summary of Notifiable Diseases—United States, 2009." *Morbidity and Mortality Weekly Report*, 58(53): 1–101. Available at http://www.cdc.gov/mmwr/PDF/wk/mm5853.pdf.

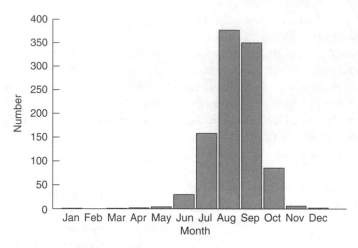

Figure 2.6 Reported cases of West Nile disease, by month—United States, 2010.
Centers for Disease Control and Prevention (2012). "Summary of Notifiable Diseases—United States, 2010." *Morbidity and Mortality Weekly Report* 59(53):1-112.

the summer months and the increase in the proportion of infected mosquitoes (see **Figure 2.6**).

Epidemic curves for single epidemics vary in appearance with each disease outbreak; however, two classic types exist. The first is the **point source epidemic curve** (see **Figure 2.7**). In a point source epidemic, each case can be traced to an exposure to the same source—spoiled food, for example. Because an epidemic curve shows cases of a disease by time or date of the onset of their symptoms, the epidemic curve for a single epidemic can be used to calculate the **incubation period**, the period of time between exposure to an infectious agent and the onset of symptoms. The incubation period, together with the symptoms, can often help epidemiologists determine the probable cause of the outbreak.

The second type of epidemic curve for a solitary outbreak is a **propagated epidemic curve**. In this type of epidemic, primary cases appear first at the end of the incubation period following exposure to an infected source. Secondary cases arise after a second incubation period, and represent exposure to the primary cases; tertiary cases appear even later as a result of exposure to secondary cases, and so on. Because new cases give rise

to more new cases, this type of epidemic is termed a propagated epidemic. Epidemics of communicable diseases such as chickenpox follow this pattern (see **Figure 2.8**).

Finally, epidemiologists must determine where the outbreak occurred. To determine where the illnesses may have originated, the residential address and travel history, including restaurants, schools, shopping trips, and vacations, of each case are recorded. This information provides a geographic distribution of cases and helps to delineate the extent of the outbreak. By plotting cases on a map, along with natural features such as streams and human-made structures such as factories, it is sometimes possible to learn something about the source of the disease.

A descriptive study is usually the first epidemiological study carried out on a disease. The data gathered should enable public health officials to plan future prevention and control programs. The data may also help investigators develop a hypothesis about the cause or source of the disease outbreak. This hypothesis can then be tested with an analytic study.

As important and useful as they are, descriptive studies have some limitations. Results from descriptive studies are usually not applicable to outbreaks elsewhere. Also, the investigation of a single epidemic cannot provide information about disease trends. Last, with few exceptions, descriptive studies by themselves rarely identify with certainty the cause of an outbreak.

incubation period
the period between exposure to a disease and the onset of symptoms
point source epidemic curve
an epidemic curve depicting a distribution of cases that all can be traced to a single source of exposure
propagated epidemic curve
an epidemic curve depicting a distribution of cases traceable to multiple sources of exposure

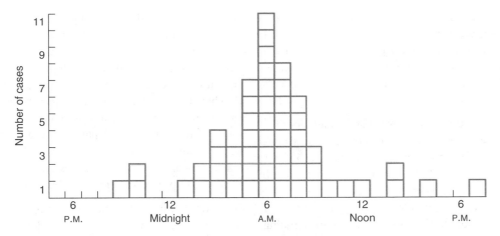

Figure 2.7 Point source epidemic curve: cases of gastroenteritis following ingestion of a common food source.
Centers for Disease Control and Prevention.

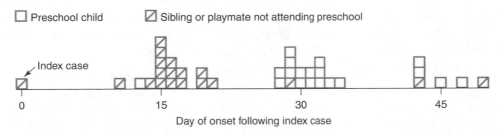

Figure 2.8 Propagated epidemic curve: cases of chickenpox during April through June.
Centers for Disease Control and Prevention.

Analytic Studies

A second type of epidemiological study is the **analytic study**. The purpose of analytic studies is to test hypotheses about associations between a disease or other health problem and possible **risk factors**, factors that increase the probability of disease. For example, one might design an analytic study to discover whether diabetes (health problem) is associated with obesity (possible risk factor), or whether lung cancer (health problem) is associated with cigarette smoking (possible risk factor). It is important to remember that the associations discovered through analytic epidemiological studies are not always cause-and-effect associations.

Observational Studies

There are two types of analytic studies—observational and experimental (interventional). These differ in the role played by the investigator. In **observational studies** the investigator simply observes the natural course of events, taking note of who is exposed or unexposed and who has

or has not developed the disease of interest. In experimental studies, the investigator actually allocates the exposure and subsequently follows the subjects for the development of disease.

Observational studies can be further divided into either case/control or cohort studies. The choice of which type of study to use to examine a particular disease–exposure relationship depends on the nature of the disease (rare or common) and the time and resources available. **Case/control studies** are analytic studies that compare people with disease (cases) to healthy people of similar age, sex, and background (controls) with respect to prior exposure to possible risk factors. These case/control studies are

analytic study an epidemiological study aimed at testing hypotheses

case/control study a study that seeks to compare those diagnosed with a disease with those who do not have the disease for prior exposure to specific risk factors

observational study an analytic, epidemiological study in which the investigator observes the natural course of events, noting exposed and unexposed subjects and disease development

risk factors factors that increase the probability of disease, injury, or death

aimed at identifying familial, environmental, or behavioral factors that are more common or more pronounced in the case group than in the control group. Such factors could be associated with the disease under study. For example, epidemiologists might wish to study the factors associated with cervical cancer in women.

To carry out this study, epidemiologists would identify a number of women with cervical cancer (cases) and an equal or larger number of healthy women (controls). Medical histories for each group would be obtained and compared. In this hypothetical example, an examination of the histories suggests that cigarette smoking is more prevalent in the case group. If exposure to the possible risk factor (smoking) is significantly greater in the cases (of cervical cancer) than in the controls, an association is said to exist. Note that this association may or may not be one of cause and effect. Further studies are usually necessary to confirm initial findings. Case/control studies almost never prove causation by themselves. Instead, they usually indicate the direction for future studies.

Cohort studies are epidemiological studies in which the researcher identifies a **cohort**, a group of healthy subjects who share a similar experience, such as year of birth or high school graduation. At the beginning of the study, the cohort must be large because of attrition over time, and the subjects must all be healthy. Subjects are then classified on the basis of their exposure to one or more possible risk factors, such as cigarette smoking, dietary habits, or other factors. The entire cohort is then observed for a number of years to determine the rate at which disease develops in each subgroup that was classified by exposure factor.

It is important to note the difference in the type of results obtained from case/control and cohort studies and the advantages and disadvantages of each type of study. In case/control studies, results obtained are not true incidence rates because disease was already present at the beginning of the study; that is, there were cases and controls to begin with, rather than a population at risk. For this reason, case/control studies cannot calculate the incidence rate of development of disease. They can only provide a probability statement about the association between factor and disease. This probability statement can be stated mathematically as an odds ratio. The following is a hypothetical example of such a probability statement: Lung cancer patients have a probability of having smoked cigarettes that is 11 times greater than that of the control group. The **odds ratio** in this case is 11:1.

In cohort studies, one begins with a population at risk, and therefore is able to calculate the incidence rate for developing disease associated with each exposure factor. This **relative risk** states the relationship between the rate of acquiring the disease in the presence of the risk factor and the rate of acquiring the disease in the absence of the risk factor. An example of a relative risk statement is as follows: Smokers are 11 times more likely to develop lung cancer than are nonsmokers.

Although cohort studies yield a relative risk, they have three distinct disadvantages. They usually: (1) are expensive, (2) take many years to complete, and (3) are not very useful for studying rare diseases because cases of disease may not develop among members of the cohort being studied. Case/control studies, on the other hand usually: (1) are less expensive to carry out, (2) can be completed more quickly, and (3) are useful for studying rare diseases because one can select the cases. Unfortunately, they cannot yield a true risk for acquiring a disease.

Experimental Studies

Experimental studies are carried out to identify the cause of a disease or to determine the effectiveness of a vaccine, therapeutic drug, or surgical procedure. The central feature of experimental (interventional) studies is that the investigator can control the intervention or variable of interest. The subjects may be humans but more often are animals such as laboratory mice, rats, or monkeys. The use of research animals in experimental studies is necessary to determine the safety and effectiveness of new therapeutic agents or medical procedures with minimum risk to human health.

Whether animals or humans are used, every effort is made to reduce unwanted variability of factors other than the risk factors under study among the experimental subjects. In the case of animal studies, the variables over which the

cohort a group of people who share some important demographic characteristic (year of birth, for example)

cohort study an epidemiological study in which a cohort is classified by exposure to one or more specific risk factors and observed to determine the rates at which disease develops in each class

experimental (interventional) studies analytic studies in which the investigator allocates exposure or intervention and follows development of disease

odds ratio a probability statement about the association between a particular disease and a specific risk factor, resulting from a case/control study

relative risk a statement of the relationship between the risk of acquiring a disease when a specific risk factor is present and the risk of acquiring that same disease when the risk factor is absent

experimenter may wish to exert control include age, sex, diet, and environmental conditions. In addition to controlling variables, three other principles are essential to properly designed experimental studies—control groups, randomization, and blinding.

The use of control groups means that the experimental treatment (intervention), such as a drug, vaccine, smoke-free environment, or special diet, is withheld from a portion of the subjects. These subjects belong to the control group, which receives blank doses or treatments, called **placebos**. For a treatment regimen to be considered effective or for a factor to be considered causally related, it must affect the treatment group significantly differently from the control group as determined by a statistical test.

Randomization refers to the practice of assigning subjects to treatments or control groups in a completely random manner. This can be accomplished by assigning numbers to subjects and then having numbers selected randomly. Numbers can be selected randomly from a table of random numbers, by drawing lots, or by using a computer-generated list of random numbers. Thus, each research subject, human or animal, has an equal chance of being placed in the treatment group.

Blinding refers to the practice in which the investigator(s) and/or subjects remain uninformed and unaware of the groups to which subjects are assigned throughout the period of experimentation and data gathering. This prevents the investigator(s) from looking favorably or unfavorably on the responses of any particular subject or group while gathering data during the experiment. Thus, the researcher can remain unbiased. When both the observer and subjects are kept ignorant, the study is referred to as a double-blind trial.

When studies involve human subjects, they normally involve the use of a placebo, such as a saline (saltwater) injection or sugar pill. The use of a placebo prevents subjects from determining by observation whether or not they are receiving treatment. This is important because human thought processes are such that some people begin to feel better if they believe they have received a treatment. For a vaccine or therapeutic drug to be labeled as effective, it must consistently perform better than a placebo.

An example of just such an experiment was performed by Tonnesen and his colleagues, who studied the effectiveness of a 16-hour nicotine patch on smoking cessation.[23] They used a double-blind randomized design to compare the effects of a nicotine skin patch with those of a placebo skin patch. Subjects were assigned to the active treatment or the placebo according to computer-generated random numbers. There were 145 subjects who received a nicotine patch and 144 who received the placebo. Subjects were scheduled for visits 1, 3, 6, 12, 26, and 52 weeks after the first visit—the day smoking cessation was to begin. Table 2.10 presents the results of cessation for each group 6, 12, 26, and 52 weeks after the study began. The results of this study indicated that there was a significant difference between the effectiveness of the nicotine patch and the placebo patch with regard to smoking cessation.

Controlling variables, the use of treatment and control groups, randomization, and blinding are techniques aimed at ensuring objectivity and avoiding bias in experimental studies. Through strict adherence to these principles, investigators hope to achieve experimental results that accurately reflect what occurs in a natural setting.

By carrying out carefully planned descriptive studies, epidemiologists define outbreaks of disease, injury, and death in specific populations and develop hypotheses about the causes of these outbreaks. By designing and carrying out analytic and experimental studies, epidemiologists test these hypotheses.

Criteria of Causation

Often, even after numerous epidemiologic studies have identified an association between exposure to a

placebo a blank treatment

Table 2.10 Percentage of Subjects Abstaining from Smoking 6, 12, 26, and 52 Weeks After the Start of the Program

Week Number	Percentage of People Remaining Abstinent	
	Nicotine Patch	Placebo Patch
6	53	17
12	41	10
26	24	5
52	17	4

Source: Tonnesen, P., J. Norregaard, K. Simonsen, and U. Sawe (1991). "A Double-Blind Trial of a 16-Hour Transdermal Nicotine Patch in Smoking Cessation." *New England Journal of Medicine*, 325(5): 311–315.

suspected risk factor (A) and the development of a specific disease (B), it may not be clear that A causes B in the same way we state that infection with the influenza virus causes the flu. In the nicotine patch study just cited, for example, researchers found an association between wearing a nicotine patch and abstaining from smoking. That is not quite the same as stating that wearing the nicotine patch *caused* smoking abstention. In 1965, this problem was addressed by Austin Bradford Hill, who laid out criteria that should be considered when deciding whether an association might be one of causation.[24] As he developed these criteria, he often cited the behavior of cigarette smoking and the development of lung cancer as examples. With minor modifications, Hill's **criteria of causation** are outlined here:

Strength: How strong is the association between the exposure and the disease? Are those exposed 3, 5, 10, or 100 times more likely to develop disease than those who are not exposed? How many times more likely are cigarette smokers to get lung cancer than nonsmokers? Also, is there a dose–response relationship? Is it the case that a greater exposure to a particular risk factor results in a higher rate of disease or death? Are those who smoke more heavily more likely to develop lung cancer than lighter smokers are?

Consistency: Has the association been reported in a variety of people exposed in a variety of settings? Are the results repeatable by other researchers?

Specificity: Is the disease or health problem associated with the exposure the only one? When someone becomes ill after exposure is it always, or almost always, the same disease? When cigarette smokers become ill, is it always, or almost always, lung cancer?

Temporality: Does A (the exposure) always precede B (the disease)? Does the behavior of cigarette smoking precede the onset of lung cancer, or do those with lung cancer take up the habit of smoking for some reason?

Biological plausibility: Does the suspected causation make sense with what we know about biology, physiology, and other medical knowledge? Does it make sense, in light of what we know about biology and physiology, that cigarette smoking could produce lung cancer?

Using these criteria together with analytic, epidemiological data, health researchers can often persuade legislatures and public officials to pass laws or alter public policies that promote health and prevent and control disease outbreaks. We often describe diseases according to organ or organ system affected—kidney disease, heart disease, respiratory infection, and so on. Another way we often describe diseases is by cause—viral disease, chemical poisoning, or a burn. Causative agents may be biological, chemical, or physical. Biological agents include viruses, rickettsiae, bacteria, protozoa, fungi, and metazoa (multicellular organisms). Chemical agents include drugs, pesticides, industrial chemicals, food additives, air pollutants, and cigarette smoke. Physical agents that can cause injury or disease include various forms of energy such as heat, ultraviolet light, radiation, noise vibrations, and speeding or falling objects.

Prevention and Control of Diseases and Other Health-Related Conditions

The goals of epidemiology are to prevent, control, and, in rare cases, eradicate diseases and injuries. **Prevention** implies the planning for and taking of action to prevent or forestall the occurrence of an undesirable event, and is therefore more desirable than **intervention**, the taking of action during an event. For example, immunization to prevent a disease is preferable to the administration of an antibiotic to cure one.

Control is a general term for the containment of a disease and can include both prevention and intervention measures. The term *control* is often used to mean the limiting of transmission of a communicable disease in a population. **Eradication** is the uprooting or total elimination of a disease from the human population. It is an elusive goal that is only rarely achieved in public health. Smallpox is the only communicable disease that has been eradicated. This was possible only because humans are the only reservoir for the smallpox virus.

Prioritizing Prevention and Control Efforts

Communities are confronted with a multitude of diseases and health-related conditions, including communicable and noncommunicable diseases, unintentional injuries,

criteria of causation criteria or factors that should be considered when deciding whether an association between a disease and possible risk factor might be one of causation

eradication the complete elimination or uprooting of a disease (e.g., smallpox eradication)

intervention efforts to control a disease in progress

prevention the planning for and taking of action to forestall the onset of a disease or other health problem

violence, alcohol and other drug abuse problems, and so on. Community leaders must decide how to allocate community resources to prevent or control these problems; that is, they must determine which problems are the most urgent and which problems are likely to benefit the most from timely intervention. Among the criteria they use to judge the relative importance of health-related conditions to their community are (1) leading causes of death, (2) years of potential life lost, and (3) economic costs to society.

Leading Causes of Death

The NCHS regularly publishes a list of the leading causes of death. For more than 80 years, the leading cause of death in the United States has been diseases of the heart. The most recent data reveal that nearly one in every four deaths can be attributed to diseases of the heart. Cancers (malignant neoplasms) represent the second leading killer; nearly one in four deaths is the result of cancer. Chronic lower respiratory disease ranks third, cerebrovascular disease (stroke) ranks fourth, and unintentional injuries rank fifth (see Table 2.7 earlier in this chapter).[11]

One might prioritize expenditures of healthcare resources solely on the basis of leading causes of death, but in doing so one would spend about two-thirds of the entire health budget on the four leading health problems alone. Few resources would remain to support infant and childhood nutrition programs, which have been shown to prevent more serious healthcare problems in later life. Likewise, few funds would be available to fight debilitating, but usually nonfatal, diseases such as chronic arthritis or mental illness.

Years of Potential Life Lost

Another approach to prioritizing a community's healthcare problems is by using the years of potential life lost (YPLL) statistic previously discussed. Using this approach, diseases of the heart would rank third in importance below malignant neoplasms (cancers) and unintentional injuries, which together account for 37% of all YPLL (refer to Table 2.9 and Figure 2.2 earlier in this chapter).[15]

Economic Cost to Society

Still another way to evaluate the impact of a particular disease or health problem is to estimate the economic cost to the country or community. Economic cost data are hard to come by, and sometimes even experts cannot agree on the estimates obtained. An example of such an estimate is the cost to our federal, state, and local governments resulting from the use and abuse of alcohol and other drugs, a whopping $467.7 billion annually, more than $1 billion per day.[25] This figure amounts to 10.7% of their entire $4.4 trillion budgets.

Levels of Prevention

There are three levels of application of preventive measures in disease control—primary, secondary, and tertiary. Applications of levels of prevention and examples are presented in Figure 2.9.

Primary prevention comprises all efforts to forestall the onset of illness or injury during the prepathogenesis period (before the disease process begins). Examples of primary prevention include health education and health promotion programs, safe-housing projects, and character-building and personality development programs. Other examples are the use of immunizations against specific diseases, the practice of personal hygiene such as hand washing, the use of rubber gloves, and the chlorination of the community's water supply.

Secondary prevention is the early diagnosis and prompt treatment of diseases before the disease becomes advanced and disability becomes severe. One of the most important secondary prevention measures is health screenings. The goal of these screenings is not to prevent the onset of disease, but rather to detect its presence during early pathogenesis, thus permitting early intervention (treatment) to limit disability. It is important to note that the purpose of a health screening is not to diagnose disease. Instead, the purpose is to economically and efficiently sort those who are probably healthy from those who could possibly be positive for a disease (see Figure 2.10). Those who screen positively can then be referred for more specific diagnostic procedures. Screenings for diabetes and high blood pressure are popular examples of health screenings, as are breast self-examination and testicular self-examination.

The goal of **tertiary prevention** is to retrain, re-educate, and rehabilitate the patient who has already incurred a disability. Tertiary preventive measures include those that are applied after significant pathogenesis has occurred. Therapy for a heart patient, including patient health education, is an example of tertiary prevention. Another example is counseling and participation in support group meetings for a recovering alcoholic.

primary prevention preventive measures that forestall the onset of illness or injury during the prepathogenesis period

secondary prevention preventive measures that lead to an early diagnosis and prompt treatment of a disease or injury to limit disability and prevent more severe pathogenesis

tertiary prevention measures aimed at rehabilitation following significant pathogenesis

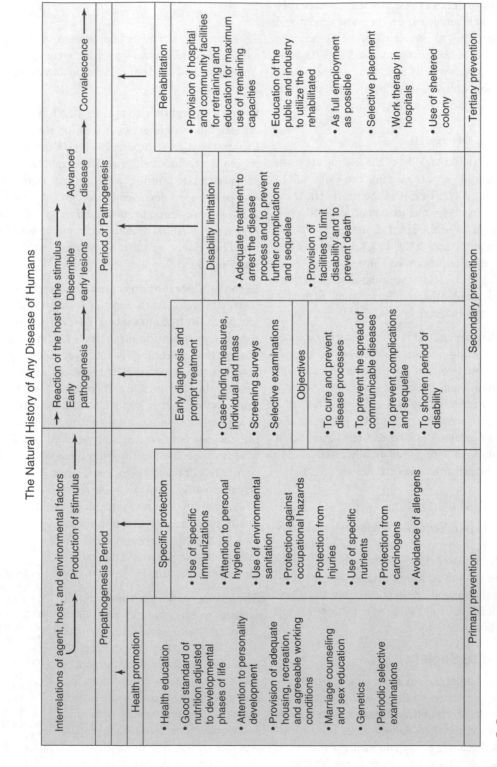

Figure 2.9 Applications of levels of prevention.

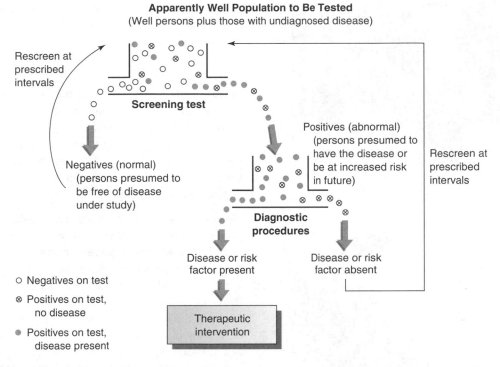

Figure 2.10 Flow diagram for a mass screening test.

Mausner, J. S., and S. Kramer (1985). *Mausner and Bahn Epidemiology—An Introductory Text*, 2nd ed. Philadelphia, PA: W.B. Saunders, p. 216.

Classification of Diseases and Health-Related Conditions

In community health, diseases and health-related conditions are usually classified as acute or chronic, or as communicable (infectious) or noncommunicable (noninfectious). **Communicable (infectious) diseases** are caused by biological agents or their products, and the agents are transmissible from a source of infection to a susceptible host. The disease process begins when the agent is able to enter and grow or reproduce within the body of the host. The entrance and growth of microorganisms or viruses in the host are called infections.

Noncommunicable (noninfectious) diseases or illnesses are those that cannot be transmitted from one person to another. Delineating the causes of noncommunicable diseases is often more difficult because several, or even many, factors may contribute to the development of a given noncommunicable health condition. These contributing factors may be genetic, environmental, or behavioral in nature. For this reason, many noncommunicable health conditions are called multicausation diseases; heart disease is an example.

Genetics, environmental factors such as stress, and behavioral choices such as poor diet and lack of exercise can all contribute to heart disease.

In the acute/chronic classification scheme, diseases are classified by their duration of symptoms. Recall that acute diseases are diseases in which the peak severity of symptoms occurs and subsides within 3 months and the recovery of those who survive is usually complete. Examples of acute communicable diseases include the common cold, influenza (flu), chickenpox, and plague. Examples of acute noncommunicable illnesses are appendicitis, injuries from motor vehicle crashes, acute alcohol intoxication or drug overdose, and sprained ankles.

Chronic diseases or conditions are those in which symptoms continue longer than 3 months, and in some cases, for the remainder of one's life and recovery is slow and sometimes incomplete (see **Figure 2.11**). These diseases can be either communicable or noncommunicable. Examples of chronic communicable diseases are

communicable (infectious) disease an illness caused by some specific biological agent or its toxic products that can be transmitted from an infected person, animal, or inanimate reservoir to a susceptible host

noncommunicable (noninfectious) disease a disease that cannot be transmitted from infected host to susceptible host

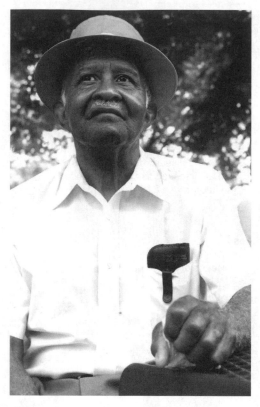

Figure 2.11 Arthritis is a noninfectious chronic condition that can persist for one's entire life.
Photographs by the U.S. Census Bureau, Public Information Office (PIO).

AIDS, tuberculosis, and herpes virus infections. Chronic noncommunicable illnesses include coronary heart disease, diabetes, and arthritis.

Communicable Diseases

Whereas **infectivity** refers to the ability of a biological agent to enter and grow in a host, the term **pathogenicity** refers to an infectious disease agent's ability to produce disease. Selected pathogenic agents and the diseases they cause are listed in Table 2.11. These agents can be transmitted from an infected individual in the community to uninfected, susceptible people.

Disease models are schematic representations that help people conceptualize disease processes. **Figure 2.12**, a simplified **communicable disease model**, depicts the essential elements necessary for the occurrence of disease—the agent, host, and environment. In this model, the **agent** is the element that must be present for disease to occur; for example, the influenza virus must be present for a person to become ill with flu. The **host** is any susceptible organism invaded by an infectious agent. The environment includes all other factors—physical, biological, or social—that inhibit or promote or permit disease transmission. Communicable disease transmission occurs when a susceptible host and a pathogenic agent exist in an environment conducive to disease transmission.

agent (pathogenic agent) the cause of the disease or health problem

communicable disease model a visual representation of the interrelationships among causative agent, host, and environment

host a person or other living organism that affords subsistence or lodgment to a communicable agent under natural conditions

infectivity the ability of a biological agent to enter and grow in the host

pathogenicity the capability of a communicable disease agent to cause disease in a susceptible host

Table 2.11 Biological Agents of Disease

Types of Agent	Name of Agent	Disease
Viruses	Varicella virus	Chickenpox
	Human immunodeficiency virus (HIV)	Acquired immune deficiency syndrome (AIDS)
	Rubella virus	German measles
Rickettsiae	*Rickettsia rickettsii*	Rocky Mountain spotted fever
Bacteria	*Vibrio cholerae*	Cholera
	Clostridium tetani	Tetanus
	Yersinia pestis	Plague
	Borrelia burgdorferi	Lyme disease
Protozoa	*Entamoeba histolytica*	Amebic dysentery
	Plasmodium falciparum	Malaria
	Trypanosoma gambiense	African sleeping sickness
Fungi and yeasts	*Tinea cruris*	Jock itch
	Tinea pedis	Athlete's foot
Nematoda (worms)	*Wuchereria bancrofti*	Filariasis (elephantiasis)
	Onchocerca volvulus	Onchocerciasis (river blindness)

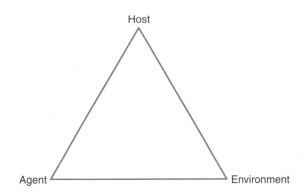

Figure 2.12 Communicable disease model.

Chain of Infection

Communicable disease transmission is a complicated but well-studied process that is best understood through a conceptual model known as the **chain of infection** (see **Figure 2.13**). Using the chain of infection model, one can visualize the step-by-step process by which communicable diseases spread from an infected person to an uninfected person in the community. The pathogenic (disease-producing) agent leaves its reservoir (infected host) via a portal of exit. Transmission occurs in either a direct or indirect manner, and the pathogenic agent enters a susceptible host through a portal of entry to establish infection.

To illustrate, using the common cold virus, the virus leaves its reservoir (the throat of an infected person), perhaps when the host sneezes (see **Figure 2.14**). The portals of exit are the nose and mouth. Transmission may be direct if saliva droplets enter the respiratory tract of a susceptible host at close range, or it may be indirect if droplets are deposited on a surface touched by others or dry and become airborne. The portal of entry could be the nose, mouth, or eye of a susceptible host. The virus enters and establishes a new infection in the new host.

There are many variations in the chain of infection, depending on the disease agent, environmental conditions,

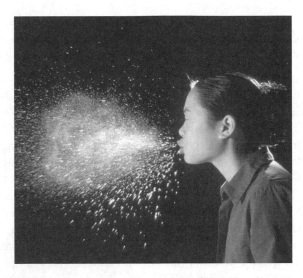

Figure 2.14 Portal of exit: The causative agents for many respiratory diseases leave their host via the mouth and nose.
© Custom Medical Stock Photo

infectivity, and host susceptibility. For example, the reservoir for a disease may be a **case**—a person who has the disease—or a **carrier**—one who is well but infected and is capable of serving as a source of infection. A (disease) carrier could be one who is incubating the disease, such as a person who is HIV positive but has no signs of AIDS, or one who has recovered from the disease (is asymptomatic), as is sometimes the case in typhoid fever. For some diseases, the reservoir is not humans but animals. Diseases for which the reservoir resides in animal populations are called **zoonoses**. Plague, rabies, Rocky Mountain spotted fever, and

carrier a person or animal that harbors a specific communicable agent in the absence of discernible clinical disease and serves as a potential source of infection to others

case a person who is sick with a disease

chain of infection a model to conceptualize the transmission of a communicable disease from its source to a susceptible host

zoonosis a communicable disease transmissible under natural conditions from vertebrate animals to humans

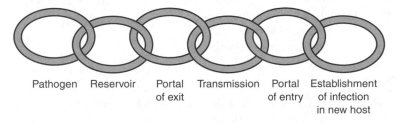

Pathogen   Reservoir   Portal of exit   Transmission   Portal of entry   Establishment of infection in new host

Figure 2.13 Chain of infection.

Lyme disease are zoonoses. Diseases for which humans are the only known reservoir, like measles, are known as **anthroponoses**.

Portals of exit and entry vary with the disease. Natural portals of exit and examples of diseases that use them are the respiratory tract (cold, influenza, measles, tuberculosis, and whooping cough), urogenital tract (gonorrhea, syphilis, herpes, and AIDS), digestive tract (amebic dysentery, shigellosis, polio, typhoid fever, and cholera), and skin (ringworm and jock itch). The skin is actually a good barrier to infection, but it can be bypassed by a hypodermic needle or when there is an open wound. Blood-sucking insects and ticks make their own portals of entry with mouth parts that penetrate the skin. Finally, many pathogenic agents can cross the placenta from mother to fetus (for example, rubella virus and hepatitis B virus).

Modes of Transmission

As noted in the previous paragraphs, communicable disease transmission may be direct or indirect. **Direct transmission** implies the immediate transfer of the disease agent between the infected and the susceptible individuals by direct contact "such as touching, biting, kissing, sexual intercourse, or by direct projection (droplet spread) of droplet spray onto the conjunctiva or onto the mucous membranes of the eye, nose or mouth during sneezing, coughing, spitting, singing or talking (usually limited to a distance of one meter or less)."[26] Examples of diseases for which transmission is usually direct are AIDS, syphilis, gonorrhea, rabies, and the common cold.

Indirect transmission includes airborne, vehicleborne, or vectorborne transmission. Airborne transmission is the dissemination of microbial aerosols to a suitable portal of entry, usually the respiratory tract. Microbial aerosols are suspensions of dust or droplet nuclei made up wholly or in part of microorganisms. These particles may remain suspended and infective for long periods of time. Tuberculosis, influenza, histoplasmosis, and legionellosis are examples of airborne diseases.

In vehicleborne transmission, contaminated materials or objects (fomites) serve as **vehicles**—nonliving objects by which communicable agents are transferred to a susceptible host. The agent may or may not have multiplied or developed on the vehicle. Examples of vehicles include toys, handkerchiefs, soiled clothes, bedding, food service utensils, and surgical instruments. Also considered vehicles are water, milk, food, or biological products such as blood, serum, plasma, organs, and tissues. Almost any disease can be transmitted by vehicles, including those for which the primary mode of transmission is direct, such as dysentery and hepatitis.

Vectorborne transmission is transmission by a living organism such as a mosquito, fly, or tick. Transmission can be mechanical, via the contaminated mouth parts or feet of the **vector**, or biological, involving multiplication or developmental changes of the agent in the vector before transmission occurs. In mechanical transmission, multiplication and development of the disease organism usually do not occur. For example, organisms that cause dysentery, polio, cholera, and typhoid fever have been isolated from insects such as cockroaches and houseflies and could presumably be deposited on food prepared for human consumption.

In biological transmission, multiplication and/or developmental changes of the disease agent occur in the vector before transmission occurs. Biological transmission is much more important than mechanical transmission in terms of its impact on community health. Examples of biological vectors include mosquitoes, fleas, lice, ticks, flies, and other insects. Mosquitoes are by far the most important vectors of human disease. They transmit more than 200 viruses, including those that cause yellow fever, dengue hemorrhagic fever, and West Nile fever. They also transmit malaria, which infects an estimated 100 million people in the world each year and kills approximately 1 million of them. Ticks, another important vector, transmit Rocky Mountain spotted fever, relapsing fever, and Lyme disease. Other vectors are flies, fleas, lice, mites, and bugs.

Prevention and Control of Communicable Diseases

In the following sections we discuss how the three levels of prevention can be applied to control communicable diseases and we give specific examples of such applications. Prevention and control of communicable diseases over the past century, resulting in unprecedented declines in morbidity and mortality from these diseases, represent one of the outstanding achievements in public health during the twentieth century.

anthroponosis a disease that infects only humans

direct transmission the immediate transfer of an infectious agent by direct contact between infected and susceptible individuals

indirect transmission communicable disease transmission involving an intermediate step

vector a living organism, usually an arthropod (e.g., mosquito, tick, louse, or flea), that can transmit a communicable agent to susceptible hosts

vehicle an inanimate material or object that can serve as a source of infection

Primary Prevention of Communicable Diseases

The primary prevention measures for communicable diseases can best be visualized using the chain of infection model described earlier in this chapter. In this model, prevention strategies are evident at each link in the chain (see Figure 2.15). Successful application of each strategy can be seen as weakening a link, with the ultimate goal of breaking the chain of infection, or interrupting disease transmission. Chlorination of the water supply to prevent outbreaks of waterborne diseases, the inspection of restaurants and retail food markets to prevent foodborne disease outbreaks, and mass immunization campaigns are examples of the primary prevention of communicable diseases. To these community efforts can be added individual actions such as hand washing, the proper cooking of food, adequate clothing and housing, and the use of condoms to prevent disease transmission.

Secondary Prevention of Communicable Diseases

Secondary preventive measures undertaken by the community against infectious diseases are usually aimed at controlling or limiting the extent of an epidemic. Examples include carefully maintaining records of cases and complying with the regulations requiring the reporting of notifiable diseases (discussed previously) and investigating cases and contacts—those who may have become infected through close contact with known cases. Secondary prevention can also include isolation and quarantine. **Isolation** is the separation, for the period of communicability, of infected persons or animals from others to prevent the transmission of a communicable agent to a susceptible host. **Quarantine** is the limitation of the freedom of movement of well persons or animals that have been exposed to a communicable disease until the incubation period has passed. Further control measures may include **disinfection**, the killing of communicable agents outside of the host, and mass treatment with antibiotics. Finally, public health education and health promotion can be a part of secondary prevention as well as primary prevention.

Individuals can initiate secondary prevention (intervention) against communicable diseases through (1) self-diagnosis and self-treatment with nonprescription medications or home remedies, and/or (2) seeking diagnosis and treatment by a physician.

Tertiary Prevention of Communicable Diseases

At the community level, tertiary preventive measures are aimed at preventing the recurrence of an epidemic. The proper removal, embalming, and burial of the dead is an example. Tertiary preventive measures might include the reapplication of such primary measures as mass immunizations to prevent further cases. Individual efforts and tertiary prevention of communicable diseases include convalescence, disinfection, recovery to full health, and return to

disinfection the killing of communicable disease agents outside the host, on countertops, for example

isolation the separation of infected persons from those who are susceptible

quarantine limitation of freedom of movement of those who have been exposed to a disease and may be incubating it

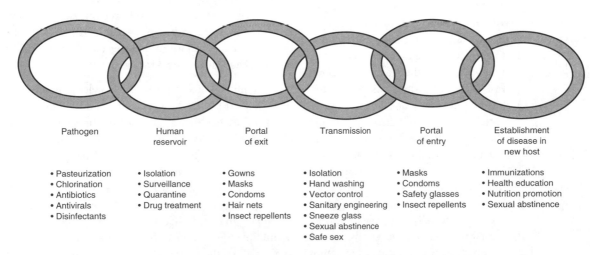

Pathogen	Human reservoir	Portal of exit	Transmission	Portal of entry	Establishment of disease in new host
• Pasteurization	• Isolation	• Gowns	• Isolation	• Masks	• Immunizations
• Chlorination	• Surveillance	• Masks	• Hand washing	• Condoms	• Health education
• Antibiotics	• Quarantine	• Condoms	• Vector control	• Safety glasses	• Nutrition promotion
• Antivirals	• Drug treatment	• Hair nets	• Sanitary engineering	• Insect repellents	• Sexual abstinence
• Disinfectants		• Insect repellents	• Sneeze glass		
			• Sexual abstinence		
			• Safe sex		

Figure 2.15 Chain of infection model showing disease prevention and control strategies.

normal activity. In some cases, such as paralytic poliomyelitis, return to the previous state of normal activity may not be possible even with extensive physical therapy.

Prevention and Control of a Communicable Disease: HIV Infection and AIDS

Human immunodeficiency virus (HIV) destroys specific blood cells (CD4+ T cells) that are crucial in fighting diseases. People can become infected when they come in contact with the virus through unprotected sexual activity, intravenous drug use, or exposure to the blood of an infected person; there is no known nonhuman reservoir of HIV. "Within a few weeks of being infected with HIV, some people develop flu-like symptoms that last for a week or two, but others experience no symptoms at all. People living with HIV may appear and feel healthy for several years. However, even if they feel healthy, HIV is still affecting their bodies."[27]

Acquired immune deficiency syndrome (AIDS) is the late stage of an infection with HIV. People with AIDS have a difficult time fighting other communicable diseases and certain cancers. In the past, it took only a few years for someone infected to develop AIDS. Now, with the development of advanced medications, people can live much longer, perhaps even decades, after acquiring an HIV infection.[27]

Despite advances in diagnosis and treatment, HIV infections and AIDS remain pandemic throughout the world. The WHO estimates that 34 million people are living with HIV/AIDS worldwide. During 2011, 2.5 million people were newly infected with HIV and 1.7 million people died of AIDS.[28] In the United States, through December 2010, a cumulative total of 1,129,127 persons with AIDS were reported to the CDC by state and territorial health departments.[29] Referring to the chain of infection, HIV normally leaves its infected host (reservoir) during sexual activity; the portal of exit is the urogenital tract. Transmission is direct and occurs when reproductive fluids or blood are exchanged with the susceptible host. In the case of injection drug users, however, transmission is indirect, by contaminated needles (vehicle). The portal of entry is usually either genital, oral, or anal in direct (sexual) transmission or transdermal in the case of injection

bloodborne pathogens disease agents, such as HIV, that are transmissible in blood and other body fluids

Bloodborne Pathogens Standard a set of regulations promulgated by OSHA that sets forth the responsibilities of employers and employees with regard to precautions to be taken concerning bloodborne pathogens in the workplace

drug users or blood transfusion recipients. Transmission can also occur during medical procedures if there is an accidental needlestick or some other type of contamination with blood or other potentially infectious material.

A closer examination of the chain of infection reveals that prevention or control measures can be identified for each link. The pathogen in the infected host can be held in check by the appropriate drug. Outside the host, measures such as sterilizing needles and other possible vehicles and disinfecting surfaces readily kill the virus and reduce the likelihood of transmission by contamination. The infected host (reservoir) can be identified through blood tests and educated to take precautions against the careless transmission of live virus through unsafe sex and needle sharing. Portals of exit (and entry) can be protected by the use of condoms.

One set of *Healthy People 2020* objectives focuses on reducing the rate of HIV transmission and, thus, the number of new cases of AIDS. One way to do this is to increase the proportion of sexually active persons using condoms. Another way is to increase the number of persons living with HIV who know their level of antibodies to HIV (their serostatus). Finally, one objective aims to increase the proportion of adolescents and adults who have been tested for HIV in the past 12 months (see **Box 2.1**).

For those working in the health professions, the risk of acquiring an HIV infection in the workplace is of particular concern. The Occupational Safety and Health Administration (OSHA) estimates that 5.6 million workers in the healthcare industry and related occupations are at risk of occupational exposure to **bloodborne pathogens**, including HIV, hepatitis B virus (HBV), hepatitis C virus (HCV), and others.[30] In 1991, recognizing that workers in the healthcare industry were at risk of occupational exposure to bloodborne pathogens, OSHA issued the **Bloodborne Pathogens Standard**.

In November 2000, Congress, acknowledging the estimates of 600,000 to 800,000 needlestick and other percutaneous injuries occurring among healthcare workers annually, passed the Needlestick Safety and Prevention Act.[31] In 2001, in response to the Needlestick Safety and Prevention Act, OSHA revised its Bloodborne Pathogens Standard. This revised standard, currently in effect, "clarifies the need for employers to select safer needle devices and to involve employees in identifying and choosing these devices" and to maintain a log of injuries from contaminated sharps.[30] The goal of all of these regulations and standards is to reduce

Box 2.1 *Healthy People 2020* Objectives

OBJECTIVES HIV-3, HIV-4, HIV-13, HIV 14.1, HIV-17.1, HIV-17.2. Reduce the number of new AIDS cases, reduce the number of deaths from AIDS, increase survivorship of those diagnosed with AIDS, increase HIV testing, and increase condom use.

Target setting method: Consistent with the National HIV/AIDS Strategy; or 10% improvement

Data Sources: HIV Surveillance System, CDC, NCHHSTP

Targets and baselines:

Objective	2006 Baseline	2020 Target
HIV-3 Reduce the rate of HIV transmission among adolescents and adults	New infections per 100 persons living with HIV	
	5.0	3.5
HIV-4 Reduce the number of new AIDS cases among adolescents and adults	New cases of AIDS per 100,000 age 13 years and older	
	13	10
HIV-13 Increase the proportion of people living with HIV who know their serostatus	Persons 13 years and older living with HIV who are aware of their HIV infection	
	79.0% (in 2006)	90.0%
HIV-14.1 Increase the proportion of adolescents and adults who have been tested for HIV in the past 12 months	Persons 15-44 years of age reporting that they had an HIV test in the past 12 months (outside of blood donation)	
	15.4%	16.9%
HIV-17.1 Increase the proportion of sexually active females using condoms	Unmarried females aged 15-44 years	
	34.5%	38.0%
HIV-17.2 Increase the proportion of sexually active males using condoms	Unmarried males aged 15-44 years	
	55.2%	60.7%

For Further Thought

Reducing the rate of HIV transmission is the best way to reduce both the number of persons living with HIV infection and the number of new AIDS cases. Reducing the number of new AIDS cases reduces the number of deaths from AIDS. Unprotected sexual contact, whether homosexual or heterosexual, with a person infected with HIV is one of the most important ways HIV infections are transmitted. An important way to slow the rate of HIV transmission and the occurrence of new AIDS cases is to increase the proportion of sexually active females and males who use condoms. Can you think of ways to increase the rate of condom use in sexually active persons in your community?

Source: Modified from U.S. Department of Health and Human Services, Office of Disease Prevention and Health Promotion (2010). *Healthy People 2020.* Available at http://www.healthypeople.gov/2020/default.aspx.

the number of HIV/AIDS cases, as well as cases of other bloodborne diseases that result from workplace exposure.

Noncommunicable Diseases and Health-Related Conditions

Although communicable diseases remain an important community health concern, noncommunicable diseases and health-related conditions currently rank high among the nation's leading causes of death. Among these are heart disease, cancer, chronic obstructive respiratory disease, and diabetes. Although not infectious, these diseases nonetheless can occur in epidemic proportions. Furthermore, the chronic nature of many of these diseases means that they place a heavy burden on a community's healthcare resources.

The complex **etiologies** (causes) of many of the noncommunicable diseases, such as coronary heart disease, are most easily conceptualized by the **multicausation disease model** (see **Figure 2.16**). In this model, the human host is pictured in the center of his or her environment. Within the host, there exists a unique, unalterable, genetic endowment. The host lives in a complex environment that includes exposures to a multitude of risk factors that can contribute to the disease process. These environmental risk factors are physical, chemical, biological, and social in nature.

etiology the cause of a disease

multicausation disease model a visual representation of the host together with various internal and external factors that promote and protect against disease

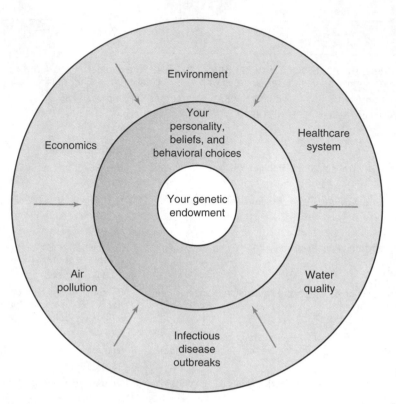

Figure 2.16 Multicausation disease model.

Physical factors in one's environment include the latitude, physical geography, and climate where one lives. Chemical factors include both natural chemical hazards and those resulting from human activities to which an individual is subjected in his or her environment. Biological factors arise from one's genetic endowment, which gives rise to one's development, biochemistry, and physiology. Social factors are those arising from one's living arrangements, interpersonal relationships, occupation, and recreational activities.

Risk factors can also be divided into unmodifiable risk factors and modifiable risk factors. **Unmodifiable risk factors** are unalterable and arise from one's genetic endowment; they include one's race, gender, personality type, age, and basic metabolic rate. **Modifiable risk factors** are those lifestyle and behavioral factors over which an individual has some control, such as one's diet, commitment to daily exercise, and decisions about smoking, drinking, and other drug use.

Poor lifestyle choices can increase the number and severity of one's risk factors and be detrimental to one's health. Because of their prominence as concerns in the United States today, diseases of the heart and blood vessels, cancer, and other selected chronic diseases are discussed in the following sections.

Diseases of the Heart and Blood Vessels

Diseases of the heart and blood vessels, cardiovascular diseases (CVDs), are a leading cause of death in the United States. **Coronary heart disease (CHD)** is the number 1 killer of Americans. In 2010 alone, more than 595,444 people died of heart disease in the United States, accounting for one in four deaths that year.[11] It is estimated that more than 74 million Americans have one or more types of CVD.[32]

The American Heart Association lists nine types of CVDs: CHD, stroke, high blood pressure, arrhythmias, diseases of the arteries, congestive heart failure, valvular heart disease, rheumatic fever/rheumatic heart disease, and congenital heart defects.[32] CHD causes more than half of all cardiovascular disease deaths. Sometimes called coronary artery disease,

coronary heart disease (CHD) a chronic disease characterized by damage to the coronary arteries in the heart

modifiable risk factors factors contributing to the development of a noncommunicable disease that can be altered by modifying one's behavior or environment

unmodifiable risk factors factors contributing to the development of a noncommunicable disease that cannot be altered by modifying one's behavior or environment

CHD is characterized by damage to the coronary arteries, the blood vessels that carry oxygen-rich blood to the heart muscle. Damage to the coronary arteries usually evolves from the condition known as atherosclerosis, a narrowing of the blood vessels. This narrowing usually results from the buildup of fatty deposits on the inner walls of arteries. When blood flow to the heart muscle is severely reduced or interrupted, a heart attack can occur. If heart damage is severe, the heart may stop beating—a condition known as cardiac arrest.

Over the past 50 years, a more complete understanding of the processes involved in CVDs has resulted in a 56% decline in deaths from heart disease and stroke. Numerous modifiable and unmodifiable risk factors for coronary artery disease have been identified. Modifiable risk factors include cigarette smoking, untreated high blood pressure, high blood cholesterol, physical inactivity, obesity, diabetes,

and stress. Unmodifiable risk factors include being male, being older, and genetic tendencies to develop CVD.

Cerebrovascular disease (stroke) is the fourth leading cause of death in the United States. Strokes killed more than 129,180 people in 2008.[11] During a stroke, or cerebrovascular accident, the blood supply to the brain is interrupted. The risk factors for developing cerebrovascular disease are similar to those for CHD and include hereditary, behavioral, and environmental factors. Hypertension, high serum cholesterol, and obesity are especially important risk factors for cerebrovascular disease. One set of *Healthy People 2020* objectives aims to reduce risk factors for and, ultimately, deaths from coronary heart disease and stroke (see **Box 2.2**).

cerebrovascular disease (stroke) a chronic disease characterized by damage to blood vessels of the brain resulting in disruption of circulation to the brain

---

Box 2.2 *Healthy People 2020* Objectives

OBJECTIVES HDS-5.1, 5.2 Reduce the proportion of adults and children and adolescents with high blood pressure.
Target-Setting Method: 10% improvement
Data Source: National Health and Nutrition Examination Survey (NHANES), CDC, NCHS
Targets and baselines:

Objective	2005-2008 Baseline	Target 2020
HDS-5.1	Reduce the proportion of adults with high blood pressure	Adults 18 years and older with high blood pressure
	29.9%	26.9%
HDS-5.2	Reduce the proportion of children and adolescents with high blood pressure	Children and adolescents aged 8-17 years with high blood pressure
	3.5%	3.2%

OBJECTIVE HDS-7 Reduce the proportion of adults with high total cholesterol.
Target-Setting Method: 10% improvement
Data Source: National Health and Nutrition Examination Survey (NHANES), CDC, NCHS
Targets and baselines:

Objective	2005-2008 Baseline	2020 Target
HDS-7	Reduce the proportion of adults with high total cholesterol	Percent of adults 20 years and older with total blood cholesterol levels of 240mg/dL or greater
	15%	13.5%

OBJECTIVE HDS-8 Reduce the mean total cholesterol levels among adults.
Target-Setting Method: 10% improvement
Data Source: National Health and Nutrition Examination Survey (NHANES), CDC, NCHS
Targets and baselines:

Objective	2005-2008 Baseline	2020 Target
HDS-8	Reduce the mean total cholesterol levels among adults	Mean total blood cholesterol level for adults 20 years and older
	197.7 mg/dL	177.9 mg/dL

For Further Thought

Cardiovascular diseases are the leading causes of deaths in the United States. Although significant progress has been made in lowering the death rate from heart attack and stroke, further progress is certainly achievable. Important contributing factors are high blood pressure, high blood cholesterol, and obesity. What can individuals and communities do to lower the average blood pressure, lower the mean level of cholesterol in the blood, and reduce obesity? Have you noticed efforts in your community to provide blood pressure screenings and cholesterol testing? If so, what agencies are offering these services?

Source: Modified from U.S. Department of Health and Human Services, Office of Disease Prevention and Health Promotion (2010). *Healthy People 2020.* Available at http://www.healthypeople.gov/2020/default.aspx.

Malignant Neoplasms (Cancer)

A total of 573,855 people died from malignant neoplasms (cancer) in 2010, making it the second leading cause of death in the United States.[11] **Malignant neoplasms** occur when cells lose control over their growth and division. Normal cells are inhibited from continual growth and division by virtue of their contact with adjacent cells. Malignant (cancerous) cells are not so inhibited; they continue to grow and divide, eventually piling up in a "new growth," a neoplasm or tumor. Early-stage tumors, sometimes called in situ cancers, are more treatable than are later-stage cancers. As tumor growth continues, parts of the neoplasm can break off and be carried to distant parts of the body, where they can lodge and continue to grow. When this occurs, the cancer is said to have **metastasized**. When malignant neoplasms have spread beyond the original cell layer where they developed, the cancer is said to be invasive.[33] The more the malignancy spreads, the more difficult it is to treat and the lower the survival rates.

Common cancer sites, in order of frequency of reported cases and deaths for both men and women, are shown in **Figure 2.17**. Cancer sites with the highest number of reported cases are the prostate gland and breast for men and women, respectively, but cancer frequently occurs in other sites, including the lungs, colon and rectum, pancreas, uterus, ovaries, mouth, bladder, and skin. Lung cancer is the leading cause of cancer deaths in both sexes. There were an estimated 226,160 new cases of lung cancer and an estimated 160,340 lung cancer deaths in 2012 alone. It has been estimated that 87% of these deaths can be attributed to smoking. Alcohol and smokeless tobacco contribute to cancers of the mouth, throat, larynx, esophagus, and liver.[33]

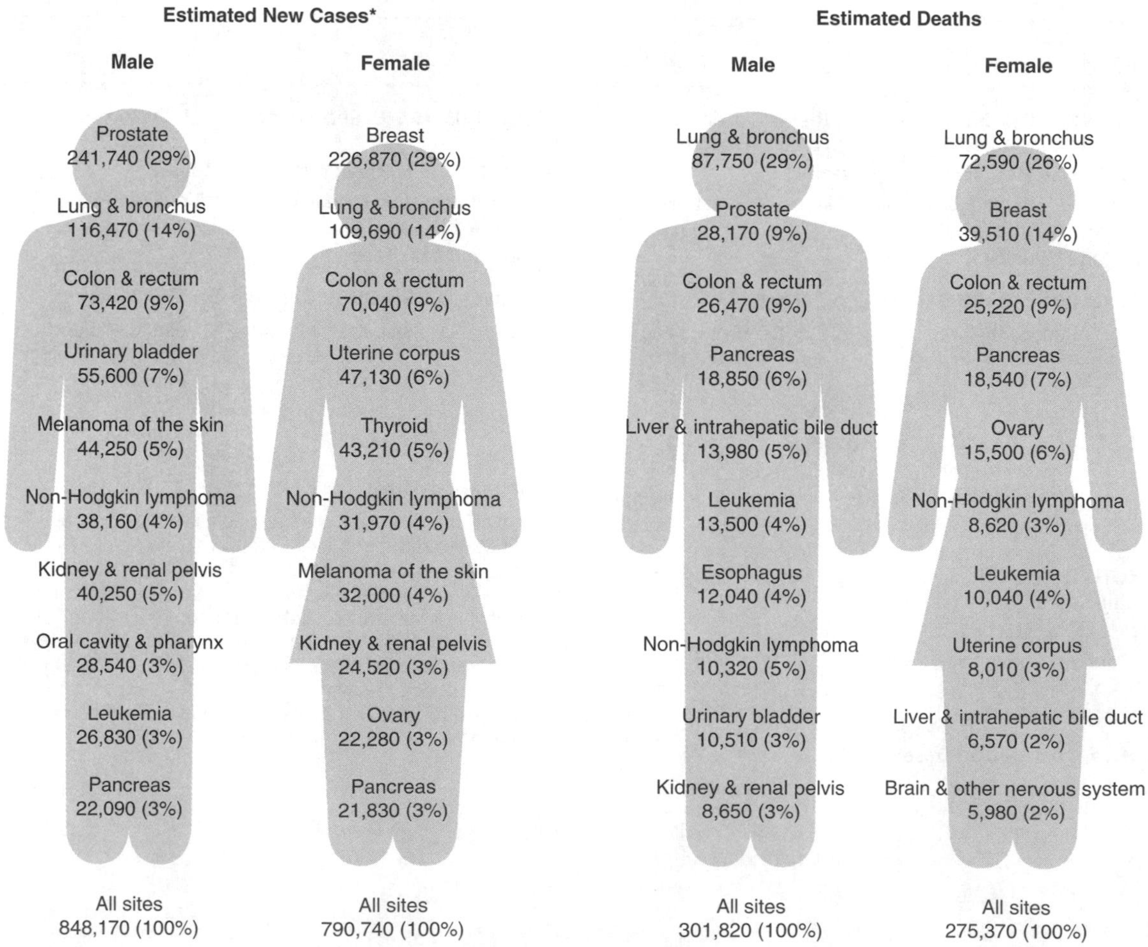

malignant neoplasm uncontrolled new tissue growth resulting from cells that have lost control over their growth and division

metastasis the spread of cancer cells to distant parts of the body by the circulatory or lymphatic system

Estimated New Cases*

Male

Prostate
241,740 (29%)

Lung & bronchus
116,470 (14%)

Colon & rectum
73,420 (9%)

Urinary bladder
55,600 (7%)

Melanoma of the skin
44,250 (5%)

Non-Hodgkin lymphoma
38,160 (4%)

Kidney & renal pelvis
40,250 (5%)

Oral cavity & pharynx
28,540 (3%)

Leukemia
26,830 (3%)

Pancreas
22,090 (3%)

All sites
848,170 (100%)

Female

Breast
226,870 (29%)

Lung & bronchus
109,690 (14%)

Colon & rectum
70,040 (9%)

Uterine corpus
47,130 (6%)

Thyroid
43,210 (5%)

Non-Hodgkin lymphoma
31,970 (4%)

Melanoma of the skin
32,000 (4%)

Kidney & renal pelvis
24,520 (3%)

Ovary
22,280 (3%)

Pancreas
21,830 (3%)

All sites
790,740 (100%)

Estimated Deaths

Male

Lung & bronchus
87,750 (29%)

Prostate
28,170 (9%)

Colon & rectum
26,470 (9%)

Pancreas
18,850 (6%)

Liver & intrahepatic bile duct
13,980 (5%)

Leukemia
13,500 (4%)

Esophagus
12,040 (4%)

Non-Hodgkin lymphoma
10,320 (5%)

Urinary bladder
10,510 (3%)

Kidney & renal pelvis
8,650 (3%)

All sites
301,820 (100%)

Female

Lung & bronchus
72,590 (26%)

Breast
39,510 (14%)

Colon & rectum
25,220 (9%)

Pancreas
18,540 (7%)

Ovary
15,500 (6%)

Non-Hodgkin lymphoma
8,620 (3%)

Leukemia
10,040 (4%)

Uterine corpus
8,010 (3%)

Liver & intrahepatic bile duct
6,570 (2%)

Brain & other nervous system
5,980 (2%)

All sites
275,370 (100%)

Figure 2.17 Leading sites of new cancer cases and deaths: 2012 estimates.

Reprinted from American Cancer Society. *Cancer Facts and Figures 2012.* Atlanta, GA: Author. Available at http://www.cancer.org.

More than 1 million new cases of basal cell or squamous cell skin cancer are detected each year in the United States. Almost all of these cases are attributable to exposure to the sun, and yet many people continue to sunbathe or use tanning salons, believing that a tanned body is a healthy one. The number of cases of nonmelanoma skin cancer is expected to rise as long as the ozone layer in the atmosphere continues to be eroded. This is an example of how environmental policy affects public health.

Other Noncommunicable Disease Problems

Other noncommunicable diseases of major concern are (1) chronic obstructive pulmonary disease and allied conditions (the fourth leading cause of death), (2) diabetes mellitus (the seventh leading cause of death), and (3) chronic liver disease and cirrhosis (the tenth leading cause of death). Each of these chronic noncommunicable diseases and those listed in Table 2.12 place a burden not only on the afflicted individuals and their families, but also on the community's health resources.

Prevention and Control of Noncommunicable Diseases

Both individuals and their communities can contribute substantially to the prevention and control of multicausation diseases and health-related conditions. The community can provide a pro-health environment—physical, economic, and social—in which it becomes easier for individuals to achieve a high level of health.

Primary Prevention of Noncommunicable Diseases and Health-Related Conditions

Primary preventive measures for noncommunicable diseases include adequate food and energy supplies; good opportunities for education, employment, and housing; and efficient community services. Beyond this foundation, a community should provide health promotion and health education programs, especially school health education, health and medical services, and protection from environmental and occupational hazards.

Primary prevention activities by individuals should include eating properly, exercising adequately, maintaining appropriate weight, and avoiding the overuse of alcohol and other drugs. Individuals can also adopt behaviors that reduce their risk of injuries, such as driving safely, wearing a safety belt while traveling in a motor vehicle, and limiting one's exposure to the sun or environmental pollutants that might cause cancer.

Secondary Prevention of Noncommunicable Diseases and Health-Related Conditions

Secondary preventive measures for communities include providing mass screening opportunities and other case-finding measures for chronic diseases and the provision of adequate health personnel, equipment, and facilities for the community. Secondary prevention responsibilities of individual citizens include personal screenings such as self-examination of breasts or testes (for cancer of these organs), colonoscopy for colorectal cancer, the Pap test for cervical cancer, and mammography for breast cancer (see Figure 2.18), as well as screenings for diabetes, glaucoma, or hypertension. Recall that health screenings are only the first step in secondary prevention of noncommunicable, chronic diseases. They must be followed by a definitive diagnosis and prompt treatment of any diseases detected.

Tertiary Prevention of Noncommunicable Diseases and Health-Related Conditions

Tertiary preventive measures for a community include adequate emergency medical personnel, services, and facilities to meet the needs of those citizens for whom primary and secondary preventive measures were unsuccessful. Examples include ambulance services, hospitals, physicians and surgeons, nurses, and other allied health professionals. Most communities are doing a more-than-adequate job in tertiary prevention and could reallocate some resources from tertiary prevention to primary and secondary preventive measures.

Tertiary prevention for the individual often requires significant behavioral or lifestyle changes. For people in recovery from mental illness or substance dependence, tertiary prevention might include a continuation of counseling or attendance at support group meetings.

Table 2.12 Some Noncommunicable Health Conditions That Affect Americans

Allergic disorders	Endogenous depression	Multiple sclerosis
Alzheimer's disease	Epilepsy	Osteoporosis
Arthritis	Fibrocystic breast condition	Premenstrual syndrome
Cerebral palsy	Lower back pain	Sickle cell trait and sickle cell disease

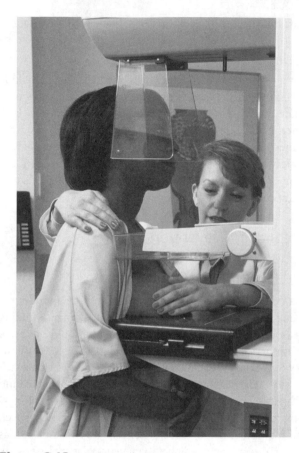

Figure 2.18 Mammography, used for screening and early detection of breast cancer, is an example of secondary prevention.
© Photodisc

Prevention and Control of a Noncommunicable Disease: CHD

One set of *Healthy People 2020* objectives aims at reducing risk factors for deaths from cardiovascular disease including coronary heart disease (refer again to Box 2.2). Modifiable risk factors that contribute to developing coronary heart disease include smoking, hypertension, and lack of exercise. Both the communities and individuals can take steps that contribute to its prevention and control.

Although individual behavioral changes hold the best prospects for reducing the prevalence of heart disease in this country, communities can provide a supporting environment for these behavioral changes. Communities can establish and enforce restricted smoking areas and can provide a clear message to youth that smoking is damaging to health. Further, communities can support healthy lifestyles by building and maintaining well-lighted sidewalks for walking, parks and recreation areas, and hiking and biking trails. Exercise reduces obesity and increases the high-density lipoproteins (HDLs) in the blood, thereby lowering risk for a heart attack. Finally, communities should promote sound nutrition throughout the life span, but particularly in schools. Insofar as these efforts forestall the initiation of harmful lifestyle choices, they can be considered primary prevention.

School systems can authorize the administration of Youth Risk Behavior Surveillance System surveys and then utilize these occasions as a springboard for discussions about the importance of healthy behavioral choices. Communities can also provide adequate opportunity for health screening for risk factors such as hypertension and serum cholesterol levels.

Chapter Summary

- Epidemiology is the study of the distribution and determinants of health-related states or events in specified populations, and the application of this study to control health problems.
- Rates of birth and death, and the incidence and prevalence of diseases and injuries are essential tools for epidemiologists.
- Notifiable diseases are those reported by doctors, clinics, medical laboratories, and hospitals to local, state, and federal health agencies.
- State and federal agencies use vital statistics and disease reports to detect trends in deaths and disease.

- Mortality rates, life expectancy, years of potential life lost (YPLL), disability-adjusted life years (DALYs), and health-adjusted life expectancy (HALE) are all measurements of the health of a community.
- Statistical data are available from the U.S. Census, the *Statistical Abstract of the United States*, the *Monthly Vital Statistics Report*, the *Morbidity and Mortality Weekly Report*, and a variety of national health surveys.
- Epidemiologists conduct descriptive and analytic studies to learn about epidemic diseases and inform public health decisions.

- There are five criteria for judging whether an association between a disease and a potential risk factor identified in epidemiological studies represents a causal relationship: (1) strength of association, (2) consistency, (3) specificity, (4) temporal correctness, and (5) biological plausibility.
- Primary prevention includes measures that forestall the onset of disease or injury, whereas secondary prevention encompasses efforts aimed at early detection and intervention to limit disease and disability. Tertiary prevention includes measures aimed at re-education and rehabilitation after significant pathogenesis has occurred.
- Diseases can be classified as communicable (infectious) or noncommunicable (noninfectious), and acute or chronic.

- The process of communicable disease transmission is best understood by the chain of infection model, in which the interruption of disease transmission can be visualized as the breaking of one or more links in the chain.
- Noncommunicable diseases are often the result of multiple risk factors that can be genetic, environmental, behavioral, and social in origin.
- The prevention and control of both communicable and noncommunicable diseases can best be accomplished by the appropriate application of primary, secondary, and tertiary preventive measures by the community and the individual.

Review Questions

1. What is an epidemic? A pandemic? Name some diseases that have caused epidemics in the past. Name some diseases that are epidemic today.
2. What do epidemiologists do?
3. What is meant by the term *endemic* disease? Give an example.
4. What is the difference between morbidity and mortality?
5. Explain why rates are important in community health.
6. What is the difference between crude and specific rates?
7. Why are prevalence rates more useful than incidence rates for measuring chronic diseases?
8. How is the infant mortality rate calculated? Why is it such an important rate in community health?
9. What are "notifiable" diseases? Give some examples.
10. Describe and explain changes in the leading causes of death in the United States between 1900 and 2010.
11. How is life expectancy calculated? What does it tell us about a population?
12. How are years of potential life lost (YPLL) calculated? What is the value of the YPLL statistic?
13. How would you define disability-adjusted life years (DALYs)? How would you define health-adjusted life expectancy (HALE)?
14. Name some sources of standardized population data and health data.

15. Describe the types of information you can obtain from each of the following: U.S. Census, *Statistical Abstract of the United States*, *Morbidity and Mortality Weekly Report*, National Center for Health Statistics.
16. List and describe five important national health surveys.
17. What types of information are gathered in a descriptive epidemiological study?
18. What is the purpose of an analytic epidemiological study? Contrast observational and experimental studies with regard to methodology and usefulness.
19. With regard to observational studies, how do case/control studies and cohort studies differ in design and in the kinds of results obtainable?
20. In experimental studies, to what principles must investigators adhere in order to properly carry out their study and assure reliable results?
21. What are Hill's criteria for judging whether an association between a risk factor and a disease can be considered causal?
22. What characteristics of a disease or health-related condition should be taken into consideration in prioritizing disease prevention and control measures?
23. Explain the difference between primary, secondary, and tertiary prevention and provide an example of each.
24. List some ways in which diseases and health problems are classified in community health. Define the

following terms and provide three examples of each: *acute disease, chronic disease, communicable disease, noncommunicable disease.*

25. What are the three components of a simplified communicable disease model?

26. What is the chain of infection model of disease transmission? Draw the model, label its parts, and indicate where in the chain prevention and control strategies could be implemented to interrupt the transmission of gonorrhea.

27. Define the following terms—*case, carrier, vector, vehicle.*

28. Explain the difference between the public health practices of isolation and quarantine.

29. Draw and explain the model for multicausation diseases.

30. Use the principles of prevention and the examples given in this chapter to outline a prevention/intervention strategy for breast cancer that includes primary, secondary, and tertiary prevention components.

Activities

1. When you hear the word *epidemic*, what disease comes to your mind first? Ask this question of 10 people you know, allowing them time to think and give you an answer. Try to find people of different ages as you complete your informal poll. List their answers on paper. Are there any answers that surprise you? Does your list include both classic and contemporary epidemic diseases?

2. Look at the data in Table 2.13. What conclusion can you draw about the risk for acquiring tuberculosis for

populations in each age group? Record your answer. Now examine Table 2.14. Which age groups exhibit the highest disease rates? Explain why it is important to calculate rates to report disease outbreaks accurately.

Table 2.13   Reported Tuberculosis Cases, by Age Group, Low Socioeconomic Area, City of Dixon, 1960

Age Group in Years	Number of Cases	Age Group in Years	Number of Cases
0-4	7	35-44	6
5-14	7	45-54	9
15-24	6	55-64	8
25-34	10	651	7

Source: Centers for Disease Control and Prevention.

Table 2.14   Reported Tuberculosis Cases and Incidence Rates per 100,000, Low Socioeconomic Area, City of Dixon, 1960

Age Group in Years	Number of Cases	Population of Age Group	Rate*
0-4	7	8,638	81.0
5-14	7	13,098	53.4
15-24	6	10,247	58.5
25-34	10	8,680	115.2
35-44	6	7,528	79.7
45-54	9	6,736	133.6
55-64	8	4,534	176.4
65+	7	4,075	171.8
Total	60	63,536	94.4

*Example: 7 cases ÷ 8,638 population × 100,000 = 81.0.
Source: Centers for Disease Control and Prevention.

Community Health on the Web

The Internet contains a wealth of information about community and public health. Increase your knowledge of some of the topics presented in this chapter by accessing the Jones & Bartlett Learning website at **go.jblearning.com/McKenzieBrief** and follow the links to complete the following Web activities.

- Epidemiology Program Office
- *Morbidity and Mortality Weekly Report*
- National Center for Health Statistics

References

1. Last, J. M., ed. (2001). *A Dictionary of Epidemiology*. New York: Oxford University Press.
2. Taubenberer, J. K., and D. M. Morens (2006). "1918 Influenza: The Mother of All Pandemics." *Emerging Infectious Diseases*, 12(1): 15-22.
3. Joint United Nations Programme on HIV/AIDS (UNAIDS) (2010). "UNAIDS Report on the Global AIDS Epidemic 2010." Available at http://www.unaids.org/globalreport/Global_report.htm.
4. Centers for Disease Control and Prevention (2012). HIV in the United States: At a Glance. Available at http://www.cdc.gov/hiv/resources/factsheets/PDF/HIV_at_a_glance.pdf.
5. Centers for Disease Control and Prevention (2011). "Lyme Disease: Lyme Disease Data." Available at http://www.cdc.gov/lyme/stats/index.html.
6. Centers for Disease Control and Prevention (2012). "2011 West Nile Virus Human Infections in the United States (Reported to CDC as of January 10, 2012)." Available at http://www.cdc.gov/ncidod/dvbid/westnile/surv&controlCaseCount11_detailed.htm.
7. Centers for Disease Control and Prevention (2010). "Update: Influenza Activity–United States, August 30, 2009-March 27, 2010, and Composition of the 2010-11 Influenza Vaccine." *Morbidity and Mortality Weekly Report*, 59(14): 423-430. Available at http://www.cdc.gov/mmwr/PDF/wk/mm5914.pdf.
8. Warner, M., L. J. Chen, D. M. Makuc, R. N. Anderson, and A. M. Miniño. (2011). *Drug Poisoning Deaths in the United States, 1980-2008*. NCHS data brief no. 81. Hyattsville, MD: National Center for Health Statistics. Available at http://www.cdc.gov/nchs/data/databriefs/db81.pdf.
9. Johnson, S. R. (2006). *The Ghost Map: The Story of London's Most Terrifying Epidemic–And How It Changed Science, Cities, and the Modern World*. New York: Riverhead Books.
10. Mausner, J. S., and S. Kramer (1985). *Mausner and Bahn Epidemiology–An Introductory Text*, 2nd ed. Philadelphia, PA: W.B. Saunders, p. 5.
11. Murphy, S. L., J. Q. Xu, and K. D. Kochanek (2012). "Deaths: Preliminary Data for 2010." *National Vital Statistics Reports*, 60(4). Hyattsville, MD: National Center for Health Statistics. Available at http://www.cdc.gov/nchs/data/nvsr/nvsr60/nvsr60_04.pdf.
12. Hamilton, B. E., J. A. Martin, and S. J. Ventura (2011). "Births: Preliminary Data for 2009." *National Vital Statistics Reports*, 60(2): 1-26. Available at http://www.cdc.gov/nchs/data/nvsr/nvsr60/nvsr60_02.pdf.
13. Centers for Disease Control and Prevention, National Center for Health Statistics (1998). "Leading Causes of Death, 1900-1998." Available at http://www.cdc.gov/nchs/data/dvs/lead1900_98.pdf.
14. Miniño, A. M., S. L. Murphy, J. Xu, and K. D. Kochaneck (2011). "Deaths 2008: Final Data." *National Vital Statistics Reports*, 59(10): 1-152.
15. National Center for Health Statistics (2011). *Health, United States, 2010: With Special Feature on Death and Dying*. Hyattsville, MD: Author. Available at http://www.cdc.gov/nchs/data/hus/hus10.pdf.
16. Murray, D. J. L., and A. D. Lopez, eds. (1996). *The Global Burden of Disease: A Comprehensive Assessment of Mortality and Disability from Diseases, Injuries and Risk Factors in 1990 and Projected to 2020. Global Burden of Disease and Injury*. Vol. 1. Cambridge, MA: Harvard School of Public Health on behalf of World Health Organization.
17. Mathers, C. C., R. Sadana, J. A. Salomon, C. J. L. Murray, and A. D. Lopez (2000). "Estimates of DALE for 191 Countries: Methods and Results." Global Programme on Evidence for Health Policy Working Paper No. 16. Geneva, Switzerland: World Health Organization. Available at http://www.who.int/healthinfo/paper16.pdf.
18. Lopez, A. S., C. D. Mathers, M. Ezzati, D. T. Jamison, and C. J. L. Murray, eds. (2006). *Global Burden of Disease and Risk Factors*. Washington, DC: World Bank and Oxford University Press.
19. Adams, P. F., M. E. Martinez, J. L. Vickerie, and W. K. Kirzinger (2011). "Summary Health Statistics for the U.S. Population: National Health Interview Survey, 2010." *Vital and Health Statistics*, 10(251): 1-117.
20. Centers for Disease Control and Prevention (2011). "National Health and Nutrition Examination Survey: About the National Health and Nutrition Examination Survey." Available at http://www.cdc.gov/nchs/nhanes/about_nhanes.htm.
21. Centers for Disease Control and Prevention (2010). "Behavioral Risk Factor Surveillance System: About the BRFSS." Available at http://www.cdc.gov/brfss/about.htm.
22. Centers for Disease Control and Prevention, Adolescent and School Health (2011). "Youth Risk Behavior Surveillance System (YRBSS)." Available at http://www.cdc.gov/HealthyYouth/yrbs/.
23. Tonnesen, P., J. Norregaard, K. Simonsen, and U. Sawe (1991). "A Double-Blind Trial of a 16-Hour Transdermal Nicotine Patch in Smoking Cessation." *New England Journal of Medicine*, 325(5): 311-315.
24. Hill, A. B. (1965). "The Environment and Disease: Association or Causation?" *Proceedings of the Royal Society of Medicine*, 58: 295-300.
25. National Center on Addiction and Substance Abuse at Columbia University (2009). *Shoveling Up II: The Impact of Substance Abuse on Federal, State and Local Budgets*. Available at http://www.casacolumbia.org/templates/Publications_Reports.aspx#rib.
26. Heymann, D. L., ed. (2008). *Control of Communicable Diseases Manual*, 19th ed. Washington, DC: American Public Health Association.
27. Centers for Disease Control and Prevention (2012). "Basic Information About HIV and AIDS." Available at http://www.cdc.gov/hiv/topics/basic/index.htm.
28. World Health Organization (2012). "HIV/AIDS: Data and Statistics. Global Summary of HIV/AIDS Epidemic, December, 2011" Available at http://www.who.int/hiv/data/en/.
29. Centers for Disease Control and Prevention (2009). "HIV in the United States: At a Glance." Available at http://www.cdc.gov/hiv/resources/factsheets/us.htm.
30. Occupational Safety and Health Administration (2009). "Bloodborne Pathogens and Needlestick Prevention: Hazard Recognition." U.S. Department of Labor. Available at http://www.osha.gov/SLTC/bloodbornepathogens/index.html.

31. U.S. Congress (2000, October 3). "An Act to Require Changes in the Bloodborne Pathogens Standard in Effect Under the Occupational Safety and Health Act of 1970." *Congressional Record*, 146.

32. American Heart Association (2010). *Heart Disease and Stroke Statistics–2010 Update: A Report of the American Heart Association*. Dallas, TX: Author. Available at http://circ.ahajournals.org/content/early/2011/12/15/CIR .0b013e31823ac046.full.pdf+html.

33. American Cancer Society (2012). *Cancer Facts and Figures–2012*. Atlanta, GA: Author. Available at http://www .cancer.org/acs/groups/content/@epidemiologysurveilance /documents/document/acspc-031941.pdf.

Chapter 3

Community Organizing/ Building and Health Promotion Programming

James F. McKenzie, PhD, MPH, MCHES

Chapter Objectives

After studying this chapter, you will be able to:

1 Define *community organizing*, *community capacity*, *community participation*, and *empowered community*.

2 Briefly explain the differences among locality development, social planning, and social action approaches to community organization.

3 Explain the difference between needs-based and strength-based community organizing models.

4 List the steps for a generalized model for community organizing/building.

5 Explain what is meant by community building.

6 Explain the difference between health education and health promotion.

7 State and summarize the steps involved in creating a health promotion program.

8 Define the term *needs assessment*.

9 Explain the difference between goals and objectives.

10 List the different types of intervention strategies.

11 Explain the differences among best practices, best experiences, and best processes.

12 Explain the purposes of pilot testing in program development.

13 State the difference between formative and summative evaluation.

Introduction

To deal with the health issues that face many communities, community health professionals must possess specific knowledge and skills. They need to be able to identify problems, develop a plan to attack each problem, gather the resources necessary to carry out that plan, implement that plan, and then evaluate the results to determine the degree of progress that has been achieved. Epidemiological methods are one essential tool of the community health professional. In this chapter, we present two other important tools: the skills to organize/build a community and to plan a health promotion program. Prior to presenting information about community organizing/building and health promotion programming, we need to introduce the concept of the social ecological approach.

Inherent in the community organizing/building and health promotion programming processes is behavior change; that is, for community organizing/building and health promotion programming efforts to be successful people must change their behavior. Some of the behaviors that need to change as part of these processes are health related and others are not. The underlying foundation of the social ecological approach is that behavior has multiple levels of influences. This approach "emphasizes the interaction between, and the interdependence of factors within and across all levels of a health problem"[1] In other words, the health behavior of individuals is shaped in part by the social context in which they live. Scholars who study and write about the levels of influence have used various labels to describe them. Commonly used labels include intrapersonal, interpersonal, institutional or organizational, community, and public policy.[2] These five levels are presented in a hierarchical order with the first level, intrapersonal, affecting a single person, and successive levels affecting greater numbers; the highest level—public policy—affects the most people. For example, to get a person to participate in a community coalition it may take someone to talk with the person (e.g., intrapersonal-level influence) about the importance of the work of the coalition, but it might also take the organization with which the person is affiliated to include the work of the coalition in its mission statement (i.e., organizational-level influence). Or, to get a person to stop smoking it may take a conversation with his or her physician (i.e., intrapersonal-level influence), a company policy (i.e., institutional- or organizational-level influence), and also a county ordinance prohibiting smoking in public places (i.e., community-level influence). Thus, a central conclusion of the social

community organizing process by which community groups are helped to identify common problems or change targets, mobilize resources, and develop and implement strategies to reach the goals

ecological approach "is that it usually takes the combination of both individual-level and environmental/policy-level interventions to achieve substantial changes in health behavior."[3]

As you read the rest of this chapter, consider the impact of the social ecological approach on both community organizing/building and health promotion programming.

Community Organizing/ Building

Community health problems can range from small and simple to large and complex. Small, simple problems that are local and involve few people can be solved with the effort of a small group of people and a minimal amount of organization. Large, complex problems that involve whole communities require significant skills and resources for their solution. For these larger problems, a considerable effort must be expended to organize the citizens of the community to work together to implement a lasting solution to their problem. For example, a trained smoking cessation facilitator could help a single person or a small group of people to stop smoking. But to reduce the smoking rates community-wide, community collaboration is needed. This more comprehensive approach to reducing smoking rates needs to bring together, in an organized and coordinated effort, the people and groups interested in the issue and the resources necessary for change. In other words, a community organization effort is needed.

"The term community organization was coined by American social workers in the late 1880s in reference to their efforts to coordinate services for newly arrived immigrants and the poor."[4] More recently, community organization has been used by a variety of professionals and refers to various methods of interventions to deal with social problems. More formally, **community organizing** has been defined as the "process by which community groups are helped to identify common problems or change targets, mobilize resources, and develop and implement strategies to reach their collective goals."[4] Community organizing is not a science, but an art of consensus building within a democratic process.[5] (See **Table 3.1** for terms associated with community organizing/building.)

The Need for Organizing Communities

In recent years, the need to organize communities seems to have increased. Advances in electronics (e.g., handheld digital devices) and communications (e.g., multifunction cell phones and the Internet), household upgrades (e.g., energy efficiency), and increased mobility (i.e., frequency of moving and ease of worldwide travel) have resulted in a loss of a sense of

Table 3.1 Terms Associated with Community Organizing/Building

Community capacity	"The characteristics of communities that affect their ability to identify, mobilize, and address social and public health problems"[6]
Empowerment	"Social action process for people to gain mastery over their lives and the lives of their communities"[7]
Participation and relevance	"Community organizing should 'start where the people are' and engage community members as equals"[4]
Social capital	"The features of social organization that facilitate coordination and cooperation for mutual benefit"[4]

community. Individuals are much more independent than ever before. The days when people knew everyone on their block are past. Today, it is not uncommon for people to never meet their neighbors. In other cases, people see or talk to their neighbors a few times each year. Because of these changes in community social structure, it now takes specific skills to organize a community to act together for the collective good.

Community Organizing Methods

There is no single, preferred method for organizing a community. In fact, a careful review reveals that several different approaches have been successful, which led Rothman and Tropman to state, "We would speak of community organization methods rather than the community organization method."[8]

The early approaches to community organization used by social workers emphasized the use of consensus and cooperation to deal with community problems.[9] However, Rothman created a typology of three primary methods of community organization.[10] Included were locality development, social planning, and social action.[8]

Although locality development, social planning, and social action methods have been the primary means by which communities have organized over the years, they do have their limitations. Maybe the greatest limitation is that they are primarily "problem-based and organizer-centered, rather than strength-based and community-centered."[11] Thus, some of the newer models are based more on collaborative empowerment and community building. However, all models—old or new—revolve around a common theme: The work and resources of many have a much better chance of solving a problem than the work and resources of a few.

Minkler and Wallerstein have done a nice job of summarizing the models, old and new, by presenting a typology that incorporates both needs- and strength-based approaches (see **Figure 3.1**).[4] Their typology is divided into four quadrants,

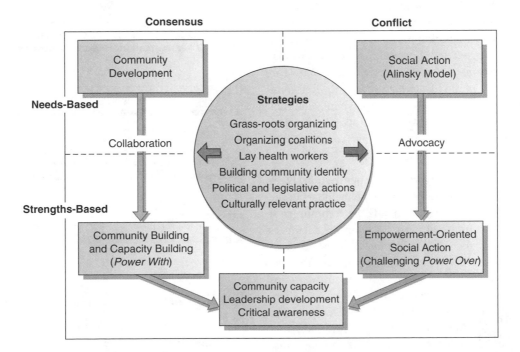

Figure 3.1 Community organization and community building typology.

with strength-based and needs-based approaches on the vertical axis and consensus and conflict on the horizontal axis.

No matter what community organizing/building approach is used, they all incorporate some fundamental principles. These include "the principle of relevance, or starting where the people are; the principle of participation; and the importance of creating environments in which individuals and communities can become empowered as they increase their community problem-solving ability."[4]

The Process of Community Organizing/Building

It is beyond the scope of this text to explain all the approaches to community organizing and building in detail. Instead, we will present a generic approach (see **Figure 3.2**) created by McKenzie, Neiger, and Thackeray that draws upon many of these other approaches.[12] The 10 steps of this generic approach are briefly reviewed in the sections that follow.

Recognizing the Issue

The process of community organizing/building begins when someone recognizes that a problem exists in a community and decides to do something about it. This person (or persons) is referred to as the initial organizer. This individual may not be the primary organizer throughout the community organizing/building process. He or she is the one who gets things started. For the purposes of this discussion, let us assume the problem is violence. People in most communities would like to have a violence-free community, but it would be most unusual to live in a community that was without at least some level of violence. How much violence is too much? At what point is a community willing to organize to deal with the problem?

The people, or organizers, who first recognize a problem in the community and decide to act can be members of the community or individuals from outside the community. If those who initiate community organization are members of the community, then the movement is referred to as being **grass-roots**, citizen initiated, or organized from the bottom up. "In grassroots organizing, community groups are built from scratch, and leadership is developed where none existed before."[13] Community members who might recognize that violence is a problem could include teachers, police officers, or other concerned citizens. When individuals

grass-roots a process that begins with those who are affected by the problem/concern

from outside of the community initiate community organization, the problem is said to be organized from the top down or outside in. Individuals from outside the community who might initiate organization could include a judge who presides over cases involving violence, a state social worker who handles cases of family violence, or a politically

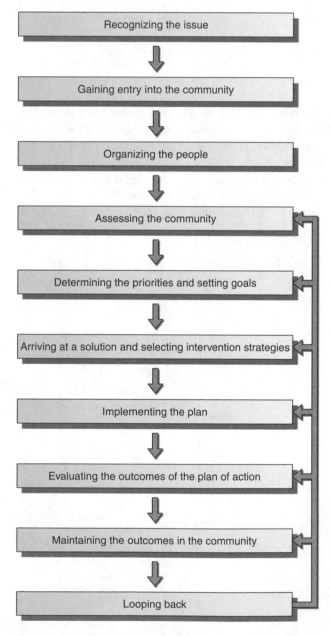

Figure 3.2 A summary of steps in community organizing and building.

McKenzie, James F., Brad L. Neiger, and Rosemary Thackeray (2013). *Planning, Implementing, and Evaluating Health Promotion Programs: A Primer,* 5th Edition. © 2009 Printed and Electronically reproduced by permission of Pearson Education, Inc., Upper Saddle River, New Jersey.

active group that is against violent behavior wherever it happens. In cases where the person who recognizes the community problem is not a community member, great care must be taken when notifying those in the community that a problem exists. "It is difficult for someone from the outside coming in and telling community members that they have problems or issues that have to be dealt with and they need to organize to take care of them."[12]

Gaining Entry into the Community

This second step in the community organizing process may or may not be needed, depending on whether the issue in step 1 was identified by someone from within the community or outside it. If the issue is identified by someone outside the community, this becomes a critical step in the process.[12]

Braithwaite and colleagues have stressed the importance of tactfully negotiating entry into a community with the individuals who control, both formally and informally, the "political climate" of the community.[14] These people are referred to as the **gatekeepers**; the term indicates that you must pass through this "gate" to get to your priority population.[15] These "power brokers" know their community, how it functions, and how to accomplish tasks within it. Long-time residents are usually able to identify the gatekeepers of their community. A gatekeeper can be a representative of an intermediary organization—such as a church or school—that has direct contact with your priority population.[15] Examples include politicians, leaders of activist groups, business and education leaders, and clergy, to name a few.

Organizers must approach such figures on the gatekeepers' own terms and play the gatekeepers' ball game. However, before approaching these important individuals, organizers must study the community well. Organizers need to know where the power lies, the community power dynamics, what type of politics must be used to solve a problem, and whether the particular problem they wish to solve has ever been dealt with before in the community.[16] In the violence example, organizers need to know (1) who is causing the violence and why, (2) how the problem has been addressed in the past, (3) who supports and who opposes the idea of addressing the problem, and (4) who could provide more insight into the problem. This is a critical step in the community organization process because failure to study the community carefully in the beginning may lead to a delay in organizing it later, a subsequent waste of time and resources, and possibly the inability to organize at all.

Once the organizers have a good understanding of the community, they are then ready to approach the gatekeepers. In keeping with the violence example, the gatekeepers would probably include the police department, elected officials, school board members, social service personnel, members of the judicial system, and possibly some of those who are creating the violence.

Organizing the People

Obtaining the support of community members to deal with the problem is the next step in the process. It is best to begin by organizing those who are already interested in seeing that the problem is solved. This core group of community members, sometimes referred to as "executive participants,"[17] will become the backbone of the workforce and will end up doing the majority of the work. For our example of community violence, the core group could include law enforcement personnel, former victims of violence and their families (or victims' support groups), parent–teacher organizations, and public health officials. It is also important to recruit people from the subpopulation that is most directly affected by the problem. For example, if most of the violence in a community is directed toward teenagers, teenagers need to be included in the core group. If elderly persons are affected, they need to be included.

"From among the core group, a leader or coordinator must be identified. If at all possible, the leader should be someone with leadership skills, good knowledge of the concern and the community, and most of all, someone from within the community. One of the early tasks of the leader will be to help build group cohesion."[12]

Although the formation of the core group is essential, this group is usually not large enough to do all the work itself. Therefore, one of the core group's tasks is to recruit more members of the community to the cause. This step can take place via a networking process, which is when organizers make personal contacts with others who might be interested. Or, the organizers can call an organizing meeting at a local school, community center, or religious organization. By broadening the constituency, the core group can spread out the workload and generate additional resources to deal with the problem. However, recruiting additional workers can often be difficult. Therefore, when organizers are expanding their constituencies, they should be sure to (1) identify people who are affected by the problem that they are trying to solve, (2) provide

gatekeepers those who control, both formally and informally, the political climate of the community

"perks" for or otherwise reward volunteers, (3) keep volunteer time short, (4) match volunteer assignments with the abilities and expertise of the volunteers, and (5) consider providing appropriate training to make sure volunteers are comfortable with their tasks. For example, if the organizers need someone to talk with law enforcement groups, it would probably be a good idea to solicit the help of someone who feels comfortable around such groups and who is respected by them, such as another law enforcement person.

When the core group has been expanded to include these other volunteers, the larger group is sometimes referred to as a task force. A **task force** has been defined as "a self-contained group of 'doers' that is not ongoing, but rather brought together due to a strong interest in an issue and for a specific purpose."[13] There may even be an occasion where a coalition is formed. A **coalition** is "a formal alliance of organizations that come together to work for a common goal"[13]—often, to compensate for deficits in power, resources, and expertise. A larger group with more resources, people, and energy has a greater chance of solving a community problem than a smaller, less powerful group. Coalitions are important to successful community organizing/building.

Assessing the Community

Earlier in this chapter we referred to Rothman and Tropman's typology for organizing a community—locality development, social planning, and social action.[8] These strategies operate "from the assumption that strategies, when appropriately matched with the situation, will rectify the challenge or problem."[18] In contrast to these strategies is community building. **Community building** is a newer and related concept that is not so much "a 'strategic framework' as an orientation to community through which people who identify as members engage together in building community capacity rather than 'fixing problems' through the application of specific and externally driven strategies."[19] Thus, one of the major differences between community organizing and community building is the type of assessment that is used to determine where to focus the community's efforts. In the community organizing approach, the assessment is focused on the needs of the community, whereas in community building

coalition formal alliance of organizations that come together to work for a common goal

community building an orientation to community through which people who identify as members engage together in building community capacity rather than 'fixing problems' through the application of specific and externally driven strategies

task force a temporary group that is brought together for dealing with a specific problem

the assessment focuses on the assets and capabilities of the community. It is assumed that a clearer picture of the community will be revealed and a stronger base will be developed for change if the assessment includes the identification of both needs and assets/capacities and involves those who live in the community. It is from these capacities and assets that communities are built.[20]

To determine the needs and assets/capacities of a community, an assessment must be completed. There are two reasons for completing an effective and comprehensive assessment: "Information is needed for change, and it is needed for empowerment."[21] This could include a traditional needs assessment and/or a newer technique called mapping community capacity. A needs assessment is a process by which data about the issues of concern are collected and analyzed. From the analyzed data, concerns or problems emerge and are prioritized so that strategies can be created to tackle them.

Traditional forms of data collection for needs assessments have included techniques such as completing written questionnaires or interviewing people in the community. Because of the importance of getting participation from community members and "starting where the people are,"[22] some organizers have used participatory data collection processes. Such processes get those from whom the data are to be collected to help with data collection. (Note: Needs assessment is discussed in greater length in the second half of this chapter, with regard to program planning.)

Mapping community capacity, on the other hand, is a process of identifying community assets, not concerns or problems. It is a process by which organizers literally use a map to identify the different assets of a community. The assets in the community then become the blocks on which other positives can be built. By knowing both the needs and assets of the community, organizers can work to identify the true concerns or problems of the community and use the assets of the community as a foundation for dealing with the concerns or problems.

Determining the Priorities and Setting Goals

An analysis of the community assessment data should result in the identification of the problems to be addressed. However, more often than not, the resources needed to solve all identified problems are not available. Therefore, the problems that have been identified must be prioritized. This prioritization is best achieved through general agreement or consensus of those who have been organized so that "ownership" can take hold. It is critical that all those working with the process feel that they "own" the problem and want to see it solved. Without this sense of ownership, they will be unwilling to give their time and energy to solve it. For example, if a few highly vocal participants intimidate people into voting for certain activities to be the top priorities before a consensus is actually reached, it is unlikely that those who disagreed on this assignment of priorities will work enthusiastically to help solve the problem. They may even drop out of the process because they feel they have no ownership in the decision-making process.

Alinsky,[23] Miller,[24] and Staples[25] (as cited in Minkler and Wallerstein[4]) have identified five criteria that community organizers need to consider when selecting a priority issue or problem. The issue or problem (1) must be winnable, ensuring that working on it does not simply reinforce fatalistic attitudes and beliefs that things cannot be improved; (2) must be simple and specific, so that any member of the organizing group can explain it clearly in a sentence or two; (3) must unite members of the organizing group and must involve them in a meaningful way in achieving resolution of the issue or problem; (4) should affect many people and build up the community; and (5) should be a part of a larger plan or strategy to enhance the community.

Once the problems have been prioritized, goals—the hoped-for results—need to be identified and written that will serve as guides for problem solving. The practice of consensus building should again be employed during the setting of goals. In the community where violence is a problem, the goal may be to reduce the number of violent crimes or eliminate them altogether. Sometimes at this point in the process, some members of the larger group drop out because they do not see their priorities or goals included on consensus lists. Unable to feel ownership, they are unwilling to expend their resources on this process. Because there is strength in numbers, efforts should be made to keep them in. One strategy for doing so is to keep the goal list as long as possible.

Arriving at a Solution and Selecting Intervention Strategies

There are alternative solutions for every community problem. The group should examine the alternatives in terms of probable outcomes, acceptability to the community, probable long- and short-term effects on the community, and the cost of resources to solve the problem.[26] A solution involves selecting one or more intervention strategies (see **Table 3.2**). Each type of intervention strategy has

Table 3.2 Intervention Strategies and Example Activities

1. *Health communication strategies:* Mass and social media, billboards, booklets, bulletin boards, flyers, direct mail, newsletters, pamphlets, posters, and video and audio materials

2. *Health education strategies:* Educational methods (such as lecture, discussion, and group work) as well as audiovisual materials, computerized instruction, laboratory exercises, and written materials (books and periodicals)

3. *Health policy/enforcement strategies:* Executive orders, laws, ordinances, policies, position statements, regulations, and formal and informal rules

4. *Environmental change strategies:* Those that are designed to change the structure of services or systems of care to improve health promotion services, such as safety belts and air bags in cars, speed bumps in parking lots, or environmental cues such as No Smoking signs

5. *Health-related community services:* The use of health risk appraisals (HRAs), community screening for health problems, and immunization clinics

6. *Other strategies:*
   a. *Behavior modification activities:* Modifying behavior to stop smoking, start to exercise, manage stress, and regulate diet
   b. *Community advocacy activities:* Mass mobilization, social action, community planning, community service development, community education, and community advocacy (such as a letter-writing campaign)
   c. *Organizational culture activities:* Activities that work to change norms and traditions
   d. *Incentives and disincentives:* Items that can either encourage or discourage people to behave a certain way, which may include money and other material items or fines
   e. *Social intervention activities:* Support groups, social activities, and social networks
   f. *Technology-delivered activities:* Educating or informing people by using technology (e.g., social media, computers and telephones)

Source: Adapted from McKenzie, J. F., B. L. Neiger, and R. Thackeray (2013). *Planning, Implementing, and Evaluating Health Promotion Programs: A Primer,* 6th ed. Boston, MA: Pearson, 205–240.

advantages and disadvantages. The group must try to agree on the best strategy and then select the most advantageous intervention activity or activities. Again, the group must work toward consensus through compromise. If the educators in the group were asked to provide a recommended strategy, they might suggest offering more preventive-education programs; law enforcement personnel might recommend more enforceable laws; judges might want more space in the jails and prisons. The protectionism of the subgroups within the larger group is often referred to as *turfism*. It is not uncommon to have turf struggles when trying to build consensus.

The Final Steps in the Community Organizing/Building Process: Implementing, Evaluating, Maintaining, and Looping Back

The last four steps in this generic approach to organizing/building a community are implementing the intervention strategy and activities that were selected in the previous step, evaluating the outcomes of the plans of action, maintaining the outcomes over time, and if necessary, going back to a previous step in the process—"looping back"—to modify or restructure the work plan to organize the community.

Implementation of the intervention strategy includes identifying and collecting the necessary resources for implementation and creating the appropriate time line for implementation. Often the resources can be found within a community, and thus horizontal relationships, the interaction of local units with one another, are needed.[27] Other times the resources must be obtained from units located outside the community; in this case, vertical relationships, those where local units interact with extra-community systems, are needed.[27] An example of this latter relationship is the interaction between a local health department and a state health department.

Evaluation of the process often involves comparing the long-term health and social outcomes of the process to the goals that were set in an earlier step. Some scholars[7] have indicated that such traditional evaluations of community organizing efforts are not easy to carry out and have some limitations. There are times when evaluations are not well planned or funded. As such they may fail to capture the shorter-term, system-level effects with which community organizing is heavily concerned, such as improvements in organizational collaboration, community involvement, capacity, and healthier public policies or environments.

Maintaining or sustaining the outcomes may be one of the most difficult steps in the entire process. It is at this point that organizers need to seriously consider the need for a long-term capacity for problem solving. Finally, through the steps

> **health education**
> any combination of planned learning experiences using evidence-based practices and/or sound theories that provide the opportunity to acquire knowledge, attitudes, and skills needed to adopt and maintain health behaviors
>
> **health promotion**
> any planned combination of educational, political, environmental, regulatory, or organizational mechanisms that support actions and conditions of living conducive to the health of individuals, groups, and communities

of implementation, evaluation, and maintenance of the outcomes, organizers may see the need to "loop back" to a previous step in the process to rethink or rework before proceeding onward in their plan.

A Special Note About Community Organizing/Building

Before we leave the processes of community organizing/building, it should be noted that regardless of the approach used, not all problems can be solved. In other cases, repeated attempts may be necessary before a solution is reached. In addition, it is important to remember that if a problem exists in a community, there are probably some people who benefit from its existence and who may work toward preventing a successful solution to the problem. Whether or not the problem is solved, the final decision facing the organized group is whether to disband the group or to reorganize in order to take on a new problem or attack the first problem from a different direction.

Health Promotion Programming

As noted earlier, being able to plan health promotion programs is an important skill for community health workers. The second half of this chapter presents the process of health promotion programming.

Basic Understanding of Program Planning

Prior to discussing the process of program planning, two relationships must be presented. These are the relationships between health education and health promotion, and program planning and community organizing/building.

Health education and *health promotion* are terms that are sometimes used interchangeably. This is incorrect because health education is only a part of health promotion. The Joint Committee on Health Education and Promotion Terminology defined the process of **health education** as "any combination of planned learning experiences using evidence based practices and/or sound theories that provide the opportunity to acquire knowledge, attitudes, and skills needed to adopt and maintain health behaviors."[28] The committee defined **health promotion** as "any planned combination of educational, political, environmental, regulatory, or organizational mechanisms that support actions and conditions of living conducive to the health of

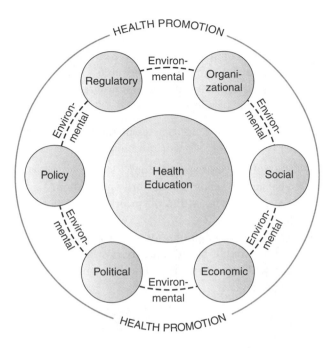

Figure 3.3 The relationship between health education and health promotion.

McKenzie, James F., Brad L. Neiger, and Rosemary Thackeray (2013). *Planning, Implementing, and Evaluating Health Promotion Programs: A Primer*, 5th Edition. © 2009 Printed and Electronically reproduced by permission of Pearson Education, Inc., Upper Saddle River, New Jersey.

individuals, groups, and communities."[28] From these definitions, it is obvious that the terms are not the same and that *health promotion* is a much more encompassing term than *health education*. **Figure 3.3** provides a graphic representation of the relationship between the terms.

The first half of this chapter described the process of community organizing/building—the process by which individuals, groups, and organizations engage in planned action to influence social problems. Program planning may or may not be associated with community organizing/building. **Program planning** is a process in which an intervention is planned to help meet the needs of a specific group of people. It may take a community organizing/building effort to be able to plan such an intervention. The antiviolence campaign used earlier in the chapter is such an example, where many resources of the community were brought together to create interventions (programs) to deal with the violence problem. However, program planning need not be connected to community organizing/building. For example, a community organizing/building effort is not needed before a company offers a smoking cessation program for its employees or a religious organization offers a stress management class for its members. In such cases, only the steps of the program planning process need to be carried out. These steps are described in the following section.

Creating a Health Promotion Program

The process of developing a health promotion program, like the process of community organizing/building, involves a series of steps. Success depends on many factors, including the assistance of a professional experienced in program planning.

Experienced program planners use models to guide their work. Planning models are the means by which structure and organization are given to the planning process. Many different planning models exist, some of which are used more often than others. Some of the more frequently used models include the PRECEDE/PROCEED model,[29] probably the best known and most often used; the Multilevel Approach to Community Health (MATCH)[30]; and the more recently developed health communication and social marketing model CDCynergy.[31] Each of these planning models has its strengths and weaknesses, and each has distinctive components that make it unique. In addition, each of the models has been used to plan health promotion programs in a variety of settings, with many successes.

It is not absolutely necessary that the student studying community health for the first time have a thorough understanding of the models mentioned here, but it is important to know the basic steps in the planning process. Therefore, we present the Generalized Model,[12] which draws on the major components of these other models (see **Figure 3.4**).

program planning
a process by which an intervention is planned to help meet the needs of a priority population

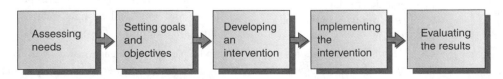

Figure 3.4 The Generalized Model.

McKenzie, James F., Brad L. Neiger, and Rosemary Thackeray (2013). *Planning, Implementing, and Evaluating Health Promotion Programs: A Primer*, 5th Edition. © 2009 Printed and Electronically reproduced by permission of Pearson Education, Inc., Upper Saddle River, New Jersey.

Prior to presenting the Generalized Model it is important to understand the community and engage the **priority population (audience)**, those whom the health promotion program is intended to serve. Understanding the community means finding out as much as possible about the priority population and the environment in which it exists. Engaging the priority population means getting those in the population involved in the early stages of the health promotion program planning process. Also, the planners should consider forming a program planning committee with representation from the various subgroups. For example, a workforce representation may come from management, labor, and clerical staff. The planning committee can help ensure that all segments of the priority population will be engaged in the planning process.

Assessing the Needs of the Priority Population

To create a useful and effective program for the priority population, planners, with the assistance of the planning committee, must determine the needs and wants of the priority population. This procedural step is referred to as a needs assessment. A **needs assessment** is the process of collecting and analyzing information to develop an understanding of the issues, resources, and constraints of the priority population, as related to the development of the health promotion program.[32] The assessment's purpose is to determine whether the needs of the people are being met.

For those interested in a detailed explanation of the process of conducting a needs assessment, extensive accounts are available.[33,34] Here is a six-step approach[12] that can be used to conduct a needs assessment:

- *Step 1: Determining the purpose and scope of the needs assessment:* What is the goal of the needs assessment and how extensive will it be?

- *Step 2: Gathering data:* What data need to be collected that will help to identify the true needs?

- *Step 3: Analyzing the data:* What problems do the data reveal? If more than one, can they be prioritized?

- *Step 4: Identifying the factors linked to the health problem:* What risk factors are linked to the prioritized problems? Can the risk factors be prioritized?

- *Step 5: Identifying the program focus:* What are the predisposing, enabling, and reinforcing factors that have a direct impact on the targeted risk factors?

- *Step 6: Validating the prioritized need:* Are you positive that the prioritized need and program focus are what should be addressed?

At the conclusion of a needs assessment, planners should be able to answer the following questions[34]:

- Who is the priority population?
- What are the needs of the priority population?
- Which subgroups within the priority population have the greatest need?
- Where are the subgroups located geographically?
- What is currently being done to resolve identified needs?
- How well have the identified needs been addressed in the past?

Setting Appropriate Goals and Objectives

Once the problem has been well defined and the needs prioritized, the planners can set goals and develop objectives for the program. The goals and objectives should be thought of as the foundation of the program and for the evaluation. The remaining portions of the programming process—intervention development, implementation, and evaluation—will be designed to achieve the goals by meeting the objectives.

The words *goals* and *objectives* are often used interchangeably, but there is really a significant difference between the two. "A goal is a future event toward which a committed endeavor is directed; objectives are the steps taken in pursuit of a goal."[35] To further distinguish between goals and objectives, McKenzie and colleagues[12] have stated that goals (1) are much more encompassing and global than objectives, (2) are written to cover all aspects of a program, (3) provide overall program direction, (4) are more general in nature, (5) usually take longer to complete, (6) do not have a deadline, (7) are usually not observed but inferred,[36] and (8) often are not measured in exact terms. Goals are easy to write and include two basic components—who will be affected and what will change because of the program. Here are some examples of program goals:

- To help employees learn how to manage their stress
- To reduce the number of teenage pregnancies in the community
- To help cardiac patients and their families deal with the lifestyle changes that occur after a heart attack

> **needs assessment** the process of collecting and analyzing information, to develop an understanding of the issues, resources, and constraints of the priority population, as related to the development of the health promotion program
>
> **priority population (audience)** those whom a program is intended to serve

Objectives are more precise and, as noted earlier, can be considered the steps to achieve the program goals. Because some program goals are more complex than others, the number and type of objectives will vary from program to program. For example, the process of getting a group of people to exercise is a more complex activity than trying to get a group to learn the four food groups. The more complex a program, the greater the number of objectives needed. Here are some example objectives:

- During a telephone interview, 35% of the residents will report having had their blood cholesterol checked in the last 6 months.
- By the end of the year, all senior citizens who requested transportation to the congregate meals will have received it.
- By the year 2015, infant mortality rates will be reduced to no more than 7 per 1,000 in Franklin County.

Close examination of the example objectives reveals that the objectives are written in specific terms. They are composed of four parts (who, what, when, and how much) and outline changes that should result from the implementation of the program.[37] As such, the objectives are written so that the level of their attainment is observable and measurable.

One final note about objectives: Selected objectives from *Healthy People 2020*, the national health goals and objectives of the nation, are presented in Box 3.1. These goals and objectives provide a good model for developing goals and objectives for a new program. In fact, these goals and objectives can be adapted for use in most community health promotion programs.

Creating an Intervention That Considers the Peculiarities of the Setting

The next step in the program planning process is to design activities that will help the priority population meet the objectives and, in the process, achieve the program goals. These activities are collectively referred to as an **intervention**, or treatment. This intervention or treatment constitutes the program that the priority population will experience.

The number of activities in an intervention may be many or only a few. Although no minimum number has been established, it has been shown that multiple activities are often more effective than a single activity. For example, if the planners wanted to change the attitudes of community members toward

> **intervention** an activity or activities designed to create change in people

---

Box 3.1   *Healthy People 2020:* Objectives

Educational and Community-Based Programs

Goal: Increase the quality, availability, and effectiveness of educational and community-based programs designed to prevent disease and injury, improve health, and enhance quality of life.

Objective: ECBP-10 Increase the number of community-based organizations (including local health departments, tribal health services, nongovernmental organizations, and state agencies) providing population-based primary prevention services in the following areas:

ECBP 10.8 Nutrition

Target: 94.7 percent.

Baseline: 86.4 percent of community-based organizations (including local health departments, tribal health services, nongovernmental organizations, and state agencies) provided population-based primary prevention services in nutrition in 2008.

Target setting method: 10 percent improvement.

Data source: National Profile of Local Health Departments, National Association of County and City Health Officials (NACCHO)

ECBP 10.9 Physical Activity

Target: 88.5 percent.

Baseline: 80.5 percent of community-based organizations (including local health departments, tribal health services, nongovernmental organizations, and state agencies) provided population-based primary prevention services in physical activity in 2008.

Target setting method: 10 percent improvement.

Data source: National Profile of Local Health Departments, National Association of County and City Health Officials (NACCHO).

Note: Other areas covered by this objective include: 10.1 Injury, 10.2 Violence, 10.3 Mental Illness, 10.4 Tobacco Use, 10.5 Substance Abuse, 10.6 Unintended Pregnancy, and 10.7 Chronic Diseases Programs.

For Further Thought

If you had the opportunity to write one more objective dealing with the implementation of health promotion programs for use in *Healthy People 2020*, what would it be? What is your rationale for selecting such an objective?

Source: Modified from U.S. Department of Health and Human Services, Office of Disease Prevention and Health Promotion (2010). *Healthy People 2020.* Available at http://www.healthypeople.gov/2020/default.aspx.

a new landfill, they would have a greater chance of doing so by distributing pamphlets door-to-door, writing articles for the local newspaper, and speaking to local service groups, than by performing any one of these activities by itself. In other words, the size and amount of intervention are important in health promotion programming. Few people change their behavior based on a single exposure; instead, multiple exposures are generally needed to change most behaviors.

Two terms that relate to the size and amount of an intervention are multiplicity and dose. **Multiplicity** refers to the number of activities that make up the intervention, and **dose** refers to the number of program units delivered. Thus, if an intervention has two activities—say, an educational workshop and a public service announcement for radio—they define multiplicity, whereas the number of times each of the activities is presented defines the dose.[12]

The actual creation of the intervention should begin by asking and answering a series of questions.[12] The first is, what needs to change? The answer to this question comes from the needs assessment and the resulting goals and objectives. The second question is, at what level of prevention (i.e., primary, secondary, or tertiary) will the program be aimed? The approach taken to a primary prevention need, that is, preventing a problem before it begins, would be different from a tertiary prevention need of managing a problem after it has existed for a while. The third question asks, at what level of influence will the intervention be focused? The various levels of influence (i.e., intrapersonal, interpersonal, institutional or organizational, community, and public policy) that were presented at the beginning of the chapter as part of the social ecological approach need to be considered. These levels provide the planners with a framework from which to think about how they will "attack" the needs of the priority population.

The fourth question asks, has an effective intervention strategy to deal with the focus of the problem already been created? There are three sources of guidance for selecting intervention strategies (see Table 3.2 for a list of strategies)—best practices, best experiences, and best processes.[29] **Best practices** refers to "recommendations for an intervention, based on critical review of multiple research and evaluation studies that substantiate the efficacy of the intervention in the populations and circumstances in which the studies were done, if not its effectiveness in other populations and situations where it might be implemented."[29] Examples of best practices related to health promotion programs are provided in *The Guide to Community Preventive Services: What Works to Promote Health*[38](see Community Health on the Web at the end of this chapter).

When best practice recommendations are not available for use, planners need to look for information on best experiences. **Best experiences** intervention strategies are those of prior or existing programs that have not gone through the critical research and evaluation studies and thus fall short of best practice criteria but nonetheless show promise in being effective. Best experiences can often be found by networking with others professionals and by reviewing the literature.

If neither best practices nor best experiences are available to planners, then the third source of guidance for selecting an intervention strategy is using best processes. **Best processes** intervention strategies are original interventions that the planners create based on their knowledge and skills of good planning processes including the involvement of those in the priority population and the theories and models used to change behaviors such as social cognitive theory[39] or the transtheoretical model.[40]

The fifth question asks, is the intervention an appropriate fit for the priority population? In other words, does the planned intervention meet the specific characteristics of the priority population such as the educational level, developmental stages, or specific cultural characteristics of the people being served?

The sixth, and final, question that needs to be asked is, are the resources available to implement the intervention selected? Planners need to evaluate the amount of money, time, personnel, and/or space that are needed to carry out the various interventions and make a determination if such resources are available to implement the intervention. Once all of these questions have been asked and answered the planners can then decide which intervention would be best for the priority population with whom they are working.

Implementing the Intervention

The moment of truth is when the intervention is implemented. **Implementation** is the actual carrying out or

best experiences intervention strategies used in prior or existing programs that have not gone through the critical research and evaluation studies and thus fall short of best practice criteria

best practices recommendations for interventions based on critical review of multiple research and evaluation studies that substantiate the efficacy of the intervention

best processes original intervention strategies that the planners create based on their knowledge and skills of good planning processes including the involvement of those in the priority population and the use of theories and models

dose the number of program units as part of the intervention

implementation putting a planned program into action

multiplicity the number of activities that make up the intervention

putting into practice the activity or activities that make up the intervention. More formally, implementation has been defined as "the act of converting planning, goals, and objectives into action through administrative structure, management activities, policies, procedures, regulations, and organizational actions of new programs."[41] It is at this point that the planners will learn whether the product (intervention) they developed will be useful in producing the measurable changes as outlined in the objectives.

To ensure a smooth-flowing implementation of the intervention, it is wise to pilot test it at least once and sometimes more. A **pilot test** is a trial run. It is when the intervention is presented to just a few individuals who are either from the intended priority population or from a very similar population. For example, if the intervention is being developed for fifth graders in a particular school, it might be pilot tested on fifth graders with similar educational backgrounds and demographic characteristics but from a different school.

The purpose of pilot testing an intervention is to determine whether there are any problems with it. Some of the more common problems that pop up are those dealing with the design or delivery of the intervention; however, any part of it could be flawed.

Once the intervention has been pilot tested and corrected as necessary, it is ready to be disseminated and implemented. If the planned program is being implemented with a large priority population and there is a lot at stake with the implementation, it is advisable that the intervention be implemented gradually rather than all at once. One way of doing so is by phasing in the intervention. **Phasing in** refers to a step-by-step implementation in which the intervention is introduced first to smaller groups instead of the entire priority population. Common criteria used for selecting participating groups for phasing in include participant ability, number of participants, program offerings, and program location.[12]

The following is an example of phasing in by location. Assume that a local health department wants to provide smoking cessation programs for all the smokers in the community (priority population). Instead of initiating one big intervention for all, planners could divide the priority population by residence location. Facilitators would begin implementation by offering the smoking cessation classes on the south side of town during the first month. During the second month, they would continue the classes on the south side and begin implementation on the west side of town. They would continue to implement this intervention until all sections of the town were included.

Evaluating the Results

The final step in the generalized planning model is the evaluation. Although evaluation is the last step in this model, it really takes place in all steps of program planning. It is very important that planning for evaluation occur during the first stages of program development, not just at the end.

Evaluation is the process in which planners determine the value or worth of the object of interest by comparing it against a **standard of acceptability**.[42] The standards of acceptability are typically the criterion of the program objectives.

Evaluation can be categorized further into summative and formative evaluation. **Formative evaluation** is done during the planning and implementing processes to improve or refine the program. For example, validating the needs assessment and pilot testing are both forms of formative evaluation. **Summative evaluation** begins with the development of goals and objectives and is conducted after implementation to determine the program's effect on the priority population. Often, the summative evaluation is broken down into two categories—impact and outcome evaluation. **Impact evaluation** focuses on immediate observable effects of a program such as changes in awareness, knowledge, attitudes, skills, environmental surroundings, and behavior of those in the priority population, whereas **outcome evaluation** focuses on the end result of the program and is generally measured by improvements in morbidity, mortality, or vital measures of symptoms, signs, or physiologic indicators.[42]

Like other steps in the planning model, the evaluation step can be broken down into smaller steps. The mini-steps of evaluation include planning the evaluation, collecting the necessary evaluative data, analyzing the data, and reporting and applying the results.

evaluation determining the value or worth of an object of interest

formative evaluation the evaluation that is conducted during the planning and implementing processes to improve or refine the program

impact evaluation focuses on the immediate observable effects of a program

outcome evaluation focuses on the end result of the program

phasing in implementation of an intervention with a series of small groups instead of the entire population

pilot test a trial run of an intervention

standard of acceptability a comparative mandate, value, norm, or group

summative evaluation the evaluation that determines the effect of a program on the priority population

Chapter Summary

- A knowledge of community organizing and program planning is essential for community health workers whose job it is to promote and protect the health of the community.
- Community organizing is the process by which community groups are helped to identify common problems or change targets, mobilize resources, and develop and implement strategies to reach the goals.
- Community building is an orientation to community that is strength-based rather than need-based and stresses the identification, nurturing, and celebration of community assets.
- The steps of the generic model for community organizing/building include recognizing the issue, gaining entry into the community, organizing the people, assessing the community, determining the priorities and setting goals, arriving at a solution and selecting the intervention strategies, implementing the plan, evaluating the outcomes of the plan of action, maintaining the outcomes in the community, and, if necessary, looping back.
- Program planning is a process in which an intervention is planned to help meet the needs of a priority population (audience).
- The steps in the program planning process include assessing the needs of the priority population, setting appropriate goals and objectives, creating an intervention that considers the peculiarities of the setting, implementing the intervention, and evaluating the results.

Review Questions

1. What is community organizing?
2. What is the difference between top-down and grass-roots community organizing?
3. What is meant by the term *gatekeepers*? Who would they be in your home community?
4. Identify the steps in the generic approach to community organizing/building presented in this chapter.
5. What is meant by community building?
6. What is a needs assessment? Why is it important in the health promotion programming process?
7. What are the five major steps in program development?
8. What are the differences between goals and objectives?
9. What are intervention strategies? Provide five examples.
10. What are best practices, best experiences, and best processes? How are they different?
11. What is meant by the term *pilot testing*? How is it useful when developing an intervention?
12. What is the difference between formative and summative evaluation? What are impact and outcome evaluation?

Activities

1. From your knowledge of the community in which you live (or from the yellow pages of the telephone book), generate a list of 7 to 10 agencies that might be interested in creating a coalition to deal with community drug problems. Provide a one-sentence rationale for why each might want to be involved.
2. Ask your instructor if he or she is aware of any community organizing/building efforts in a local community.

If you are able to identify such an effort, make an appointment—either by yourself or with some of your classmates—to meet with the person who is leading the effort and ask the following questions:

a. What is the problem that faces the community?
b. What is the goal of the group?
c. What steps have been taken so far to organize/build the community, and what steps are yet to be taken?

d. Who is active in the core group?

e. Did the group conduct a community assessment?

f. What intervention will be/has been used?

g. Is it anticipated that the problem will be solved?

3. Visit a voluntary health agency in your community, either by yourself or with classmates. Ask employees if you may review any of the standard health promotion programs the agency offers to the community. Examine the program materials, locating the five major components of program development discussed in this chapter. Then, in a two-page paper, summarize your findings.

Community Health on the Web

The Internet contains a wealth of information about community and public health. Increase your knowledge of some of the topics presented in this chapter by accessing the Jones & Bartlett Learning website at **go.jblearning .com/McKenzieBrief** and follow the links to complete the following Web activities:

- MAPP
- CDC's Healthy Communities Program
- The Guide to Community Preventive Services—The Community Guide: What Works to Promote Health

References

1. Rimer, B. K., and K. Glanz (2005). *Theory at a Glance: A Guide for Health Promotion Practice*, 2nd ed. NIH Pub. No. 05-3896. Washington, DC: National Cancer Institute.
2. McLeroy, K. R., D. Bibeau, A. Steckler, and K. Glanz (1988). "An Ecological Perspective for Health Promotion Programs." *Health Education Quarterly*, 15(4): 351-378.
3. Sallis, J. F., N. Owen, and E. B. Fisher (2008). "Ecological Models of Health Behavior." In K. Glanz, B. K. Rimer, and K. Viswanath, eds., *Health Behavior and Health Education Practice: Theory, Research, and Practice*, 4th ed. San Francisco, CA: Jossey-Bass, 465-485.
4. Minkler, M., and N. Wallerstein (2012). "Improving Health through Community Organization and Community Building: Perspectives from Health Education and Social Work." In M. Minkler, ed., *Community Organizing and Community Building for Health and Welfare*, 3rd ed. New Brunswick, NJ: Rutgers University Press, 37-58.
5. Ross, M. G. (1967). *Community Organization: Theory, Principles, and Practice*. New York: Harper and Row, 86-92.
6. Goodman, R. M., M. A. Speers, K. McLeroy, S. Fawcett, M. Kegler, E. Parker, S. R. Smith, T. D. Sterling, and N. Wallerstein (1998). "Identifying and Defining the Dimensions of Community Capacity to Provide a Basis for Measurement." *Health Education and Behavior*, 25(3): 258-278.
7. Minkler, M., N. Wallerstein, and N. Wilson (2008). "Improving Health Through Community Organizing and Community Building." In K. Glanz, B. K. Rimer, and K. Viswanath, eds., *Health Behavior and Health Education Practice: Theory, Research, and Practice*, 4th ed. San Francisco, CA: Jossey-Bass, 287-312.
8. Rothman, J., and J. E. Tropman (1987). "Models of Community Organization and Macro Practice Perspectives: Their Mixing and Phasing." In F. M. Cox, J. L. Erlich, J. Rothman, and J. E. Tropman, eds., *Strategies of Community Organization: Macro Practice*. Itasca, IL: Peacock, 3-26.
9. Garvin, C. D., and F. M. Cox (2001). "A History of Community Organizing Since the Civil War with Special Reference to Oppressed Communities." In J. Rothman, J. L. Erlich, and J. E. Tropman, eds., *Strategies of Community Intervention*, 5th ed. Itasca, IL: Peacock, 65-100.
10. Rothman, J. (2001). "Approaches to Community Intervention." In J. Rothman, J. L. Erlich, and J. E. Tropman, eds., *Strategies of Community Intervention*, 6th ed. Itasca, IL: Peacock.
11. Checkoway, B. (1989). "Community Participation for Health Promotion: Prescription for Public Policy." *Wellness Perspectives: Research, Theory, and Practice*, 6(1): 18-26.
12. McKenzie, J. F., B. L. Neiger, and R. Thackeray (2013). *Planning, Implementing, and Evaluating Health Promotion Programs: A Primer*, 6th ed. Boston, MA: Pearson.
13. Butterfoss, F. D. (2007). *Coalitions and Partnerships in Community Health*. San Francisco, CA: Jossey-Bass.
14. Braithwaite, R. L., F. Murphy, N. Lythcott, and D. S. Blumenthal (1989). "Community Organization and Development for Health Promotion Within an Urban Black Community: A Conceptual Model." *Health Education*, 20(5): 56-60.
15. Wright, P. A. (1994). *A Key Step in Developing Prevention Materials Is to Obtain Expert and Gatekeepers' Reviews* (Technical Assistance Bulletin). Bethesda, MD: Center for Substance Abuse Prevention (CSAP) Communications Team, 1-6.
16. Perlman, J. (1978). "Grassroots Participation from Neighborhood to Nation." In S. Langton, ed., *Citizen Participation in America*. Lexington, MA: Lexington Books, 65-79.
17. Brager, G., H. Specht, and J. L. Torczyner (1987). *Community Organizing*. New York: Columbia University Press, 55.
18. Walter, C. L., and C. A. Hyde (2012). "Community Building Practice: An Expanded Conceptual Framework." In M. Minkler, ed., *Community Organizing and Community Building for Health and Welfare*, 3rd ed. New Brunswick, NJ: Rutgers University Press, 78-90.

19. Minkler, M. (2012). "Introduction to Community Organizing and Community Building." In M. Minkler, ed., *Community Organizing and Community Building for Health and Welfare*, 3rd ed. New Brunswick, NJ: Rutgers University Press, 5–26.

20. McKnight, J. L., and J. P. Kretzmann (2012). "Mapping Community Capacity." In M. Minkler, ed., *Community Organizing and Community Building for Health and Welfare*, 3rd ed. New Brunswick, NJ: Rutgers University Press, 171–186.

21. Hancock, T., and M. Minkler (2012). "Community Health Assessment or Healthy Community Assessment." In M. Minkler, ed., *Community Organizing and Community Building for Health and Welfare*, 3rd ed. New Brunswick, NJ: Rutgers University Press, 153–170.

22. Nyswander, D. B. (1956). "Education for Health: Some Principles and Their Application." *Health Education Monographs*, 14: 65–70.

23. Alinsky, S. D. (1972). *Rules for Radicals: A Primer for Realistic Radicals*. New York: Random House.

24. Miller, M. (2009). *A Community Organizer's Tale: People and Power in San Francisco*. Berkley, CA: Heyday Books.

25. Staples, L. (2004). *Roots to Power: A Manual for Grassroots Organizing*, 2nd ed. Westport, CT: Praeger.

26. Archer, S. E., and R. P. Fleshman (1985). *Community Health Nursing*. Monterey, CA: Wadsworth Health Sciences.

27. Warren, R. L. (1963). *The Community in America*. Chicago: Rand-McNally.

28. Joint Committee on Health Education and Promotion Terminology (2012). *Report of the 2011 Joint Committee on Health Education and Promotion Terminology*. Reston, VA: American Association of Health Education.

29. Green, L. W., and M. W. Kreuter (2005). *Health Program Planning: An Educational and Ecological Approach*, 4th ed. Boston: McGraw-Hill.

30. Simons-Morton, D. G., W. H. Greene, and N. H. Gottlieb (1995). *Introduction to Health Education and Health Promotion*, 2nd ed. Prospect Heights, IL: Waveland Press.

31. Centers for Disease Control and Prevention, U.S. Department of Health and Human Services (2003). *CDCynergy 3.0: Your Guide to Effective Health Communication* [CD-ROM Version 3.0]. Atlanta, GA: Author.

32. Anspaugh, D. J., M. B. Dignan, and S. L. Anspaugh (2000). *Developing Health Promotion Programs*. Boston: McGraw-Hill Higher Education.

33. Gilmore, G. D. (2012). *Needs and Capacity Assessment Strategies for Health Education and Health Promotion*, 4th ed. Burlington, MA: Jones & Bartlett Learning.

34. Peterson, D. J., and G. R. Alexander (2001). *Needs Assessment in Public Health: A Practical Guide for Students and Professionals*. New York, NY: Kluwer Academic/Plenum.

35. Ross, H. S., and P. R. Mico (1980). *Theory and Practice in Health Education*. Palo Alto, CA: Mayfield, 219.

36. Jacobsen, D., P. Eggen, and D. Kauchak (1989). *Methods for Teaching: A Skills Approach*, 3rd ed. Columbus, OH: Merrill.

37. McKenzie, J. F. (2005). "Planning and Evaluating Interventions." In J. Kerr, R. Weitkunat, and M. Moretti, eds., *ABC of Behavior Change: A Guide to Successful Disease Prevention and Health Promotion*. Oxford, England: Elsevier, 41–54.

38. Centers for Disease Control and Prevention (2012). *The Guide to Community Preventive Services–The Community Guide: What Works to Promote Health*. Available at http://www.thecommunityguide.org/index.html.

39. McAlister, A. L., C. L. Perry, and G. S. Parcel (2008). "How Individuals, Environments, and Health Behaviors Interact: Social Cognitive Theory." In K. Glanz, B. K. Rimer, and K. Viswanath, eds., *Health Behavior and Health Education: Theory, Research, and Practice*, 4th ed. San Francisco, CA: Jossey-Bass, 167–188.

40. Prochaska, J. O., C. A. Redding, and K. E. Evers (2008). "The Transtheoretical Model and Stages of Change." In K. Glanz, B. K. Rimer, and K. Viswanath, eds., *Health Behavior and Health Education: Theory, Research, and Practice*, 4th ed. San Francisco, CA: Jossey-Bass, 97–121.

41. Timmreck, T. C. (1997). *Health Services Cyclopedic Dictionary*, 3rd ed. Sudbury, MA: Jones & Bartlett.

42. Green, L. W., and F. M. Lewis (1986). *Measurement and Evaluation in Health Education and Health Promotion*. Palo Alto, CA: Mayfield.

Chapter 4

The School Health Program: A Component of Community Health

James F. McKenzie, PhD, MPH, MCHES

Chapter Objectives

After studying this chapter, you will be able to:

1 Define *coordinated school health program*.

2 List the ideal members of a school health advisory council.

3 Explain why a school health program is important.

4 Identify the major foundations of a coordinated school health program.

5 Define *written school health policies* and explain their importance to the school health program.

6 List the eight components of a coordinated school health program.

7 Describe the role of the school health coordinator.

8 Identify those services offered as part of school health services and explain why schools are logical places to offer such services.

9 Explain what is meant by a *healthy school environment* and discuss the two major environments.

10 Define *school health education*.

11 Identify the eight National Health Education Standards.

12 Identify and briefly explain two issues that school health advocates face.

Introduction

The school health program is an important component of community health. Although the primary responsibility for the health of school-aged children lies with their parents/guardians, the schools have immeasurable potential for affecting the health of children, their families, and the community. As former U.S. Surgeon General David Satcher states, "The school setting is a great equalizer, providing all students and families—regardless of ethnicity, socioeconomic status or level of education—with the same access to good nutrition and physical activity. Because children also teach their parents, important lessons learned at school can help the entire family,"[1] thus improving the health of the entire community.

In this chapter, we define *coordinated school health program*, explain who is involved in school health programs, explore the reasons why school health is important, discuss the components of school health, and present some of the issues facing school health programs today.

Coordinated School Health Program Defined

A **coordinated school health program (CSHP)** has been defined as an organized set of policies, procedures, and activities designed to protect, promote, and improve the health and well-being of pre-K through grade 12 students and staff, thus improving a student's ability to learn. It includes, but is not limited to, comprehensive school health education, school health services, a healthy school environment, school counseling, psychological and social services, physical education, school nutrition services, family and community involvement in school health, and school-site health promotion for staff.[2] This definition is based on the work of Allensworth and Kolbe,[3] and is represented in **Figure 4.1**.

The school health program has great potential for affecting the health of many. An estimated 55.5 million school-aged children attend more than 132,000 schools, and there are more than 7.2 million instructional and noninstructional employees in the United States.[4] This represents about one-fifth of the entire U.S. population. "The knowledge, attitudes, behavior, and skills developed as a result of effective school health programs enable individuals to make informed

> **coordinated school health program (CSHP)** an organized set of policies, procedures, and activities designed to protect, promote, and improve the health and well-being of pre-K through grade 12 students and staff, thus improving a student's ability to learn. It includes, but is not limited to, comprehensive school health education, school health services, a healthy school environment, school counseling, psychological and social services, physical education, school nutrition services, family and community involvement in school health, and school-site health promotion for staff

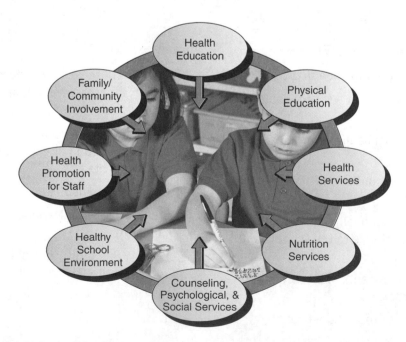

Figure 4.1 The coordinated school health program.

Division of Adolescent and School Health, Centers for Disease Control and Prevention (2008). "Coordinated School Health Program." Available at http://www.cdc.gov/healthyyouth/CSHP. Photo: © Photodisc

choices about behavior that will affect their own health throughout their lives, as well as the health of the families for which they are responsible, and the health of the communities in which they live."[5] However, in practice, the quality and quantity of CSHPs in school districts throughout the United States vary greatly. Most likely, every school has some elements of a coordinated school health program. Significant improvements would be seen if energy and resources were dedicated to coordinating these services.[6,7] For example, it is not unusual for a health teacher to talk about the importance of aerobic exercise but to never tell the physical education teacher. Similarly, a science teacher may teach about pathogens and the prevention of communicable diseases, but yet the restrooms in a school are not properly equipped for adequate hand washing. Additionally, there may be little coordination between school districts and community health agencies to improve the health of the school-aged child.

School Health Advisory Council

For CSHPs to fulfill their potential, a great deal of time and effort must be expended by those involved in the program's various components. When these individuals work together to plan and implement a school health program, they are referred to as the **school health advisory council**, or sometimes the school wellness council. The primary role of this council is to provide coordination of the various components of the CSHP to help students reach and maintain high-quality health. An ideal council would include representation from administrators, food service workers, counseling personnel, maintenance workers, medical personnel (especially a school nurse and school physician), social workers, parents and other caregivers, students, teachers (especially those who teach health, physical education, and family and consumer science classes), and personnel from appropriate community health agencies. From this group must come a leader or coordinator. This coordinator should have an educational background that includes training in school health. In addition, the coordinator should "be able to plan, implement, and evaluate a coordinated school health program; be familiar with existing community resources; and have connections to local, state, and national health and education organizations."[8,9] Most often the coordinator of the school health council is a health education specialist or school nurse.

Key Personnel

The school nurse and the classroom teachers are key to successful school health programs. As previously noted, the school nurse is one of several people who is positioned

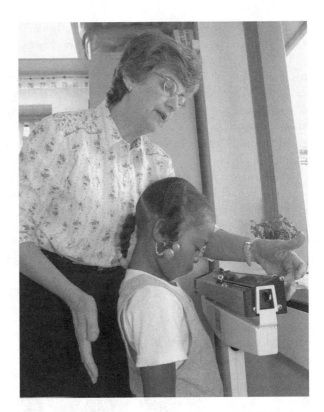

Figure 4.2 The school nurse is in a good position to guide the school health program.
© Steve Miller/AP Photos

to provide leadership for a CSHP (**Figure 4.2**). The nurse not only has medical knowledge, but also should have formal training in health education and an understanding of the health needs of all children in kindergarten through the twelfth grade.

Note that even though school nurses are in a good position to provide leadership to the school health council, many school districts do not have the resources to hire a full-time school nurse. It is not uncommon for a school district to contract with an outside health agency such as a local health department or hospital for nursing services. When this scenario occurs, it is normal for the contracted nurse to complete only the nursing tasks required by state law and not to take on the leadership responsibilities for the school health council. This task may then be fulfilled by a health education teacher. In fact, the health teacher may even be responsible when a full-time nurse is present.

school health advisory committee school, health, and community representatives who act collectively to advise the school district or school on aspects of coordinated school health

Although the school nurse might provide the leadership for a CSHP, the classroom teachers carry a heavy responsibility for seeing that the program works (see Figure 4.3). On the average school day, teachers spend more waking hours with school-aged children than do the parents of many children. A teacher may spend 6 to 8 hours a day with any given child, whereas the parents spend an hour with that child before school and maybe 4 to 5 hours with the child after school and before bedtime. Teachers are also in a position to make observations on the "normal and abnormal" behaviors and conditions of children because they are able to compare the students in their classroom each day. Furthermore, many health teachers are receiving leadership training regarding CSHPs in their undergraduate or postgraduate coursework, thus making them ideal individuals to lead the coordination.

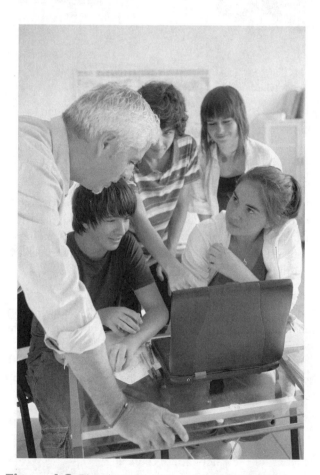

Figure 4.3 The classroom teacher's participation is essential for a successful school health program.
© auremar/ShutterStock, Inc.

The Need for School Health

The primary role of schools is to educate. However, an unhealthy child has a difficult time learning. Consider, for example, a student who arrives at school without having breakfast, with poor hygiene, and without adequate sleep. This student will be unable to concentrate on schoolwork and may distract others. As a reader, you know how difficult it is to study for a test or even to read this textbook when you do not feel well or are sleepy or hungry.

"Health and success in school are interrelated. Schools cannot achieve their primary mission of education if students and staff are not healthy and fit physically, mentally, and socially."[10] More specifically,

> [a] student who is not healthy, who suffers from an undetected vision or hearing defect, or who is hungry, or who is impaired by drugs or alcohol, is not a student who will profit from the educational process. Likewise, an individual who has not been provided assistance in the shaping of healthy attitudes, beliefs, and habits early in life, will be more likely to suffer the consequences of reduced productivity in later years.[11]

A CSHP provides the integration of education and health.

The importance of the school health program is also evident by its inclusion in the national health objectives for the year 2020. Of all the objectives listed in the publication *Healthy People 2020: Understanding and Improving Health*, a significant number can either be directly attained by schools or their attainment can be influenced in important ways by schools (see Box 4.1).

Nevertheless, a CSHP is not a cure-all. There are no quick and easy solutions to improving the overall health of a community. However, a CSHP provides a strong base on which to build.

Foundations of the School Health Program

The true foundations of any school health program are (1) a school administration that supports such an effort; (2) a well-organized school health council that is genuinely interested in providing a coordinated program for the students, families, and staff; and (3) written school health policies. A highly supportive administration is a must for a quality CSHP. In almost all organizations—and schools are no different—the administration controls resources. Without leadership and support from top school

---

Box 4.1 *Healthy People 2020:* Objectives

Educational and Community-Based Programs

Goal: Increase the quality, availability, and effectiveness of educational and community-based programs designed to prevent disease and injury, improve health, and enhance quality of life.

Objective: ECBP-2. Increase the proportion of elementary, middle, and senior high schools that provide comprehensive school health education to prevent health problems in the following areas: unintentional injury; violence; suicide; tobacco use and addiction; alcohol or other drug use; unintended pregnancy, HIV/AIDS, and STD infection; unhealthy dietary patterns; and inadequate physical activity.

ECBP 2.2 Unintentional Injury

Target: 89.9 percent.

Baseline: 81.7 percent of elementary, middle, and senior high schools provided comprehensive school health education to prevent unintentional injury in 2006.

Target setting method: 10 percent improvement.

Data source: School Health Policies and Programs Study (SHPPS), CDC, NCCDPHP.

ECBP 2.6 Alcohol and Other Drug Use

Target: 90.0 percent.

Baseline: 81.8 percent of elementary, middle, and senior high schools provided comprehensive school health education to prevent alcohol and other drug use in 2006.

Target setting method: 10 percent improvement.

Data source: School Health Policies and Programs Study (SHPPS), CDC, NCCDPHP.

ECBP 2.8 Unhealthy Dietary Patterns

Target: 92.7 percent.

Baseline: 84.3 percent of elementary, middle, and senior high schools provided comprehensive school health education to prevent unhealthy dietary patterns in 2006.

Target setting method: 10 percent improvement.

Data source: School Health Policies and Programs Study (SHPPS), CDC, NCCDPHP.

Note: Other areas covered by this objective include: 2.1 All Priority Areas; 2.3 Violence; 2.4 Suicide; 2.5 Tobacco Use and Addiction; 2.7 Unintended Pregnancy; HIV/AIDS, and STD Infection; and 2.9 Inadequate Physical Activity.

For Further Thought

Assuming money is available, why doesn't every school district in the nation have a coordinated school health program?

Source: U.S. Department of Health and Human Services, Office of Disease Prevention and Health Promotion (2010). *Healthy People 2020.* Available at http://www.healthypeople.gov/2020/default.aspx.

---

administrators, it will be an ongoing struggle to provide a quality program. Furthermore, every effort should be made to employ personnel who are appropriately trained to carry out their responsibilities as members of the school health council. For example, the National Association of School Nurses has taken the position that "every school-aged child deserves a school nurse who is a graduate of a baccalaureate degree program from an accredited college or university and licensed by that state as a registered nurse,"[12] yet many school nurses without college degrees and training in health education are asked to provide health education. Conversely, certified teachers who lack preparation in school health are required to teach health to secure a job.[13] Qualified personnel are a must.

School Health Policies

School health policies, which include "laws, mandates, regulations, standards, resolutions, and guidelines—provide a foundation for school district practices and procedures."[14] The written policies also describe the nature of the program and the procedure for its implementation to those outside the program.[15] Sound school health policies:

- Inform, support, and direct individuals throughout the school system
- Reassure families, students, and school staff that safety and health protection measures are in place
- Provide legal protection for schools
- Help contain or prevent controversy[14]

Sound school health policies are not easy to create and take much time and effort. Steps for creating local health-related policies include the following[16,17]:

1. Identify the policy development team.
2. Assess the district's needs.
3. Prioritize needs and develop an action plan.
4. Draft a policy.
5. Build awareness and support.
6. Adopt and implement the policy.
7. Maintain, measure, and evaluate.

The development of a set of written policies is not an easy task. This challenging and time-consuming task should be executed by the school health advisory council because the council includes those most knowledgeable about the school health program in addition to

school health policies written statements that describe the nature and procedures of a school health program representing many different constituencies in the school community.

Monitoring the Status of School Health Policy in the United States

Because school health policy is an important foundation for CSHPs, the Division of Adolescent Health at the Centers for Disease Control and Prevention (CDC) conducts a national survey to assess school health policies and practices at the state, district, school, and classroom levels. The survey, which is titled the School Health Policies and Practices Study (SHPPS), has been conducted every 6 years since 1994. Specifically, SHPPS is used to do the following[18]:

- Describe characteristics of each component of school health at various levels and across elementary, middle, and high schools.
- Describe the professional background of the personnel who deliver each component of the school health program.
- Describe collaboration among components of school health programs.
- Describe how key policies and practices have changed over time.

Results of these national surveys are available at the Division of Adolescent and School Health's website.

Components of a Coordinated School Health Program

If implemented appropriately, a coordinated approach to school health can have a significant positive impact on the overall health status of students, staff, and the community, which, in turn, can be linked to higher academic achievement for students. To do so, all eight components illustrated in Figure 4.1 need to be provided in a coordinated fashion. Because of the limitation of space, we discuss the importance of the administration and organization of the eight components, provide an overview of the three traditional components of the school health program—(1) school health services, (2) healthy school environment, and (3) health education—and provide a brief explanation of the five additional components.

school health coordinator a professional at the district (or school) level responsible for management and coordination of all school health policies, activities, and resources

school health services health services provided by school health workers to appraise, protect, and promote the health of students

Administration and Organization

Effective administration and organization of the school health program ensure that the people and activities that constitute the program work in a coordinated manner to meet the program's goals. As previously noted, the responsibility for coordinating the program in each school district should be delegated to a properly trained and knowledgeable individual. Logical choices for this position of **school health coordinator** are a trained school nurse or a health education specialist.[6] Whereas nearly two-thirds of school districts in the United States employ school health coordinators, there are only a few states that require such a person.[18,19]

The following are responsibilities common to school health coordinators[20]:

- Ensuring that the instruction and services provided through various components of the school health program are mutually reinforcing and present consistent messages
- Facilitating collaboration among school health program personnel and between them and other school staff
- Assisting the superintendent/school principal and other administrative staff with the integration, management, and supervision of the school health program
- Providing or arranging for necessary technical assistance
- Identifying necessary resources
- Facilitating collaboration between the district/school and other agencies and organizations in the community that have an interest in the health and well-being of children and their families
- Conducting evaluation activities that assess the implementation and results of the school health program, as well as assisting with reporting evaluation results

School Health Services

School health services are those health "services provided for students to appraise, protect, and promote health."[21] Specifically, those services offered by schools include health appraisals (screenings and examinations), emergency care for injury and sudden illness, management of chronic disease, prevention and control of communicable disease, provisions for special needs students, health counseling, and remediation of detected health problems within the limits of state laws through referral and follow-up by the school nurse and teachers (see **Figure 4.4**). Originally, the intent of school health services was to supplement rather than to supplant the family's responsibility for meeting the health-care needs of its children. However, because of the poorer health status of youth, the involvement of youth in high-risk behaviors (such as smoking, drinking, substance abuse, and unprotected sexual intercourse), and such barriers to health care as inadequate health insurance and lack of providers, there has been a broadening of the role of schools in providing health care.

Because school attendance is required throughout the United States, schools represent our best opportunity to reach many of those children in need of proper health care. More than 95% of all youths ages 5 to 17 years are enrolled in schools.[22] "The school's ability to reach children and youth slipping through the cracks of the healthcare system and at highest risk for poor health and potentially health-threatening behaviors is unmatched."[23]

The American Academy of Pediatrics (AAP) recommends that at minimum schools should provide the following three types of services: (1) state-mandated services, including health screenings, verification of immunization status, and infectious disease reporting; (2) assessment of minor health complaints, medication administration, and care for students with special needs; and (3) management of emergencies and other urgent situations.[24] When resources permit, more comprehensive services may be offered, such as administration of immunizations, case management, wellness promotion, and patient education.[24]

Expanded services are increasingly being offered through school-based, mobile, and school-linked programs. School-based health centers (SBHCs) have been defined as "a health center located in a school or on school grounds that provides, at a minimum, on-site primary and preventive health care, mental health counseling, health promotion, referral and follow-up services for young people enrolled."[25] Mobile programs are those "without a fixed site that rotate a health care team through a number of schools."[26] School-linked health centers (SLHCs) are typically coordinated at the school but delivered off campus through collaborations with community clinics, hospitals, or other healthcare professionals and agencies.[27] A number of healthcare professionals are employed on a full-time basis for these programs to function successfully. The idea of young people receiving more comprehensive health care within the context of the school setting is gaining momentum throughout the country.

Healthy School Environment

The term *healthy school environment* designates the part of a CSHP that provides for a safe—both physically and emotionally—learning environment (see **Figure 4.5**). If children are not placed in a safe environment, learning becomes difficult at best. The most comprehensive definition of **healthy school environment** was provided by the 1972–1973 Joint Committee on Health Education Terminology.

> **healthy school environment**
> the promotion, maintenance, and utilization of safe and wholesome surroundings in a school

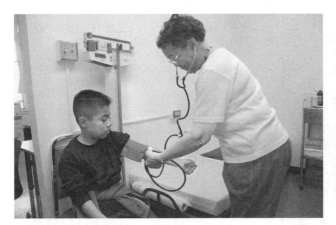

Figure 4.4 Health screenings are important components of school health services.
© Bill Aron/PhotoEdit, Inc.

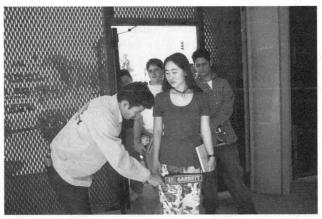

Figure 4.5 The school should be a safe and healthy place to learn.
© Michael Newman/PhotoEdit, Inc.

It stated that providing a healthy school environment includes "the promotion, maintenance, and utilization of safe and wholesome surroundings, organization of day-by-day experiences and planned learning procedures to influence favorable emotional, physical and social health."[28] The CDC, although brief, expands the definition to include school culture, defining the healthy school environment as "the physical and aesthetic surroundings and the psychosocial climate and culture of the school."[21]

By law, school districts are required to provide a safe school environment. However, the responsibility for maintaining this safe environment should rest with all who use it. Everyone, including those on the board of education, administrators, teachers, custodial staff, and students, must contribute to make a school a safer place through their daily actions. An unsafe school environment can exist only if those responsible for it and those who use it allow it to exist.

Implementing a school crisis plan can assist with addressing situations that affect the school environment. A clear, written plan that includes procedures for handling various emergencies (e.g., fire, tornado, death of a student or staff member, mass illness, person with a gun, terrorism, suicide attempt), communication procedures, staff training, practice drills, and coordination with local public safety agencies, among other procedures, can help ensure that safe practices are implemented when threats occur.[18,29]

School Health Education

School health education provides students with a "planned, sequential, K–12 curriculum that addresses the physical, mental, emotional and social dimensions of health. The curriculum is designed to motivate and assist students to maintain and improve their health, prevent disease, and reduce health-related risk behaviors."[21] If designed properly, school health education could be one of the most effective means to reduce serious health problems in the United States.

School health education includes all health education in the school. It includes health education that takes place in the classroom as well as any other activities designed to positively influence the health knowledge and skills of students, parents, and school staff. For example, health education can take place when the school nurse gives a vision-screening test

curriculum a written plan for instruction
school health education the development, delivery, and evaluation of a planned curriculum, kindergarten through grade 12
scope part of the curriculum that outlines what will be taught
sequence part of the curriculum that states in what order the content will be taught

to a student or when coaches talk with their teams about good nutrition.

For health education to be effective, it should be well conceived and carefully planned. The written plan for school health education is referred to as the health **curriculum**. The curriculum not only outlines the **scope** (what will be taught) and the **sequence** (when it will be taught), but also provides (1) learning objectives, (2) standards (see Box 4.2), (3) learning activities, (4) possible instructional resources, and (5) methods for assessment to determine the extent to which the objectives and standards are met. If health instruction is to be effective, the health curriculum should include lessons of appropriate scope and sequence for all grades from kindergarten through the twelfth grade.

As with the CSHP, results from CDC's School Health Policies and Practices Study (SHPPS) show that good school health instruction is not widespread. To enhance the state of health instruction in schools, the National Health Education Standards[30] have been developed. The National Health Education Standards delineate the essential knowledge and skills that every student should know and be able to do following the completion of quality school health education. The standards are not a federal

---

Box 4.2   National Health Education Standards

1. Students will comprehend concepts related to health promotion and disease prevention to enhance health.
2. Students will analyze the influence of family, peers, culture, media, technology, and other factors on health behaviors.
3. Students will demonstrate the ability to access valid information and products and services to enhance health.
4. Students will demonstrate the ability to use interpersonal communication skills to enhance health and avoid or reduce health risks.
5. Students will demonstrate the ability to use decision-making skills to enhance health.
6. Students will demonstrate the ability to use goal setting to enhance health.
7. Students will demonstrate the ability to practice health-enhancing behaviors to avoid or reduce health risks.
8. Students will demonstrate the ability to advocate for personal, family, and community health.

Source: Reprinted, with permission, from the American Cancer Society. (2007). *National Health Education Standards: Achieving Excellence,* 2nd ed. Atlanta, GA: American Cancer Society, 2007. http://www.cancer.org/bookstore.

mandate or national curriculum, but rather provide a foundation for curriculum development, instructional delivery, and assessment of student knowledge and skills for students in grades pre-K–12.[30] There are eight standards (see Box 4.2), and each standard has grade-level performance indicators set for grades pre-K–2, 3–5, 6–8, and 9–12. "The standards evolved from the health education profession's current thinking about what constitutes grade-appropriate and challenging content and performance expectations for students."[31] Currently, 72% of states mandating standards-based health education have used the National Health Education Standards as their basis for requirements and recommendations[18] (see Box 4.3).

Counseling, Psychological, and Social Services

Counseling, psychological, and social services are services provided to improve students' mental, emotional, and social health. These services can include individual and group assessments, interventions, and referrals. Professionals such as certified school counselors, psychologists, and social workers provide these services.[21]

Physical Education

Physical education is defined as a "planned, sequential K–12 curriculum that provides cognitive content and learning experiences in a variety of activity areas."[21] Emphasis is placed on physical fitness and skill development that lead to lifelong physical activity. Physical education should be taught by qualified teachers.[21]

School Nutrition Services

School nutrition services should provide access to a variety of nutritious and appealing meals that accommodate the health and nutrition needs of all students in a school district. Additionally, the school nutrition services program should offer students a learning laboratory for classroom nutrition and health education. The program should also serve as a resource for links with nutrition-related community services.[21]

Family/Community Involvement for School Health

Family/community involvement allows for an "integrated school, parent, and community approach for enhancing the health and well-being of students."[21] The school is an agency within a community that cannot function in isolation. Schools that actively engage parents and community resources in their school health councils, curriculum committees, and other health-related programming respond more effectively to the health-related needs of students.[21]

Box 4.3   Barriers to School Health Education

Although the importance of school health education is being recognized more and more, there are several barriers to its implementation. Research by various authors has informed health education specialists of barriers to establishing effective health instruction. Those barriers include the following:

1. Lack of local administrative commitment
2. Lack of adequately prepared teachers
3. Lack of time in the school day/year
4. Lack of money/funds
5. Health education's lack of credibility as an academic subject
6. Lack of community/parental support for controversial topics
7. Policy constraints
8. Teacher priorities
9. Pressure to focus on subjects included in high-stakes tests
10. General lack of reinforcement by state and local education policymakers

The top three barriers tend to be seen as the most significant. Recommendations to address them include the following:

1. Inviting administrators to workshops and conferences dealing with current health issues
2. Conducting quality in-service programs
3. Advocacy to school administrators and professors of education

Sources: Bender, S. J., J. J. Neutens, S. Skonie-Hardin, and W. D. Sorochan (1997). *Teaching Health Science: Elementary and Middle School*, 4th ed. Sudbury, MA: Jones & Bartlett, 32; Butler, S. C. (1993). "Chief State School Officers Rank Barriers to Implementing Comprehensive School Health Education." *Journal of School Health*, 63(3): 130–132; Telljohann, S. K., C. W. Symons, B. Pateman, and D. M. Seabert (2012). *Health Education: Elementary and Middle School Applications*, 7th ed. New York, NY: McGraw-Hill; Thackeray, R., B. L. Neiger, H. Bartle, S. C. Hill, and M. D. Barnes (2002). "Elementary School Teachers' Perspectives on Health Instruction: Implications for Health Education." *American Journal of Health Education*, 33(2): 77–82; and Sy, A., and K. Glanz (2008). "Factors Influencing Teachers' Implementation of an Innovative Tobacco Prevention Curriculum for Multiethnic Youth: Project SPLASH." *Journal of School Health*, 78(5): 264–273.

School-Site Health Promotion for Staff

School-site health promotion for staff includes "opportunities for school staff to improve their health status" through health-related assessments and activities.[21] These opportunities encourage staff to engage in healthy behaviors, resulting in improved health status, improved morale, positive health role modeling, reduced health insurance costs, and decreased absenteeism.[21]

Issues and Concerns Facing the School Health Program

Like most other community health programs, the school health program is not without its issues and concerns. "In the 1940s, the three leading school discipline problems were talking, chewing gum, and making noise."[32] Today, many of the leading school discipline problems are related to health, such as bullying and the consequences of low self-esteem. In the remainder of this chapter, we summarize two of the challenges that still lie ahead for those who work in school health—lack of support for coordinated school health and violence in the schools.

Lack of Support for Coordinated School Health Programs

"Schools offer the most systematic and efficient means available to improve the health of youth and enable young people to avoid health risks,"[33] yet, ironically, school health advocates have had limited success in getting a CSHP implemented in school districts across the country.

We have already pointed out that healthy children are better learners and that a CSHP can contribute to the health of children. A CSHP "can provide a safe haven for teaching and learning by addressing the immediate needs of the whole child. In the long term, it can have a significant effect on youth development and academic achievement."[8]

Although many Americans support the idea that everyone is entitled to good health, we have not supported through legislation the notion that everyone is entitled to a CSHP. Obviously, getting legislation passed is a complicated process and is dependent on a number of different circumstances, including, but not limited to, economics, social action, and politics. Additionally, limited resources, lack of buy-in and investment, the inability of schools to demonstrate competence and effectiveness to stakeholders, lack of organizational capacity, leadership support, and continued emphasis on high-stakes testing have made it difficult for

school districts to make a CSHP a priority.[34,35] This difficult task should not deter those who feel coordinated school health is vital. It is becoming clearer that many of the answers to current and future health problems lie with the resources found in the school—the one institution of society through which all of us must pass. The following are a few examples of the impact coordinated school health can have:

- At the present time, the key to dealing with the AIDS problem is education.
- The biggest stride in improving the health of the country will not come from new technology, but from the health behavior in which we engage.
- Many of the primary healthcare services needed by the children of this country are not available because of the barriers of the healthcare system.[36]
- Effective school-based prevention programs have been estimated to save society $18 per $1 invested. "If effective prevention programs were implemented nationwide, substance abuse initiation would decline for 1.5 million youth and be delayed for 2 years on average."[37]

The need for coordinated school health should be obvious to all. We have taken the liberty to rephrase a quote from a group of school health experts who say it best: Society should not be as concerned with what happens when we implement a CSHP as about what is likely to happen if we do not.[38] Although garnering support for CSHPs has been an uphill battle, we are moving in the right direction. With the passing of the Child Nutrition and WIC Reauthorization Act of 2004,[39] school districts are now required to institute local wellness policies promoting better nutrition, physical activity, and wellness. Some states have taken this one step further by passing state legislation requiring districts to institute coordinated school health advisory councils.[40] The inclusion of "coordinated school health" in the title of these councils encourages many districts to begin talking about, developing, and/or implementing a CSHP.

Violence in Schools

Our nation's schools should be safe havens for teaching and learning, free of crime and violence.[41] But more recently, there have been a number of high-profile incidents of violence in schools (e.g., Newtown, Connecticut; Paducah, Kentucky; Pearl, Missouri; Moses Lake, Washington; Springfield, Oregon; Littleton, Colorado; and San Diego, California) that have made the general public more aware of the violence in schools. "Any instance of crime or violence at school not only affects the individuals involved, but also may disrupt the educational process and affect bystanders, the school itself, and the surrounding community."[42] CDC Youth Risk Behavior data indicate that 5.9% of U.S. high school students had missed at least one day of school in the preceding month because that student felt unsafe either being at school or going to and from school; 7.4% had been threatened or injured with a weapon on school property during the preceding year; and 12% had been in a physical fight on school property.[43]

We know that males are involved in more violent acts than are females.[43] We also know that certain racial and ethnic groups participate and are victims of violence at school more often than other students are.[43] Yet, it is close to impossible to predict who will be next to commit a violent act in a school.

Another form of violence that has received significant attention recently is bullying. Bullying can be defined as "unwanted, aggressive behavior among school aged children that involves a real or perceived power imbalance. The behavior is repeated, or has the potential to be repeated, over time. Bullying includes actions such as making threats, spreading rumors, attacking someone physically or verbally, and excluding someone from a group on purpose."[41] In 2011, 20% of students in grades 9–12 experienced bullying.[43] Being bullied can affect academic achievement and self-esteem. Bullying can also affect bystanders by creating a climate of fear and disrespect in schools. Furthermore, bullying behavior can be a sign of other serious antisocial or violent behavior by those who bully their peers.[44]

With the technologic advances of late, concern has increased about the connection between electronic media and youth violence. Electronic aggression, which has been defined as "any kind of aggression perpetrated through technology—any type of harassment or bullying that occurs through email, a chat room, instant messaging, a Web site (including blogs), or text messaging,"[45] is a recent phenomenon among youth. Because electronic aggression is fairly new, limited information is available. However, 9% to 35% of young people say they have been a victim of electronic aggression. Some evidence suggests that electronic aggression may peak around the end of middle school/beginning of high school.[45] Instant messaging appears to be the most common way electronic aggression is perpetrated, and it is most often experienced between a victim and perpetrator who know each other. Whether electronic aggression occurs at home or at school, it has implications for school. "Young people who were harassed on-line were more likely to get a detention or be suspended, to skip school, and to

experience emotional distress than those who were not harassed."[45] This behavior also influences students' sense of safety at school.[45]

Like most other health problems, risk factors need to be identified and steps taken to reduce the risk of violent acts occurring in the schools.

> Generally, children who are bullied have one or more of the following risk factors: Are perceived as different from their peers, such as being overweight or underweight, wearing glasses or different clothing, being new to a school, or being unable to afford what kids consider 'cool;' are perceived as weak or unable to defend themselves; are depressed, anxious, or have low self esteem; are less popular than others and have few friends; and/or do not get along well with others, seen as annoying or provoking, or antagonize others for attention. However, even if a child has these risk factors, it doesn't mean that they will be bullied.[46]

Many schools have taken steps to try to reduce the chances for violence, yet many more have stated that violence is not a problem at "our school." These are the schools that are most vulnerable to such a problem. The CDC makes the following recommendations for educators and educational policymakers for improving the school climate as it relates to violence, bullying, and electronic aggression[45]:

- Explore current bullying prevention policies. Determine if they need to be modified to reflect electronic aggression.
- Work collaboratively to develop policies. States, school districts, and boards of education must work in conjunction with other stakeholders to meet the needs of the state or district and those it serves.
- Explore current programs to prevent bullying and youth violence. A number of evidence-based programs exist.
- Offer training on electronic aggression for educators and administrators.
- Talk to teens. Provide opportunities for students to discuss their concerns.
- Work with technology staff. Ensure that all involved are aware and working on strategies for minimizing risk.
- Create a positive school atmosphere. Students who feel connected to their school are less likely to perpetrate any type of violence or aggression.
- Have a plan in place for what should happen if an incident is brought to the attention of school officials.

With the new phenomenon of electronic aggression, it becomes clear that violence is not a problem that will go away soon. Many school personnel do not believe it is a problem in their schools. As life has shown us, it can happen anywhere. Violence is an issue that all schools need to face and something for which they need to plan to reduce the risks to schoolchildren and personnel. "We send our children out into the world every day to explore and learn, and we hope that they will approach a trusted adult if they encounter a challenge; now, we need to apply this message to the virtual world."[45]

Chapter Summary

- The potential impact of a coordinated school health program on the health of children, their families, and the community is great because the school is the one institution through which most pass.
- To date, the full potential of school health has not been reached because of lack of support and interest.
- If implemented properly, coordinated school health programs can improve access to health services, educate students about pressing health issues, and provide a safe and healthy environment in which students can learn and grow.
- The foundations of the school health program include (1) a school administration that supports such an effort, (2) a well-organized school health council that is genuinely interested in providing a coordinated program for the students, and (3) written school health policies.
- School health policies are critical for ensuring accountability, credibility, and the institutionalization of programs and efforts to make schools a healthy learning environment.

- The components of a coordinated school health program include (1) school health services; (2) a healthy school environment; (3) school health education; (4) counseling, psychological, and social services; (5) physical education; (6) school nutrition services; (7) family/community involvement for school health; and (8) school-site health promotion for staff.
- The eight National Health Education Standards emphasize a skills-based curriculum focusing on the following: (1) core concepts; (2) analyzing influences; (3) accessing valid health information, products, and services; (4) demonstrating interpersonal communication skills; (5) utilizing decision-making skills; (6) utilizing goal-setting skills; (7) practicing health-enhancing behaviors; and (8) advocating for personal, family, and community health.
- A number of issues face school health advocates, including a lack of support for coordinated school health and violence in schools.

Review Questions

1. What is meant by the term *coordinated school health program*?
2. Which individuals (name by position) should be considered for inclusion on the school health advisory council?
3. What foundations are needed to ensure a coordinated school health program? Why?
4. Why are written school health policies needed?
5. What are the eight components of a coordinated school health program?

6. The American Academy of Pediatrics recommends that at minimum schools should provide three types of services. What are the three types of services?
7. Explain the importance of using a standards-based health curriculum.
8. State two issues facing school health advocates and explain why they are issues.

Activities

1. Make arrangements to observe an elementary classroom in your town for a half day. While observing, keep a chart of all the activities that take place in the classroom that relate to a coordinated school health program. Select one activity from your list and write a one-page paper describing the activity, why it was health related, how the teacher handled it, and what could have been done differently to improve the situation.

2. Visit a voluntary health agency in your community and ask the employees to describe the organization's philosophy on health education. Inquire if their health education materials are available for use in a school health program. Summarize your visit with a one-page reaction paper.

3. Make an appointment to interview either a school nurse or a school health coordinator. During your interview, ask the person to provide an overview of what his or her school offers in the way of a coordinated school health program. Ask specifically about the eight components of the school health program and the issues of controversy presented in this chapter. Summarize your visit with a two-page written paper.

Community Health on the Web

The Internet contains a wealth of information about community and public health. Increase your knowledge of some of the topics presented in this chapter by accessing the Jones & Bartlett Learning website at **go.jblearning. com/McKenzieBrief** and follow the links to complete the following Web activities:

- American School Health Association
- Action for Healthy Kids
- Division of Adolescent and School Health

References

1. Satcher, D. (2005). "Healthy and Ready to Learn." *Educational Leadership*, 63(1): 26-30.
2. Joint Committee on Health Education and Promotion Terminology (2012). *Report of the 2011 Joint Committee on Health Education and Promotion Terminology*. Reston, VA: American Association of Health Education.
3. Allensworth, D. D., and L. J. Kolbe (1987). "The Comprehensive School Health Program: Exploring an Expanded Concept." *Journal of School Health*, 57(10): 409-412.
4. U.S. Census Bureau (2011). "Back to School: 2011-2012." In *U.S. Census Bureau News: Facts for Features*. Washington, DC: U.S. Department of Commerce. Available at http://www.census .gov/newsroom/releases/archives/facts_for_features_ special_editions/cb11-ff15.html.
5. McGinnis, J. M., and C. DeGraw (1991). "Healthy Schools 2000: Creating Partnerships for the Decade." *Journal of School Health*, 61(7): 292-296.
6. American Cancer Society (2012). *School Health Programs Elements of Excellence: Helping Children to Grow Up Healthy and Able to Learn*. Available at http://www.cancer.org/acs /groups/content/@nho/documents/document /elementsofexcellencepdf.pdf.
7. Fetro, J. V., C. Givens, and K. Carroll (2010). "Coordinated School Health: Getting It All Together." *Educational Leadership*, 67(4): 32-37.
8. Fetro, J. V. (1998). "Implementing Coordinated School Health Programs in Local Schools." In E. Marx, S. F. Wooley, and D. Northrop, eds., *Health Is Academic: A Guide to Coordinated School Health Programs*. New York, NY: Teachers College Press, 15-42.
9. Ottoson, J., G. Streib, J. Thomas, M. Rivera, and B. Stevenson (2004). "Evaluation of the National School Health Coordinator Leadership Institute." *Journal of School Health*, 74(5): 170-176.
10. National Association of State Boards of Education (2000). *Fit, Healthy, and Ready to Learn: Part 1: Physical Activity, Healthy Eating, and Tobacco-Use Prevention*. Alexandria, VA: Author.
11. McGinnis, J. M. (1981). "Health Problems of Children and Youth: A Challenge for Schools." *Health Education Quarterly*, 8(1): 11-14.
12. National Association of School Nurses (2012). "Position Statement: Education, Licensure, and Certification of School Nurses." Available at http://www.nasn.org /PolicyAdvocacy/PositionPapersandReports /NASNPositionStatementsFullView/tabid/462/ArticleId/26

/Education-Licensure-and-Certification-of-School-Nurses-Revised-January-2012.

13. Kann, L., S. Telljohann, and S. Wooley (2007). "Health Education: Results from the School Health Policies and Programs Study 2006." *Journal of School Health*, 77(8): 408-434.

14. Centers for Disease Control and Prevention (2012). "School Health Policy." Available at http://www.cdc.gov/healthyyouth /policy/index.htm.

15. McKenzie, J. F. (1983). "Written Policies: Developing a Solid Foundation for a Comprehensive School Health Program." *Future Focus: Ohio Journal of Health, Physical Education, Recreation, and Dance*, 4(3): 9-11.

16. Bureau of Health and Nutrition Services and Child/Family /School Partnerships (2009). *Action Guide for School Nutrition and Physical Activity Policies*. Middletown: Connecticut State Department of Education.

17. U.S. Department of Agriculture, Food and Nutrition Service (2004). "The Local Process: How to Create and Implement a Local Wellness Policy." Available at http://www.fns.usda.gov /TN/Healthy/wellnesspolicy2004_process.html.

18. Division of Adolescent and School Health, Centers for Disease Control and Prevention (2010). "School Health Policies and Practices Study (SHPPS)." Available at http://www.cdc.gov /healthyyouth/shpps/index.htm.

19. National Association of State Boards of Education (2010). "State-by-State School Health Program Coordinators." Available at http://nasbe.org/healthy_schools/hs /bytopics.php.

20. American Cancer Society (2010). "The Role of the School Health Coordinator." Available at http://www.cancer .org/healthy/morewaysacshelpsyoustaywell/schoolhealth /whatsschoolhealthallabout/the-role-of-the-school-health-coordinator.

21. Division of Adolescent and School Health, Centers for Disease Control and Prevention (2008). "Coordinated School Health." Available at http://www.cdc.gov/healthyyouth/CSHP/.

22. U.S. Department of Commerce, Census Bureau (2010). *Digest of Education Statistics: 2010*. Available at http://nces.ed.gov /programs/digest/d10.

23. Schlitt, J. J. (June 1991). *Issue Brief–Bringing Health to School: Policy Implications for Southern States*. Washington, DC: Southern Center on Adolescent Pregnancy Prevention and Southern Regional Project on Infant Mortality. Printed in *Journal of School Health*, 62(2): 60a-60h.

24. American Academy of Pediatrics (2004). *School Health: Policy and Practice*. Elk Grove Village, IL: Author.

25. National Health and Education Consortium (1995). *Starting Young: School-Based Health Centers at the Elementary Level*. Washington, DC: Author.

26. Strozer, J., L. Juszczak, and A. Ammerman (2010). *2007-2008 National School-Based Health Care Census*. Washington, DC: National Assembly on School-Based Health Care.

27. Committee on School Health (2001). "School Health Centers and Other Integrated School Health Services." *Pediatrics*, 107(1): 198-201.

28. Joint Committee on Health Education Terminology (1974). "New Definitions: Report of the 1972-73 Joint Committee on Health Education Terminology." *Journal of School Health*, 44(1): 33-37.

29. Centers for Disease Control and Prevention (2005). *School Health Index: A Self-Assessment and Planning Guide*. Atlanta, GA: Author. Available at http://www.cdc.gov /healthyyouth/shi.

30. Joint Committee on National Health Education Standards (2007). *National Health Education Standards*, 2nd ed. Atlanta, GA: Author.

31. Joint Committee on National Health Education Standards (1995). *National Health Education Standards*. Atlanta, GA: American Cancer Society.

32. U.S. Department of Health and Human Services, Office for Substance Abuse Prevention (1989). *Drug-Free Committees: Turning Awareness into Action* (DHHS pub. no. ADM 89-1562). Washington, DC: U.S. Government Printing Office.

33. "Healthy People 2000: National Health Promotion and Disease Prevention Objectives and Healthy Schools." (1991). *Journal of School Health*, 61(7): 298-299.

34. Rosas, S., J. Case, and L. Tholstrup (2009). "A Retrospective Examination of the Relationship Between Implementation Quality of the Coordinated School Health Program Model and School-Level Academic Indicators Over Time." *Journal of School Health*, 79(3): 108-115.

35. Weiler, R., R. M. Pigg, and R. McDermott (2003). "Evaluation of the Florida Coordinated School Health Program Pilot Project." *Journal of School Health*, 73(1): 3-8.

36. Centers for Disease Control and Prevention, Division of Adolescent and School Health (1997). "Is School Health Education Cost-Effective? An Exploratory Analysis of Selected Exemplary Components." As quoted in F. D. McKenzie and J. B. Richmond (1998). "Linking Health and Learning: An Overview of Coordinated School Health Programs." In E. Marx, S. F. Wooley, and D. Northrop, eds., *Health Is Academic: A Guide to Coordinated School Health Programs*. New York, NY: Teachers College Press, 1-14.

37. Miller, T. and D. Hendrie (2009). *Substance Abuse Prevention Dollars and Cents: A Cost-Benefit Analysis* (DHHS pub. no. [SMA] 07-4298). Rockville, MD: Center for Substance Abuse Prevention, Substance Abuse and Mental Health Services Administration.

38. Gold, R. S., G. S. Parcel, H. J. Walberg, R. V. Luepker, B. Portnoy, and E. J. Stone (1991). "Summary and Conclusions of the THTM Evaluation: The Expert Work Group Perspective." *Journal of School Health*, 61(1): 39-42.

39. Child Nutrition and WIC Reauthorization Act of 2004, Pub. L. No. 108-265, § 204 (2004). Available at http://www.fns.usda .gov/TN/Healthy/108-265.pdf.

40. Student Nutrition and Physical Activity. S. Enrolled Act No. 111, 114th Gen. Assem., 2d Reg. Sess. (Ind. 2006). Available at http://www.in.gov/legislative/bills/2006/SE /SE0111.1.html.

41. National Center for Education Statistics (2011). "Indicators of School Crime and Safety: 2011." Available at http://nces .ed.gov/programs/crimeindicators/crimeindicators2011 /key.asp.

42. National Center for Education Statistics (2009). *Indicators of School Crime and Safety: 2009*. Available at http://nces .ed.gov/programs/crimeindicators/crimeindicators2009/.

43. Centers for Disease Control and Prevention (2012). "Youth Risk Behavior Surveillance–United States, 2011." *MMWR Surveillance Summaries*, 61(SS-4): 1-168.

44. U. S. Department of Health and Human Services. (n.d.). "Roles for Health and Safety Professionals in Bullying Prevention and Intervention." Available at www.stopbullying.gov. /resources-files/roles-for-health-professionals-tipsheet.pdf.

45. Hertz, M. F. and C. David-Ferdon (2008). *Electronic Media and Youth Violence: A CDC Issue Brief for Educators and Caregivers*. Atlanta, GA: Centers for Disease Control and Prevention. Available at *www.cdc.gov/violenceprevention/pdf /ea-brief-a.pdf*.

46. Health Resources and Services Administration (2012). "Risk Factors." Available at http://www.stopbullying.gov/at-risk /factors/index.html.

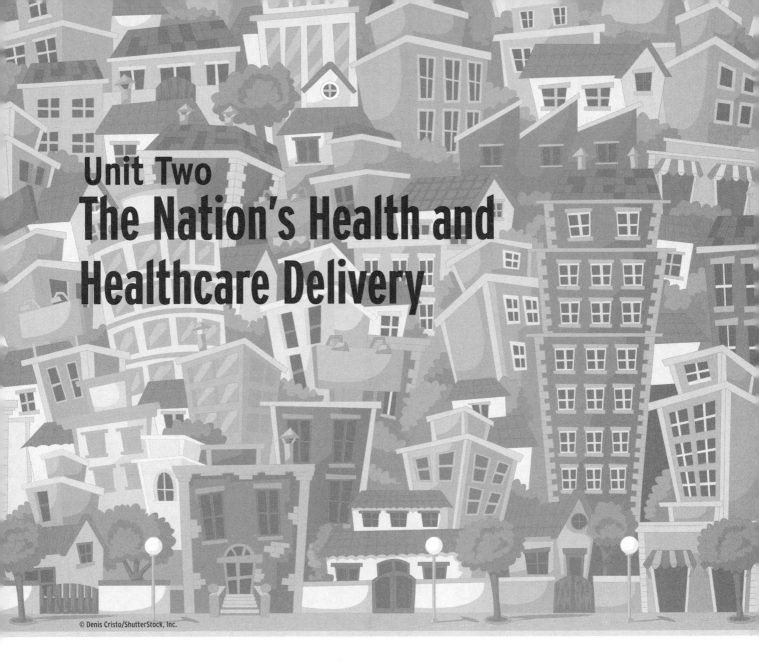

Unit Two
The Nation's Health and Healthcare Delivery

© Denis Cristo/ShutterStock, Inc.

Maternal, Infant, and Child Health

Chapter Objectives

After studying this chapter, you will be able to:

1. Define *maternal, infant, and child health*.

2. Explain the importance of maternal, infant, and child health as indicators of a society's health.

3. Define *family planning* and explain why it is important.

4. Identity consequences of teenage pregnancies.

5. Define *legalized abortion* and discuss *Roe v. Wade* and the pro-life and pro-choice movements.

6. Define *maternal mortality rate*.

7. Define *prenatal care* and *preconception care* and how they might influence pregnancy outcomes.

8. List the major factors that contribute to infant health and mortality.

9. Explain the differences among infant mortality, neonatal mortality, and postneonatal mortality.

10. Identify the leading causes of childhood morbidity and mortality.

11. List the immunizations required for a 2-year-old child to be considered fully immunized.

12. Explain how health insurance and healthcare services affect childhood health.

13. Identify important governmental programs developed to improve maternal and child health.

14. Briefly explain what WIC programs are and who they serve.

15. Identify the major groups that are recognized as advocates for children.

Introduction

A clear understanding of the health-related problems and opportunities of all Americans is necessary to create a health profile for just one American. Age is the first and perhaps the most important population characteristic to consider when describing the occurrence of disease, injury, and/or death in a population. Almost every health-related event or state has greater differences with age than any other population characteristic. For this reason, community health professionals use age-specific rates when comparing the amount of disease between populations. When they analyze data by age, they use groups that are narrow enough to detect any age-related patterns, which may be present as a result of either the natural life cycle or behavioral patterns. Viewing age-group profiles in this manner enables community health workers to identify risk factors for specific age groups within the population and to develop and propose interventions aimed at reducing these risk factors. Health promotion and disease prevention programs successful at reducing the exposure of specific age groups to such risk factors can improve the health status of the entire population.

In this chapter, we present a health profile of mothers, infants (those younger than 1 year), and children (ages 1–14 years). Other important age groups are adolescents and young adults (15–24 years), adults (25–64 years), and older adults or seniors (65 years or older). These same age subgroupings are used by the *Healthy People 2020* report and many other documents produced by the National Center for Health Statistics (NCHS) to describe and measure the health status of Americans.

Maternal, infant, and child health encompasses the health of women of childbearing age (18–45 years) from pre-pregnancy through pregnancy, labor, delivery, and the postpartum period and the health of the child prior to birth through adolescence.[1] In this chapter, we define and discuss commonly used indicators for measuring maternal, infant, and child health; examine the risk factors associated with maternal, infant, and child morbidity and mortality; and review selected community-based programs aimed at improving the health of women of childbearing age, infants, and children in the United States.

> **maternal, infant, and child health** the health of women of childbearing age and that of the child through adolescence

Maternal, infant, and child health is important to a community for several reasons. First, maternal, infant, and child health statistics are regarded as important indicators of the effectiveness of the disease prevention and health promotion services in a community. It is known that unintended pregnancies, lack of prenatal care, poor maternal and child nutrition, maternal substance use and abuse, low immunization rates, poverty, limited education, and unsafe child care—combined with a lack of knowledge of or access to healthcare services in a community—are precursors to increased rates of maternal, infant, and childhood morbidity and mortality. Second, we now know that many of these risk factors can be reduced or prevented with the early intervention of educational programs and preventive medical services for women, infants, and children. These early community-based efforts can provide a positive environment that supports the physical and emotional needs of the woman, infant, and family, reducing the need for more costly medical or social assistance to these same members of society later in their lives (see **Figure 5.1**).

During the past several decades the United States has made important progress in reducing infant and maternal mortality. However, despite these declines in mortality rates, serious challenges remain. Possibly the most important concern is that infant and maternal mortality data for the United States are characterized by a continual and substantial disparity between mortality rates for whites and blacks. In 2006, the mortality rate among non-Hispanic black

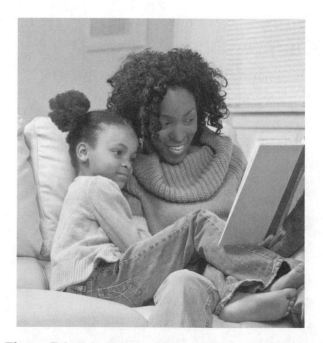

Figure 5.1 The health of a nation is often judged by the health of its mothers and children.
© Anthony Harris/ShutterStock, Inc.

infants (13.8 per 1,000 live births) was about 2.5 times the rate among non-Hispanic white and Hispanic infants (5.6 and 5.5 per 1,000 live births, respectively) (see Figure 5.2). That same year, the mortality rate among black mothers (34.8 per 100,000 births) was about four times the rate among white mothers (9.1 per 100,000 live births) (see Figure 5.3). These disparities are not directly attributable to race or ethnicity, although certain diseases occur more often in certain races or ethnicities. Rather, the disparity can be traced to differences in the socioeconomic status between segments of the U.S. population.

For example, research indicates that low income and limited education correlate very highly with poor health status.[2] A second concern is that the United States has higher infant and maternal mortality rates than other industrialized nations. It ranked thirtieth in infant mortality (see Figure 5.4) and twentieth in maternal mortality in 2005.[2] These differences among industrialized nations mirror differences in the health status of women before, during, and after pregnancy as well as the ease of access to and quality and quantity of primary care for women of childbearing age and their infants.

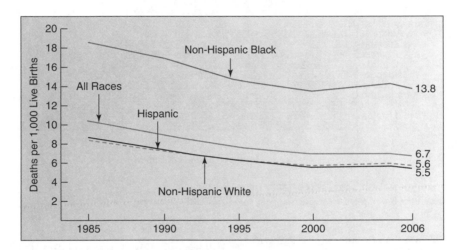

Figure 5.2 U.S. mortality rates among infants younger than 1 year, by maternal race/ethnicity, 1985–2006.

U.S. Department of Health and Human Services, Health Resources and Services Administration, Maternal and Child Health Bureau (2009). *Child Health USA 2008–2009*. Rockville, MD: U.S. Department of Health and Human Services.

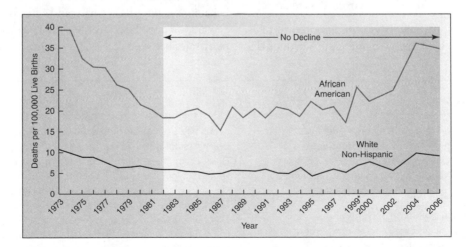

Figure 5.3 African American and white women who died of pregnancy-related complications: United States, 1973–2006 (annual number of deaths during pregnancy or within 42 days after delivery, per 100,000 live births).

* The apparent increase in the number of maternal deaths between 1998 and 1999 is the result of changes in how maternal deaths are classified and coded.

U.S. Department of Health and Human Services, Health Resources and Services Administration, Maternal and Child Health Bureau (2009). *Child Health USA 2008–2009*. Rockville, MD: U.S. Department of Health and Human Services.

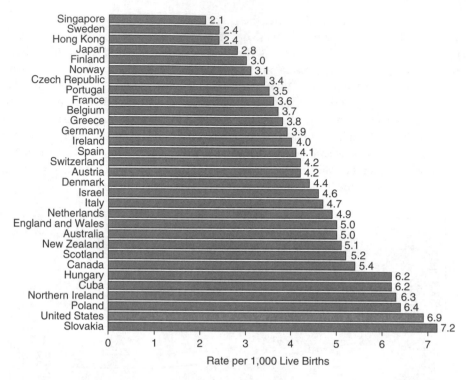

Figure 5.4 Comparison of national infant mortality rates, 2005.

National Center for Health Statistics (2009). *Health, United States, 2008 With Special Feature on the Health of Young Adults.* Hyattsville, MD.

Similar to the decline in infant and maternal mortality rates, the mortality rates of children (ages 1–14) have decreased significantly in the past few decades. The death rate declined by more than one-half for 1- to 4-year-old children and by nearly one-half for 5- to 14-year-old children from 1980 to 2006.[2]

Even with these improvements in child mortality rates, there is still much to be done to improve the health of U.S. children. First, we must recognize that children face other issues that can put them at significant risk for poor health. These concerns have been referred to as the "new morbidities" and include their family and social environments, behaviors, economic security, and education (see Box 5.1).[2] Second, we must be concerned about the difference in mortality rates between races. The young are the hope for every

---

Box 5.1   Moments in the United States for *All* Children

Every second a public school student is suspended.*

Every 11 seconds a high school student drops out.*

Every 19 seconds a child is arrested.

Every 19 seconds a baby is born to an unmarried mother.

Every 20 seconds a public school student is corporally punished.*

Every 32 seconds a baby is born into poverty.

Every 41 seconds a child is confirmed as abused or neglected.

Every 42 seconds a baby is born without health insurance.

Every minute a baby is born to a teen mother.

Every minute a baby is born at low birth weight.

Every 4 minutes a child is arrested for a drug offense.

Every 7 minutes a child is arrested for a violent crime.

Every 18 minutes a baby dies before his or her first birthday.

Every 45 minutes a child or teen dies from an accident.

Every 3 hours a child or teen is killed by a firearm.

Every 5 hours a child or teen commits suicide.

Every 6 hours a child is killed by abuse or neglect.

Every 15 hours a mother dies from complications of childbirth or pregnancy.

*Based on calculations per school day (180 days of 7 hours each).

Source: Children's Defense Fund (2010). *The State of America's Children 2010.* Reprinted with permission. Available at http://www.childrensdefense.org/child-research-data-publications/data/state-of-americas-children-2010-report.html.

country's future, and the United States is no different. Thus, the United States must continue to work hard to improve and ensure the health of each infant and child, regardless of race or socioeconomic status.

Many factors affecting the health of infants and children are reflected in or are related to the health status of mothers and their immediate environments. One of the first steps to ensure healthy children is to ensure the health of women of childbearing age, because many pregnancies are unplanned or unintended. Thus, although it remains important for pregnant women to have access to quality prenatal care early in and throughout pregnancy, it is, perhaps, more important for women of childbearing age to have access to quality preventive primary medical care. Therefore, we begin by looking at the health status of women in their childbearing years and the family structure.

Family and Women's Health

The family is the foundation of society. It is the primary social group for most people and it influences and is influenced by other people and societal institutions. Families are the primary unit in which infants and children are nurtured and supported so that they may experience healthy development.[1] The U.S. Census Bureau defines a family as "a group of two people or more... related by birth, marriage, or adoption and residing together; all such people (including related subfamily members) are considered as members of one family."[3] However, this definition does not include a variety of family structures that exist in our society today. Friedman broadens the definition of family to include "two or more persons who are joined together by bonds of sharing and emotional closeness and who identify themselves as being part of the family."[4] These definitions not only provide a basis for describing a family, but also are important to consider because most people, at some point in their life, will consider becoming a parent.

From a community health perspective, having two parents serves as an important family characteristic in relation to a child's health and well-being. Research shows that there are increased health risks for infants and children who are raised in single-parent families, including adverse birth outcomes, low birth weight, and infant mortality, and that these children are more likely to live in poverty than children of married mothers.[5,6] Additionally, unmarried mothers generally have lower education, lower incomes, and greater dependence on welfare assistance than do married mothers. Teenage women who give birth are substantially

more likely than women age 20 or older to have that birth outside of marriage.[6]

Teenage Pregnancy

Teenage pregnancy and childbearing represents a significant social and financial burden on both the family and the community. Teenage girls who become pregnant and have a child are more likely than their peers who are not mothers to (1) drop out of school, (2) not get married or to have a marriage end in divorce, (3) rely on public assistance, and (4) live in poverty.[5,7] Teenage pregnancy and childbearing also have substantial economic consequences for society in the form of increased public welfare costs. Each year teenage childbearing costs taxpayers at least $9 billion in direct costs associated with health care, foster care, criminal justice, and public assistance, as well as lost tax revenues.[8] Furthermore, teenage pregnancy and childbearing have considerable long-term consequences for teenage parents, particularly for young mothers, and their children. For instance, teenagers who give birth are less likely to graduate from high school and more likely to have a larger number of children in poverty than are teenagers who never become pregnant. Also, children born to teenage mothers may experience lower educational attainment and higher rates of teenage childbearing themselves when compared with children born to older mothers.

Teenage pregnancies also result in serious health consequences for young women and their babies. Teenage mothers are much less likely than women older than the age of 20 to receive early prenatal care and are more likely to smoke during pregnancy and have a preterm birth and low-birthweight baby.[7] As a consequence of these and other factors, babies born to teenagers are more likely to die in infancy and are more likely to suffer certain serious health problems than babies born to women in their twenties and thirties. A teenage mother is at greater risk than a woman older than the age of 20 for pregnancy complications (such as premature labor, anemia, and high blood pressure).[7] Therefore, teenage pregnancies are a significant public health concern in the United States.

In large part, as a result of effective community and public health campaigns aimed at reducing teenage pregnancies, teen pregnancy and birth rates have declined steadily in recent years. Between 1991 and 2010, the teenage birth rate in the United States declined by 44.6% to 34.2 births per 1,000 teenage girls.[6] Despite the recently declining rates, one-third of teenage girls get pregnant at least once before they reach age 20, resulting in approximately 754,000

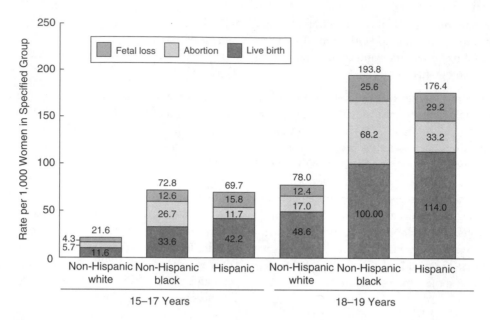

Figure 5.5 Teen pregnancy rates by outcome, by age, race, and Hispanic origin: United States, 2008.

Reproduced from Ventura, S. J., S. C. Curtin, and J. C. Abma. "Estimated Pregnancy Rates and Rates of Pregnancy Outcomes for the United States, 1990-2008." [Figure 2]. *National Vital Statistics Reports*, 60(07). Available at http://www.cdc.gov/nchs/data/nvsr/nvsr60/nvsr60_07.pdf.

teen pregnancies a year.[9] In fact, the United States still leads the industrialized world in teen pregnancy and birth rates by a large margin. U.S. rates are at least double those of other Western countries, placing the United States at a significant competitive disadvantage in the global economy.[10]

As stated in the introduction, the future of all nations depends on its children. The extent to which society believes and values this could be measured by the degree to which we plan, provide for, educate, and protect our children. Yet, *every day* in the United States, 4,498 babies are born to unmarried mothers; 2,692 babies are born into poverty; 2,222 are born to mothers who are not high school graduates; 2,175 are confirmed abused or neglected; 2,062 babies are born without health insurance; 1,200 babies are born to teenage mothers; 964 babies are born at low birth weight; and 78 babies die before their first birthday.[11] The need to plan a pregnancy and thereby place children first in families and in communities must be reemphasized. Unwanted and unplanned childbearing has long been linked to adverse outcomes for mothers, couples, and families, as well as for the children themselves.[12]

The choice to become a parent is a critical decision that affects the individual, the family, and the community. People who become parents acquire the major responsibility for another human being. They must provide an

environment conducive to child development, which is one that protects and promotes health and well-being. However, the broader community and environment also contribute to this growth and development.[12] This is best illustrated by an African proverb, "It takes an entire village to educate and raise a child."[13] Therefore, the community must also make provisions for each child's care, nurturance, and socialization.

Family Planning

Planning for the birth of a child, or the arrival of an adopted child, can be one of life's splendid experiences. Ideally, the first step is making a conscious decision on whether or not to become a parent. This determination will perhaps be one of the most important and consequential decisions a woman, or a couple, will make during her or their lifetime. Parenthood requires enormous amounts of time, energy, and financial commitment, but most notably it requires the willingness to take full responsibility for a child's growth and development.

It is important that a pregnancy be planned to ensure the best health for the mother and fetus during the pregnancy. However, approximately one-half of pregnancies in the United States are unintended, and 40% of those end in abortion.[14] Of particular importance is ensuring good health nationwide for women of childbearing age, or pre- and interconceptional women, because these women could become unintentionally pregnant. Preconceptional women are those who have never conceived, and interconceptional women are those who are in between pregnancies. The United States has set a national goal of increasing intended pregnancies to 56% by 2020.[12]

An unintended pregnancy is a pregnancy that is either mistimed (the woman did not want to be pregnant until later) or unwanted (the woman did not want to be pregnant at any time) at the time of conception. Unintended pregnancy is associated with a range of behaviors that can adversely affect the health of pregnant women and their babies. Risky behaviors include delayed entry into prenatal care, inadequate weight gain, cigarette smoking, and the use of alcohol and other drugs.[15] Any woman in the childbearing years may have an unintended pregnancy, but some groups are at higher risk, including teenagers, those living in poverty, and those with limited education.[15,16]

The most important approach to reducing unintended pregnancies and their adverse consequences is effective family planning.[12] **Family planning** is defined as the process of determining the preferred number and spacing of children in one's family and choosing the appropriate means of contraception to achieve this preference. Although many maternal, infant, and child morbidity and mortality outcomes cannot be completely prevented by effective family planning, the frequency of occurrence can be reduced. Thus, preconception health

care and education and quality gynecological, maternal, and child health care are required for effective family planning.[12] All women in their childbearing years should seek quality preventive primary medical care, and **preconception health care (pre- or inter-conception health)** should begin when a woman is considering becoming pregnant.

In the United States, family planning programs at the community level have historically included both governmental and nongovernmental health organizations (see **Box 5.2**). The federal and state governments provide funding assistance through a myriad of funds, the Maternal and Child Health Bureau, and Social Service block grants. Of these, **Title X**, or the Family Planning Act, is the only federal program dedicated solely to funding family planning and related reproductive healthcare services through the National Family Planning Program (PL 91-572).[17] Title X of the Public Health Service Act was signed into law by President Nixon in 1970 to provide family planning services and help to all who wanted, but could not afford them. For more than three decades, Title X has been this nation's major program to reduce unintended pregnancy by providing contraceptive and other reproductive healthcare services to low-income women.

family planning determining the preferred number and spacing of children and choosing the appropriate means to accomplish it

preconception health care (pre- or inter-conception health) health care that begins before pregnancy, or in between pregnancies, when a woman is considering becoming pregnant.

Title X a portion of the Public Health Service Act of 1970 that provides funds for family planning services for low-income people

---

Box 5.2 Ten Great Public Health Achievements, 1900–1999: Family Planning

Changes in Family Planning

In 1900, the average life span was 47 years, and 10% of infants died during their first year of life. The average woman had 3.5 children, and 6 to 9 women per 1,000 died in childbirth. Distribution of information regarding contraception and contraceptive devices was generally illegal under federal and state Comstock laws, which were enacted in the late 1800s. In 1900, the most common methods of contraception included withdrawal before ejaculation, rhythm, contraceptive douches, and vaginal pessaries (diaphragms, for example).

Milestones in Family Planning, United States, 1900-1999

1914 Margaret Sanger arrested for distributing information regarding birth control
1916 First birth control clinic, Brooklyn, New York; closed after 10 days by the New York City Vice Squad
1917 Federal registration of birth certificates

1928 Timing of ovulation during the menstrual cycle established
1955 First national fertility survey
1960 First licensure of birth control pills
1960 Modern intrauterine device licensed
1965 *Griswold v. Connecticut*; Supreme Court legalizes contraception
1970 Title X created
1972 Medicaid funding for family planning services authorized
1972 *Roe v. Wade*; Supreme Court legalizes abortion
1973 First National Survey of Family Growth taken
1990 Norplant licensed
1992 Depo-Provera licensed
1993 Female condom licensed

Source: Centers for Disease Control and Prevention (1999). "Ten Great Public Health Achievements—United States, 1900–1999." *Morbidity and Mortality Weekly Report*, 48(12): 241–242. Available at http://www.cdc.gov/mmwr/PDF/wk/mm4812.pdf.

Currently, it provides funding support to approximately 61% of the 4,000-plus family planning clinics nationwide. Every year more than 5 million women receive healthcare services at family planning clinics funded by Title X.[18,19] Those served are predominantly young, poor, uninsured, and have never had a child.[20]

Family planning clinics funded by Title X are located in every state and in 85% of all counties. The administration of all Title X grants is through state health departments or regional agencies that subcontract with local agencies and clinics. Currently, slightly more than half of the grants are administered by state and local health departments, one-fifth by Planned Parenthood affiliates, and the remaining one-fourth by regional or local family planning councils located in community organizations and hospitals.[20]

For clinics to receive funding under the Title X program, they must offer a broad range of acceptable family planning methods (oral contraceptives, condoms, sterilization, and abstinence), they must encourage family participation, they must give priority to low-income families, and they must not use abortion as a method of family planning.[17] In addition to contraceptive methods, clinics also provide a comprehensive group of other health services critical to their consumers' sexual and reproductive health.

In 1981, family planning clinics that received federal funds were required to provide counseling on all options open to a pregnant woman, including abortion, as outlined in Title X. However, these facilities were not allowed to perform abortions. In 1984, the **gag rule** regulations were enacted. These regulations barred healthcare providers in clinics receiving federal funds from counseling consumers about abortions. Family planning providers challenged this legislation on the grounds that it denied women their right to information that was needed to make an informed decision. Many healthcare providers believed that the gag rule restricted their obligations to counsel a consumer even when childbirth could be detrimental to her health.[17] Supporters of the gag rule regulation believed that Title X was created to help prevent unwanted pregnancy by providing education and contraception services and was not intended to provide services related to pregnancy options.

gag rule regulations that barred physicians and nurses in clinics receiving federal funds from counseling clients about abortions

In 1992, congressional action loosened the gag rule and allowed for all pregnancy options, including abortion, to be discussed between a consumer and her physician at Title X facilities. Although this may appear to be a reasonable compromise, in reality most women who visit family planning clinics are served by a nurse or nurse-practitioner and never see a physician. Therefore, this change in the gag rule still did not permit the free exchange of information between consumers and all healthcare providers in the clinic. In 1993, President William Clinton signed a presidential memorandum to reverse the gag rule regulations. This change enabled Title X facilities to discuss abortion as a pregnancy option. In 2003, President George W. Bush reimposed the gag rule to cover State Department family planning grants. President Barack Obama then rescinded the gag rule in 2009. This tug of war over the gag rule is expected to continue for as long as abortion remains politically controversial in the United States.

Controversy regarding acceptable family planning methods is not new in our country. In the early 1900s, a maternity nurse by the name of Margaret Sanger delivered babies in the homes of poor, mostly immigrant women. The women Sanger cared for knew nothing of how to prevent pregnancy and because of the Comstock laws (i.e., laws that prevented sending contraceptive information through the U.S. mail), they could get no information from their doctors. Disheartened by her inability to fully care for these women, Sanger decided to try to prevent the condition of unintended pregnancy in the first place.[21]

In 1914, Sanger, with the help of funds from numerous supporters worldwide, founded the National Birth Control League. The establishment of this organization is credited with starting the birth control movement in the United States. The purpose of this organization was to win greater public support for birth control by demonstrating the association between a woman's ability to limit her fertility and the improvement of both her health and the health of her children. In 1942, the National Birth Control League joined with hundreds of family planning clinics nationwide and formed the Planned Parenthood Federation of America.

Today, Planned Parenthood Federation of America, Inc., has grown to be the largest voluntary reproductive healthcare organization in the world and is still dedicated to the principle that every woman has the fundamental right to choose when or whether to have children.[22] Currently, Planned Parenthood operates nearly 900 health centers, which are located in every state and the District of Columbia. This not-for-profit organization serves nearly 5 million women and men each year.[22]

Evaluating the Success of Community Health Family Planning Programs

The establishment of local family planning clinics, many of which receive funding through Title X, has resulted in an improvement in maternal and child health indicators for the communities served.[20] Many people in need of family planning services are uninsured, and private health insurance often does not provide coverage for contraceptive services. By providing access to contraceptive methods and instructions on how to use them effectively as well as counseling about the health concerns of women of childbearing age, community family planning clinics are able to show large reductions in unintended pregnancies, abortions, and births. Each year, publicly subsidized family planning services help prevent 1.9 million unplanned pregnancies, which would otherwise result in 860,000 unintended births, 810,000 abortions, and 270,000 miscarriages.[20]

Publicly funded family planning services are vital to enabling low-income women to avoid unintended pregnancy. From an economic perspective, each public health dollar spent by federal and state governments to provide family planning services saves $4 in Medicaid costs for pregnancy-related and newborn care.[23] The total annual savings is estimated at nearly $5 billion, which represents money currently being spent on welfare, medical, and nutritional services as required by law. A 2010 report showed that more women are in need of publicly funded family services.[23] This is due in large part to the increase in the number of poor women needing publicly funded contraceptive services and supplies.

Abortion

One of the most important outcomes of community family planning programs is preventing abortions. Abortion has been legal throughout the United States since 1973 when the Supreme Court ruled in the **Roe v. Wade** case that women, in consultation with their physician, have a constitutionally protected right to have an abortion in the early stages of pregnancy free from government interference.[24] Since the early 1970s, the Centers for Disease Control and Prevention (CDC) has been documenting the number and characteristics of women obtaining legal induced abortions to monitor unintended pregnancy and to assist with efforts to identify and reduce preventable causes of morbidity and mortality associated with abortions.[25] As a result of the *Roe v. Wade* decision, the number of women dying from illegal abortions has diminished sharply during the last three decades in the United States. However, doubters remain, largely among those whose main strategy for reducing abortion is to outlaw it. However, although it may seem paradoxical, the legal status of abortion appears to have relatively little connection to its overall prevalence.

The fate of legalized abortion itself is as unclear as the right of a consumer to discuss abortion options in federally funded clinics. The Hyde Amendment of 1976 made it illegal to use federal funds to perform an abortion except in cases where the woman's life was in danger. In 1992, the Supreme Court was asked to rule on the constitutionality of the landmark court decision of *Roe v. Wade*. The *Roe v. Wade* Supreme Court ruling made it unconstitutional for state laws to prohibit abortions. In effect, this decision concluded that an unborn child is not a person and therefore has no rights under the law. The decision of whether to have an abortion or not was left up to the woman until she was 12 weeks pregnant. After the twelfth week, an abortion was permissible only when the health of the mother was in question. In 1989, the Supreme Court appeared to reverse this decision. It ruled that the individual states could place restrictions on a woman's right to obtain an abortion. Some states now have a 24-hour waiting period after counseling before permitting an abortion.

The issue of abortion has become a hotly debated topic. Political appointments can be won or lost depending on a candidate's stance as "pro-life" or "pro-choice" on the abortion issue (see **Figure 5.6**).

> **Roe v. Wade** a 1973 Supreme Court decision that made it unconstitutional for state laws to prohibit abortions

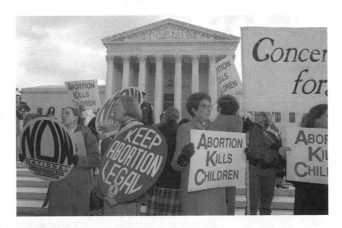

Figure 5.6 Political appointments and elections can be won or lost on the issue of abortion.
© Joe Marquette/AP Photos

Pro-life groups argue that performing an abortion is an act of murder. Generally, pro-life individuals believe that life begins at conception and that an embryo is a person. The **pro-choice** position is that women have a right to reproductive freedom. Pro-choice advocates believe that the government should not be allowed to force a woman to carry a pregnancy to term and give birth to an unwanted child. The question of when life begins can only be decided by each individual based on his or her own values and beliefs.[21]

Maternal Health

Maternal health encompasses the health of women in the childbearing years, including those in the preconceptional, or pre-pregnancy, period; those who are pregnant; and those who are caring for young children and may be interconceptional, or between pregnancies. The effect of pregnancy and childbirth on women is an important indicator of their health. Pregnancy and delivery can lead to serious health problems. Maternal mortality rates are the most severe measure of ill health for pregnant women.

The Tenth Revision of the *International Statistical Classification of Diseases and Related Health Problems* (ICD-10) defines a *maternal death* (maternal mortality) as "the death of a woman while pregnant or within 42 days of termination of pregnancy, irrespective of the duration and site of the pregnancy, from any cause related to or aggravated by the pregnancy or its management but not from accidental or incidental causes."[26] The *maternal mortality rate* is the number of mothers dying per 100,000 live births in a given year. The number of live births is used in the denominator because the total number of pregnant women is unknown.

In the United States, two to three women die of pregnancy-related complications every day. Between 1970 and 1982, maternal mortality decreased from 21.5 deaths per 100,000 live births to 9.1 deaths per 100,000 live births, more than a 50% decline. However, since 1982 the risk of dying has remained relatively stable. This is disturbing because many studies indicate that as many as half of all maternal deaths could be prevented if women had better access to health care and better quality of care, and made changes in health and lifestyle behaviors. Causes of maternal death are classified as direct, indirect, or unspecified. The most common direct causes include complications related to the puerperium (period of time after delivery), eclampsia and preeclampsia, and hemorrhage. Indirect causes comprise deaths from preexisting conditions complicated by pregnancy. The optimal time to medically treat most preexisting health conditions is before a woman becomes pregnant.

Additionally, the gap between death rates for black and white women remains, with black women being four times more likely than white women to die from pregnancy and its complications. Ensuring early initiation of prenatal care during maternity greatly contributes to reductions in perinatal illness, disability, and death for both the mother and the infant.[27] In addition, a number of underlying causes of high maternal morbidity and mortality rates include poverty, the sociocultural factor, and a limited education.

Preconception and Prenatal Health Care

High-quality **prenatal health care** is one of the fundamentals of a safe motherhood program and includes three major components—risk assessment, treatment for medical conditions or risk reduction, and education.[12,27] Health care that occurs before pregnancy that is health improving and risk reducing is referred to as *preconception health care*. Prenatal care should begin when a woman becomes pregnant and should continue at regular intervals throughout pregnancy (see **Box 5.3**). The goals of prenatal care include providing the best care for the pregnant woman and the fetus as well as preparing the mother-to-be for the delivery of a healthy baby. During prenatal visits, tests are performed on both the mother and fetus to assess any potential risks, to treat any maternal or fetal complications, and to monitor the growth and development of the fetus. In addition, counseling and guidance are provided regarding the various aspects of pregnancy, including recommended weight gain, exercise, nutrition, and overall health.

Prenatal care is essential to maternal and infant health. Women who receive early and continuous prenatal health care have better pregnancy outcomes than women who do not. A pregnant woman who receives no prenatal care is three times as likely to give birth to a **low-birth-weight infant** (one who weighs less than 5.5 pounds or 2,500 grams) as one who receives the appropriate care, and she is four times as likely to have her baby die in infancy. Getting pregnant women into prenatal care early (during the first

low-birth-weight infant one that weighs less than 2,500 grams, or 5.5 pounds, at birth

prenatal health care (prenatal care) one of the fundamentals of a healthy pregnancy program that includes three major components: risk assessment, treatment for medical conditions or risk reduction, and education. Prenatal health care should begin *preconceptionally* (before pregnancy) when a woman is considering becoming pregnant and should continue throughout pregnancy.

pro-choice a medical/ethical position that holds that women have a right to reproductive freedom

pro-life a medical/ethical position that holds that performing an abortion is an act of murder

---

Box 5.3 Opportunities to Reduce Maternal and Infant Mortality

Prevention measures that reduce maternal and infant mortality and promote the health of all childbearing women and their newborns should start before conception and continue through the postpartum period. Some of these prevention measures include the following.

Before Conception

- Screen women for health risks and preexisting chronic conditions such as diabetes, hypertension, and sexually transmitted diseases.
- Counsel women about contraception and provide access to effective family planning services (to prevent unintended pregnancies and unnecessary abortions).
- Counsel women about the benefits of good nutrition; encourage women especially to consume adequate amounts of folic acid supplements (to prevent neural tube defects) and iron.
- Advise women to avoid alcohol, tobacco, and illicit drugs.
- Advise women about the value of regular physical exercise.

During Pregnancy

- Provide women with early access to high-quality care throughout the phases of pregnancy, labor, and delivery. Such care includes risk-appropriate care, treatment for complications, and use of antenatal corticosteroids when appropriate.
- Monitor and, when appropriate, treat preexisting chronic conditions.
- Screen for and, when appropriate, treat reproductive tract infections, including bacterial vaginosis, group B streptococcus, and human immunodeficiency virus.
- Vaccinate women against influenza, if appropriate.
- Continue counseling against use of alcohol, tobacco, and illicit drugs.
- Continue counseling about nutrition and physical exercise.
- Educate women about the early signs of pregnancy-related problems.

During Postpartum Period

- Vaccinate newborns at age-appropriate times.
- Provide information about well-baby care and the benefits of breastfeeding.
- Warn parents about exposing infants to secondhand smoke.
- Counsel parents about placing infants to sleep on their backs.
- Educate parents about how to protect their infants from exposure to infectious diseases and harmful substances.

Source: Centers for Disease Control and Prevention (1999). "Ten Great Public Health Achievements—United States, 1900–1999." *Morbidity and Mortality Weekly Report,* 48(12): 241–242. Available at www.cdc.gov/mmwr/PDF/wk/mm4812.pdf.

---

3 months of pregnancy) is the main policy goal of most publicly funded programs designed to reduce the incidence of low birth weight and infant mortality in the United States. The percentage of women receiving prenatal care during the first trimester was 70.5% in 2007. The target goal for 2020 was 77.6%.[12] Non-Hispanic black, Hispanic, and American Indian/Alaskan Native women were 2.5 to 3.5 times more likely to begin care late or to receive no prenatal care at all in 2006 (see **Figure 5.7**). Black, Native American, Hispanic, and poorly educated women, and those most likely to be poor and without health insurance are significantly less likely to receive early and comprehensive prenatal care.[27]

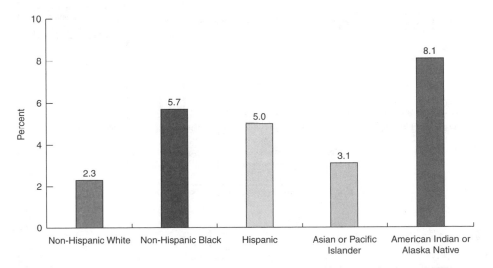

Figure 5.7 Percentage of mothers receiving late or no prenatal care by race and Hispanic origin, 2006.

National Center for Health Statistics, National Vital Statistics System. "Prenatal Care—2006." Available at http://205.207.175.93/VitalStats/TableViewer/tableView.aspx?Reportid=15101.

Infant Health

An infant's health depends on many factors, which include the mother's health and her health behavior prior to (preconceptionally) and during pregnancy, her engagement in prenatal care, the quality of her delivery, and the infant's environment after birth. The infant's environment includes not only the home and family environment, but also the availability of essential medical services, such as a postnatal physical examination by a neonatologist (a medical doctor who specializes in the care of newborn children up to 2 months of age), regular visits to a pediatrician or family physician, and the appropriate immunizations. The infant's health also depends on proper nutrition and other nurturing care in the home environment. Shortcomings in these areas can result in illness, developmental problems, and even the death of the child.

Infant Mortality

Infant death is an important measure of a nation's health because it is associated with a variety of factors, such as maternal health, access to quality medical care, socioeconomic conditions, and public health practices.[12] An infant death (infant mortality) is the death of a child younger than 1 year (see **Figure 5.8**). The infant mortality rate is expressed as the number of deaths of children younger than 1 year per 1,000 live births.

The infant mortality rate gradually declined from 1980 to 2000 (see Figure 5.2). Decreases in the infant mortality rate during this period have been attributed to improved disease surveillance, advanced clinical care, improved access to health care, better nutrition, the recommendation that infants be placed on their backs when sleeping, and increased educational levels of the population.[12] Since 2000, the infant mortality rate in the United States has shown no further significant decline, maintaining a rate of between 6.7 and 7.0 deaths per 1,000 live births (see Figure 5.2).[28] This is disturbing because many of the causes of infant deaths could be eliminated by modifying the behaviors, lifestyles, and conditions that affect birth outcomes. These include smoking, substance use and abuse, poor nutrition, lack of prenatal care, medical problems, and chronic disease.

The leading causes of infant death include congenital abnormalities, preterm/low birth weight, sudden infant death syndrome (SIDS), problems related to complications of pregnancy, and respiratory distress syndrome.[28]

Infant deaths, or infant mortality, can be further divided into neonatal mortality and postneonatal mortality (see Figure 5.8). Neonatal mortality is deaths that occur during the first 28 days after birth. Approximately two-thirds of all infant deaths take place during this period. The most common causes of neonatal death are disorders related to short gestation (premature births) and low birth weight and

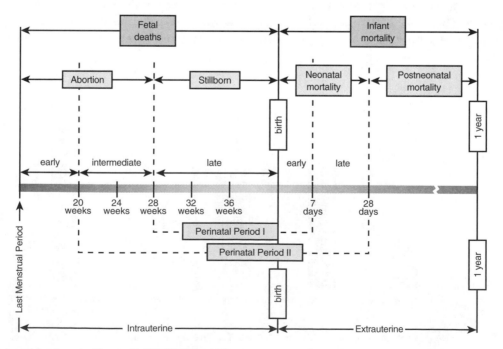

Figure 5.8 Important early-life mortality time periods.

congenital birth defects. These causes currently account for approximately one-half of all neonatal deaths. Postneonatal mortality is deaths that occur between 28 days and 365 days after birth. The most common causes of postneonatal deaths are sudden infant death syndrome and congenital birth defects.

Improving Infant Health

In part because of medical research and public health and social services supported by both public and private organizations, infant mortality has declined considerably during the past couple of decades. However, there are many opportunities for decreasing infant deaths and improving infant health even further through reducing risk factors associated with these conditions.

Premature Births

Premature (or preterm) babies are born prior to 37 weeks of gestation. The average length of gestation is 40 weeks, and normal gestation is considered 38 to 42 weeks. The number of babies born prematurely in the United States has risen steadily since 1980, and only recently leveled off to 12.3% of all births in 2008.[29,30] Disorders related to short gestation and low birth weight are the leading causes of neonatal death in the United States. Premature babies usually have less developed organs than full-term babies, so they are more likely to face serious multiple health problems following delivery. Premature babies often require neonatal intensive care, which utilizes specialized medical personnel and equipment. In 2005, the economic burden of preterm births was $26.2 billion, or $51,600 per infant. The majority of the expense was for medical care provided in infancy. Other factors that contribute to the economic burden are maternal care services, early intervention services, special education for preterm infants with learning difficulties, and lost work productivity of parents.[29,30]

Approximately half of all premature births have no known cause. Known major risk factors associated with preterm labor and birth include a woman's past history of preterm delivery; multiple fetuses; late or no prenatal care; cigarette smoking; using substances, including alcohol; exposure to domestic violence; lack of social support; low income; diabetes; anemia; high blood pressure; obesity; and women younger than 17 or older than 35.[29]

Therefore, although a number of causes of premature birth may have eluded researchers and are currently beyond our control, preconception and prenatal health care and lifestyle changes can help women reduce their risk of having a premature delivery. Consequently, there is a lot that community health programs can do to assist a woman in reducing her risk of having a premature baby. Specifically, community health programs can educate parents about premature labor and what can be done to prevent it as well as expanding access to healthcare coverage so that more women can get prenatal care.

Low Birth Weight

Today, it is widely accepted that low birth weight (LBW) is the single most important factor in neonatal death, as well as being a significant predictor of postneonatal mortality and infant and later childhood morbidity. The majority of infants weigh around 3,400 grams (7 pounds) at birth. LBW infants are those that weigh 2,500 grams, or about 5.5 pounds at birth. LBW infants are 40 times more likely to die in their first year of life than normal-weight babies. LBW babies often require extensive medical attention early in life and subsequently may suffer from a variety of physical, emotional, and intellectual problems. LBW babies have a higher incidence of cerebral palsy, deafness, blindness, epilepsy, chronic lung disease, learning disabilities, and attention deficit disorder.[31]

The percentage of U.S. infants born at LBW has remained relatively stable (between 7.0% and 8.3%) in the last two decades. LBW must continually be targeted aggressively by public health researchers as well as community-based public health programs, especially among various racial/ethnic groups, because significant disparities exist among these groups.

The two factors that are generally recognized to govern infant birth weight are the duration of gestation (premature births) and intrauterine growth rate. Approximately two-thirds of LBW infants are born premature. Therefore, reduction in premature births holds the most potential for overall reduction in LBW. Research on the causes of intrauterine growth retardation (IUGR) leading to LBW babies finds that maternal cigarette smoking during pregnancy is by far the most important risk factor. Other maternal characteristics that are risk factors connected with IUGR include maternal LBW, prior LBW history, low pre-pregnancy weight, drinking alcohol, prior birth of multiples, and low pregnancy weight gain.[12] Therefore, all pregnant women should (1) get early, regular prenatal care; (2) eat a balanced diet, including adequate amounts of folic acid; (3) gain the recommended amount of weight; and (4) not smoke, drink alcohol, or use other substances.[32]

Cigarette Smoking

Research has shown that maternal cigarette smoking during pregnancy is the leading modifiable cause of LBW in the United States, therefore making it an ideal target for intervention. Researchers estimate that smoking during pregnancy is linked to 20% to 30% of LBW infants and 10% of infant deaths.[33] The incidence of LBW infants among mothers who smoke is more than twice that of nonsmokers. The good news is that the percentage of births to women who smoked during pregnancy has been dropping, from 19.5% in 1989 to 10% in 2006 (see Figure 5.9). This seems to indicate that the United States is definitely progressing in the right direction when it comes to reaching its goal of 98.6% of females abstaining from smoking cigarettes during pregnancy by 2020.[12]

fetal alcohol syndrome (FAS) a group of abnormalities that may include growth retardation, abnormal appearance of face and head, and deficits of central nervous system function including mental retardation in babies born to mothers who have consumed heavy amounts of alcohol during their pregnancies

Alcohol and Other Substances

Prenatal exposure to alcohol can cause a range of disorders, known as fetal alcohol spectrum disorders (FASDs). FASD refers to conditions such as **fetal alcohol syndrome (FAS)**, fetal alcohol effects (FAE), alcohol-related neurodevelopmental disorder (ARND), and alcohol-related birth defects (ARBD). A safe level of alcohol consumption during pregnancy has not been

determined, but adverse effects are associated with heavy consumption during the first few months of pregnancy.[33] In general, no alcohol during pregnancy is strongly recommended.

Other drug use can also result in a number of deleterious effects on the developing fetus, including impaired fetal growth that can lead to congenital defects. Crack cocaine use during pregnancy can result in genital and urinary tract malformations in the baby. Marijuana use also has been associated with an increased risk of birth defects. A study showed that infants born to women using marijuana and/or cocaine were significantly smaller than infants of nonusers. Marijuana's effects of increasing maternal heart rate, blood pressure, and carbon monoxide levels may be responsible for impairing the growth of the fetus. Maternal use of cocaine results in lower fetal oxygen levels by inducing uterine contractions.[33]

Breastfeeding

The American Academy of Pediatrics (AAP) recommends that babies be breastfed for the first year of life. Breast milk is the ideal food for babies, newborn through 4 to 6 months of age. Breastfeeding has many advantages for both baby and mother. Breast milk contains substances that help babies resist infections and other diseases. Breastfed babies have fewer ear infections and colds, less diarrhea, and vomit less often. In addition, breastfeeding has been shown to improve maternal health by reducing postpartum bleeding, allowing for an earlier return to prepregnancy weight, and reducing the risk of osteoporosis later in life.[12]

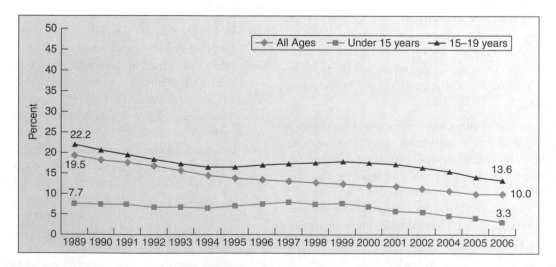

Figure 5.9 Percentage of mothers who smoked during pregnancy, by age: 1989-2006.

National Center for Health Statistics (2008). *Table 11. Mothers Who Smoked Cigarettes During Pregnancy, by Selected Characteristics: United States, Selected Years 1990-2000 and Selected States, 2005-2006. Health, United States, 2008 with Special Feature on the Health of Young Adults.* Hyattsville, MD: Author. Available at http://ftp.cdc.gov/pub/Health_Statistics/NCHS/Publications/Health_US/hus99/Excel/table011.xls.

Breastfeeding rates for women of all races have increased in the last decade. The *Healthy People 2020* objectives for breastfeeding are to increase the percentage of women ever breastfeeding to 82% and those still breastfeeding at 6 months to 60% (see **Box 5.4**). Breastfeeding rates are highest among those who are college educated (see **Figure 5.10**), among women 35 years or older, and among women participating in the Women, Infants, and Children (WIC) supplemental nutrition program. Women least likely to breastfeed were those younger than 20 years of age, those

---

Box 5.4   *Healthy People 2020:* Objectives

Objective MICH-21: Increase the proportion of infants who are breastfed.
Target and baseline:

Objective	Increase in Mothers Who Breastfeed	2005-2007 Status	2020 Target
21.1	Ever breastfed	74%	82%
21.2	At 6 months	43%	61%
21.3	At 1 year	23%	34%
21.5	Exclusively through 6 months	12%	24%

Source: U.S. Department of Health and Human Services, Health Resources and Services Administration, Maternal and Child Health Bureau (2009). *Women's Health USA 2009.* Rockville, MD: U.S. Department of Health and Human Services.

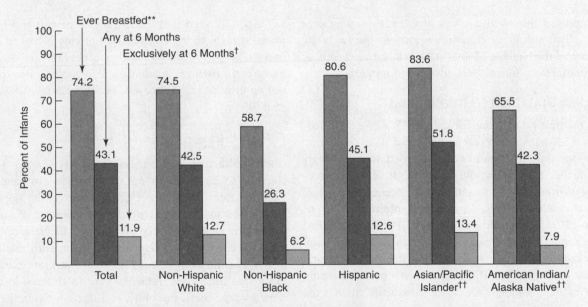

Infants* who are breastfed, by race/ethnicity and duration, 2005-2007.

* Includes only infants born in 2005; data are provisional. ** Reported that child was ever breastfed or fed human breastmilk. † Exclusive breastfeeding is defined as only human breastmilk—no solids, water, or other liquids. †† Includes Hispanics.

Centers for Disease Control and Prevention, National Immunization Survey.

For Further Thought

An important public health goal is to increase the number of mothers who breastfeed. Human milk is acknowledged by the American Academy of Pediatrics as the most complete form of nutrition for infants, with a broad realm of benefits for infants' growth and development. What types of programs would you recommend to educate new mothers and their partners and to educate healthcare providers?

Source: U.S. Department of Health and Human Services, Office of Disease Prevention and Health Promotion (2010). *Healthy People 2020.* Available at http://www.healthypeople.gov/2020/default.aspx.

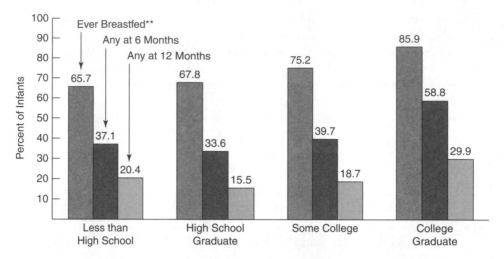

Figure 5.10 Infants* who are breastfed, by maternal education and duration, 2005-2007.

* Includes only infants born in 2005; data are provisional. ** Reported that child was ever breastfed or fed human breastmilk.

U.S. Department of Health and Human Services, Health Resources and Services Administration, Maternal and Child Health Bureau (2009). *Women's Health USA 2009*. Rockville, MD: U.S. Department of Health and Human Services.

not employed, those with a low income, and those who were black.[12] Two voluntary community groups, the La Leche League and the Nursing Mother's Council, are good sources for breastfeeding information, advice, and support.

Sudden Unexpected Infant Death

Sudden unexpected infant death (SUID) strikes approximately 4,500 babies each year in the United States. SUIDs are "deaths in infants less than 1 year of age that occur suddenly and unexpectedly, and whose cause of death are not immediately obvious prior to investigation."[34] Approximately half of these deaths are caused by **sudden infant death syndrome (SIDS)**, the leading cause of SUID. SIDS is defined as the sudden unanticipated death of an infant in whom, after examination, there is no recognizable cause of death. Because most cases of SIDS occur when a baby is sleeping in a crib, SIDS is sometimes called "crib death." SIDS is the third leading cause of infant death. Moreover, after the first month of life, it is the leading cause of infant death (post-neonatal mortality), accounting for one-third of deaths during the period of 1 month to 12 months of age.[12,34]

sudden infant death syndrome (SIDS) sudden unanticipated death of an infant in whom, after examination, there is no recognized cause of death

There is currently no way of predicting which infants will die because of SIDS. However, research has shown that sleeping on the back rather than the side or stomach greatly decreases the risk of SIDS among healthy full-term infants.[35] In response to this research, the federal government initiated a national "Back

to Sleep" campaign in 1992 to educate parents and health professionals with the message that placing babies on their backs to sleep can reduce the risk of SIDS. Since the dissemination of the recommendation, more infants have been put to bed on their backs, and the rate of SIDS has fallen by more than 50%.

Child Health

Good health during the childhood years (ages 1–14) is essential to each child's optimal development and the United States' future. The United States cannot hope for every child to become a productive member of society if children in this country are allowed to grow up with poverty or live in a violent environment, with mediocre or unsafe child care, or with no health insurance. Failure to provide timely and remedial care to children leads to unnecessary illness, disability, and death—events that are associated with much greater costs to society than provision of timely care. The cost of not providing prenatal care, mentioned earlier in this chapter, presents a vivid example. For those who believe that access to basic care is a standard of justness and fairness in any socialized society, the United States lingers sadly behind many other nations in the health of its children (see **Box 5.5**).

Childhood Mortality

Childhood mortality rates are the most severe measure of health in children. The death of a child is an enormous tragedy for family and friends, as well as a loss to the

Box 5.5 How the United States Ranks Among Industrialized Countries in Investing in and Protecting Children

1st in gross domestic product
1st in number of billionaires
1st in number of persons incarcerated
1st in health expenditures
1st in military technology
1st in defense expenditures
1st in military weapons exports
21st in 15-year-olds' science scores

21st in low-birth-weight rates
25th in 15-year-olds' math scores
28th in infant mortality rates
Last in relative child poverty
Last in the gap between the rich and the poor
Last in adolescent birth rates (ages 15 to 19)
Last in protecting our children against gun violence

Source: Children's Defense Fund (2010). *The State of America's Children 2010.* Reprinted with permission. Available at http://www.childrensdefense.org/child-research-data-publications/data/state-of-americas-children-2010-report.html.

community. As mentioned in the introduction of this chapter, the mortality rates of children have generally declined over the past couple of decades. Unintentional injuries are the leading cause of mortality in children (see **Figure 5.11**).

In fact, unintentional injuries kill more children than all diseases combined. The overwhelming majority of unintentional injury deaths in children are the result of motor vehicle crashes. Moreover, the majority of children killed in

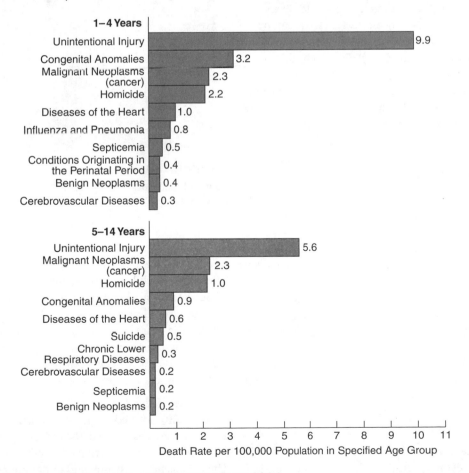

Figure 5.11 Leading causes of death in children ages 1 to 14: 2006.

U.S. Department of Health and Human Services, Health Resources and Services Administration, Maternal and Child Health Bureau (2009). *Child Health USA 2008–2009.* Rockville, MD: U.S. Department of Health and Human Services.

such accidents were not wearing a seat belt or other child safety restraint.[36] All 50 states have primary child restraint laws. They allow law enforcement officers to stop a driver if a child is not restrained according to the state law. However, the regulations of these laws vary from state to state.

Childhood Morbidity

Although for many children childhood represents a time of relatively good overall health, it is a time when far too many suffer from acute illness, chronic disease, and disabilities. Morbidity statistics on children are more difficult to calculate because they consist of a variety of perspectives. These include unintentional injuries, child maltreatment, and infectious diseases.

Unintentional Injuries

The United States needs to do a better job of protecting its children from unintentional injuries. Even though unintentional injuries are the leading cause of death among children in the United States, deaths are a rare event; however, injury-related morbidity is much more prevalent among children (see **Figure 5.12**). For each childhood death by injury, there are approximately 25 hospitalizations and 925 emergency department visits.[37] Each year about one-fourth of all children sustain an injury severe enough to require medical attention, missed school, or bed rest. Moreover, injuries are the leading cause of disability in children, with approximately 100,000 children becoming permanently disabled annually.[37]

In addition to the physical and emotional effects on children and their families, these injuries have enormous financial costs. Injuries requiring medical attention or resulting in restricted activity cost $17 billion annually for medical treatment.[38] Estimates are that 90% of the more than 4,000 unintentional injuries suffered by children each day in a manner serious enough to require medical treatment could be prevented. Childhood injuries can deprive the country of the child's potential contributions to their community and society. The injuries incurred in 2000 by children age 14 or younger will have lasting effects, including total lifetime economic costs, of more than $50 billion in medical expenses and lost productivity.[38]

Child Maltreatment

Child maltreatment is another source of injury to children. Child maltreatment includes physical abuse, neglect (physical, educational, emotional, and/or medical), sexual abuse, emotional abuse (psychological/verbal abuse and/

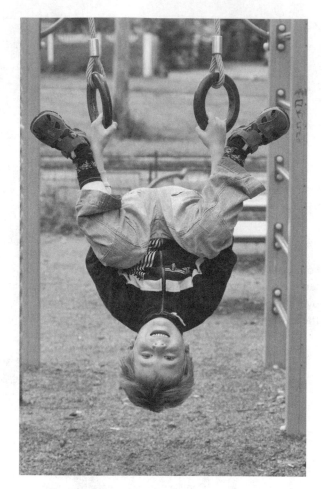

Figure 5.12 Unintentional injuries are the leading cause of childhood morbidity and mortality.
© Kitti/ShutterStock, Inc.

or mental injury), and other types of maltreatment such as abandonment, exploitation, and/or threats to harm the child. The causes of child maltreatment are not well understood. Child abuse or neglect is often associated with physical injuries and delayed physical growth. However child abuse and neglect also is associated with psychological problems such as aggression and depression. The rate of children maltreated annually has remained between 10 and 15 per 1,000 children over the past decade (see **Table 5.1**).[39]

The oldest federal agency for children, the Children's Bureau (CB), located in the Administration for Children and Families, has worked to lead the public in taking a more informed and active part in child abuse prevention. The CB has been instrumental in defining the scope of the problem of child maltreatment and in promoting community responsibility for child protection. The CB believes

Table 5.1   Child Maltreatment: Rate of Substantiated Maltreatment Reports of Children Ages 0–17 by Selected Characteristics, 1998–2007

Characteristic	(Substantiated Maltreatment Reports per 1,000 Children Ages 0–17)									
	1998	1999	2000	2001	2002	2003	2004	2005	2006	2007[a]
Total	12.9	11.8	12.2	12.5	12.3	12.2	12.0	12.1	12.1	10.6
Gender										
Male	–	–	11.4	11.7	11.5	11.5	11.3	11.3	11.4	10.0
Female	–	–	12.9	13.2	13.0	12.9	12.7	12.7	12.7	11.2
Race and Hispanic Origin[b]										
White, non-Hispanic	–	–	10.7	10.9	10.9	11.0	10.9	10.8	10.7	9.1
Black, non-Hispanic	–	–	21.5	21.8	20.8	20.7	20.1	19.5	19.8	16.7
Asian	–	–	2.0	3.7	3.2	3.0	2.9	2.5	2.5	14.1
Native Hawaiian or Other Pacific Islander	–	–	21.7	20.7	18.6	18.6	18.0	16.1	14.3	2.4
American Indian or Alaska Native	–	–	20.5	26.5	21.8	21.5	16.5	16.5	15.9	13.6
Multiple races	–	–	12.3	11.1	13.0	12.9	14.5	15.0	15.4	14.0
Hispanic	–	–	10.2	10.3	8.2	10.2	10.1	10.7	10.8	10.3
Age	–	–	15.7	16.1	16.1	16.1	16.0	16.5	16.8	15.0
Ages 0–3	–	–	–	–	21.6	21.7	22.0	23.4	23.9	22.0
Age <1	–	–	–	–	14.2	14.2	13.9	14.1	14.2	12.6
Ages 1–3	–	–	13.4	13.8	13.6	13.7	13.5	13.5	13.5	11.6
Ages 4–7	–	–	11.8	12.2	11.9	11.6	11.1	10.9	10.8	9.4
Ages 8–11	–	–	10.4	10.8	10.7	10.6	10.3	10.2	10.2	8.7
Ages 12–15	–	–	5.8	6.0	6.0	6.0	6.1	6.2	6.3	5.4
Ages 16–17	–	–	12.3	11.1	13.0	12.9	14.5	15.0	15.4	14.0

—Not available.

[a]Data since 2007 are not directly comparable with prior years because differences may be partially attributed to changes in one state's procedures for determination of maltreatment. Other reasons include the increase in children who received an "other" disposition, the decrease in the percentage of children who received a substantiated or indicated disposition, and the decrease in the number of children who received an investigation or assessment.

[b]The revised 1997 OMB standards were used for Race and Hispanic origin, where respondents could choose one or more of five racial groups: White, Black or African American, Asian, Native Hawaiian or Other Pacific Islander, or American Indian or Alaska Native. Those reporting more than one race were classified as "Two or more races." In addition, data on race and Hispanic origin are collected separately, but are combined for reporting. Persons of Hispanic origin may be of any race.

Note: The count of child victims is based on the number of investigations by Child Protective Services that found the child to be a victim of one or more types of maltreatment. The count of victims is, therefore, a report-based count and is a "duplicated count," because an individual child may have been maltreated more than once. Substantiated maltreatment includes the dispositions of substantiated, indicated, or alternative response-victim. Rates are based on the number of states submitting data to the National Child Abuse and Neglect Data System (NCANDS) each year; states include the District of Columbia and Puerto Rico. The overall rate of maltreatment is based on the following number of states for each year: 51 in 1998, 50 in 1999, 50 in 2000, 51 in 2001, 51 in 2002, 51 in 2003, 50 in 2004, 52 in 2005, 51 in 2006, 50 in 2007, and 51 in 2008. The number of states reporting on sex for each year from 2000 to the present was 50 in 2000, 51 in 2001, 51 in 2002, 51 in 2003, 50 in 2004, 51 in 2005, 51 in 2006, 50 in 2007, and 51 in 2008. The number of states reporting on race and Hispanic origin for each year from 2000 to the present was 48 in 2000, 49 in 2001, 50 in 2002, 50 in 2003, 49 in 2004, 50 in 2005, 49 in 2006, 46 in 2007, and 47 in 2008. The number of states reporting on age for each year from 2000 to the present was 50 in 2000, 51 in 2001, 51 in 2002, 51 in 2003, 50 in 2004, 51 in 2005, 51 in 2006, 50 in 2007, and 51 in 2008. Rates from 1998 to 1999 are based on aggregated data submitted by states; rates from 2000 to 2008 are based on case-level data submitted by the states. The reporting year changed in 2003 from the calendar year to the federal fiscal year. Additional technical notes are available in the annual reports entitled *Child Maltreatment*. These reports are available on the Internet at http://www.acf.hhs.gov/programs/cb/stats_research/index.htm#can.

Source: Federal Interagency Forum on Child and Family Statistics. "National Child Abuse and Neglect Data System." Available at http://www.childstats.gov/americaschildren/tables.asp.

that parents have a right to raise their children as long as they are willing to protect them. When parents cannot meet their children's needs and keep them from harm, the community has a responsibility to act on behalf of the child. If one suspects a child is being abused or neglected, it is important to call the proper authorities. According to the CB, the community's responsibility for child protection is based on the following[40]:

- Communities should develop and implement programs to strengthen families and prevent the likelihood of child abuse and neglect.
- Child maltreatment is a community problem; no single agency or individual has the necessary knowledge, skills, resources, or societal mandate to provide assistance to abused and neglected children and their families.
- Intervention must be sensitive to culture, values, religion, and other differences.
- Professionals must recognize that most parents do not intend to harm their children. Rather, abuse and neglect may be the result of a combination of psychological, social, situational, and societal factors.
- Service providers should recognize that many maltreating adults have the capacity to change their abusive/neglectful behavior, when given sufficient help and resources to do so.
- To help families protect their children and meet their basic needs, the community's response should be nonpunitive, noncritical, and conducted in the least intrusive manner possible.
- Growing up in their own family is optimal for children, as long as the children's safety can be assured.

- When parents cannot or will not meet their child's needs, removal from the home may be necessary. All efforts to develop a permanent plan for a child should be made as quickly as possible.

Infectious Diseases

In the past, infectious diseases were the leading health concern among children, but increased public health action has resulted in a substantial reduction in both morbidity and mortality rates. Infectious disease control resulted from improvements in sanitation and hygiene and the implementation of universal vaccination programs. Because many vaccine-preventable diseases are more common and more deadly among infants and children, the federal Centers for Disease Control and Prevention (CDC) recommends vaccinating children against most vaccine-preventable diseases early in life. The 2010 recommended immunization schedule is shown in **Figure 5.13**.

Immunization rates are considered an important indicator of the adequacy of health care for children and of the level of protection a community values related to preventable infectious diseases. The proportion of children ages 19 to 35 months receiving the recommended combined series of immunizations has increased from 69% in 1994 to 80% in 2008 (see **Figure 5.14**).

All children should be immunized at regular healthcare visits, beginning at birth and continuing to age 6.[41] By immunizing, the community safeguards its children against the potentially devastating effects of vaccine-preventable diseases. No child should ever have to endure the effects of these diseases simply because he or she was not vaccinated on time.

Vaccine ▼ Age ▶	Birth	1 month	2 months	4 months	6 months	12 months	15 months	18 months	19–23 months	2–3 years	4–6 years
Hepatitis B	HepB	HepB			HepB						
Rotavirus			RV	RV	RV						
Diphtheria, Tetanus, Pertussis			DTaP	DTaP	DTaP		DTaP				DTaP
Haemophilus influenzae type b			Hib	Hib	Hib	Hib					
Pneumococcal			PCV	PCV	PCV	PCV					
Inactivated Poliovirus			IPV	IPV	IPV						IPV
Influenza					Influenza (Yearly)						
Measles, Mumps, Rubella						MMR					MMR
Varicella						Varicella					Varicella
Hepatitis A						HepA (2 doses)					
Meningococcal											

Range of recommended ages for all children except certain high-risk groups

Figure 5.13 Recommended 2012 immunization schedule for ages 0–6 years.
Centers for Disease Control and Prevention. "Recommended Immunization Schedules for Persons Aged 0 Through 18 Years –United States, 2010." *Morbidity and Mortality Weekly Report*, 58(51&52):1-4.

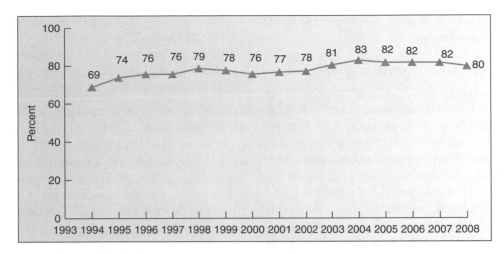

Figure 5.14 Percentage of children ages 19 to 35 months receiving the combined series vaccination (4:3:1:3), 1994-2008.

Data for 1994: Eberhardt, M. S., D. D. Ingram, D. M. Makuc, et al. (2001). *Urban and Rural Health Chartbook:Health, United States, 2001.* Hyattsville, MD: National Center for Health Statistics. Data for 1995-2001: National Center for Health Statistics (2003). *Health, United States 2003 with Chartbook on Trends in the Health of Americans.* Hyattsville, MD: Author. Data for 2002: National Immunization Program (2003). *Immunization Coverage in the U.S. Results from National Immunization Survey, Centers for Disease Control and Prevention.* Data for 2003: National Immunization Program (2004). Immunization Coverage.

Although progress in improving immunization rates has been substantial, about 1 million children in the United States under 2 years of age have not been fully vaccinated with the most critical vaccines. In addition, the National Immunization Survey data showed considerable variation between states and urban areas, indicating that children are not equally well protected in all parts of the United States. This large number of unvaccinated children has been attributed to cost, lack of access to medical care, uneducated parents, and confusion on when to vaccinate children. The U.S. government's Childhood Immunization Initiative includes five strategies: (1) improving immunization services for needy families, especially in public health clinics; (2) reducing vaccine costs for lower-income and uninsured families, especially for vaccines provided in private physicians' offices; (3) building community networks to reach out to families and ensure that young children are vaccinated as needed; (4) improving systems for monitoring diseases and vaccinations; and (5) improving vaccines and vaccine use.[41]

More stringent measures by the medical community are needed to ensure that all children are immunized. Opportunities to vaccinate are frequently missed by healthcare practitioners in primary care settings who do not routinely inquire about the immunization status of the child. Parents and health practitioners need to work together to ensure that youth are protected from communicable diseases. Timely immunization of children must be accepted as a national obligation because the United States cannot afford the waste that results from unnecessary illness, disability, and death.[41]

Community Programs for Women, Infants, and Children

In the preceding pages, many problems associated with maternal, infant, and child health were identified. Solutions to many of these problems have been proposed, and in many cases programs are already in place. Some of these programs are aimed at preventing or reducing the levels of maternal and infant morbidity and mortality, whereas others are aimed at the prevention or reduction of childhood morbidity and mortality.

The federal government has more than 35 health programs in 16 different agencies to serve the needs of our nation's children. The majority of these programs are well respected and help meet the needs of many children. However, others are **categorical programs**, meaning they are only available to people who can be categorized into a specific group based on disease, age, family means, geography, financial need, or other variables. This means too many children fall through the cracks and are not served. Some children require services from multiple programs, which complicates the eligibility determination of each child. At times, this can lead to an inefficient system of child health care. Nonetheless, federal programs have contributed to a monumental improvement in maternal, infant, and child health. We discuss some of the more consequential

categorical programs programs available only to people who can be categorized into a group based on specific variables

government programs and their past successes and future objectives in the following text.

Maternal and Child Health Bureau

In 1935, Congress enacted Title V of the Social Security Act. Title V is the only federal legislation dedicated to promoting and improving the health of our nation's mothers and children. Since its enactment, Title V–sponsored projects have been incorporated into the ongoing healthcare system for children and families. Although Title V has been modified frequently over the last couple of decades, the fundamental goal has remained constant: continued progress in the health, safety, and well-being of mothers and children. The most notable landmark achievements of Title V are projects that have produced "guidelines for child health supervision from infancy through adolescence; influenced the nature of nutrition care during pregnancy and lactation; recommended standards for prenatal care; identified successful strategies for the prevention of childhood injuries; and developed health safety standards for out-of-home child care facilities."[42]

In 1990, the Maternal and Child Health Bureau (MCHB) was established as part of the Health Resources and Services Administration in the Department of Health and Human Services to administer Title V funding. This means the MCHB is charged with the responsibility for promoting and improving the health of our nation's mothers and children. MCHB's mission is "to provide leadership, in partnership with key stakeholders, to improve the physical and mental health, safety and well-being of the maternal and child health (MCH) population, which includes all of the nation's women, infants, children, adolescents, and their families, including fathers and children with special healthcare needs."[43] To fulfill its mission, the MCHB has maternal and child health programs that accomplish the following in 2009[43]:

- 2,513,320 pregnant women were served by the MCH Block Grant and an additional 118,258 served, mostly through Healthy Start
- 4,134,329 infants were screened through the Title V Block. Services were provided to an additional 62,125 infants through Healthy Start and early identification services through such programs as LEND
- 27,611,884 children were served through the MCH Block Grant and an additional 89,654 mostly through Healthy Start and LEND
- 1,944,766 children with special healthcare needs received services

through the MCH Block Grant and an additional 148,761 mostly through LEND.
- 3,132,908 women and men were served through the MCH Block Grant and an additional 485,809 mostly through the first Time Motherhood/New Parents.

The MCHB works on accomplishing its goals through the administration of four core public health services: (1) infrastructure-building services, (2) population-based services, (3) enabling services, and (4) direct healthcare (gap-filling) services. MCHB uses the construct of a pyramid to provide a useful framework for understanding programmatic directions and resource allocation by the bureau and its partners (see **Figure 5.15**).

Special Supplemental Food Program for Women, Infants, and Children

The Special Supplemental Food Program for Women, Infants, and Children (**WIC**) is a clinic-based program designed to provide a variety of nutritional and health-related goods and services to pregnant, postpartum, and breastfeeding women, infants, and children under the age of 5. The WIC program began as a pilot in 1972 and received permanent federal funding in 1974, in response to growing evidence linking nutritional inadequacies to mental and physical health defects. Congress intended that WIC, unlike other food programs, would serve as "an adjunct to good health care, during critical times of growth and development, to prevent the occurrence of health problems."[44]

The U.S. Department of Agriculture (USDA) administers WIC. The USDA administers grants to the states, where the WIC programs are most often offered through local health departments or state health and welfare agencies (see **Figure 5.16**). Pregnant or postpartum women, infants, and children up to age 5 are eligible if they meet the following three criteria: (1) residency in the state in which they are applying, (2) income requirements (applicant must have a household income at or below 185% of the federal poverty income guidelines), and (3) determination to be at "nutritional risk" by a health professional.

Since WIC's inception as a national nutrition program, it has grown dramatically. In 1974, the average number of monthly WIC participants was 88,000; in 2008 that number was more than 9.5 million women, infants, and children. Among WIC participants, children make up half, infants one-quarter, and women one-quarter (see **Figure 5.17**). This constitutes nearly half of all infants born in the United

WIC a special supplemental food program for women, infants, and children, sponsored by the USDA

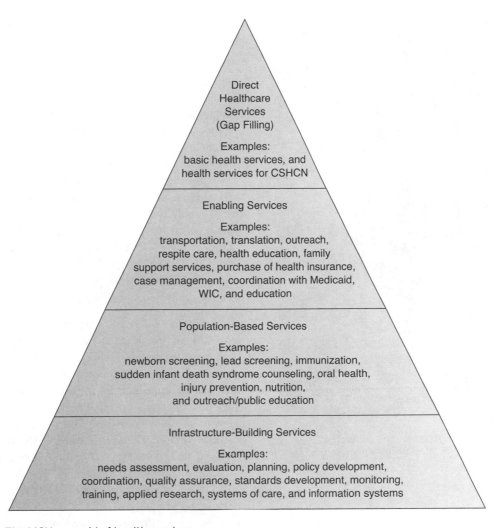

Figure 5.15 The MCH pyramid of health services.

U.S. Department of Health and Human Services (2003). *Understanding Title V of the Social Security Act.* Washington, DC: Health Resources and Service Administration, Maternal and Child Health Bureau.

States and approximately one-quarter of children between 1 and 5 years of age.

The WIC program has proved to be one of the most effective ways to improve the health of mothers, infants, and young children. Research indicates that participation in the WIC program during pregnancy provides women with a number of positive outcomes, some of which include birth to babies with higher birth weights and fewer fetal and infant deaths. The WIC program is also cost effective. USDA research has shown that for every dollar spent on WIC, the taxpayer saves $4 in future expenditures on Medicaid.[45] For this reason, the WIC program continues to possess strong bipartisan support in Congress.

Providing Health Insurance for Women, Infants, and Children

All children deserve to start life on the right track and to have access to comprehensive health services that provide preventive care when they are well and treatment when they are ill or injured. Health insurance provides access to critical preventive medical services as well as acute medical care in the case of illness or injury. When compared with children who are privately insured or have governmental insurance, children without health insurance are much more likely to have necessary care delayed or receive no care for health problems, putting them at greater risk for

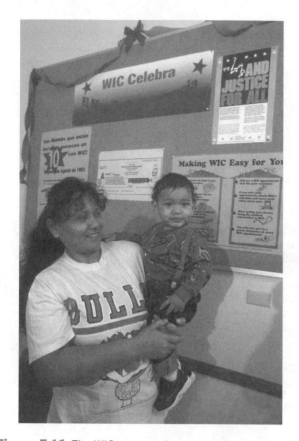

Figure 5.16 The WIC program has proven to be extremely effective in improving the health of woman, infants, and children in the United States.
© A. Ramey/PhotoEdit, Inc.

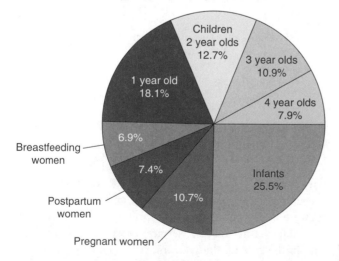

Figure 5.17 Distribution of individuals enrolled in the WIC program.

Conner, P., S. Bartlett, M. Mendelson, K. Condon, J. Sutcliffe, et al. (January 2010). *WIC Participant and Program Characteristics, 2008* (WIC-08-PC). Alexandria, VA: U.S. Department of Agriculture, Food and Nutrition Service, Office of Research and Analysis.

hospitalization.[46] Therefore, providing health insurance to low-income children is a critical healthcare safety net.

The government has two principal programs aimed at providing healthcare coverage to low-income children: the Medicaid program and the State Children's Health Insurance Program (formerly called SCHIP, now called CHIP). Medicaid, created in 1965, provides medical assistance for certain low-income individuals and families, mostly women and children. Children represent slightly more than half of all Medicaid beneficiaries, yet account for only 17% of program spending. A major reason that Medicaid is working well for U.S. children is the multiphase program for preventive health called the Early and Periodic Screening, Diagnosis, and Treatment (EPSDT) for individuals younger than the age of 21. The Medicaid EPSDT provisions entitle poor children to a comprehensive package of preventive health care and medically necessary diagnosis and treatment.

Although the Medicaid program is a critical healthcare program for low-income children, being poor does not automatically qualify a child for Medicaid. Medicaid eligibility is determined by each state based on various age and income requirements. As a result, Medicaid coverage varies across the states and leaves a significant number of poor children uninsured. To broaden coverage to low-income children, Congress created CHIP under provisions in the Balanced Budget Act of 1997. The program targets uninsured children younger than 19 with family incomes below 200% of poverty who are not eligible for Medicaid or covered by private insurance. Government-funded health insurance is an important source of coverage for children, and its significance has been growing. Medicaid coverage for children increased from 20% of all children in 2000 to 30% in 2008 (see **Figure 5.18**). During the same time period, the percentage of children with private health insurance coverage decreased from 71% in 2000 to 63% in 2008 (see Figure 5.18). The success in increasing the number of children with coverage is attributable not just to Medicaid, but also to the combined effects of Medicaid and CHIP. However, despite these programs, approximately 10% of youth younger than the age of 19 were uninsured in 2008. Advocates have encouraged state and community decision makers to continue the expansion of Medicaid and CHIP programs to cover as many uninsured children as possible.

Providing Child Care

Experiences during the first years of childhood significantly influence the health of a child. Research shows that early investments in the nurturing of children provides

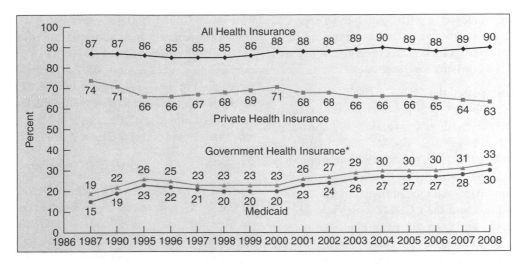

Figure 5.18 Percentage of children covered by health insurance, by type of insurance, selected years, 1987–2008.

* Government health insurance consists primarily of Medicaid but also includes such coverage as Medicare, State Children's Health Insurance Programs (SCHIP), and Medical Care Program of the Uniformed Services (CHAMPUS/Tricare).

U.S. Census Bureau (2009). *Income, Poverty, and Health Insurance Coverage in the United States, 2008. Current Population Reports, Consumer Income* (P60-236).Washington, DC: U.S. Government Printing Office.

major advantages for families and society later. Whereas parents should accept the primary responsibility for raising their children, the government can assist families who need help making important investments. Two important investments in the health and welfare of America's children are parenting during the first months of life and the accompanying need for secure relationships with a small number of adults in safe settings as they develop during the first few years of life.

To support new parents, the **Family and Medical Leave Act (FMLA)** was signed into law in 1993. The FMLA grants 12 weeks of unpaid job-protected leave to men or women after the birth of a child, an adoption, or in the event of illness in the immediate family.[47] This legislation has provided employed parents with the time to nurture their children and develop their parenting skills. However, the FMLA only affects businesses with 50 or more employees. Those employees covered by the law include those who have worked 1,250 hours for an employer over a 12-month period (an average of 25 hours per week). This excludes about 40% of American employees who work in small businesses that do not fall under the law's guidelines. Also, employers covered by the FMLA can exempt key salaried employees who are among their highest paid 10%, if they are needed to prevent "substantial and grievous" economic harm to the employer. Some experts feel the law divides people by class, helping those who can afford the 3 months without pay, and bypassing those who cannot. Experts have recommended a 6- to 12-month family care leave program

with partial pay for at least 3 months. The United States is the only industrialized nation that has not enacted a paid infant-care leave.

Today more families are in need of child care than ever before. Estimates are that as many as 13 million children younger than age 6 are in child care every day. The need for increased use of professional child care has come about as women increasingly are working outside the home and as more children grow up in single-parent households. However, for many families, especially those with low and moderate incomes, high-quality, affordable child care is simply not available. According to a recent study, much of the care we offer children is inadequate, yet a full day of child care costs an average of $4,000 to $10,000 annually per child.[11] These costs are beyond the reach of many working parents, half of whom earn $35,000 or less a year. The lack of high-quality child care prevents children from entering school ready to learn, hinders their success in school, and limits the ability of their parents to be productive workers. Furthermore, after-school care is crucial because juvenile crime peaks between the hours of 3 p.m. and 7 p.m., and school-aged children may be at greater risk of engaging in activities that lead to problems such as violence and teen pregnancy.

In 1988, Congress passed the Family Support Act, which provided funding for child care assistance to welfare

Family and Medical Leave Act (FMLA) federal law that provides up to a 12-week unpaid leave to men and women after the birth of a child, an adoption, or an event of illness in the immediate family

parents who are employed or participating in an approved training program. Unfortunately, states must match federal funds for this program, which makes meeting the needs of eligible participants difficult for poor states.

In 1990, Congress passed the Child Care and Development Block Grant (CCDBG), which provides child care subsidies for low-income children and funding to improve the quality of child care services. The "At Risk" Child Care Program, also passed in 1990, provides additional funding to support child care assistance to low-income families at risk of going on welfare. With the initiation of the "At Risk" Child Care Program and the CCDBG, states were able to provide additional assistance to many more low-income families. However, according to state-reported statistics, of the 15 million children eligible for federal support, only 12% are receiving federal help because of limited federal funding.[48] This means that only 1 of 10 children who are eligible for child care assistance under federal law receives any help. Not one state is currently serving all eligible families. This means that too many parents are unable to obtain necessary child care assistance.

Other Advocates for Children

Numerous groups advocate for children's health and welfare. Among them are the Children's Defense Fund, UNICEF, and the American Academy of Pediatrics.

Children's Defense Fund

Since 1973, the Children's Defense Fund (CDF) has been working to create a nation in which the network of family, community, private-sector, and government supports for children is so tightly intertwined that no child can slip through the cracks. The CDF is a private, nonprofit organization headquartered in Washington, D.C., and it is dedicated to providing a voice for U.S. children. It has never accepted government funds and supports its programs through donations from foundations, corporate grants, and individuals. The CDF focuses on the needs of poor, minority, and handicapped children and their families. The aim of the CDF is to educate the nation about the needs of children and to encourage preventive investment in children before they get sick or suffer. It provides information and technical assistance to state and local child advocates.

United Nations Children's Fund

Founded in 1946, the United Nations Children's Fund (UNICEF) is the only organization of the United Nations assigned exclusively to children. This organization works with other United Nations' members, governments, and nongovernmental organizations to improve child conditions through community-based services in primary health care, basic education, and safe water and sanitation in more than 140 developing countries. UNICEF gathers data on the health of children throughout the world. UNICEF has assisted in mass vaccinations and has been involved in other international health efforts to protect children.

American Academy of Pediatrics

The American Academy of Pediatrics (AAP) was founded in 1930 by 35 pediatricians who felt the need for an independent pediatric forum to address children's needs. When the Academy was established, the idea that children have special developmental and health needs was a new one. Preventive health practices now associated with child care, including immunizations and regular health exams, were only just beginning to change the custom of treating children as "miniature adults." The AAP is committed to the attainment of optimal physical, mental, and social health and well-being for all infants, children, adolescents, and young adults. The activities and efforts of the AAP include research, advocacy for children and youth, and public and professional education.

An example of a program that the AAP coordinates is the Healthy Child Care America (HCCA) program. HCCA is partly funded by the Child Care Bureau (CCB), Office of Family Assistance (OFA), Administration for Children and Families (ACF), the Maternal and Child Health Bureau, HRSA, and the U.S. Department of Health and Human Services. The specific goals of the HCCA program are the following:

- To promote the healthy development and school readiness of children in early education and child care by strengthening partnerships between health- and child care professionals
- To provide information and support necessary to strengthen children's access to health services
- To promote the cognitive, social, and physical development of children in early education and child care
- To provide technical assistance regarding health and safety for health professionals and the early childhood community
- To enhance the quality of early education and child care with health and safety resources
- To support the needs of health professionals interested in promoting healthy and safe early education and child care programs

Since the Healthy Child Care America program was launched in 1995, many communities around the country have been promoting collaborative partnerships between health- and child care professionals to ensure that children receive the best and highest-quality care possible. By expanding and creating partnerships among families, child care providers, and government, the best care for millions of children continues to occur.

Chapter Summary

- Maternal, infant, and child health are important indicators of a community's overall health. Maternal health encompasses the health of women of childbearing age from pre-pregnancy through pregnancy, labor, and delivery, and in the postpartum period. Infant and child health refers to the health of individuals through 14 years of age.
- Families are the primary unit in which infants and children are nurtured and supported regarding healthy development. Significant increases in births to unmarried women in the last two decades, especially among teenagers, are among the many changes in U.S. society that have affected family structure and the economic security of children. Teenage childbearing represents a significant social and financial burden on both the family and the community.
- The establishment of local family planning clinics with Title X funding has resulted in an improvement in maternal and child health indicators for the communities served.
- High-quality prenatal care is one of the fundamentals of a safe motherhood program. Ensuring early initiation of prenatal care during pregnancy greatly contributes to reductions in perinatal illness, disability, and death for the mother and the infant.
- An infant's health depends on many factors, such as the mother's health and her health behavior prior to and during pregnancy, her engagement in prenatal care, the quality of her delivery, and the infant's environment after birth.
- Good health during the childhood years (ages 1–14) is essential to each child's optimal development and the United States' future.
- The federal government offers many health programs through a variety of agencies to serve the needs of our nation's children. Two of the more successful ones are the Women, Infant, and Children (WIC) program, and the Children's Health Insurance Program (CHIP).

Review Questions

1. What has been the trend in infant mortality rates in the United States in the last 30 years? What is the current rate? How does this rate compare with that of other industrial countries?
2. What has been the trend in maternal mortality rates in the United States in the last 30 years? What factors have influenced this trend?
3. Why is prenatal care so important for mothers and infants? What types of services are included?
4. What are the consequences of teen pregnancy to the mother? To the infant? To the community?
5. What is included in family planning? Why is family planning important?
6. Discuss the pro-life and pro-choice positions on the abortion issue.
7. Why was the *Roe v. Wade* court decision so important?
8. What are the leading causes of death in children ages 1 to 4 and ages 5 to 14 years?
9. Why are childhood immunizations so important?
10. What is the WIC program?
11. Why is health insurance important for women, infants, and children?
12. Name three groups that are advocates for the health of children and what they have done to show their support.

Activities

Write a two-page paper summarizing the results and/or information you gain from one of the following activities:

1. Survey 10 classmates and friends and ask them what leads to teen pregnancy. What prompts adolescents to risk pregnancy when they have adequate knowledge of contraception? Ask if they know anyone who became pregnant as an adolescent. Are the reasons given the same as your own? Divide your list into categories of personal beliefs, barriers to action, and social pressure. For example, a comment that might fit under beliefs is "they don't think they can get pregnant the first time"; under barriers, "they are too embarrassed to buy contraception"; and under social pressure, "all the messages in society promoting sex." Which of the three categories had the most responses? Does this surprise you? What implications does this have for programs trying to reduce the incidence of teen pregnancy?

2. Call your local health department and ask for information about the local WIC program. Ask permission to visit and talk to a representative about the program and clientele.

3. Visit, call, or get on the website of your state health department and obtain information concerning the number of childhood communicable diseases reported in your state. What are your state laws concerning immunization of children? Does your state provide immunizations free of charge? What qualifications must a person meet to receive free immunizations?

4. Call a local obstetrician's office and ask if he or she accepts Medicaid reimbursement. What is the normal fee for prenatal care and delivery? If he or she does not take Medicaid, ask the obstetrician to whom he or she would refer a pregnant woman with no private insurance.

Community Health on the Web

The Internet contains a wealth of information about community and public health. Increase your knowledge of some of the topics presented in this chapter by accessing the Jones & Bartlett Learning website at **go.jblearning.com/McKenzieBrief** and follow the links to complete the following Web activities.

- Maternal and Child Health Bureau
- Women, Infants, and Children Program
- Insure Kids Now!

References

1. Pillitteri, A. (2010). *Maternal and Child Health Nursing: Care of the Childbearing and Childrearing Family*, 6th ed. Philadelphia, PA: J. B. Lippincott.
2. U.S. Department of Health and Human Services (2009). *Child Health–USA 2009*. Washington, DC: U.S. Government Printing Office.
3. U.S. Census Bureau, Population Division, Fertility and Family Statistics Branch (2010). "Current Population Survey (CPS), Definitions and Explanations." Available at http://www.census.gov/cps/about.
4. Friedman, M. (2003). *Family Nursing: Research, Theory and Practice*, 5th ed. Stamford, CT: Appleton & Lange.
5. Terry-Humen, E., J. Manlove, and K. A. Moore (2001). "Births Outside of Marriage: Perceptions vs. Reality." In *Child Trends Research Brief*. Washington, DC: Child Trends.
6. Martin, J. A., B. E. Hamilton, S. J. Ventura, M. J. K. Osterman, E. C. Wilson, and T. J. Mathews (2012). "Births: Final Data for 2010." *National Vital Statistics Reports*, 61(1):1-72.
7. Ventura, S. J., T. J. Mathew, and B. E. Hamilton (2001). "Births to Teenagers in the United States, 1940-2000." *National Vital Statistics Reports*, 57(12): 1-24.
8. National Campaign to Prevent Teen and Unplanned Pregnancy (2010). "The Public Costs of Teen Childbearing."

Available at http://www.thenationalcampaign.org/costs/pdf/resources/key_data.pdf.

9. Ventura, S. J., S. C. Curtin, J. C. Abam, and S. K. Henshaw (2012). "Estimated Pregnancy Rates and Rates of Pregnancy Outcomes for the United States, 1990-2008." *National Vital Statistics Reports*, 60(7):1-22.

10. United Nations (2010). *Demographic Yearbook, 2006*. New York, NY: Author. Available at http://unstats.un.org/unsd/demographic/products/dyb/.

11. Children's Defense Fund (2010). *The State of America's Children 2010*. Washington, DC: Author.

12. U.S. Department of Health and Human Services, Office of Disease Prevention and Health Promotion (2010). *Healthy People 2020*. Available at http://www.healthypeople.gov/2020/default.aspx.

13. Jackson, S. (1993). "Opening Session Comments: Laying the Groundwork for Working Together for the Future." *Journal of School Health*, 63(1): 11.

14. Finer, L. B., and S. K. Henshaw (2006). "Disparities in Rates of Unintended Pregnancy in the United States, 1994 and 2001." *Perspectives on Sexual and Reproductive Health*, 38(2): 90-96.

15. Sonfield, A., C. Alrich, and R. B. Gold (2008). *Public Funding for Family Planning, Sterilization, and Abortion Services, FY 1980-2006* (Occasional Report no. 38). New York, NY: Guttmacher Institute.

16. Sonfield, A. (2003). "Preventing Unintended Pregnancy: The Need and the Means." *Guttmacher Report on Public Policy*, 6(5): 7 11.

17. "Title X Pregnancy Counseling Act." (1991). *Congressional Digest*, 70(8,9): 195-224.

18. Frost, J. J., L. Frohwirth, and A. Purcell (2004). "The Availability and Use of Publicly Funded Family Planning Clinics: U.S. Trends, 1994-2001." *Perspectives on Sexual and Reproductive Health*, 36(5): 206-215.

19. Alan Guttmacher Institute (2005). *Family Planning Annual Report: 2004 Summary*. Submitted to the Office of Population Affairs, Department of Health and Human Services. Available at http://www.guttmacher.org/search/index.jsp.

20. R. B. Gold, A. Sonfield, C. L. Richards, and J. J. Frost (2009). *Next Steps for America's Family Planning Program: Leveraging the Potential of Medicaid and Title X in an Evolving Health Care System*. New York, NY: Guttmacher Institute. Available at http://www.guttmacher.org/pubs/summaries/NextStepsExec.pdf.

21. Hyde, J., and J. DeLamater (2003). *Understanding Human Sexuality*, 8th ed. Boston, MA: McGraw-Hill.

22. Planned Parenthood Federation of America (2009). *2007-2008 Annual Report*. New York, NY: Author. Available at http://www.plannedparenthood.org/about-us/annual-report-4661.htm.

23. Frost J., S. Henshaw, and A. Sonfield (2010). *Contraceptive Needs and Services: National and State Data, 2008 Update*. New York, NY: Guttmacher Institute.

24. "Court Reaffirms Roe but Upholds Restrictions." (1992). *Family Planning Perspectives*, 24: 174-185.

25. Pazol, K., S. Gamble, W. Parker, D. Cook, S. Zane, and S. Hamdan (2009). "Abortion Surveillance—United States, 2006." *Morbidity and Mortality Weekly Report*, 58(SS 08): 1-35.

26. World Health Organization (1992). *International Statistical Classification of Diseases and Related Health Problems*, 10th Revision. Geneva, Switzerland: Author.

27. Centers for Disease Control and Prevention (2000). "Entry into Prenatal Care—United States, 1989-1997." *Morbidity and Mortality Weekly Report*, 49(18): 393-398.

28. Xu, J., K. Kochanek, S. Murphy, and B. Fejada-Vera (2010). "Deaths: Final Data for 2007." *National Vital Statistics Reports*, 58(19): 1-31.

29. Behrman, R. E., and A. Stith Buter, eds. (2006). *Preterm Birth: Causes, Consequences, and Prevention*. Washington, DC: National Academies Press.

30. Martin, J., J. K. Michelle, M. H. S. Osterman, and P. D. Sutton (2010). "Are Preterm Births on the Decline in the United States? Recent Data from the National Vital Statistics System." Available at http://www.cdc.gov/nchs/data/databriefs/db39.pdf.

31. S. Nigel Paneth (1995). "The Problem of Low Birth Weight." *Future of Children*, 5(1): 35-56.

32. Chomitz, O. R., L. W. Cheung, and E. Lieberman (1995). "The Role of Lifestyle in Preventing Low Birthweight." *Future of Children*, 5(1): 162-175.

33. Centers for Disease Control and Prevention (1998). "Trends in Infant Mortality Attributable to Birth Defects—United States, 1980-1995." *Morbidity and Mortality Weekly Report*, 47(37): 773-778.

34. Centers for Disease Control and Prevention (2012). "Sudden Unexpected Infant Death." Available at http://www.cdc.gov/SIDS/.

35. Willinger, M., M. J. Hoffman, K. T. Wu, J. R. Hou, R. C. Kessler, S. L. Ward, T. G. Keens, and M. J. Corwin (1998). "Factors Associated with the Transition to Non-prone Sleep Positions of Infants in the United States. The National Infant Sleep Position Study." *Journal of the American Medical Association*, 280: 329-335.

36. National Highway Traffic Safety Administration (2009). *Traffic Safety Facts 2008: Occupant Protection*. Washington, DC: U.S. Department of Transportation.

37. Centers for Disease Control and Prevention (2012). "Child Injury." Available at http://www.cdc.gov/vitalsigns/ChildInjury/index.html.

38. Finkelstein, E. A., P. S. Corso, and T. R. Miller (2006). *Incidence and Economic Burden of Injuries in the United States*. New York, NY: Oxford University Press.

39. U.S. Department of Health and Human Services, Administration for Children and Families (2009). *Child Maltreatment 2007*. Washington, DC: U.S. Government Printing Office.

40. U.S. Department of Health and Human Services, Administration for Children and Families (2004). "Community Responsibility for Child Protection." Available at http://www.acf.hhs.gov/programs/cb/.

41. Centers for Disease Control and Prevention (2000). *Immunization 2000: A History of Achievement, a Future of Promise*. Atlanta, GA: Author.

42. U.S. Department of Health and Human Services, Health Resources and Services Administration (2003). *Understanding Title V of the Social Security Act*. Rockville, MD: Author.

43. U.S. Department of Health and Human Services, Health Resources and Services Administration (2012). "About Us." Available at http://mchb.hrsa.gov/about/index.html.

44. Special Supplemental Nutrition Program for Women, Infants, and Children (7CFR246) (January 1, 2002). "WIC Regulations." Available at www.fns.usda.gov/wic/.../wicregulations-7cfr246.pdf.

45. U.S. Department of Agriculture, Food and Nutrition Service (2010). "About WIC." Available at http://www.fns.usda.gov/wic/aboutwic/.

46. Institute of Medicine (2002). *Health Insurance Is a Family Matter*. Washington, DC: National Academies Press. Available at http://nap.edu/books/0309085187/html/.

47. Ruhm, C. J. (1997). "The Family and Medical Leave Act." *Journal of Economic Perspectives*, 3: 10-14.

48. U.S. Department of Health and Human Services (2000). "National Study of Child Care for Low-Income Families, State, and Community Substudy." Available at http://www.acf.hhs.gov/programs/opre/resource/national-study-of-child-care-for-low-income-families-state-and-community.

Chapter 6

Adolescents, Young Adults, and Adults

Denise M. Seabert, PhD, MCHES

Chapter Objectives

After studying this chapter, you will be able to:

1 Explain why it is important for community health workers to be aware of the different health concerns of the various age groups in the United States.

2 Outline the health profiles for the various age groups—adolescents and young adults, and adults—listing the major causes of mortality, morbidity, and risk factors for each group.

3 Identify key data sources used to help community health professionals understand the behaviors of adolescents, young adults, and adults.

4 Give examples of community health strategies for improving the health status of adolescents, young adults, and adults.

Introduction

In this chapter, we present a profile of the health of Americans in two different groups—adolescents and young adults (15 to 24 years of age) and adults (25 to 64 years of age). Each of these groups has its own set of health risks and problems. Viewing these age group profiles enables public health workers to detect the sources of diseases, injury, and death for specific priority populations and to propose programs to reduce those sources. Effective programs aimed at specific population age groups can reduce the risk factors that contribute to disease, injury, and death for the entire population.

The years of life between the ages of 15 and 64 are some of the most productive, if not the most productive, of people's lives. Most people complete their formal education, meet and commit to their lifelong partners, become parents and raise a family, find and develop their vocation, become owners of property, earn their greatest amount of wealth, actively engage in the development of their community, travel more than during any other time in their lives, become aunts or uncles and grandparents, become valued employees, serve as role models and mentors, and plan and save for retirement. This is also a time when individuals enjoy some of the best health of their lives as well as shape their health (through their lifestyle and health behavior) for their later years.

Adolescents and Young Adults

Adolescents and young adults are considered to be those people who fall into the 15- to 24-year-old age range. The individuals in this age group are considered very important by our society because they represent the future of our nation. If the United States is going to maintain its standard of living and preeminent position among the countries of the world that it enjoys today, it will depend in large part on these young people.[1]

This period of development of adolescence and young adulthood, often combined when reporting data about young people, can be further split into two subgroups. "Adolescence is generally regarded as the period of life from puberty to maturity,"[2] and includes the transition from childhood to adulthood. Like adolescents, young adults face many physical, emotional, and educational changes. Couple the demands of the personal changes experienced in

> **adolescents and young adults** those people who fall into the 15- to 24-year-old age range

this phase of life with the demands of a fast-paced, ever-changing society and it is easy to see why this stage in life is considered one of the most difficult.[1]

The combined period of adolescence and young adulthood is a critical one healthwise. It is during this period in one's life that many health-related beliefs, attitudes, and behaviors are adopted and consolidated.[2-4] In this stage of life, young people have increased freedom and access to health-compromising substances and experiences—such as alcohol, tobacco, other drugs, and sexual risk taking—as well as opportunities for health-enhancing experiences such as regularly scheduled exercise and healthful diets.[2-4] Additionally, certain lifestyle decisions are made during this stage that will have long-term influences on health in later years of life.

Demography

Several demographic variables affect the health of this age group, but the three variables most important to community health are the number of young people, their living arrangements, and their employment status.

Number of Adolescents and Young Adults

The number of adolescents and young adults peaked in 1979, when the baby boomers swelled their ranks to about 21% of the total population. Since 1979, the proportion of 15- to 24-year-olds has declined. Thus, in 2010 they made up 14% of the population, roughly the same proportion they made up in 1960.[5-7]

As we look to the future, the proportion of adolescents and young adults in the general population will continue to increase, and at the same time the racial and ethnic makeup will become increasingly more diverse. In 2008, approximately 60% of adolescents were non-Hispanic white. It is estimated that in 2050, this percentage will decrease to 44%.[2,7,8]

Living Arrangements

The percentage of children younger than the age of 18 living in a single-parent family has been on the rise since 1965. In fact, the percentage increased sharply in the 1970s and continued to rise slowly through the 1990s. The sharp rise in the 1970s can be attributed to the great increase in the divorce rate.[1] In 2010, one-third (34%)[9] of all children lived in single-parent families versus approximately one-tenth (11%) in 1970.[6] Additionally, more black children (66%) lived in a single-parent home than did white children (24%) or Hispanic children (41%).[9]

Family household statistics on single-parent families are only a snapshot of children's living status during a single year. Unfortunately, many children are affected over their lifetimes by growing up in single-parent families. Although the psychological and emotional consequences of single-parent families are not clear, the economic consequences are indeed visible. Children living in single-parent families are more likely to experience severe economic disadvantages,[1] with more than one in five youths under age 18 living below the Federal Poverty Line.[10] These economic disadvantages adversely affect health.

Employment Status

Since the years of the 1960s and the early 1980s, when there were significant increases in the participation of young women in the labor force, the proportion of all adolescents and young adults in the labor force has remained relatively constant. However, this age group has seen some significant declines in its labor-force participation, particularly 16- to 19-year-old males, mainly because of an increase in school attendance including summer school over the past decade, and the two recessions that have occurred since 2000.[11] The youth labor force, composed of 16- to 24-year-olds, makes up nearly 14% of the overall labor force.[11] When the unemployment rates of this age group are separated by race and ethnicity, differences appear. Regardless of sex, black adolescents and young adults are more likely to be unemployed than are whites or Hispanics. White adolescents and young adults have the lowest proportion of unemployment.[12] These proportions, like so many others already discussed, are disproportionate by race/ethnicity. These figures are important to community health because most health insurance, and thus access to health care, is connected to employment status.

A Health Profile

With regard to the health profile of this age group, three major areas stand out—mortality, morbidity from specific infectious diseases, and health behavior and lifestyle choices.

Mortality

Although, on average, Americans live longer than ever before, adolescents and young adults suffer their share of life-threatening problems.[1] As is true for most other age groups, the death rate for adolescents and young adults has significantly declined. Between 1950 and 2008, the death rate of adolescents and young adults declined by 41%, from 128.1 to 75.6 per 100,000.[13] This decline in the death rate for adolescents and young adults, like that for children, can be attributed to advances in medicine and injury and disease prevention.[1,13]

Regardless of race or ethnicity, men have a higher mortality rate than women.[13] Mortality rates for men and women were highest among blacks. The lowest mortality rates for both men and women belong to Asian/Pacific Islanders.[13]

Much of the physical threat to adolescents and young adults stems from their behavior rather than from disease.[1] For young people overall, approximately three-fourths of all mortality can be attributed to three causes—unintentional injuries (mainly motor vehicle crashes) (44%), homicide (16%), and suicide (13%).[13] Although mortality from unintentional injuries in this age group has declined over recent years, it still remains the leading cause of death in adolescents and young adults, accounting for almost half of all deaths in this age group (see **Figure 6.1**).

Deaths from motor vehicle–related injuries account for nearly one-fifth of all deaths for young people in this age group, with alcohol being a significant contributing factor.[13,14] Unlike other mortality data in this age group, white males have a higher rate of death in motor vehicles than do black males. Motor vehicle–related death rates of Native American males are the highest for this age group.

The most alarming mortality trend in this age group is the growing number of homicides and suicides. Over the last 50 years, homicide and suicide rates increased between 200% and 300%.[13] Homicide is the second leading cause of death in the 15- to 24-year age group, and it is the leading cause of death among black Americans.[13] Differences in homicide rates between races are significantly reduced when socioeconomic and environmental factors are taken into account.[14]

Suicide is the third leading cause of death in adolescents and young adults; it is the second leading cause of death of white males in this age group, but the rate among American Indian males is more than double that of white males.[13] The suicide rate in females is significantly lower than that for males, although young women attempt suicide more frequently than do young men.[13,15]

Although the number of completed suicides by adolescents and young adults is alarming, it represents only a fraction of all the suicides contemplated. Data from the 2011 Centers for Disease Control and Prevention's Youth Risk Behavior Surveillance System (YRBSS) indicate that nearly

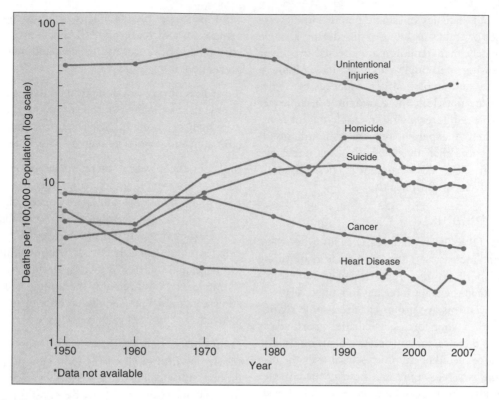

Figure 6.1 Death rates for leading causes of death for ages 15 to 24, 1950-2007.

Data from Fried, V. M., K. Prager, A. P. MacKay, and H. Xia (2003). *Health, United States, 2003, with Chartbook on Trends in Health of Americans.* Hyattsville, MD: National Center for Health Statistics, 50; National Center for Health Statistics (2006). *Health, United States, 2006, with Chartbook on Trends in the Health of Americans.* Hyattsville, MD: Author; and National Center for Health Statistics (2012). *Health, United States, 2011, with Special Feature on Socioeconomic Status and Health.* Hyattsville, MD: Author.

one in seven ninth to twelfth graders in the United States have thought seriously about attempting suicide (13.8%), 10.9% have made a specific plan to attempt suicide, and 6.3% have actually attempted suicide.[15]

Morbidity

Sexually transmitted diseases (STDs) cause considerable morbidity in adolescents and young adults. "Compared with older adults, sexually-active adolescents 15–19 years of age and young adults 20–24 years of age are at higher risk of acquiring STDs for a combination of behavioral, biological, and cultural reasons."[16] Whereas many STDs are completely curable with antibiotics, some viral infections, such as hepatitis, human immunodeficiency virus (HIV), and human papillomavirus (HPV), can be treated but never cured.[17] The effects of some STDs can last a lifetime. For example, some forms of HPV are the precursor to cervical cancer, and the effects of chlamydia, if untreated, can lead to infertility. In the case of HIV, the precursor to AIDS, the result may even be death.[17] Chlamydia and gonorrhea are the most common curable STDs among this age group.[16]

Estimates suggest that although they represent 25% of the sexually experienced population, 15- to 24-year-olds acquire nearly half of all new STDs.[16]

Health Behaviors and Lifestyle Choices of High School Students

Whereas many behavioral patterns begin during the childhood years (ages 1–14), others begin in adolescence and young adulthood. During this period of experimentation, young people are susceptible to developing deleterious behaviors such as the abuse of alcohol and/or tobacco and other drugs, fighting, and weapon carrying.

In 1990, the Centers for Disease Control and Prevention (CDC) initiated the Youth Risk Behavior Surveillance System (YRBSS) to better track selected health behaviors among young people. The YRBSS includes a national school-based survey, as well as state, territorial, tribal, and district surveys. The CDC conducted the first Youth Risk Behavior Survey (YRBS) in 1991 and it continues to be conducted biennially during odd-numbered years among national probability samples of ninth- through twelfth-grade students from private and public schools. During 2011, 47 state, 6 territory, 2 tribal government, and 22 local surveys were conducted.[15] In the time the YRBSS has been in operation, it has proved to be very helpful at both the state and local levels. Specifically, data are used to set and track progress toward meeting school health goals, support curriculum modification, and support new legislation and policies that promote the health of youth.

Behaviors That Contribute to Unintentional Injuries

Five different behaviors of high school students that relate to unintentional injuries are monitored as part of the YRBSS: bicycle helmet use, seat belt use, riding with a driver who has been drinking alcohol, driving after drinking alcohol, and texting or e-mailing while driving. Since 1991, the numbers of students engaging in these risk behaviors have declined. Yet in 2011, nearly one-fourth of students nationwide had, in the 30 days preceding the survey, ridden with a driver who had been drinking alcohol and one-third of students (32.8%) had texted or e-mailed while driving a car or other vehicle at least one time in the 30 days preceding the survey.[15]

Behaviors That Contribute to Violence

Behaviors that contribute to violence-related injuries of high school students include carrying a weapon (e.g., gun, knife, or club), engaging in a physical fight, engaging in dating violence, having been forced to have sexual intercourse, engaging in school-related violence including bullying, suicide ideation, and suicide attempts. Nationwide nearly one-sixth (16.6%) of high school students reported having carried a weapon during the 30 days prior to the survey, and about one-third (32.8%) of all high school students reported having been in a fight in the past 12 months. Additionally, one in five students (20.1%) had been bullied on school property in the past 12 months before the survey. It is no wonder that many school districts around the country are taking steps to reduce violent behavior in school. Males are more likely than females are to get in a fight or carry a weapon. However, females are more likely than males to have been forced to have sexual intercourse and to report sadness, suicide ideation, and suicide attempts.[15]

Tobacco Use

The use of tobacco products represents one of the most widespread, high-risk health behaviors for this group. In 2011, more than one-sixth of high school students (18.1%) nationwide were current smokers—that is, smoked on at least one day in the past 30 days—which is a significant decrease from 1997, when 36.4% of students were current smokers. Overall, white students (20.3%) were significantly more likely to report current cigarette use than were Hispanic (17.5%) or black (10.5%) students.[15] The vast majority of people who become dependent on nicotine do so between the ages of 15 and 24, because nearly 60% of new smokers are under the age of 18 when they smoke their first cigarette.[18]

Because use of tobacco that begins during adolescence can lead to a lifetime of nicotine dependence and a variety of negative health consequences, the federal government has exerted considerable effort to keep tobacco out of the hands of adolescents. Many believed, and data from the YRBSS verified, that most adolescents have had easy access to tobacco products. During his term of office, President Clinton was proactive in trying to restrict the distribution of tobacco to youth. One piece of legislation that was approved during President Clinton's term included a requirement that retailers must verify the age of persons who purchase cigarettes or smokeless tobacco products.[19] That guideline stated that anyone who appears to be 27 years of age or younger must be "carded" by retailers.

The Congress and President Obama have continued to positively affect the number of children who begin smoking. In 2009, an increase in federal tobacco taxes, including a 62-cent increase in the cigarette tax, was passed, which will help fund the Children's Health Insurance Program (CHIP).[20] More recently, legislation was passed to require large, graphic health warnings on cigarette packs and 20% of advertisements.[21]

Alcohol and Other Drugs

Although, for some, the first use of alcohol or other drugs begins during the childhood years, for most people experimentation with these substances occurs between the ages of 15 and 24 years. YRBSS data from 2011 indicate that 38.7% of all high school students reported drinking during the previous month. Further, the data indicate that 21.9% have experienced episodic heavy drinking, and 23.1% have used marijuana at least once in the preceding month.[15]

Although more than one-fifth of all high school students have used marijuana during the preceding month, alcohol use and abuse continue to be major problems for adolescents, particularly among high school dropouts, and contributes significantly to motor vehicle crashes and violence in this age group.[13-15]

Sexual Behaviors That Contribute to Unintended Pregnancy and Sexually Transmitted Diseases

Since the early 1980s, adolescents in the United States have experienced high rates of unintended pregnancies and STDs, including HIV infection.[22,23] YRBSS data from 2011 show that almost half (47.4%) of all high school students have engaged in sexual intercourse sometime in their lifetime. The prevalence of sexual intercourse ranged between 27.8% for ninth-grade girls to 62.6% for high school senior boys. Furthermore, it was much more likely for black students (60.0%) to have engaged in sexual intercourse than for Hispanic (48.6%) and white (44.3%) students.[15] Table 6.1 shows the trends of selected sexual risk behaviors for high school students since 1991.

Each year nearly 750,000 women in the United States between the ages of 15 and 19 become pregnant.[24] In 2008, the U.S. teenage pregnancy rate was a record low, down 42% since its peak in 1990,[24] yet more than 80% of these pregnancies were unintended.[25] In addition to the health risks associated with teenage pregnancies for both mother and child, there are educational, economic, and psychosocial risks as well. Teenage mothers are less likely to get or stay married, less likely to complete high school or college, and more likely to require public assistance and to live in poverty than their peers who are not mothers.[26]

Physical Activity

Lack of physical activity by young people has increasingly become a concern. In 2011, half (51.5%) of students had not been physically active for at least 60 minutes per day on 5 or more days during the 7 days prior to the survey. Males (59.9%) were more likely than females (38.5%) to engage in sufficient physical activity. The prevalence of not having participated in at least 60 minutes of physical activity on any day was highest among black and Hispanic students. Nationally, 13.8% of students had not participated in 60 minutes of any kind of physical activity that increased their heart rate or made them breathe hard some of the time on at least 1 day during the 7 days preceding the survey.[15]

Overweight and Weight Control

Much like the concern for insufficient physical activity, the concern regarding students becoming overweight has received significant attention recently (see Figure 6.2). In 2011, approximately one-quarter of students were obese (13.0%) or overweight (15.2%), and 29.2% described themselves as slightly or very overweight. Almost one-half of students were trying to lose weight (46.0%). The prevalence for engaging in weight loss behaviors was higher among females (61.2%) than males (31.6%). Nationally, 12.2% of students had gone without eating for 24 hours or more to lose weight or to keep from gaining weight during the 30 days preceding the survey.[15]

Health Behaviors and Lifestyle Choices of College Students

Two currently available data sources regarding the health behaviors of college students are the National College Health Assessment (NCHA)[27] and Monitoring the Future.[28] The NCHA is a national, nonprofit research effort organized by the American College Health Association.[27] Monitoring the Future, conducted at the University of

Table 6.1 Percentage of High School Students Who Reported Selected Sexual Risk Behaviors, by Year—Youth Risk Behavior Survey, United States, 1991, 2001, and 2011

Behavior	1991	2001	2011
Ever had sexual intercourse	54.1	45.6	47.4
Ever had sexual intercourse with four or more partners	18.7	14.2	15.3
Had sexual intercourse during the 3 months preceding the survey	37.5	33.4	33.7
Used alcohol or drugs before last sexual intercourse	21.6	25.6	22.1
Used or partner used condom at last sexual intercourse	46.2	57.9	60.2
Did not use any method to prevent pregnancy during last sexual intercourse	16.5	13.3	12.9

Source: Data from Centers for Disease Control and Prevention (2012). "Trends in the Prevalence of Sexual Behaviors and HIV Testing. National YRBS: 1991–2011." Available at http://www.cdc.gov/healthyyouth/yrbs/index.htm.

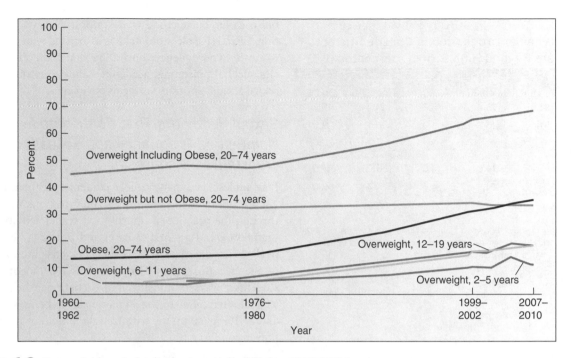

Figure 6.2 Overweight and obesity by age: United States, 1960–2006.

Data from National Center for Health Statistics (2012). *Health, United States, 2011, with Special Feature on Socioeconomic Status and Health.* Hyattsville, MD: Author; Odgen, C. and M. Carroll. (2010). *Prevalence of Obesity Among Children and Adolescents: United States, Trends 1963-1965 Through 2007-2008.* Atlanta, GA: Centers for Disease Control and Prevention.

Michigan's Institute for Social Research, is funded by the National Institute on Drug Abuse. Monitoring the Future specifically examines drug behaviors and related attitudes of a broad participant age range: eighth, tenth, and twelfth graders to adults through age 40,[28] whereas the NCHA examines a wide range of health behaviors in college students. These data sources, among others, can be helpful to those responsible for delivering health promotion education and services to many of the over 21 million students enrolled in the nation's colleges and universities.[29]

Behaviors That Contribute to Unintentional Injuries

Motor vehicle crashes, operating motor vehicles after consuming alcohol, riding with a driver who has consumed alcohol, swimming or boating while using alcohol, and not wearing seat belts are common incidences causing unintentional injuries to college-aged students.[15] Unintentional injuries have been the leading cause of death for young adults throughout the past 50 years (see Figure 6.1 presented earlier).[13]

Behaviors That Contribute to Violence

College campuses are communities just like small towns or neighborhoods in large cities. Thus, they have their share

of violence. Knowing this, most colleges and universities have programs in place to address issues of violence with a particular emphasis on sexual assault. Collectively, approximately one-fourth of female college students reported experiencing some form of sexual abuse/assault in the past school year—sexual touching (6.8%), verbal threats (15.3%), attempted penetration (3.2%), or sexual penetration (1.8%).[27] Although not all the reasons for these sexual assaults are clear, alcohol is a contributing factor in many of these episodes.

Tobacco Use

Statistics indicate that the more education a person has, the less likely he or she is to use tobacco. In 2010, the prevalence of daily smoking for college students was 7.6% versus 22.6% for age-mates not enrolled full-time in college.[28]

Alcohol and Other Drug Use

College and university campuses have long been thought of as places where alcohol and other drugs have been abused. Table 6.2 shows that alcohol is the drug of choice on college campuses, with 65% of students reporting that they had consumed alcohol in the previous 30 days. Table 6.2 also shows that illicit drug use continues to be a concern

Table 6.2 Trends in 30-Day Prevalence of Various Types of Drugs Among College Students 1 to 4 Years Beyond High School (percentage)

	1980	1990	2000	2010
Any illicit drug[a]	38.4	15.2	21.5	19.2
Any illicit drug other than marijuana	20.7	4.4	6.9	8.1
Marijuana	34.0	14.0	20.0	17.5
Alcohol	81.8	74.5	67.4	65.0
Cigarettes	25.8	21.5	28.2	16.4

[a]"Any illicit drug" includes use of marijuana, hallucinogens, cocaine, or heroin, or other narcotics, amphetamines, sedatives (barbiturates), methaqualone (until 1990), or tranquilizers not under a doctor's orders.
Source: Data from Johnston, L. D., P. M. O'Malley, J. G. Bachman, and J. E. Schulenberg (2011). *Monitoring the Future National Survey Results on Drug Use, 1975–2010.* Vol. II: College Students and Adults Ages 19–50. Bethesda, MD: National Institute on Drug Abuse.

with nearly one in six college students using marijuana in the past 30 days.[28] Although the number of individuals consuming alcohol has decreased over the past 30 years, **Figure 6.3** demonstrates the need for concern regarding the number of college students participating in binge drinking, which is commonly defined as consuming five or more drinks in a row.

According to the National College Health Association, 39.7% of males and 27.3% of females binge drank on at least one occasion during the 2 weeks prior to survey administration.[27] Excessive alcohol intake is associated with a number of adverse consequences, including fatal and nonfatal injuries, alcohol poisoning, academic failure, unprotected sex, sexual assault, and various forms of violence.[30,31]

Sexual Behaviors That Contribute to Unintended Pregnancy and Sexually Transmitted Diseases

Like adolescents, many college students put themselves at risk for unintended pregnancies and infections with STDs through the practice of unprotected sexual activity. More than 60% of all gonorrhea cases and nearly three-fourths of all chlamydia cases occur among persons under 25 years of age (see **Box 6.1**).[32] Only one-half (50.9%) of college students always or mostly used a condom when having vaginal intercourse in the 30 days prior to being surveyed, and 27.1% relied on the withdrawal method for pregnancy prevention.[27]

Community Health Strategies for Improving the Health of Adolescents and Young Adults

There are no easy, simple, or immediate solutions for reducing or eliminating the health problems of adolescents and young adults. Many health problems originate from the social and cultural environments in which people have been raised and live, and the culture and social norms

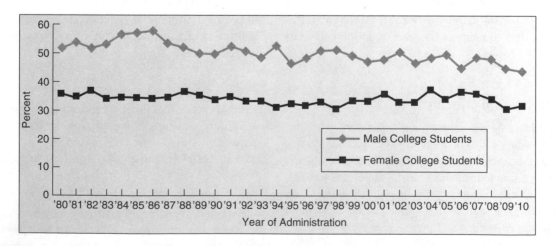

Figure 6.3 Alcohol: trends in two-week prevalence of five or more drinks in a row among male and female college students.
Reproduced from Johnston, L. D., P. M. O'Malley, and J. G. Bachman (2011). *Monitoring the Future National Survey Results on Drug Use, 1975–2010. Vol. II: College Students and Adults Ages 19–50.* Bethesda, MD: National Institute on Drug Abuse.

Box 6.1 *Healthy People 2020:* Objectives

Sexually Transmitted Diseases
Goal: Promote healthy sexual behaviors, strengthen community capacity, and increase access to quality services to prevent STDs and their complications.
Objective: STD-1 Reduce the proportion of adolescents and young adults with *Chlamydia trachomatis* infections.
STD 1.1 Among females aged 15 to 24 years attending family planning clinics:
Target: 6.7 percent.
Baseline: 7.4 percent of females aged 15 to 24 years who attended family planning clinics in the past 12 months tested positive for *Chlamydia trachomatis* infections in 2008.
Target setting method: 10 percent improvement.
Data source: STD Surveillance System (STDSS), CDC, NCHHSTP.
For Further Thought
If you were given the responsibility of lowering the incidence of chlamydia in the United States, what community health activities would you recommend?
Source: U.S. Department of Health and Human Services, Office of Disease Prevention and Health Promotion (2010). *Healthy People 2020.* Available at http://www.healthypeople.gov/2020/default.aspx.

that have been with us in some cases for many years. For example, alcohol contributes to all the leading causes of mortality and morbidity in these age groups. If the norm of a community is to turn its back on adolescents consuming alcohol or young adults (of legal age) abusing alcohol, efforts need to be made to change the culture. However, in most communities, culture and social norms do not change quickly. Efforts to turn these health problems around will need to be community-wide in nature and sustained over a long period of time. For examples of programs that have been effective, visit the SAMHSA (Substance Abuse and Mental Health Services Administration) National Registry of Evidence-Based Programs and Practices (NREPP) website at http://nrepp.samhsa.gov, which includes a searchable online registry of mental health and substance abuse interventions that have been reviewed and rated by independent reviewers.[33]

To change the culture, adolescent alcohol prevention efforts need to be a part of a comprehensive school health education effort and should include components outside the classroom. Thus, prevention programs need to include components that focus on changing norms, interaction among peers, social skills training, and developmental and cultural appropriateness.[34–36]

Many colleges and universities are trying to change the culture on campus as it relates to the use of alcohol. Research strongly supports an integrated approach to programming that targets: (1) individuals, including at-risk or alcohol-dependent drinkers; (2) the student population as a whole; and (3) the college and the surrounding community. Strategies such as cognitive-behavioral skills training, norms or values clarification, strengthening of students' intrinsic desire to change behavior, and challenging alcohol expectations have proved effective in changing the culture with college students.[37]

Adults

The adult age group (those 25 to 64 years old) represents slightly more than half of the U.S. population. The size of this segment of the overall population is expected to remain stable over the next couple of decades, but in proportion to the rest of the population this segment will become smaller. Therefore, provisions to deal with the health concerns of this age group will need to be maintained.

A Health Profile

The health profile of this age group of adults is characterized primarily by mortality from chronic diseases stemming from poor health behavior and poor lifestyle choices made during the earlier years of life.

Mortality

With life expectancy at birth between 75 and 80 years,[13] most Americans can expect to live beyond their 65th birthday. However, many do not. During the 1950s and 1960s, it was revealed that many of the leading causes of death in this age group resulted from preventable conditions associated with unhealthy behaviors and lifestyles. As such, many adults have quit smoking, and more Americans than ever before are exercising regularly and eating healthier diets. These lifestyle improvements, along with successes in public health and advances in medicine, have resulted in a significant decline in the death rate for adults.

In 2008, the leading causes of death for those in the 25–44 age group were unintentional injuries, malignant neoplasms (cancer), heart disease, suicide, homicide, and HIV. With the exception of HIV, the current leading causes of death were also at the top of the list in 1980.[13] When these mortality data were broken down in 2006 by age, sex, and ethnicity, some differences appear. For 25- to 34-year-olds, with the exception of diabetes mellitus for whites and HIV among blacks and Hispanics, the six leading causes of death are the same, but differ in rank order by race and ethnic group. For 35- to 44-year-olds, diabetes mellitus is among the six leading causes for whites, replacing homicide; liver disease and cirrhosis replaces suicide among Hispanics; and among blacks, the six leading causes include cerebrovascular disease (stroke) rather than suicide (see Table 6.3).[38]

For individuals in the 45–64 age group, the majority of deaths were the result of noncommunicable health problems. They include cancer; heart disease; unintentional injuries; chronic lower respiratory disease, which includes emphysema, asthma, and bronchitis; diabetes; chronic liver disease; and stroke.[13] Like with the 25- to 44-year-olds, there are racial and ethnic disparities. Although cancer and heart disease are the first and second causes of death for all three groups presented in Table 6.4, chronic lower respiratory disease appears in the list of the six leading causes for whites, HIV appears in the list for blacks, and liver disease and cirrhosis appears in the Hispanic list.[38]

Cancer

Since 1983, the number one cause of death in the adult age group has been cancer (malignant neoplasms). Age-adjusted cancer death rates have remained relatively steady since 1950 (193.9 per 100,000 in 1950 compared to 175.3 per 100,000 in 2008). However, the crude death rates have jumped from 139.8 per 100,000 to 186.0 per 100,000 during that same time, reflecting an aging U.S. population.[13]

Four types of cancers account for these large numbers—prostate, lung, and colorectal for men; and breast, lung, and colorectal for women. The leading cause of cancer deaths and the most preventable type of cancer for both men and women is lung cancer. This trend is expected to continue as large numbers of smokers continue to age. Cigarette smoking continues to be the most significant risk factor for lung cancer.[39] The second leading cause of cancer death is colorectal cancer, of which the risk increases with age. Modifiable factors associated with an increased risk include obesity, lack of physical activity, alcohol consumption, long-term smoking, a diet high in red or processed meats, and possibly inadequate intake of fruits and vegetables.[39] Breast cancer is the other cancer of much concern. Although it is less deadly than lung cancer, the number of cases of breast cancer is more than twice that of lung cancer in women.[39] Because of increased community awareness

Table 6.3 2006 Death Rates, Adults, Ages 25-34 and 35-44 (rate per 100,000 population)

	Non-Hispanic White		Non-Hispanic Black		Hispanic	
Cause	**25-34 (102.1)**	**35-44 (184.8)**	**25-34 (185.7)**	**35-44 (325.2)**	**25-34 (81.5)**	**35-44 (134.4)**
Unintentional injuries	41.8	43.6	35.6	42.4	29.7	31.6
Cancer	9.2	32.4	11.9	45.8	7.2	21.6
Heart disease	7.4	27.6	19.1	55.8	4.6	14.0
Suicide	15.3	19.1	8.7	7.5	7.1	6.6
Homicide	3.9	3.6	49.3	24.5	12.3	8.1
HIV	0.9	4.1	14.3	39.7	2.4	8.8
Liver disease and cirrhosis	0.7	5.9	–	4.6	1.1	6.7
Diabetes mellitus	1.4	4.4	4.4	10.6	0.9	2.8
Stroke	1.0	3.8	2.8	12.7	1.2	4.6

Source: Heron, M. (2010). "Deaths: Leading Causes for 2006." *National Vital Statistics Reports,* 58(14). Hyattsville, MD: National Center for Health Statistics.

Table 6.4   2006 Death Rates, Adults, Ages 45–54 and 55–64 (rate per 100,000 population)

Cause	Non-Hispanic White 45-54 (406.6)	Non-Hispanic White 55-64 (861.2)	Non-Hispanic Black 45-54 (738.5)	Non-Hispanic Black 55-64 (1,472.4)	Hispanic 45-54 (310.7)	Hispanic 55-64 (657.6)
Cancer	115.8	325.1	174.0	450.1	74.7	198.6
Heart disease	83.1	196.8	170.1	382.6	51.7	142.2
Unintentional injuries	46.5	35.4	56.2	49.5	35.6	33.2
Diabetes mellitus	11.0	30.3	28.0	79.3	13.2	42.6
Stroke	11.1	29.8	37.9	83.0	14.4	34.2
Chronic lower respiratory disease	9.9	43.7	12.3	38.1	2.6	12.0
Liver disease and cirrhosis	17.6	22.1	15.8	22.4	23.7	34.2
Suicide	21.0	17.1	6.0	–	6.5	6.0
Kidney disease	3.5	10.3	16.7	42.7	4.9	14.4
Septicemia	4.2	11.0	13.4	31.6	4.0	9.9

Source: Heron, M. (2010). "Deaths: Leading Causes for 2006." *National Vital Statistics Reports*, 58(14). Hyattsville, MD: National Center for Health Statistics.

and the availability of diagnostic screening for breast cancer, survival rates are much higher than for lung cancer. However, breast cancer rates could be reduced even further if a higher percentage of women 40 and over received regular mammograms.[39]

Cardiovascular Diseases

Some of the greatest changes in cause-specific mortality rates in adults are those for the cardiovascular diseases. Age-adjusted mortality rates from diseases of the heart dropped from 588.8 per 100,000 in 1950 to 186.5 per 100,000 in 2008, and deaths from strokes dropped from 180.7 per 100,000 to 40.7 per 100,000 during the same period of time.[13] These figures represent drops of about 70% and 75%, respectively. These changes are primarily the result of public health efforts that have encouraged people to stop smoking, increase their physical activity, and eat more nutritionally.

Health Behaviors and Lifestyle Choices

Many of the risk factors associated with the leading causes of morbidity and mortality in U.S. adults are associated with health behavior and lifestyle choices. Today, more than ever before, adults are watching what they eat, wearing their seat belts, controlling their blood pressure, and exercising with regularity. The prevalence of smoking among adults has declined, as has the incidence of drinking and driving. Although these are encouraging signs, much more still can be done.

Risk Factors for Chronic Disease

The best single behavioral change Americans can make to reduce morbidity and mortality is to stop smoking. Smoking is responsible for 30% of deaths in the United States[40] and is associated with many of the leading causes of death.[38] Three other interrelated risk factors that contribute to disease and death in this age group are lack of exercise, failure to maintain an appropriate body weight, and alcohol consumption. Although U.S. adults are exercising more than ever before, few are exercising on a regular basis. Less than 10% of U.S. adults are getting the recommended amount of moderate to vigorous physical activity each day.[41] Being overweight increases one's chances of encountering a number of health problems, including heart disease, some cancers, hypertension, elevated blood cholesterol, diabetes, stroke, gallbladder disease, and osteoarthritis. Results from the 2007–2008 National Health and Nutrition Examination Surveys (NHANES) indicate that 73% of 20- to 74-year-olds were overweight (including obese and extremely obese), with nearly 34% being obese and almost 6% being extremely obese as defined by **body mass index (BMI)**.[42] Obesity in the United States is truly an epidemic

body mass index (BMI) the ratio of weight (in kilograms) to height (in meters, squared)

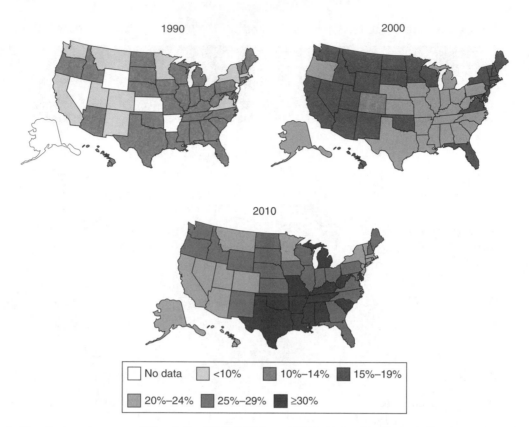

Figure 6.4 Obesity trends among U.S. adults: 1990, 2000, and 2010. Note: Obesity is defined as a BMI > 30, or about 30 pounds overweight for a five-foot, four-inch person.

Reproduced from Centers for Disease Control and Prevention. *Obesity Trends Among U.S. Adults, BRFSS, 1990, 2000, 2010.* Behavioral Risk Factor Surveillance System.

(see Figure 6.4).[43] The key to maintaining an appropriate weight throughout life is a combination of diet and exercise; total reliance on either factor alone makes it a difficult process.[43]

As with other age groups, alcohol consumption often places adults at greater health risk. Approximately 65% of adult Americans consume alcohol.[44] Although most do so in moderation, a relatively small percentage develop serious problems with their alcohol use. In 2010, 15% of adults reported binge drinking (males having five or more drinks on one occasion, females having four or more drinks on one occasion) in the previous month.[42] It has been estimated that the 5% who consume the greatest amount of alcohol consume about 36% of all the alcohol consumed in the United States.[45] These people are at greatest risk for developing a dependence on alcohol and for developing such alcohol-related health problems as cirrhosis and alcoholism.

One does not have to become dependent on alcohol to have a drinking problem. Alcohol contributes to society's problems in a great many other ways. Alcohol increases the rates of homicide, suicide, family violence, and unintentional injuries such as those from motor vehicle crashes, boating incidents, and falls. The use of alcohol by pregnant women can cause fetal alcohol spectrum disorder, one of the most common causes of mental retardation in children.[46] Clearly, alcohol consumption adversely affects the health and well-being of Americans.

Risk Factors for Personal Injury

Like individuals in the other age groups, adults also put themselves at risk for personal injury by the way they behave. Two such areas of concerns are both related to the operation of motor vehicles—the use of seat belts and the operation of a motor vehicle after drinking alcohol. Most Americans (84%) report wearing seat belts when driving or riding in a motor vehicle, which is an improvement from 15 years ago, when approximately 60% of the population reported wearing a seat belt when in a motor vehicle.[47] Among drivers 21 years or older, an estimated 15% drive under the influence of alcohol annually.[48] The data on both of these behaviors are interesting because both behaviors are regulated by public health laws. This suggests that a society can be controlled by regulations only to the extent that it wants to be.

Awareness and Screening of Certain Medical Conditions

A number of regular, noninvasive or minimally invasive health screenings are recommended for adults to participate in, such as screenings for hypertension, diabetes, high blood cholesterol, and cancer.

There is no "ideal" blood pressure. Instead, the acceptable blood pressure falls within a range considered healthy. **Hypertension** exists when systolic pressure is equal to or greater than 140 mm of mercury (Hg) and/or diastolic pressure is equal to or greater than 90 mm Hg for extended periods of time. Statistics show that hypertension is found in about one in three adults in the United States, with one-third of those unaware they have it, making it the most prevalent risk factor for cardiovascular disease in the United States.[49] Fortunately, once detected, hypertension is a risk factor that is highly modifiable (see **Figure 6.5**). The most desirable means of controlling hypertension is through a combination of diet modification, appropriate physical exercise, and weight management.[49]

Diabetes results from failure of the pancreas to make or use a sufficient amount of insulin. Without insulin, food cannot be properly used by the body. Diabetes cannot be cured, but it can be controlled through a combination of diet, exercise, medications, and insulin injections. The percentage of

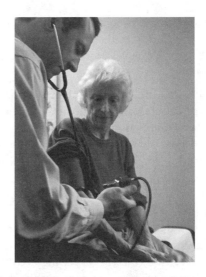

Figure 6.5 Hypertension is a highly modifiable risk factor.
© Photodisc

adults with diagnosed diabetes has increased significantly over the past 20 years (see **Figure 6.6**).[42] Furthermore, many individuals with diabetes are unaware they have the disease.[50] Early detection and treatment could greatly decrease the number of deaths associated with diabetes.

Cholesterol is a soft, fatlike substance that is necessary to build cell membranes. About 75% of cholesterol is produced by the liver and other cells in the body, with the other 25% coming from the foods we eat, specifically animal products. Elevated cholesterol

> **hypertension** systolic pressure equal to or greater than 140 mm of mercury (Hg) and/or diastolic pressure equal to or greater than 90 mm Hg for extended periods of time

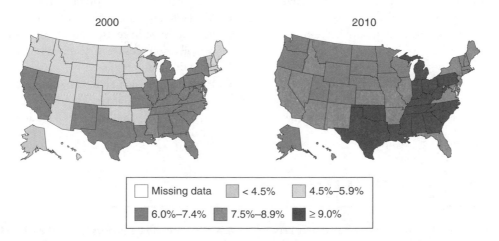

Figure 6.6 Age-adjusted percentage of U.S. adults who had diagnosed diabetes, 2000 and 2010.

Reproduced from Centers for Disease Control and Prevention: National Diabetes Surveillance System. Available at http://apps.nccd.cdc.gov/ddtstrs/default.aspx. Accessed July 15, 2012.

levels in blood can put people at greater risk for heart disease and stroke. The higher the cholesterol level, the greater the risk.[51] A person's cholesterol level is affected by age, heredity, and diet.

Dietary factors are associated with 4 of the 10 leading causes of death in this age group. Many dietary components are involved in the diet–health relationship, but chief among them is the disproportionate consumption of foods high in fat, often at the expense of foods high in complex carbohydrates and dietary fiber. Total dietary fat (saturated and unsaturated) accounts for too many total calories consumed in the United States.[51] Blood cholesterol levels less than 200 mg/dL in middle-aged adults seem to indicate a relatively low risk of coronary heart disease. In contrast, people with a blood cholesterol level of 240 mg/dL have twice the risk of having a coronary heart attack as do people who have a cholesterol level of 200 mg/dL.[51] **Hypercholesterolemia** is the term used for high levels of cholesterol in the blood. Like diabetes, the key to controlling hypercholesterolemia is screening and treatment.

The other prevalent medical condition in this age group that should be screened for on a regular basis is cancer. As noted earlier, malignant neoplasms are the leading cause of death in 45- to 64-year-olds. The American Cancer Society recommends a number of

hypercholesterol-emia high levels of cholesterol in the blood

screenings for various age groups. The earlier that cancer is detected, the greater the chance for successful treatment.

Community Health Strategies for Improving the Health of Adults

Adults in the United States face a number of health issues. Even so, for most individuals the years between 25 and 64 are some of the healthiest of their lifetime. A key to keeping these people healthy is to reemphasize the importance of individual responsibility for health; that is, individuals must engage in behaviors that are health enhancing. From a community health perspective, this means that community health workers must continue to offer primary, secondary, and tertiary prevention programs that are aimed at the needs of this age group. For example, primary prevention programs could include exercise and nutrition programs that help reduce the risks of cancer and cardiovascular disease. Secondary prevention programs that emphasize self or clinical screenings to identify and control disease processes in their early stages, such as mammography, self-testicular exams, and cholesterol screenings, are also appropriate for this age group. In addition, tertiary prevention programs such as medication compliance to prevent disability by restoring individuals to their optimal level of functioning after the onset of disease or injury could also be useful.

Chapter Summary

- The overall health status of 15 to 64 year olds could be improved by reducing the prevalence of high-risk behaviors (e.g., cigarette smoking, excessive alcohol consumption, and physical inactivity) and by increasing participation in health screenings and institutionalizing preventive health care in our society.
- Adolescents and young adults are at risk of early death due to motor vehicle crashes and other unintentional injuries and remain at considerable risk for STD morbidity.

- College students put themselves at considerable risk through unprotected sexual activity and the use of alcohol, tobacco, and other drugs.
- Mortality rates for older adults (45 to 64 years old) have declined in recent years, but cancer is still the overall leading cause of death, followed by cardiovascular disease.
- Health problems in adults resulting from unhealthy behaviors—such as smoking, poor diet, and physical inactivity—can be reduced if adults are willing to modify their behavior.

Review Questions

1. Why it is important for community health workers to be aware of the significant health problems of the various age groups in the United States?

2. What are the behaviors that put each of these cohorts—adolescents, college students, and adults—at greatest risk?

3. What are key data sources used by community health professionals to assess the needs of adolescents, young adults, and adults?
4. How would you summarize the health profile of the two cohorts (adolescents and young adults, and adults) presented in this chapter?

5. What are recommended community health strategies for improving the health status of adolescents and young adults, and adults?

Activities

1. Obtain data presenting the 10 leading causes of death according to age and race for the age groups presented in this chapter. Review the data, and prepare to lead a discussion on the conclusions that can be drawn about race, the leading causes of death, and age.

2. Interview a small group (about 10) of adults (ages 45 to 64) about their present health status. Ask them questions about their health behavior and health problems. Then, summarize the data you collect in writing and compare them to the information in this chapter on this age group. How are the data similar? How do they differ?

Community Health on the Web

The Internet contains a wealth of information about community and public health. Increase your knowledge of some of the topics presented in this chapter by accessing the Jones & Bartlett Learning website at **go.jblearning.com/McKenzieBrief** and follow the links to complete the following Web activities:

- Youth Risk Behavior Surveillance System
- Vital Statistics

References

1. Snyder, T., and L. Shafer (1996). *Youth Indicators, 1996* (NCES 96-027). Washington, DC: U.S. Department of Education, National Center for Education Statistics.
2. MacKay, A. P., L. A. Fingerhut, and C. R. Duran (2000). *Health, United States, 2000 with Adolescent Health Chartbook.* Hyattsville, MD: National Center for Health Statistics.
3. Seffrin, J. R. (1990). "The Comprehensive School Health Curriculum: Closing the Gap Between State-of-the-Art and State-of-the-Practice." *Journal of School Health,* 60(4): 151-156.
4. Valois, R. F., W. G. Thatcher, J. W. Drane, and B. M. Reininger (1997). "Comparison of Selected Health Risk Behaviors Between Adolescents in Public and Private High Schools in South Carolina." *Journal of School Health,* 67(10): 434-440.
5. Hobbs, F., and N. Stoops (2002). *Demographic Trends in the 20th Century* (Census 2000 Special Reports, Series CENSR-4). Washington, DC: U.S. Government Printing Office.
6. U.S. Bureau of the Census (1999). *Statistical Abstract of the United States, 1999,* 119th ed. Washington, DC: Author.
7. U.S. Census Bureau (2010). *The 2010 Statistical Abstract.* Available at http://www.census.gov/compendia/statab/2010/2010edition.html.
8. Howden, L., and J. Meyer. (2011). *Age and Sex Composition: 2010.* 2010 Census Briefs, May 2011. Washington, DC: U.S. Census Bureau. Available at http://www.census.gov/prod/cen2010/briefs/c2010br-03.pdf.
9. Annie E. Casey Foundation (2010). "Children in Single-Parent Families by Race (Percent)–2010." Available at http://datacenter.kidscount.org/data/acrossstates/Rankings.aspx?ind=107.
10. Annie E. Casey Foundation (2012). "2012 Kids Count Data Book." Available at http://datacenter.kidscount.org/DataBook/2012/OnlineBooks/KIDSCOUNT2012DataBookFullReport.pdf.
11. Toosi, M. (2012, January). "Labor Force Projections to 2020: A More Slowly Growing Workforce." *Monthly Labor Review* pp. 43-64.
12. U.S. Department of Labor, Bureau of Labor Statistics (2010). "Labor Force Statistics from the Current Population Survey." Available at http://data.bls.gov/cgi-bin/surveymost?ln.

13. National Center for Health Statistics (2012). *Health, United States, 2011 with Special Feature on Socioeconomic Status and Health*. Hyattsville, MD: Author.

14. U.S. Department of Health and Human Services (2012). *Healthy People 2020: Social Determinants of Health*. Washington, DC: Author. Available at http://www.healthypeople.gov/2020 /default.aspx.

15. Centers for Disease Control and Prevention (2012). "Youth Risk Behavior Surveillance–United States, 2011." *MMWR Surveillance Summaries*, 61(SS-4).

16. Centers for Disease Control and Prevention (2011). *Sexually Transmitted Disease Surveillance, 2010*. Atlanta, GA: U.S. Department of Health and Human Services.

17. Centers for Disease Control and Prevention (2012). "Sexually Transmitted Diseases. CDC Fact Sheets." Available at http://www.cdc.gov/std/healthcomm/fact_sheets.htm.

18. National Institute on Drug Abuse (2009). *Research Report Series: Tobacco Addiction*. Washington, DC: U.S. Department of Health and Human Services.

19. American Heart Association, American Cancer Society, Campaign for Tobacco-Free Kids, and American Lung Association (2006). "A Broken Promise to Our Children: The 1998 State Tobacco Settlement Eight Years Later." Available at http://www.tobaccofreekids.org/what_we_do/state_local /tobacco_settlement/.

20. Campaign for Tobacco-Free Kids (2009, February 4). "Congress, President Deliver Historic Victory for Children's Health by Increasing Tobacco Taxes to Fund SCHIP Program." Available at http://www.tobaccofreekids.org.

21. Campaign for Tobacco-Free Kids (2009, June 22). "New Law Protects Kids, Will Save Lives." Available at http://www .tobaccofreekids.org.

22. Centers for Disease Control and Prevention (1996). "Trends in Sexual Risk Behavior Among High School Students–United States–1990, 1991, and 1993." *Morbidity and Mortality Weekly Report*, 44(7): 124-125, 131-132.

23. Centers for Disease Control and Prevention (2012). "Sexual Risk Behavior: HIV, STD, and Teen Pregnancy Prevention." Available at http://www.cdc.gov/HealthyYouth/sexualbehaviors /index.htm.

24. Kost, K., S. Henshaw, and L. Carlin (2010). *U.S. Teenage Pregnancies, Births and Abortions: National and State Trends and Trends by Race and Ethnicity*. Available at http://www .guttmacher.org/pubs/USTPtrends.pdf.

25. The National Campaign to Prevent Teen and Unplanned Pregnancy (2008). "Briefly . . . Unplanned Pregnancy in the United States." Available at http://www.thenationalcampaign .org/resources/pdf/briefly-unplanned-in-the-united-states.pdf.

26. The National Campaign to Prevent Teen and Unplanned Pregnancy (2009). "Briefly...Unplanned Pregnancy and Community College." Available at http://www.thenational campaign.org/colleges/publications.aspx.

27. American College Health Association (2011, Fall). "National College Health Assessment, Reference Group Executive Summary." Available at http://www.achancha.org/docs /ACHA-NCHA-II_ReferenceGroup_ExecutiveSummary_Fall2011 .pdf.

28. Johnston, L. D., P. M. O'Malley, and J. E. Schulenberg (2011). *Monitoring the Future National Survey Results on Drug Use, 1975-2010*. Vol. II: College Students and Adults Ages 19-50. Bethesda, MD: National Institute on Drug Abuse.

29. U.S. Department of Education Statistics (2011). *Digest of Education Statistics: 2010*. Available at http://nces.ed.gov /programs/digest/.

30. Gealt, R., W. Gunter, S. Martin, D. O'Connell, and C. Visher (2011). *Binge Drinking and Other Risk Behaviors Among College Students*. Newark, DE: University of Delaware Center for Drug and Alcohol Studies.

31. Goldman, M. S., G. M. Boyd, and V. Faden, eds. (2002, March). "College Drinking, What It Is, and What to Do About It: A Review of the State of the Science" [Special issue]. *Journal of Studies on Alcohol* (Suppl. 14).

32. Centers for Disease Control and Prevention (2010). *Sexually Transmitted Disease Surveillance, 2009*. Atlanta, GA: Author.

33. Substance Abuse and Mental Health Services Administration (2012). "SAMHSA National Registry of Evidence-Based Programs and Practices." Available at http://www.nrepp .samhsa.gov.

34. Dusenbury, L., and M. Falco (1995). "Eleven Components of Effective Drug Abuse Prevention Curricula." *Journal of School Health*, 65: 420-425.

35. Joint Committee on National Health Education Standards (2007). *National Health Education Standards*, 2nd ed. Atlanta, GA: ACS.

36. Centers for Disease Control and Prevention (2007). *Health Education Curriculum Analysis Tool (HECAT)*. Atlanta, GA: Author. Available at http://www.cdc.gov/healthyyouth/HECAT /index.htm.

37. National Institute on Alcohol Abuse and Alcoholism (2007). *A Call to Action: Changing the Culture of Drinking at U.S. Colleges*. Washington, DC: Author.

38. Heron, M. (2010). "Deaths: Leading Causes for 2006." *National Vital Statistics Reports*, 58(14). Hyattsville, MD: National Center for Health Statistics.

39. American Cancer Society (2012). *Cancer Facts and Figures 2012*. Atlanta, GA: Author.

40. Mokdad, A. H., J. S. Marks, D. F. Stroup, and J. L. Gerberding (2004). "Actual Causes of Death in the United States, 2000." *Journal of the American Medical Association*, 291(10): 1238-1245.

41. American Heart Association (2010). "Obesity, Nutrition, and Physical Activity." Available at http://www.heart.org /obesitypolicy.

42. Centers for Disease Control and Prevention (2010). "Behavioral Risk Factor Surveillance System." Available at http://www.cdc.gov/brfss/index.htm.

43. Centers for Disease Control and Prevention (2012). "Overweight and Obesity." Available at http://www.cdc.gov /obesity/.

44. Pleis, J. R., J. W. Lucas, and B. W. Ward (2009). "Summary Health Statistics for U.S. Adults: National Health Interview Survey, 2008." *Vital and Health Statistics*, 10(242). Available at http://www.cdc.gov/nchs/data/series/sr_10/sr10_242.pdf.

45. Manning, W. G., L. Blumberg, and L. H. Moulton (1995). "The Demand for Alcohol: The Differential Response to Price." *Journal of Health Economics*, 14(2): 123-145.

46. March of Dimes (2012). "Alcohol During Pregnancy." Available at http://www.marchofdimes.com/pregnancy/alcohol_indepth .html.

47. Chen, Y., and T. Jianqiang (2010). *Seat Belt Use in 2009–Use Rates in the States and Territories*. Washington, DC: NHTSA National Center for Statistics and Analysis. Available at http://www-nrd.nhtsa.dot.gov/Pubs/811324.pdf.

48. Substance Abuse and Mental Health Services Administration (2006). *The NSDUH Report: Driving Under the Influence Among Adult Drivers*. Available at http://www.oas.samhsa.gov/2K5/DUI/DUI.cfm.

49. American Heart Association (2012). "High Blood Pressure". Available at http://www.heart.org/HEARTORG/Conditions/HighBloodPressure/High-Blood-Pressure_UCM_002020_SubHomePage.jsp.

50. American Diabetes Association (2012). "Diabetes Basics." Available at http://www.diabetes.org/diabetes-basics.

51. American Heart Association (2012). "Cholesterol Levels." Available at http://www.heart.org/HEARTORG/Conditions/Cholesterol/Cholesterol_UCM_001089_SubHomePage.jsp.

Chapter 7

Elders

Charity Bishop, MA, CHES

Chapter Objectives

After studying this chapter, you will be able to:

1. Identify the characteristics of an aging population.

2. Define the terms associated with elders.

3. Describe demographic characteristics of elders.

4. Explain how health behaviors can improve the quality of later life.

5. Briefly outline elder abuse and neglect in the United States.

6. Identify the instrumental needs of older adults.

7. Briefly summarize the Older Americans Act of 1965.

8. List the services provided for older adults in most communities.

Introduction

The U.S. population is growing older. The number of **elders** in the United States and their proportion of the total population increased dramatically during the twentieth and early twenty-first centuries. In 1950, there were 12 million people (8% of the population) age 65 years or older; by 2008, that number had increased to 38.9 million. "They represented 12.8% of the U.S. population, over one in every eight Americans."[1] For the first time in U.S. history, a significant number of Americans will achieve elder status and, in doing so, live long enough to assume some responsibilities for the care of their aging parents. In the twenty-first century, the economic, social, and health issues associated with the growing proportion of people older than age 65 in the United States have become major political concerns. In this chapter, we will define terminology, describe the demographics, and discuss the special needs of and community service for the aging.

Definitions

A person's age might depend on who measures it and how they define it. For example, whereas demographers might define old according to chronological years, clinicians might define it by stages of physiological development, and psychologists by developmental stages. Children might see their 35-year-old teacher as old, whereas the 35-year-old teacher might regard her 61-year-old principal as old. Age is and always will be a relative concept.

In the United States and other developed countries, people are considered old once they reach the age of 65. But because there are a number of people who are very active and healthy at age 65 and will live a number of productive years after 65, researchers have subdivided old into the young old (65–74), the middle old (75–84), and the old old (85 or over). Interestingly enough, it is this latter group, the old old, that makes up the fastest-growing segment of the elder population.

Also for the purposes of our discussion in this chapter, we use terms that are associated with aging. They include the following:

> **demography** the study of a population and those variables bringing about change in that population
>
> **elders** those 65 years of age or older

aged: The state of being old. A person may be defined as aged on the basis of having reached a specific age; for example, 65 years is often used for social or legislative policies, whereas 75 years is used for physiological evaluations by geriatricians.[2]

aging: The changes that occur normally in plants and animals as they grow older. Some age changes begin at birth and continue until death; other changes begin at maturity and end at death.[2]

geriatrics: The branch of medicine concerned with medical problems and care of the elderly.[3]

geriatrician: A physician specializing in the care of patients with multiple chronic diseases who may not be able to be cured but whose care can be managed.[3]

gerontology: The multidisciplinary study of the biological, psychological, and social processes of aging and the elderly.[3]

Many terms have been used to describe individuals who are 65 years of age or older, including seniors, "senior citizens, golden agers, retired persons, mature adults, elderly, aged, and old people. There is no clear preference among older people for any of these terms."[4] As Ferrini and Ferrini have stated, "Many gerontologists have chosen to adopt the term 'elder' to describe those 65 and older. This term is an attempt to redefine aging in a more positive way that connotes wisdom, respect, leadership, and accumulated knowledge."[4]

Demography of Aging

Demography is "the study of a population (an aggregate of individuals) and those variables bringing about change in that population."[2] The demography of aging is typically defined as a study of those who are 65 years or older and of the variables that bring about change in their lives. In the following paragraphs, we review some of the demographic features of the elder population, including size, growth rate, and the factors that contribute to this growth. We also discuss other demographic characteristics of this population, such as living arrangements, racial and ethnic composition, geographic distribution, economic status, and housing.

Size and Growth of the Elder Population

The aging of any population can be graphically illustrated with a symbolic age pyramid[5] (see **Figure 7.1**). The base of this pyramid represents the youngest and largest segment of the population. The sloping sides indicate higher mortality rates and limited life expectancy. Until the mid-1950s, the population pyramid for the United States was not so very different from the traditional age pyramid.

Since the mid-1950s, however, the shape of the United States' population pyramid has changed. As noted earlier

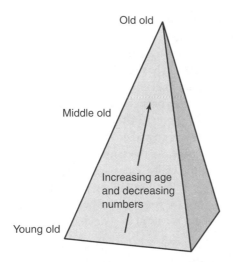

Figure 7.1 Symbolic age pyramid.

in the chapter, both the number of elders and the proportion of the total population made up of elders grew significantly during the twentieth and early twenty-first centuries. Demographers' projections suggest that populations will continue to age, not only in this country, but also in most other countries. In 2011, the baby boom generation began to turn 65, and it is projected that by 2030, 71.5 million people (1 in 5) will be age 65 or older.[1] The population aged 85 or older is currently the fastest-growing segment of the older population. It will double in size by 2030.[6] During this same time, it is expected that the percentage of people age 18 or younger will decrease slightly to around 24%. These

changes will alter the shape of the population pyramid and make it more like the shape of a population rectangle. **Figure 7.2** shows the difference in the population pyramid of 2000 and the projections for 2030.

As one might guess, the projected growth of the elder population is expected to raise the **median age** of the U.S. population. In 2000, the median age was 35.3 years.[7] Projections put the median age at 36.9 years in 2010, and then continue up to 39 years by 2035 and stay right around that number until 2050.[7]

Factors That Affect Population Size and Age

Three factors affect the size and age of a population: its fertility rates, its mortality rates, and its gain or loss from migration of individuals into or out of that population.[2] Although one might assume that all populations will age with time, that is not necessarily true. In fact, a population could get younger with time.[2] If fertility rates and mortality rates are both high, life expectancy would be low, and the age of a population could grow younger. However, this has not been the case in the United States.

Fertility Rates

The fertility rate is an expression of the number of births per 1,000 women of childbearing age (15–44 years) in the population during a specific time period. Fertility rates in the United

> **median age** the age at which half of the population is older and half is younger

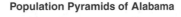

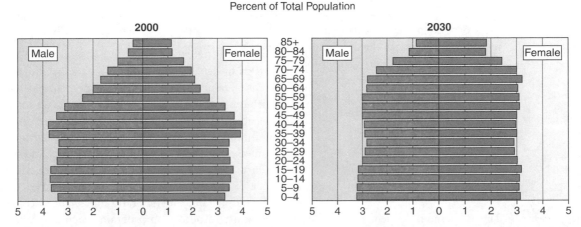

Figure 7.2 Population pyramid for 2000 and the projected pyramid for 2030: Percentage of total population.

U.S. Census Bureau, Population Division. (2005). Interim State Population Projections, 2005.

States were at their highest at the beginning of the twentieth century. Those rates dipped during the Depression years but rebounded after World War II. The period of consistently high fertility rates immediately following World War II has become known as the "baby boom years," hence the name *baby boomers* for those born between 1946 and 1964. During those years, 76 million babies were born. U.S. society has tried to adjust to the size and needs of the baby boom generation throughout the stages of the life cycle. Just as this generation had a dramatic impact on expanding obstetrics and pediatrics, creating split shifts for students in public schools, and disrupting government policy toward the Vietnam War, the baby boom cohorts will also place tremendous strain on programs and services (e.g., Social Security and Medicare) required by an elderly population.[8]

Mortality Rates

The mortality or death rate (usually expressed in deaths per 100,000 population) also has an impact on the aging population. The annual crude mortality rate in the United States in 1900 was 1,720 per 100,000. Recent data show that figure has dropped by more than half to 810.[9] The decrease in the annual mortality rate achieved over the twentieth century was the result of triumphs in medical science and public health practice.

Another demographic variable that interacts with the mortality rate is life expectancy. Although the mortality rate in the United States has been fairly constant for 20+ years, life expectancy has continued to increase. During the twentieth and early twenty-first centuries, there was an overall jump in life expectancy at birth from 47.3 years in 1900 to 77.9 years in 2007.[9] The life expectancy of men and black Americans has always trailed those of women and white Americans, respectively. Whereas the increase in life expectancy in the first half of the twentieth century could be attributed to the decrease in infant and early childhood deaths, the increase in life expectancy since 1970 can be traced to the postponement of death among the middle-aged and elder population.

Migration

The movement of people from one country to another, migration, has also contributed to the aging of the population. **Net migration** is the population gain or loss from the movement of migrants into (immigration) and out of (emigration) a country. Historically in the United States, net migration has resulted in population gain; more people immigrate than emigrate. The greatest immigration in the United States occurred between the end of the Civil War and the beginning of the Great Depression. Most of the immigrants were between the ages of 18 and 35 years—of childbearing age. As these immigrants had children, the population of the United States remained young. However, the decline in immigration following the Depression led to the aging of the U.S. populace as the early immigrants grew old and were not replaced by younger immigrants.

Fortunately, however, the United States continued to absorb young immigrants during the closing decades of the twentieth century. As a consequence, the dependency ratio of workers to older adults in the United States is declining more slowly than in many other developed countries.

Dependency and Labor-Force Ratios

Other demographic signs of an aging population are changes in dependency and labor-force ratios. The **dependency ratio** is a comparison between those individuals whom society considers economically unproductive (the nonworking or dependent population) and those it considers economically productive (the working population). Traditionally, the productive and nonproductive populations have been defined by age; the productive population includes those who are 19 to 64 years of age. The unproductive population includes both youth (0–19 years old) and the old (65+ years). When the dependency ratio includes both youth and elders, it is referred to as a **total dependency ratio**. When only the youth are compared to the productive group, the term used is **youth dependency ratio**; when only the old are compared, it is called **old-age dependency ratio**.

Changes in dependency ratios "provide an indirect broad indication of periods when we can expect the particular age distribution of the country to affect the need for distinct types of social services, housing, and consumer products."[10] Communities can refer to dependency ratio data as a guide for making the best social policy decisions and as a way to allocate resources. For example, leaders in a community with a relatively high youth dependency ratio compared to the old-age dependency ratio may want to concentrate community resources on programs such as education for the young, health promotion programs for children, special programs for working parents, and other youth-associated

---

dependency ratio a ratio that compares the number of individuals whom society considers economically unproductive to the number it considers economically productive

net migration the population gain or loss resulting from migration

old-age dependency ratio the dependency ratio that includes only old-age dependency

total dependency ratio the dependency ratio that includes both youth and old-age dependency

youth dependency ratio the dependency ratio that includes only youth dependency

concerns. Communities with high old-age dependency ratios might increase programs for elders, including programs to reengage retirees into **encore careers**.

The total dependency ratio (DR) is calculated by adding the number of youth and elders, divided by the number of persons 20 to 64 years of age, times 100. In the twentieth century, the lowest DR (70.5) was recorded in 1900. The DR in 2010 was 67, but projections have it climbing to a peak of 85 in 2040 and staying steady through 2050[11] (see **Figure 7.3**). This increase over the next 30 to 40 years will be driven by the old-age dependency ratio and thus will guide future social policy.

Such an increase in the old-age dependency ratio provides an interesting political scenario because the costs to support youth and the old are not the same. Parents pay directly for most of the expenditures to support their children, with the primary exception being public education, which is paid for by taxes. In contrast, much of the support for elders comes from tax-supported programs such as Social Security, Medicare, and Medicaid. To meet the impending burden of the elderly, taxes will most certainly need to be raised or benefits reduced. Therefore, the two questions for the future are: Will the productive population be willing to pay increased taxes to support elders? Will services to the elderly be drastically reduced?

Although dependency ratio data clearly show one trend, they are merely an estimate and should not be the only accepted estimate. Actually, the dependency ratios presented in Figure 7.3 are based on the assumption that everyone of productive age supports all members of the nonproductive age group. Obviously, this is not the case. Many of those in the productive age group (for instance, homemakers, those who are unemployed, and those who are disabled) do not participate in the paid labor force. Conversely, many teenagers and elders do. Thus, dependency ratios, in some situations, could provide misleading figures for decision makers.

Other experts believe that labor-force ratios also need to be considered. **Labor-force ratios** differ from dependency ratios in that they are based on the number of people who are actually working and those who are not, independent of their ages. When labor-force participation rates

encore careers when individuals transition out of their work careers and into jobs and volunteer opportunities in nonprofit and public sectors

labor-force ratio compares the total number of those individuals who are not working (regardless of age) to the number of those who are

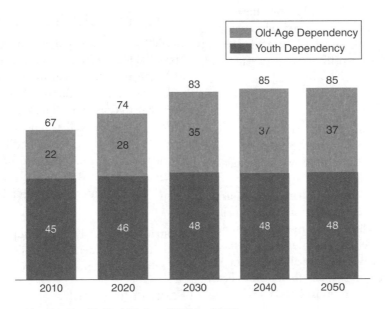

Figure 7.3 Dependency ratios for the United States: 2010 to 2050.

Note: Total dependency = ((Population under age 20 + Population age 65 years or over)/(Population ages 20 to 64 years)) × 100. Old-age dependency = (Population age 65 years or over/Population ages 20 to 64 years) × 100. Youth dependency = (Population under age 20 / Population ages 20 to 64 years) × 100.

U.S. Census Bureau (2010). "The Next Four Decades, The Older Population in the United States: 2010 to 2050, Current Population Reports" (#P25-1138). Available at http://www.census.gov/newsroom/releases/archives/aging_population/cb10-72.html.

are used to calculate the labor-force ratios, it is projected that the burden of support for the labor force in the future will be somewhat lighter than that projected through dependency ratios. This is because baby boomers plan to work longer than did members of the previous generations.[12]

Other Demographic Variables Affecting Elders

Other demographic variables that affect the community health programs of older Americans include marital status, living arrangements, racial and ethnic composition, geographic distribution, economic status, and housing.

Marital Status

Approximately three-fourths of elder men are married, whereas just over half of elder women are married. In addition, elder women are three times more likely than men to be widowed.[8] There are three primary reasons for these differences. First, men have shorter average life expectancies than women (75.7 vs. 80.8 years in 2010)[7] and thus tend to precede their wives in death. Second, men tend to marry women who are younger than themselves. Finally, men who lose a spouse through death or divorce are more likely to remarry than women in the same situation. These statistics reveal that most elder men have a spouse for assistance, especially when health fails, whereas most elder women do not.

As the baby boomers move into their older years, the number of divorced elders will grow. These divorced elders represent a new type of need group—those who lack the retirement benefits, insurance, and net worth assets associated with being married.

Living Arrangements

"Like marital status, the living arrangements of America's older population are important because they are closely linked to income, health status, and the availability of caregivers. Older persons who live alone are more likely to be in poverty than older persons who live with their spouses."[8]

assisted-living facility a special combination of housing, personalized supportive services, and health care designed to meet the needs—both scheduled and unscheduled—of those who need help with activities of daily living

Two-thirds of noninstitutionalized elders live with someone else (spouse, relative, or other nonrelatives), and the remainder live alone.[8] Women are much more likely than men to be living alone (almost 2 to 1).

Only a small percentage of the elderly population in the United States resides in nursing homes. About 1.8 million of those age 65 years or older are in nursing homes, representing 5% of the elder population.[7] This percentage is down from previous years, in part as a result of the increase in **assisted-living facilities**, which provide an alternative to long-term care in a nursing home. Approximately three-fourths of nursing home residents are women, and more than half of all nursing home residents are older than 85 years. The proportion of elders living in a nursing home increases with age.[8]

Racial and Ethnic Composition

As the elder population grows larger, it will also grow more diverse, reflecting the demographic changes in the U.S. population as a whole. In 2010, the elder population was predominately white. Of the total elder population in 2010, it was estimated that about 80% were white; 9% were black; 7% were of Hispanic origin; 3% were Asian; and less than 1% were Pacific Islanders, American Indians, or Alaska Natives.[1] By 2050, the white population is expected to decline to 58%, whereas Americans of Hispanic origin will increase to 15%, black Americans will increase to 11%, Asian Americans will increase to 8%, and Pacific Islanders, American Indians, and Alaska Natives will stay at less than 1% but still continue to grow in numbers.[1]

As the older population becomes more ethnically diverse, health professionals will need to become more knowledgeable about the cultural backgrounds of their elder clients.

Geographic Distribution

In 2008, it was estimated that about two-fifths of the United States' elders lived in southern states (see **Figure 7.4**), and just more than half lived in the following 10 states: California, Florida, Illinois, Michigan, New Jersey, New York, North Carolina, Ohio, Pennsylvania, and Texas. Each of these states, as well as nine other states, had more than 1 million elders. California had the greatest number, and Florida had the greatest proportion.[1] Some states, including many in the Midwest, have a small total number of elders, but the elders make up a large percentage of their total population.

From an ethnic and racial standpoint, the regional concentrations of the elderly are similar to the concentrations of the total population of each group.[11]

Economic Status

In 1970, about 25% of the elderly lived in poverty, whereas in 2006 the figure had dropped to just less than 9%.[8] Today, a smaller percentage of the elderly are impoverished than among those under age 18.[13]

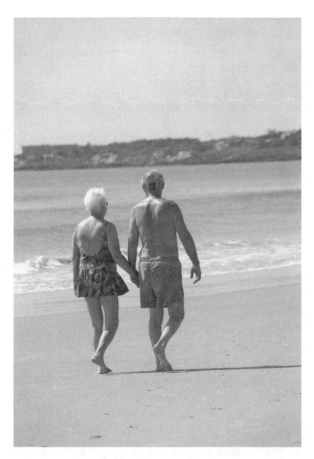

Figure 7.4 Many elders choose to spend their retirement years in states with warm weather.
© Elena Elisseeva/ShutterStock, Inc.

When the sources of income of elders are examined, it is found that 37% of elder income comes from Social Security, 28% comes from earnings, almost equal percentages come from asset income (15%) and pensions (18%), and a small percentage (2%) comes from other miscellaneous sources.[8] Because just more than one-fourth of elder income comes from work earnings, they are economically more vulnerable to circumstances beyond their control, such as the loss of a spouse; deteriorating health and self-sufficiency; changes in Social Security, Medicare, and Medicaid legislation; and inflation.[14]

Housing

In general, most older Americans live in adequate, affordable housing.[8] Of the almost 3 million households headed by older Americans in 2007, 80% were owners and 20% were renters.[15] Characteristics of the homes of elders versus those of younger people are that elders have (1) older homes, (2) homes of lower value, (3) homes in greater need of repair, and (4) homes less likely to have central heating and air conditioning.[15]

For most elders, housing represents an asset because they have no mortgage or rental payments, or they can sell their home for a profit. But for others with low incomes, housing becomes a heavy burden. Approximately 30% of all elderly households pay more for housing than they can afford.[16] The cost of utilities, real estate taxes, insurance, repairs, and maintenance have forced many to sell their property or live in a less-desirable residence.

A Health Profile of Elders

The health status of elders has improved over the years, in terms of both living longer and remaining functional. The percentage of chronically disabled older persons—those with impairments for 3 months or longer that impede daily activities—has been slowly falling. However, we do know that the most consistent risk factor of illness and death across the total population is age, and that, in general, the health status of elders is not as good as for their younger counterparts. In this section of the chapter, we examine some of the health concerns of aging, including mortality, morbidity, and health behaviors and lifestyle choices.

Mortality

In 2007, the top five causes of death for elders, in order of number of deaths, were heart disease, cancer, stroke, chronic lower respiratory disease (CLRD), and Alzheimer's disease.[17] These five causes of death were responsible for two-thirds of elder deaths.[17] Over the past 50 years, the overall age-adjusted mortality rate for elders has continued to fall. The primary reason for this has been the declining death rates for heart disease and stroke. Despite such drops, heart disease remains the leading cause of death in this age group, and it is responsible for almost one-third of the deaths.[17] Unlike the death rates for heart disease and stroke, the cancer death rate has stayed about the same in recent years. The biggest jump in death rates for elders has occurred with diabetes and CLRD (see **Box 7.1**).

Morbidity

Among Medicare enrollees age 65 or older, about one in five men and one in three women are unable to perform at least one of five physical activities (walking two to three blocks, writing, stooping or kneeling, reaching up overhead, or lifting something as heavy as 10 pounds).[8] Activity limitations increase with age, and women are more likely than men to have physical limitations.[8] The causes of this reduced activity can be classified into two types—chronic conditions and impairments.

Chronic Conditions

Chronic conditions are systemic health problems that persist longer than 3 months, such as hypertension, arthritis, heart disease, diabetes, and emphysema. The actual number of chronic conditions increases with age; therefore, limitations from activities become increasingly prevalent with age. About one-third of elders reported a limitation of activity as a result of chronic conditions.[1] Furthermore, many chronic conditions can result in impairments, such as the loss of sight from diabetes. Chronic conditions of elders vary by gender and race. More men experience life-threatening acute illnesses (e.g., heart disease and hypertension-induced stroke), whereas more women experience physically limiting chronic illness (e.g., osteoporosis and arthritis).[8]

Impairments

Impairments are deficits in the functioning of one's sense organs or limitations in one's mobility or range of motion. Like chronic conditions, impairments are far more prevalent in older adults. The primary impairments that affect elders are sensory impairments (i.e., vision, hearing, postural balance, or loss of feeling in the feet), physical limitations, and memory impairments[18] (see Box 7.2). "Memory skills are important to general cognitive functioning, and declining scores on tests of memory are indicators of general cognitive loss for older adults. Low cognitive functioning (i.e., memory impairment) is a major risk factor for entering a nursing home."[19]

Sensory impairments increase with age, and the prevalence of them will increase as life expectancy increases. Currently, one in six elders has impaired vision, one in four has loss of feeling in the feet, one in four has impaired hearing, and three in four have balance impairment.[20] The balance impairment may be in part why so many elders have physical limitations. Like sensory impairments, physical limitations increase with age. One in four elders ages 60–69 years has at least one physical limitation, and two in five of those 80 years of age or older have at least one.[21]

Like rates for chronic conditions, rates for impairments differ by gender and race. But unlike chronic conditions, impairments are affected by two other variables—previous income level and previous occupational exposure. The smaller the income and the more occupational exposure to health hazards, the greater the number of impairments.

Health Behaviors and Lifestyle Choices

There is no question that health behavior and social factors play significant roles in helping elders maintain health in later life. In interviews, elders generally report more favorable health behaviors than their younger counterparts. They are less likely to (1) consume large amounts of alcohol, (2) smoke cigarettes, and (3) be overweight or obese. However, it should be noted that many of those who abused alcoholic beverages, smoked cigarettes, and were overweight or obese died before age 65 and thus were unavailable for interview.

The health behaviors that can most positively affect the health of elders are healthy eating, exercise, and immunizations. Healthy eating plays a major role in preventing or delaying the onset of chronic diseases. The quality of elders' dietary habits is better than their younger counterparts', but they still leave room for improvement.[21]

The 1996 *Surgeon General's Report on Physical Activity and Health*—still the most definitive assessment of activity and age in the United States—reported that inactivity increased with age. Whereas a substantial majority of adults at all age levels did not achieve the recommended level of physical activity, the number of sedentary persons—those who engage in no discretionary physical activity at all—increased with age. Only 22% of those age 65 or older report engaging in regular leisure-time physical activity, and that percentage drops to 10% for those age 85 or older.[8]

Influenza and pneumonia are a leading cause of death in elders. Vaccinations against these diseases are recommended for elders, especially those who are at increased risk for complications from influenza and pneumonia. Influenza vaccinations are given annually, whereas pneumococcal vaccinations are usually given once in a lifetime, with possible revaccination with severe comorbidity after 5 years.

In large measure because of the onset of Medicare reimbursement, the pneumococcal vaccination rate increased dramatically, from 10% in 1989 to 57% in 2006.[8] Nonetheless, many elders remained unvaccinated, and there is considerable racial disparity. In 2006, 62% of whites received pneumonia vaccination, compared with 36% of blacks and 33% of Hispanics.[8] The influenza vaccination rate also increased dramatically, from 20% in 1989 to 64% in 2006.[8] Although this improvement is dramatic and gratifying to public health officials, more than a third of elders are still not getting an annual flu shot. And among older blacks, the influenza vaccination rate was about 20% lower than among older whites.[8]

Elder Abuse and Neglect

Reports of elder abuse and neglect have increased greatly in recent years. Perhaps a substantial part of the increase in these numbers was the result of all 50 states having passed some form of elder abuse prevention laws. Although the laws and definitions of terms vary from state to state, all states have set up reporting systems. Prior to the reporting systems, many incidences of abuse were never recorded. "Generally, adult protective service (APS) agencies receive and investigate reports of suspected elder abuse."[20] According to the first-ever National Elder Abuse Incidence Study, released in 1998, an estimated total of 551,000 elderly persons older than age 60 had experienced abuse (physical, emotional/psychological), neglect, or self-neglect in a domestic setting during the year of the study.[22] This study also revealed the following:

- Female elders are abused at a higher rate than are men.
- Elders 80 years or older are abused or neglected at two to three times the rate of their proportion of the elderly population.
- In almost 90% of all elder abuse and neglect incidents where a perpetrator is identified, the perpetrator is a family member, and two-thirds of the perpetrators are adult children or spouses.
- Victims of self-neglect are usually depressed, confused, or extremely frail.

Elder abuse and neglect are special problems for elders because they are (1) frail, (2) unable to defend themselves, (3) vulnerable to telemarketing scams and mail-order swindles, and (4) the most common victims of theft of their benefit checks. On a positive note, elder abuse is a problem that has responded well to community monitoring. However, there is still much need for improvement because one in four vulnerable elders is at risk of abuse and only a small portion of these incidents is detected and reported.[23]

Instrumental Needs of Elders

Atchley lists six instrumental needs that determine lifestyles for people of all ages.[24] These are income, housing, personal care, health care, transportation, and community facilities and services. The aging process can alter these needs in unpredictable ways. Whereas those elders in the young old group (65–74 years) usually do not experience appreciable changes in their lifestyles relative to these six needs, elders in the middle old group (75–84 years) and the old old group (85 years or older) eventually do. The rest of this chapter explores these six needs, discusses their implications for elders, and describes community services for elders.

Income

Although the need for income continues throughout one's life, achieving elder status often reduces the income needs. Perhaps the major reduction occurs with one's retirement. Retirees do not need to purchase job-related items such as special clothing or tools, pay union dues, or join professional associations. Expenses are further reduced because retirees no longer commute every day, buy as many meals away from home, or spend money on business travel. Reaching elder status also usually means that children are grown and no longer dependent, and, as noted earlier, the home mortgage has often been retired. Taxes are usually lower because income is lower. In addition, many community services are offered at reduced prices for elders.

However, aging usually means increased expenses for health care and for home maintenance and repairs that aging homeowners can no longer do themselves. Despite these increased costs, the overall need for income seems to decrease slightly for people after retirement.

Social Security benefits account for about two-fifths of income for elders, and asset income, pensions, and personal earnings each provide about one-fifth of total income.

The average monthly Social Security benefit for a retired worker was about $1,230 at the beginning of 2012.[25] This amounts to an average of $14,760 per year. About 87% of all people older than age 65 years receive Social Security benefits.[26] Further, Social Security was the major source of income (providing at least 50% of total income) for about two-thirds of the recipients and it was 90% or more of the income for about one-third of the recipients.[26]

In recent years, the income of elders has improved significantly. When income and other assets of elders are combined, the economic status of elders and those younger than 65 is not that far apart. However, the fact remains that 9% of the elder population lives in poverty. Certain subgroups of elders have higher rates. Unmarried women and minorities have the highest poverty rates, ranging from 12% to 23%. Married persons have the lowest poverty rates.[8]

Housing

When housing for the elderly is examined, four major needs are discussed: appropriateness, accessibility, adequacy, and affordability.[8] These needs are not independent of each other; they are closely intertwined. Elders may live in affordable housing, but the housing may not be appropriate for their special needs. Or, certain housing may be accessible to the elderly, but it may not be affordable, or there may not be an adequate number available to meet demand.

The single biggest change in the housing needs of elders is the need for special modifications because of physical disabilities. Such modifications can be very simple—such as handrails for support in bathrooms—or more complex—such as chair lifts for stairs. Sometimes there is a need for live-in help, whereas at other times disabilities may force seniors to leave their homes and seek specialized housing.

Because of the psychological and social value of the home, changing an elder's place of residence has negative effects for both the elder and the family members who help make the arrangements for the move. Recognizing the importance of a home and independence, families often feel tremendous conflict and guilt in deciding to move an elder relative. Although moving an elder is very difficult, it is often best for all involved. For example, moving a frail person from a two-story to a one-story home makes good sense, and moving an elder from a very large home to a smaller home or an apartment is logical.

One of the biggest fears associated with relocating an elder is the move to group housing, especially a nursing home.

The stereotype that many people have about group housing is not very positive, and most know it can be very expensive. However, just like any other consumer product, good group homes are available.

Perhaps the ideal model for large-scale long-term care facilities is the Eden Alternative, founded by William Thomas, M.D., in 1991. The basic premise of the Eden Alternative is that nursing homes should treat residents as people who need attentive care in a homelike setting. To accomplish this goal, nursing homes need to contain pets, plants, children, and other amenities that make life worth living.[27] Three hundred nursing homes around the country have incorporated the Eden Alternative into their facilities.

William Thomas went one step further than the Eden Alternative; he created the Green House. These houses avoid the institutionalization of larger nursing homes—including those based on the Eden Alternative—by limiting residents in number to about 10 and creating a large home for them rather than a facility. The first Green House, about 6,400 square feet, was constructed in Tupelo, Mississippi, in 2003. Each resident had a private room and bath, and access to a central kitchen where cooking and socializing was done. There was a surrounding garden for contemplative walks and for growing vegetables and flowers.

Green Houses promote autonomy. Residents get up, eat, and go to bed when they want. They decide on which foods to eat. Medications are locked in individual rooms, rather than distributed by a cart that is wheeled from room to room. There are few features that are different from the typical home. Green House workers are paid more and are better trained, but the extra costs are offset by employee empowerment that reduces staff turnover and additional training expenses.

The relocation of elders is not always traumatic or done against their will. Many elders are finding housing in communities that have been planned as **retirement communities**. Although these communities are available in all areas of the country, they are most popular in areas with temperate climates (see **Figure 7.5**). Some of the communities are built as private associations, whereas others are developed as special areas within larger, already established communities. Legally, the private associations are able to adopt by-laws that put restrictions on the residents, such

retirement communities residential communities that have been specifically developed for those in their retirement years

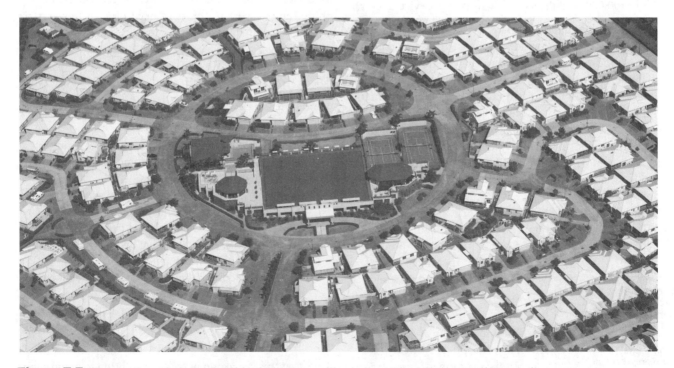

Figure 7.5 The number of planned retirement communities in the United States continues to increase.
© Brisbane/ShutterStock, Inc.

as a minimum age to move into the area, no children under a certain age living in the residence, and no pets. Retirement communities usually offer a variety of housing alternatives ranging from home or condominium ownership to apartment living. Because these communities are developed to meet the needs of elders, special accommodations are usually made for socializing, recreation, shopping, transportation, and selected educational programs.

Two other housing options for elders are **continuing-care retirement communities (CCRCs)** and assisted-living residences. CCRCs guarantee the residents a lifelong residence and health care. They work in the following way: The retirees either purchase or term lease (sometimes lifelong) a living unit on a campus-like setting. The living unit could be a single-family dwelling, an apartment, or a room, as in a nursing home. In addition to the living units, the campus usually includes a health clinic and often has either a nursing home or a healthcare center. These other facilities are available to the residents for an additional fee. Residents of the CCRCs can live as independently as they wish, but have available to them a variety of services, including housekeeping, meals, transportation, organized recreational and social activities, health care, and security. CCRCs are a housing alternative for well-to-do seniors. Unfortunately, CCRCs are beyond the reach of many elders; the purchase or lifelong lease is more than $100,000, and the fee for many of the services is extra.

An assisted-living residence is a more recent housing option than CCRCs, but it includes many of the same concepts. It is a model of residential care that blends many of the characteristics of the nursing home and community-based long-term care. The Assisted Living Federation of America (ALFA) has defined assisted living "as a long-term care option that combines housing, support services and health care, as needed. Assisted living is designed for individuals who require assistance with everyday activities such as meals, medication management or assistance, bathing, dressing and transportation."[28] Such facilities may range from high-rise buildings to one-story Victorian mansions to large multi-acre campuses.[28] They are regulated in all 50 states and may be operated by nonprofit or for-profit companies. Most of these facilities offer a variety of amenities and personal care services, including the following[28]:

- Three meals a day served in a common dining area
- Housekeeping services
- Transportation
- 24-hour security

- Exercise and wellness programs
- Personal laundry services
- Social and recreational activities
- Staff available to respond to both scheduled and unscheduled needs
- Assistance with eating, bathing, dressing, toileting, and walking
- Access to health and medical services, such as physical therapy and hospice
- Emergency call systems for each resident's apartment
- Medication management
- Care for residents with cognitive impairments

Costs for assisted living vary according to facility and parts of the county. "They offer a less-expensive, residential approach to delivering many of the same services available in skilled nursing, either by employing personal care staff or contracting with home health agencies and other outside professionals."[28] According to data collected by several different nonprofit senior living organizations, including ALFA, "the median rate for a private one-bedroom apartment in an assisted living residence is $2,575 per month."[28] It has been estimated that there are about 36,000+ assisted-living facilities nationwide.[28]

Of all the housing problems that confront seniors, the availability of affordable housing is the biggest. Unfortunately, those seniors who are most in need of such housing are often frail and disabled, have low incomes, and live in rural areas.

Personal Care

Four different levels of tasks have been identified with which seniors may need assistance:

1. *Instrumental tasks:* Such as housekeeping, transportation, maintenance on the automobile or yard, and assistance with business affairs
2. *Expressive tasks:* Including emotional support, socializing and inclusion in social gatherings, and trying to prevent feelings of loneliness and isolation
3. *Cognitive tasks:* Assistance that involves scheduling appointments, monitoring health conditions, reminding elders of the need to take medications, and in general acting as a backup memory
4. *Tasks of daily living:* Such as eating, bathing, dressing, toileting, walking, getting in and out of bed or a chair, and getting outside

Note that this last group of tasks, in addition to being a part of this listing, has special significance. These items have

continuing-care retirement communities (CCRCs) planned communities for seniors that guarantee a lifelong residence and health care

been used to develop a scale, called **activities of daily living (ADLs)**, to measure **functional limitations**. *Functional limitation* refers to the difficulty in performing personal care and home management tasks. However, ADLs do not cover all aspects of disability and are not sufficient by themselves to estimate the need for long-term care. As previously noted, some elders have cognitive impairments that are not measured by ADLs. An additional, commonly used measure called **instrumental activities of daily living (IADLs)** measures more complex tasks such as handling personal finances, preparing meals, shopping, doing housework, traveling, using the telephone, and taking medications.[14]

When elders begin to need help with one or more of these tasks, it is usually a spouse, adult children, or other family members who first provide the help, thus assuming the role of informal caregivers. An **informal caregiver** has been defined as one who provides unpaid care or assistance to someone who has some physical, mental, emotional, or financial need that limits his or her independence. "There is wide latitude in the estimates of the number of informal caregivers in the U.S., depending on the definitions and criteria used."[29] Estimates range from about 6 to 52 million.[30] An informal caregiver can be either a care provider or care manager. The **care provider** helps identify the needs of the individual and personally performs the caregiving service. Obviously, this can only be done if the person in need and the caregiver live in close proximity to each other. The **care manager** also helps to identify needs, but as a result of living some distance away or for other reasons, does not provide the service. The care manager makes arrangements for someone else (volunteer or paid) to provide the services. With the aging of the population, it is now highly probable that many, if not most, adults can expect to have some responsibility as caregivers for their parents (see **Figure 7.6**).

Caregivers for elders face a number of problems, including decreased personal freedom, lack of privacy, constant demands on their time and energy, resentment that siblings do not share in the caregiving, and an increased financial burden. Many experience feelings of guilt for asking a spouse to help with the care of an in-law or in knowing that the end of caregiving responsibilities usually means either the elder person's death or placement in a group home. Caregivers often experience a change in lifestyle, especially associated with time for leisure and recreation. Caregiving can also lead to a negative impact on health.[13]

To assist caregivers, federal legislation was passed called the Older Americans Act Amendments of 2000 (Public Law 106-501). This law established the National Family Caregiver

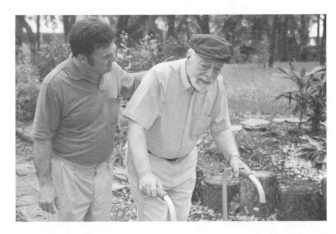

Figure 7.6 Adult children are gaining greater responsibility as caregivers.
© Lisa F. Young/Fotolia.com

Support Program (NFCSP), which is administered by the Administration on Aging (AoA) of the U.S. Department of Health and Human Services. It was modeled in large part after successful state long-term care programs in California, New Jersey, Wisconsin, Pennsylvania, and other states and after listening to the needs expressed by hundreds of family caregivers in discussions held across the country. The program calls for all states, working in partnership with area agencies on aging and local community-service providers, to have the following five basic services for family caregivers:

- Information for caregivers about available services
- Assistance to caregivers in gaining access to services
- Individual counseling, organization of support groups, and caregiver training to assist them in making decisions and solving problems relating to their caregiving roles
- Respite care to enable caregivers to be temporarily relieved from their caregiving responsibilities
- Supplemental services, on a limited basis, to complement the care provided by caregivers

activities of daily living (ADLs) eating, toileting, dressing, bathing, walking, getting into and out of a bed or chair, and getting outside

care manager one who helps identify the healthcare needs of an individual but does not actually provide the healthcare services

care provider one who helps identify the healthcare needs of an individual and also personally performs the caregiving service

functional limitations difficulty in performing personal care and home management tasks

informal caregiver one who provides unpaid assistance to someone who has some physical, mental, emotional, or financial need limiting his or her independence

instrumental activities of daily living (IADLs) more complex tasks such as handling personal finances, preparing meals, shopping, doing housework, traveling, using the telephone, and taking medications

Further assistance for long-term care became available in January 2011. A part of the Patient Protection and Affordable Care Act (P.L. 111-148), signed into law by President Obama on March 23, 2010, was the Community Living Assistance Services and Supports (CLASS) program. It is a voluntary program that employers can choose to offer employees. If offered, it will be a premium-funded (through payroll deductions) government insurance program in which all adult-age employees with functional limitations will become eligible for a cash benefit of not less than an average of $50 per day (to purchase nonmedical services and supports necessary to maintain community residence) after paying into the program for 5 years. Also, if offered by the employer, employees are automatically enrolled in the program, unless they choose to opt out.[31,32] The CLASS program was one of the last legislative efforts of the late Senator Edward Kennedy (D-MA) when he had it added to the health bill in the summer prior to his death.[31]

Health Care

Elders are the heaviest users of healthcare services. Approximately 20% of elders have 10 or more visits a year to a physician, compared with 13% for all people in the United States.[7] They are also hospitalized more often and for longer stays. Although persons 65 years of age or older only represented approximately 13% of the total population in 2007, they accounted for almost 37% of the roughly 35 million patient discharges from nonfederal short-stay hospitals,[7] and they spend over twice as much per person on prescription drugs as those younger than 65 years of age. In addition, elders have higher usage rates for professional dental care, vision aids, and medical equipment and supplies than people younger than age 65. Usage of healthcare services increases with age, and much of the money spent on health care is spent in the last year of life.

Whereas private sources, such as employer-paid insurance, are the major sources of healthcare payment for people younger than age 65, public funds are used to pay for the majority of the healthcare expenses for elders. Medicare, which was enacted in 1965 and became effective July 1, 1966, provides almost universal health insurance coverage for elders. Medicare coverage, however, is biased toward hospital care; chronic care health needs such as eyeglasses, hearing aids, and most long-term services are not covered. In 2010, the Medicare program had 47.5 million enrollees[33] and expenditures of $524.6 billion.[34]

In addition, Medicaid, a federal–state program that was also approved in 1965, helps to cover the healthcare costs of poor elders, primarily for nursing home care (continuing care), home health care, and prescription drugs. In 2006, almost 8 million elders were covered by Medicaid.[9]

All indications are that the healthcare costs for elders will continue to escalate because of the aging population and rising healthcare costs. The first of the baby boomers (those born in 1946) turned 65 years old, and thus became eligible for Medicare, in 2011. Therefore, future legislators will be forced to choose from among the following alternatives: (1) raising taxes to pay for the care, (2) reallocating tax dollars from other programs to pay for care, (3) cutting back on coverage presently offered, (4) offering care to only those who truly cannot afford it otherwise (also known as means testing), or (5) completely revamping the present system under which the care is funded.

In the meantime, the importance of instilling in Americans the value of preventing the onset of chronic diseases through healthy living cannot be overstated. Although it is not possible to prevent all chronic health problems, encouraging healthy behaviors is a step in the right direction.

Transportation

The National Institute on Aging estimates that 600,000 people age 70 or older give up their driving each year. On average, elders live about 10 years after they stop driving.[35] There is little guidance, however, not only on when to stop driving, but also on how to compensate for no longer having personal control over one's transportation.

Transportation is of prime importance to elders because it enables them to remain independent. "Housing, medical, financial and social services are useful only to the extent that transportation can make them accessible to those in need."[36] The two factors that have the greatest effect on the transportation needs of elders are income and health status. Some elders who have always driven their own automobiles eventually find that they are no longer able to do so. The ever-increasing costs of purchasing and maintaining an automobile sometimes become prohibitive on a fixed income. Also, with age comes physical problems that restrict one's ability to operate an automobile safely. In addition, those with extreme disabilities may find that they will need a modified automobile (to accommodate their disability) or specialized transportation (e.g., a vehicle that can accommodate a wheelchair) to be transported.

With regard to transportation needs, elders can be categorized into three different groups: (1) those who can use the present forms of transportation, whether it be their own vehicle or public transportation; (2) those who could use public transportation if the barriers of cost and access (no service available) were removed; and (3) those who need special services beyond what is available through public transportation.[24]

The unavailability of transportation services has stimulated a number of private and public organizations that serve elders (e.g., churches, community services, and local area agencies on aging) to provide these services. Some communities even subsidize the cost of public transportation by offering reduced rates for elders. Although these services have been helpful to elders, mobility is still more difficult for elders than for other adults.

The ideal solution to the transportation needs of elders, according to Atchley, would include four components: (1) fare reductions or discounts for all public transportation, including that for interstate travel; (2) subsidies to ensure adequate scheduling and routing of present public transportation; (3) subsidized taxi fares for the disabled and infirm; and (4) funds for senior centers to purchase and equip vehicles to transport seniors properly, especially in rural areas.[24]

Community Facilities and Services

Because of the limitations of elders and the barriers they must face, they have special needs in regard to community facilities and services. If these needs are met, the lifestyles of elders are greatly enhanced. If not, they are confronted with anything from a slight inconvenience to a very poor quality of life.

With a view toward improving the lives of elders, Congress enacted the **Older Americans Act of 1965 (OAA)** and has amended it several times. Among the programs created by key amendments are the national nutrition program for elders, the State and Area Agencies on Aging, and other programs (e.g., the caregiver program discussed earlier) to increase the services and protect the rights of elders.

Though the initial act was important, the services and facilities available to elders were greatly improved after the passage of the 1973 amendments, which established the State Departments on Aging and Area Agencies on Aging. These systems inform, guide, and link older persons to available, appropriate, and acceptable services to meet their needs. The amendments were written to provide the state and area

agencies with the flexibility to develop plans that allow for local variations. In 2010, there were 56 State Units on Aging (covering all 50 states and 6 territories). "Most states are divided into planning and service areas (PSAs), so that programs can be tailored to meet the specific needs of older persons residing in those areas. Area Agencies on Aging are the agencies designated by the state to be the focal point for OAA programs within a PSA."[36]

With each part of the country—and for that matter each community—having its own peculiarities, the services available to elders can vary greatly from one community to another. It may require a phone call to the National Association of Area Agencies on Aging (202-872-0888) to locate your local Area Agency on Aging and the services it provides. In the following text, we provide brief descriptions of facilities and services available in many communities.

Meal Service

The 1972 amendments to the Older Americans Act outlined a national nutrition program for elders and provided funds for communities to establish meal services. Today's meal services are provided through home-delivered meal and congregate meal programs. The concept of the home-delivered meal programs (often known as **Meals on Wheels**) is the regular delivery of meals—usually once a day, 5 days per week—to elders in their homes. These meals are prepared in a central location, sometimes in a hospital, school, or senior center, and are delivered by community volunteers.

Congregate meal programs are provided for individuals who can travel to a central site, often within senior centers or publicly funded housing units. Usually, it is the noon meal that is provided. Generally, these meals are funded by federal and state monies and make use of commodity food services. In recent years, congregate meal programs seem to be gaining favor over home-delivered meal programs because they also provide social interaction (see **Figure 7.7**) and the opportunity to tie in with other social services.[24]

Both types of meal programs are strictly regulated by federal and state guidelines to ensure that the meals meet standard nutritional requirements. The cost of the meals varies by site and client income level. Elders may

congregate meal programs community-sponsored nutrition programs that provide meals at a central site, such as a senior center

Meals on Wheels a community-supported nutrition program in which prepared meals are delivered to elders in their homes, usually by volunteers

Older Americans Act of 1965 (OAA) federal legislation to improve the lives of elders

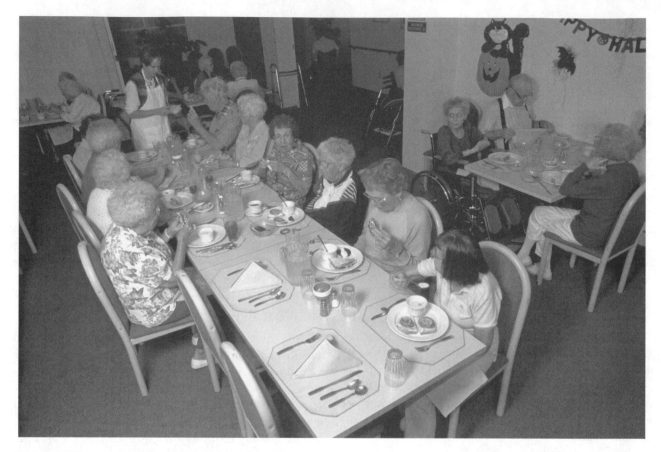

Figure 7.7 Congregate meals programs are valuable not only because of the enhanced nutrition, but also because of the social interaction.
© Ken Hammond/USDA

pay full price, pay a portion of the cost, or just make a voluntary contribution.

Homemaker Service

For a number of elders, periodic homemaker services can be the critical factor enabling them to remain in their own homes. For these elders, physical impairment restricts their ability to carry out normal housekeeping activities such as house cleaning, laundry, and meal preparation.

Chore and Home Maintenance Service

Chore and home maintenance service includes such services as yard work, cleaning gutters and windows, installing screens and storm windows, making minor plumbing and electrical

repairs, maintaining furnaces and air conditioners, and helping to adapt a home to any impairments seniors might have. This adaptation may include provisions for wheelchairs and installing ramps or special railings to assist elders to move from one area to another.

Visitor Service

Social interaction and social contacts are an important need for every human being, regardless of age. **Visitor services** amount to one individual taking time to visit with another person who is **homebound**, or unable to leave his or her residence. This service is usually done on a voluntary basis, many times with elders doing the visiting, and serves both the homebound and those who are institutionalized. It is not uncommon for church or social organizations to conduct a visitor program for homebound members.

homebound a person unable to leave home for normal activities
visitor services one individual taking time to visit with another who is unable to leave his or her residence

Adult Day Care

Adult day care programs provide care during the daytime hours for elders who are unable to be left alone. These services are modeled after child day care. Most programs offer meals, snacks, and social activities for the clients. Some either provide or make arrangements for the clients to receive therapy, counseling, health education, or other health services. Other day care programs are designed for elders with special needs, such as Alzheimer clients, those who are blind, or veterans. Adult day care programs allow families to continue with daytime activities while still providing the primary care for a family member.

Respite Care

Respite care is planned, short-term care. Such care allows families who provide primary care for an elder family member to leave their elder in a supervised care setting for anywhere from a day to a few weeks. Respite services provide full care, including sleeping quarters, meals, bathing facilities, social activities, and the monitoring of medications.[2] Such a program allows primary caregivers to take a vacation, visit other relatives, or be otherwise relieved from their constant caregiving responsibilities.

Home Health Care

Home health care "is an important alternative to traditional institutional care. Services such as medical treatment, physical therapy, and homemaker services often allow patients to be cared for at lower cost than a nursing home or hospital and in familiar surroundings of their home."[14] These programs, run by official health agencies like the local health department, hospitals, or private companies, provide a full range of services, including preventive, primary, rehabilitative, and therapeutic services, in the client's home. The care is often provided by nurses, home health aides, and personal care workers (licensed healthcare workers). A decreasing percentage of home healthcare expenditures have been paid for by Medicare over the past decade, and a significant portion is being paid for by families out of pocket.

Senior Centers

The enactment of the Older Americans Act of 1965 provided funds to develop multipurpose senior centers, facilities where elders can congregate for fellowship, meals, education, and recreation. More recently, a number of communities have built additional senior centers with local tax dollars. There are about 13,000 senior centers in the United States and they are the most common community facility aimed at serving seniors.[21] They are found much less commonly in rural areas.

In addition to the traditional services (meals, fellowship, and recreation) offered at senior centers, some communities use the centers to serve as a central location for offering a variety of other senior services, including legal assistance, income counseling, income tax return assistance, program referrals, employment services, and other appropriate services and information.

> **adult day care programs** daytime care provided to elders who are unable to be left alone
> **home health care** healthcare services provided in the patient's place of residence
> **respite care** planned short-term care, usually for the purpose of relieving a full-time informal caregiver

Chapter Summary

- The median age of the U.S. population is at an all-time high and will continue to increase through the first third of this century.
- The increasing median age is affected by decreasing fertility rates, declining mortality rates, and the decline in immigration.
- We are now at a point in history when a significant portion of Americans will assume some responsibility for the care of their aging parents.
- An aging population presents the community with several concerns, which means legislators and taxpayers will be faced with decisions about how best to afford the costs (Social Security, government employee pensions, Medicare, etc.) of an ever-increasing old-age dependency ratio.
- Communities will need to deal with the special needs of income, housing, personal care, health care, transportation, and community facilities and services for elders.
- All projections indicate that the incomes of seniors will remain lower than those of the general population, that the need for affordable and accessible housing will increase, that there will be increased needs for personal services and care, that healthcare needs and costs will increase, and that the demand for barrier-free transportation will increase for elders.

Review Questions

1. What years of life are defined by each of the following groups—old, young old, middle old, and old old?
2. What is meant by the terms *aged*, *aging*, *elder*, *gerontology*, *geriatrician*, and *geriatrics*?
3. Why did a pyramid represent the age characteristics of the U.S. population of the 1950s, but in 2030 it will be a rectangle?
4. What are the three factors that affect the size and age of a population?
5. Why are dependency and labor-force ratios so important?
6. How do the income needs of people change in retirement?
7. What are some of the major problems caregivers face?
8. Why are continuing-care retirement communities attractive to elders?
9. What is an assisted-living residence?
10. What is the difference between activities of daily living and instrumental activities of daily living?
11. What are the most frequently occurring health problems of elders?
12. From what financial sources do elders normally pay for health care?
13. How do income and health status affect the transportation needs of elders?
14. What are Area Agencies on Aging?
15. What is the difference between adult day care and respite care?

Activities

1. Interview a retired person over the age of 65. In your interview, include the following questions. Write a two-page paper about this interview.
   - What are your greatest needs as an elder?
   - What are your greatest fears connected with aging?
   - What are your greatest joys at this stage in your life?
   - If you could have done anything differently when you were younger to affect your life now, what would it have been?
   - Have you had any problems getting health care with Medicare? If so, what were they?
   - In what ways are you able to contribute to your community in retirement?
   - Are there any barriers to seeking volunteer opportunities in your community? What do you think about paid part-time work in retirement?
2. Review a newspaper obituary column for 7 consecutive days. Using the information provided in the obituaries: (a) demographically describe those who died, (b) keep track of what community services are noted, and (c) consider what generalizations can be made from the group as a whole.

Community Health on the Web

The Internet contains a wealth of information about community and public health. Increase your knowledge of some of the topics presented in this chapter by accessing the Jones & Bartlett Learning website at **go.jblearning.com/McKenzieBrief** and follow the links to complete the following Web activities:

- Administration on Aging
- National Institute on Aging

References   **181**

References

1. Administration on Aging (2010). *A Profile of Older Americans: 2009*. Available at http://www.aoa.gov/AoAroot/Aging_Statistics/Profile/2009/index.aspx.
2. U.S. Department of Health and Human Services (1986). *Age Words: A Glossary on Health and Aging* (NIH pub. no. 86-1849). Washington, DC: U.S. Government Printing Office.
3. Slee, D. A., V. N. Slee, and H. J. Schmidt (2008). *Slee's Health Care Terms*, 5th ed. Sudbury, MA: Jones & Bartlett.
4. Ferrini, A. F., and R. L. Ferrini (2000). *Health in the Later Years*, 3rd ed. Boston, MA: McGraw-Hill Higher Education.
5. Thomlinson, R. (1976). *Population Dynamics: Causes and Consequences of World Demographic Change*. New York, NY: Random House.
6. U.S. Census Bureau (2010). *U.S. Population Projections*. Available at http://www.census.gov/population/socdemo/statbriefs/agebrief.html.
7. U.S. Census Bureau (2010). *The 2010 Statistical Abstract: The National Data Book–Population*. Available at http://www.census.gov/compendia/statab/.
8. Federal Interagency Forum on Aging Related Statistics (2008). *Older Americans 2008: Key Indicators of Well-Being*. Available at http://www.agingstats.gov/Main_Site/Data/Data_2008.aspx.
9. National Center for Health Statistics (2010). *Health, United States, 2009: With Special Feature on Medical Technology*. Hyattsville, MD: Author.
10. U.S. Bureau of the Census (1996). *65 in the United States* (Current Population Reports P23-190). Washington, DC: U.S. Government Printing Office.
11. Vincent, G. K., and V. A. Velkoff (2010). *The Next Four Decades–The Older Population in the United States: 2010 to 2050* (Current Population Reports P25-1138). Washington, DC: U.S. Census Bureau.
12. Mermin, G., R. W. Johnson, and D. P. Murphy. (2007). "Why Do Boomers Plan to Work Longer?" *Journal of Gerontology: Social Sciences*, 62B: S286–S294.
13. Hooyman, N., and H. Kiyak (2008). *Social Gerontology: A Multidisciplinary Perspective*, 8th ed. Boston, MA: Allyn and Bacon.
14. Kramarow, E. H., H. Lentzner, R. Rooks, J. Weeks, and S. Saydah (1999). *Health and Aging Chartbook: Health United States, 1999* (HHS pub. no. PHS-99-123-1). Hyattsville, MD: National Center for Health Statistics.
15. U.S. Census Bureau (2008). *American Housing Survey for the United States: 2007* (Current Housing Reports, Series H150/07). Washington, DC: U.S. Government Printing Office.
16. U.S. Department of Housing and Urban Development, Office of Policy Development and Research (1999). *Housing Our Elders*. Washington, DC: Author.
17. Xu, J. Q., K. D. Kochanek, S. L. Murphy, and B. Tejada-Vera (2010). "Deaths: Final Data for 2007." *National Vital Statistics Reports*, 58(19). Hyattsville, MD: National Center for Health Statistics.
18. Dillon, C. F., G. Qiuping, J. J. Hoffman, and C.-W. Ko. (2010). *Vision, Hearing, Balance, and Sensory Impairment in Americans Aged 70 and Over: United States 1999-2006* (NCHS Data Brief no. 31). Hyattsville, MD: National Center for Health Statistics.
19. Federal Interagency Forum on Aging-Related Statistics (2001). *Older Americans 2000: Key Indicators of Well-Being*. Available at http://www.agingstats.gov/Main_Site/Data/2000_Documents/entire_report.pdf.
20. Administration on Aging (2006). "Elder Abuse Prevention." Available at http://www.aoa.gov/press/fact/alpha/fact_elder_abuse_pf.asp.
21. Haber, D. (2010). *Health Promotion and Aging: Practical Applications for Health Professionals*, 5th ed. New York, NY: Springer.
22. National Center on Elder Abuse, Administration on Aging (2005). *Fact Sheet: Elder Abuse Prevalence and Incidence*. Washington, DC: Author. Available at http://www.ncea.aoa.gov/ncearoot/main_site/pdf/publication/FinalStatistics050331.pdf.
23. Cooper, C., A. Selwood, and G. Livingston. (2008). "The Prevalence of Elder Abuse and Neglect: A Systematic Review." *Age and Ageing*, 37(2): 151-160.
24. Atchley, R. C. (1994). *Social Forces and Aging: An Introduction to Social Gerontology*, 7th ed. Belmont, CA: Wadsworth.
25. Social Security Administration (2012). "Average Monthly Social Security Benefit for a Retired Worker." Available at http://ssa-custhelp.ssa.gov/app/answers/detail/a_id/.
26. Social Security Administration (2010). *Fast Facts and Figures About Social Security, 2009*. Available at http://www.socialsecurity.gov/policy/docs/chartbooks/fast_facts/2009/index.html.
27. Thomas, W. (1995). *The Eden Alternative*. Acton, MA: VanderWyk & Burnham.
28. Assisted Living Federation of America (2010). "What Is Assisted Living?" Available at http://www.alfa.org/alfa/Assisted_Living_Information.asp?SnID=1383416766.
29. Family Caregiver Alliance (2010). "Selective Caregiver Statistics." Available at http://www.caregiver.org/caregiver/jsp/content_node.jsp?nodeid=439.
30. Cohen, C., A. Colantonio, and L. Vernich. (2002). "Positive Aspects of Caregiving: Rounding Out the Caregiver Support System." *The Gerontologist*, 35: 489-497.
31. National Public Radio (2010). "Long-Term Care Program Debuts in New Health Law." Available at http://www.npr.org/templates/story/story.php?storyId=125461417.
32. Henry J. Kaiser Family Foundation (2010). "Summary of New Health Reform Law." Available at http://www.kff.org/healthreform/8061.cfm.
33. U.S. Census Bureau (2012). *The 2012 Statistical Abstract: The National Data Book–Health and Nutrition*. Available at http://www.census.gov/compendia/statab/cats/health_nutrition.html.
34. Centers for Medicare and Medicaid Services (2012). "Quick Reference: National Health Expenditure Category Definitions." Available at https://www.cms.gov/Research-Statistics-Data-and-Systems/Statistics-Trends-and-Reports/NationalHealthExpendData/Downloads/quickref.pdf.
35. Foley, D., H. K. Heimovitz, J. M. Guralnik, D. B. Brock. (2002). "Driving Life Expectancy of Persons Aged 70 Years and Older in the United States." *American Journal of Public Health*, 92: 1284-1289.
36. Administration on Aging (2007). "How to Find Help." Available at http://www.aoa.gov/eldfam/How_To_Find/Agencies/Agencies.asp.

Chapter 8

Community Health and Minorities

Miguel A. Perez, PhD, MCHES

Chapter Objectives

After studying this chapter, you should be able to:

1. Explain the concept of diversity as it describes the American people.

2. Explain the impact of a more diverse population in the United States as it relates to community health efforts.

3. Explain the importance of the 1985 landmark report *The Secretary's Task Force Report on Black and Minority Health*.

4. List the racial and ethnic categories currently used by the U.S. government in statistical activities and program administration reporting.

5. List some limitations related to collecting racial and ethnic health data.

6. Identify some of the sociodemographic and socioeconomic characteristics of minority groups in the United States.

7. List some of the beliefs and values of minority groups in the United States.

8. List and describe the six priority areas of the Race and Health Initiative.

9. Explain the role socioeconomic status plays in health disparities among racial and ethnic minority groups.

10. Define *cultural sensitivity* and *cultural and linguistic competence* and the importance of each related to minority community health.

11. Identify the three kinds of power associated with empowerment and explain the importance of each related to minority community health.

Introduction

Over the centuries, wave after wave of immigrants has come to the United States to start anew, and they have brought with them many of their traditions and cultures. However, it is recognized that even as the United States' demographic profile changes, race relations remains an issue that too often divides the nation. In 1997, then-President Bill Clinton announced "One America in the 21st Century: The President's Initiative on Race." The goal of the Initiative on Race was to strengthen our shared foundation as Americans so we can all live in an atmosphere of trust and understanding.

majority those with characteristics that are found in more than 50% of a population
minority groups subgroups of the population that consist of fewer than 50% of the population
minority health refers to the morbidity and mortality of American Indians/ Alaska natives, Americans of Hispanic origin, Asians and Pacific Islanders, and black Americans in the United States

In 2010, 64% of Americans, the **majority,** self-identified as "white, non-Hispanic." The remaining 36% of the U.S. population are members of what are traditionally viewed as racial or ethnic **minorities**[1] (see **Figure 8.1**). This represents a 2% decrease among non-Hispanic whites from the 2000 census.

Minority health refers to the morbidity and mortality of American Indians/ Alaska Natives, Asian Americans and Pacific Islanders, black Americans, and Hispanics in the United States. It is estimated that by 2050, nearly one-half of the U.S. population will be composed of racial minorities (see **Figure 8.2**).[2] As the racial and ethnic minority groups currently experiencing poorer health status grow in proportion to the total U.S. population, the future health of all Americans will be influenced by the success in improving the health of these groups.[3] The nature of health disparities among the least empowered (primarily minorities) is the main focus of this chapter.

The 1985 report, *Secretary's Task Force Report on Black and Minority Health*, first documented the health status disparities of minority groups in the United States.[4] This report provided substantial documentation about health disparities experienced by members of under-represented groups. Specifically, the report identified six causes of death that accounted for more than 80% of the excess mortality observed among black Americans and other groups. The *Secretary's Task Force Report on Black and Minority Health* contributed significantly to the development of a number of *Healthy People 2000* objectives,[5] which resulted in some measurable decreases in age-adjusted death rates for seven specific causes of death.

In 1998, then-President Clinton declared that the United States would continue to commit to a national goal of eliminating racial and ethnic health disparities by the year 2010,[6] and launched the Initiative to Eliminate Racial and Ethnic Disparities in Health, or the Race and Health Initiative. The purpose of this national effort was to enhance efforts in (1) preventing disease, (2) promoting

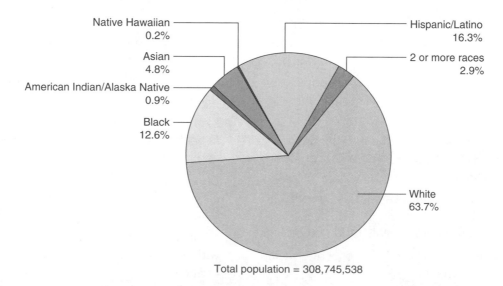

Figure 8.1 Percent Distribution of the U.S. population in 2010.

Note: Percentages do not add up to 100% due to rounding and because Hispanics may be any race and are therefore counted under more than one category.

Data from U.S. Census Bureau (2011). "State and County Quick Facts." Available at http://quickfacts.census.gov/qfd/states/00000.html.

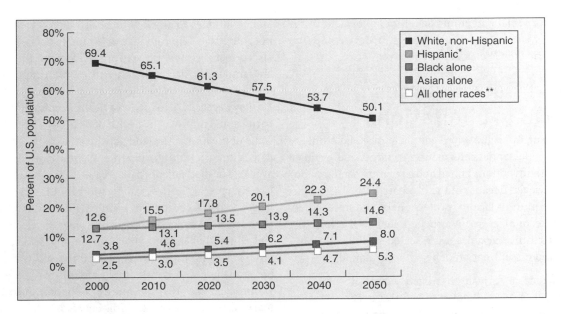

Figure 8.2 Projected U.S. population by race and Hispanic origin, selected years.

Note: Percentages for 2000 are actual. * Hispanics can be of any race. Totals do not equal 100% for this reason. ** "All other races" includes American Indian and Alaska Native alone, Native Hawaiian and Other Pacific Islander alone, and two or more races.

U.S. Census Bureau, Population Division (2004). "U.S. Interim Projections by Age, Sex, Race, and Hispanic Origin." Available at http://www.census.gov/ipc/www/usinterimproj/.

health, and (3) delivering care to racial and ethnic minority communities. One of the primary aims of this initiative consists of consultation and collaboration among federal agencies; state, local, and tribal governments; and community professionals to research and address issues that affect health outcomes. Accordingly, the Race and Health Initiative is a paramount part of *Healthy People 2020*'s broad health goal to "achieve health equity, eliminate disparities, and improve the health of all groups."[7]

Racial and Ethnic Classifications

It is standard practice for healthcare and public health professionals to describe participants and populations in terms of "race" or "ethnicity." The racial and ethnic categories are used in statistical activities and program administration reporting, including the monitoring and enforcement of civil rights. In the 1980s, the regulations used for the statistical classification of racial and ethnic groups by federal agencies were based on the 1978 publication by the Office of Management and Budget (OMB) of Directive 15 titled "Race and Ethnic Standards for Federal Statistics and Administrative Reporting."[8] This directive presented brief rules for classifying persons into four racial categories (American Indian or Alaska Native, Asian or Pacific Islander, black, and white) and two ethnic categories (of Hispanic origin or not of Hispanic origin). Directive 15 was not intended to be scientific or anthropological in nature, but rather a way to **operationalize** race and ethnicity, and its guidelines provided the standards by which federal government agencies collected and classified racial and ethnic data in the 1980s and 1990s.

As a result of criticism leveled against Directive 15, new standards were issued in 1997. The new classification standards expanded race from four to five categories by separating the "Asian or Pacific Islander" category into two categories—"Asian" and "Native Hawaiian or Other Pacific Islander." Additionally, the term "Hispanic" was changed to "Hispanic or Latino" and "Negro" can be used in addition to "Black or African American." Finally, the reporting of more than one race for multiracial persons was strongly encouraged, along with specifying that the Hispanic origin question should precede the race question.[9]

In October 1997, the Department of Health and Human Services (HHS) adopted a policy supporting the inclusion of the new revised federal

operationalize (operational definition) provide working definitions

standards for racial and ethnic data for employment in the HHS data systems, and consequently in developing and measuring *Healthy People 2010* objectives.

Health Data Sources and Their Limitations

The reporting of accurate and complete race and ethnicity data provides essential information to target and evaluate public health inventions aimed at under-represented populations. However, because of the diversity in the U.S. population, community health professionals and researchers have long recognized many crucial issues in the way that racial and ethnic variables are assessed in the collection, analysis, and dissemination of health information.

Although race historically has been viewed as a biological construct, it is now known to be more accurately characterized as a social category that has changed over time and varies across societies and cultures.[10–12] Similarly, self-reported data regarding race and ethnicity may be unreliable because individuals of varied cultures and heritage and multiple races can have difficulty classifying their racial or ethnic identity on standardized forms. Finally, many non-federal health data systems do not collect self-reported race or ethnicity data, or in some cases, it may be uncertain who recorded the race and ethnicity data. This can make analyzing health information concerning the health status of minorities a challenging task. According to the authors of the National Electronic Telecommunications System for Surveillance study, race and ethnicity may not be reported by healthcare providers for at least four reasons including not knowing the standards for data collection, failing to ask the patient, and clinical staff not having access to the information.[13,14]

In addition to these issues, there are many cases of bias analysis that occur when two separate data reporting systems are used to obtain rates by race and Hispanic origin. It has been estimated that death rates are overestimated by about 1% for the white population and by 5% for the black population in the United States. At the same time, death rates are underestimated for the American Indian or Alaska Native population by nearly 21%, by 11% for Asian or Pacific Islanders, and by 2% for Hispanics.[15]

One national health objective for 2020 is the continued upgrading of data collection on race and ethnicity in public health surveys. In addition,

acculturated cultural modification of an individual or group by adapting to or borrowing traits from another culture

HHS continues to work with health data systems that do not collect self-reported race or ethnicity data on individuals, so that they will do so. Increasing both the reliability and amount of data will assist in monitoring and assessing the outcomes related to meeting the proposed goal of *Healthy People 2020* to "achieve health equity, eliminate disparities, and improve the health of all groups."[7] Recognizing some of the limitations and gaps in collecting racial/ethnic data is important. Knowing that in some cases data are not available or the available data are not as precise as we would like, we present the best information about the community health issues faced by the primary minority groups. The next section provides a broad overview of selected health and illness beliefs and practices among selected ethnic groups. However, caution is needed to avoid stereotyping because there is a considerable amount of heterogeneity within each racial/ethnic group; therefore, making summary statements about cultural beliefs is difficult and can be questionable. Additionally, members of a cultural or ethnic group who are younger or more **acculturated** into mainstream U.S. society may not adhere to popular and traditional health beliefs.

Americans of Hispanic Origin

The term *Hispanic* was introduced by the OMB in 1977, creating an ethnic category that included persons of Mexican, Puerto Rican, Cuban, Central American, South American, or some other Spanish origin regardless of race.[8] In 1997, the term *Hispanic* was changed to *Hispanic or Latino*.[9] For the purposes of data collection, the only ethnic distinction that the U.S. government makes is "Hispanic" or "non-Hispanic"; therefore, nearly all Americans of Hispanic origin are racially classified as white.

Since 1990, the Hispanic population has been the most rapidly growing ethnic group in the United States. In 2010, Americans of Hispanic origin constituted 16.3% of the total U.S. population, making them the largest minority group in the nation. People of Mexican origin are the largest Hispanic group in the United States (63%), followed by Puerto Ricans (9.2%) and Salvadorans (3.3%). The remaining are of some other Central American, South American, or other Hispanic or Latino origins.[16]

Although a high school education is considered an essential basic training requirement to enter the labor force, the high school educational attainment level of Hispanic youth has been consistently lower when compared to other groups (see **Figure 8.3**).[17] Linked with education is earning power. The median income of Hispanic families is significantly lower than that of Asian/Pacific Islanders and whites.[18] The poverty rate for persons of Hispanic origin was 26.7% in 2010 , nearly three times the rate for white Americans (see **Figure 8.4**). The poverty rate of foreign-born Hispanics was higher than for those who were born in the United States.[19]

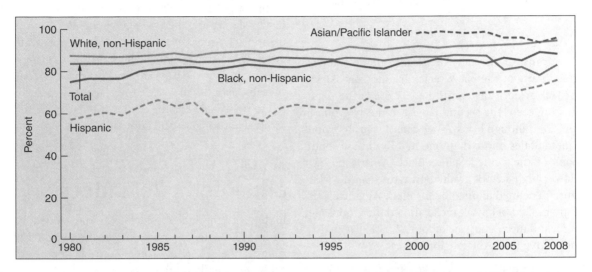

Figure 8.3 Percentage of adults ages 18 to 24 who have completed high school, by race and Hispanic origin, 1980-2008.

Note: Percentages are based only on those not currently enrolled in high school or below. Prior to 1992, this indicator was measured as completing 4 or more years of high school rather than the actual attainment of a high school diploma or equivalent.

U.S. Census Bureau (2010). Current Population Survey, School Enrollment Supplement. Tabulated by the U.S. Department of Education, National Center for Education Statistics.

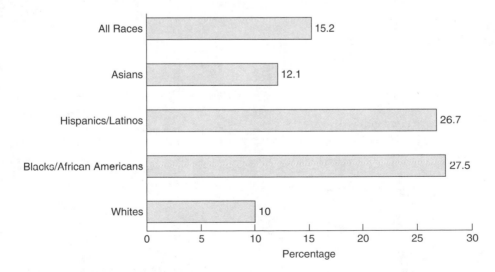

Figure 8.4 Poverty rates by race and Hispanic origin: 2010.

Note: Federal surveys now give respondents the option of reporting more than one race. Therefore, two basic ways of defining a race group are possible. A group such as Asian may be defined as those who reported Asian and no other race (the race-alone or single-race concept) or as those who reported Asian regardless of whether they also reported another race (the race-alone-or-in-combination concept). This figure shows data using the first approach (race alone).

Data from DeNavas-Walt, C., B. D. Proctor, and J. C. Smith (2011). *U.S. Census Bureau, Current Population Reports, P60-236, Income, Poverty, and Health Insurance Coverage in the United States, 2008.* Washington, DC: U.S. Government Printing Office.

Traditional health beliefs perceive good health as a matter of fortune or reward from God for good behavior. *Curanderismo* is a very common form of Hispanic folk medicine.[20] A *curandera*'s, or healer's, ability includes a varied repertoire of religious belief systems (mainly Catholicism), herbal knowledge, witchcraft, and scientific medicine.

Black Americans

Black Americans, or African Americans, are people having origins in any of the black racial groups from Africa. In 2010, black Americans constituted 12.6% of the population, making them the second largest minority group in the nation. Even though black Americans live in all regions of the United States, more than one-half live in the southern regions of the United States. Black Americans have slightly lower high school graduation rates than do white Americans.[17] The median income for black Americans has consistently ranked below all racial and ethnic groups (see **Figure 8.5**), and more than one in four (27.5%) live in poverty, almost three times the rate for whites.[18–20]

When discussing black American culture, it is important to mention the effect of slavery.[21] Laws that forbade slaves from providing health care to each other, under the threat of death, led to an underground system of health care by mostly untrained providers because health care available through slave owners was often inadequate.

After the Civil War, poverty, discrimination, and poor living conditions led to a high prevalence of disease, disability, and death among black Americans, a legacy that continues to this day.[22] Lacking access to more formalized health care, first by slavery and then by segregation and discrimination, many black Americans depend on traditional health methods.[23] These traditional methods include curing illnesses with roots, herbs, barks, and teas by an individual knowledgeable about their use. Many black Americans continue to use traditional healing methods today because they are acceptable, available, and affordable.

Asian Americans and Pacific Islanders

In June 1999, then-President Clinton signed Executive Order 13125 to improve the quality of life of Asian Americans and Pacific Islanders through increased participation in federal programs where they may be underserved and by collecting separate data on each group to decrease the concealment of substantial socioeconomic and health differences among the two groups.[24,25] However, even by

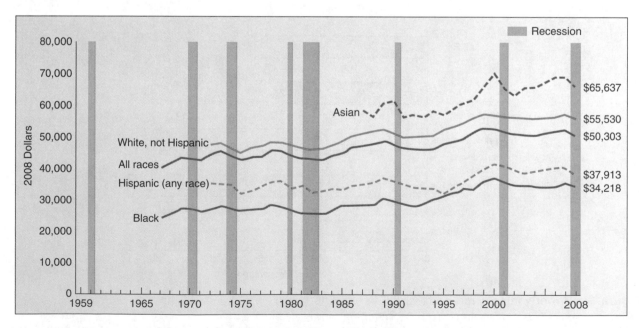

Figure 8.5 Real median income by race and Hispanic origin: 1967–2008.

Note: Median household income data are not available prior to 1967.

U.S. Census Bureau. *Current Population Survey, 1968 to 2009 Annual Social And Economic Supplements.* Washington, DC: U.S. Government Printing Office. Available at http://www.census.gov/prod/2009pubs/p60-236.pdf.

2001, most federal agencies were still not collecting separate data on these two groups, citing methodological and funding constraints.[26]

Asian American populations are generally concentrated in the western states, the Northeast, and parts of the South. Native Hawaiian and other Pacific Islanders (NHOPIs) live throughout the United States, but their populations are most concentrated in the western mainland states and Hawaii. In 2010, Asians constituted 4.8% of the population, and native Hawaiians and other Pacific Islanders numbered 0.2% of the population.

When education and income are reported in aggregate for Asians and NHOPIs, they appear well off. The high school completion rates of 18- through 24-year-olds and the median incomes were the highest compared with all other racial and ethnic groups. Unfortunately, these aggregated data mask the large variation within this population group.[27,28]

As mentioned previously, Asian Americans and Pacific Islanders are two discrete groups. The term *Asian American* refers to people of Asian descent who trace their roots to more than 20 different Asian countries, including Cambodia, China, India, Japan, Korea, Malaysia, Pakistan, the Philippine Islands, Thailand, and Vietnam.[29] Immigration is an integral part of Asian American community growth, because many are seeking better economic and employment opportunities and/or are reuniting with family members. Even among those who have come from the same country, immigration to the United States may have occurred at different times, and thus there are generational differences. For example, some families may have immigrated well over a hundred years ago as laborers, whereas those coming today carry with them professional degrees.[30] These differences contribute to a substantial diversity in socioeconomic status among these groups.

Although variations among Asian Americans is the norm, many share similarities based on their religious background and the belief of equilibrium or balance.[31] The concept of balance is related to health, and imbalance is related to disease. This balance or imbalance is highly related to diet, which influences people's daily activities of living within their environment. Therefore, to achieve health and avoid illness, people must adjust to the environment in a holistic manner.

The term *Pacific Islander (PI)* includes peoples of Hawaii, Guam, Samoa, or other Pacific Islands and their descendants,[29] with the Native Hawaiian population forming the majority of PIs. In contrast to Asian Americans, there is no large-scale immigration of PIs into the continental United States.

Approximately 20% of Native Hawaiians live in rural Hawaii. However, the majority of the state's healthcare resources are fixed in the capital city of Honolulu. As a result of this imbalance of healthcare resource allocation, there is an inadequate number of healthcare professionals on the neighboring islands.[32,33] Transportation between the islands makes it difficult to access healthcare services for the native population. The second medical care issue deals with a Native Hawaiian health belief, which suggests that the healer cannot be reimbursed directly for his or her therapeutic work. According to Blaisdell,[34] such healer skill is not a question of learning but rather a question of righteousness. Therefore, it is not considered appropriate to be paid for doing what is right.

American Indians and Alaska Natives

The American Indian and Alaska Native (AI/AN) population, the original inhabitants of America, account for 0.09% of the total population. It has been estimated that prior to the arrival of European explorers, 12 million AI/ANs lived and flourished throughout what is now the United States. Exposure to non-native diseases and ecological changes introduced by explorers and colonists decimated the AI/AN population. Although many of the descendants were assimilated by intermarriages or successfully adapted to the new culture, as a group, the AI/ANs became economically and socially disadvantaged, and this status is reflected in their relatively poor health status.[35,36] The 2008 average poverty rate for AI/ANs was 25.7%, which is the highest among all racial and ethnic groups (see Figure 8.5).[37] Similarly, their median income and high school completion rates were among the lowest of any racial and ethnic group.

The Native American community is composed of many different American Indian tribal groups and Alaskan villages. Each of these tribes/villages has distinct customs, language, and beliefs; however, the majority share similar cultural values including an emphasis on an individual's right to freedom, autonomy, and respect as well as respect for all living things, and an expectation that tribal/village members will bring honor and respect to their families, clans, and tribes.[38]

Central to Native American culture is that the people "strive for a close integration within the family, clan and tribe and live in harmony with their environment. This occurs simultaneously on physical, mental, and spiritual levels; thus, individual wellness is considered as harmony and balance among mind, body, spirit and the environment."[38] This concept is not congruent with the medical model approach or public health. As a result, in many Native American communities there is conflict between the medical/public health approach and the approaches used by Native American healers. Providing appropriate health care for Native Americans usually involves resolving conflicts between the two approaches in such a way that they complement each other.

U.S. Government, Native Americans, and the Provision of Health Care

Although classified by definition and for statistical purposes as a minority group, Native Americans are unlike any other ethnic or racial group in the United States. Some tribes are sovereign nations, based on their treaties with the U.S. government. Tribal sovereignty, which came about when the tribes transferred virtually all the land in the United States to the federal government in return for the provision of certain services, creates a distinct and special relationship between various tribes and the U.S. government.

Provisions of health services to Native Americans began in 1832.[35] The first medical efforts were carried out by Army physicians who vaccinated Native Americans against smallpox and applied sanitary procedures to curb other communicable diseases among tribes living in the vicinity of military posts. The health services provided for Native Americans after the signing of the early treaties were limited. It was not until 1921, when the Snyder Act created the Bureau of Indian Affairs (BIA) Health Division, that more emphasis was given to providing health services to Native Americans. In 1954 with the passage of Public Law 83-568, known as the Transfer Act, the responsibility of health care for Native Americans was transferred from the Department of the Interior's BIA to the Public Health Service (PHS). It was at this time that the Indian Health Service (IHS) was created.

Indian Health Service

In keeping with the concept of tribal sovereignty, the Indian Self-Determination and Education Assistance Act (PL 93-63) of 1975 authorized the IHS to involve tribes in the administration and operation of all or certain programs under a special contract. It authorized the IHS to provide grants to tribes, on request,

alien a person born in and owing allegiance to a country other than the one in which he or she lives

immigrant individual who migrates from one country to another for the purpose of seeking permanent residence

refugee a person who flees one area or country to seek shelter or protection from danger in another

unauthorized immigrant an individual who entered a country without permission

for planning, development, and operation of health programs.[35] Today, a number of programs are managed and operated under contract by individual tribes.[36]

The IHS is responsible for providing federal health services to Native Americans and Alaska Natives.[36] This agency operates hospitals, clinics and health stations, and a variety of other programs. The goal of the IHS is to raise the health status of American Indians and Alaska Natives to the highest possible level.[36]

The New Immigrants

Refugees are defined as people who flee one area, usually their home country, to seek shelter or protection from danger. Refugees arriving in the United States may be seeking political asylum, refuge from war, or escape from famine or another environmental disaster. The term **immigrants** describes individuals who migrate from another country for the purpose of seeking permanent residence and hopefully a better life. **Aliens** are defined as people born in and owing allegiance to a country other than the one in which they live. Thus, aliens are not citizens and are only allowed to stay in a foreign country for a specified period of time defined by law or policy. Sometimes, however, they violate this provision and find employment illegally. Finally, **unauthorized immigrants** are those who enter a country without any permission whatsoever.[39]

Although all refugees who enter this country can be classified into one of the existing racial/ethnic categories used by our government, as a single group they present many special concerns not seen in minorities who are born and raised in the United States. Most of the refugees currently entering the United States arrive from developing countries, and many refugees are poor, have low levels of formal education, and have few marketable work skills. Many arrive with serious health problems, including undernourishment or starvation, physical and emotional injuries from hostile action or confinement in refugee camps, poor health care, and overcrowding.[40] A majority of the refugees are young, many of the women are of childbearing age, and most come from Latin American and Southeast Asian countries.

The difficulties facing refugees in the United States, including finding employment and obtaining access to education and appropriate human, health, and mental health services, represent significant barriers to the social integration of refugees into U.S. society. Like most of the other minority groups in the United States, refugees may become a part of those disadvantaged in this country.

There is, however, one bright note to the increase of refugees in this country—the enrichment of the U.S. culture. Until 1970, cultural diversity in the United States was limited; today, however, the minority groups are the fastest-growing segments of the U.S. population.[41]

Race and Health Initiative

The Race and Health Initiative committed the nation to the ambitious goal of eliminating health disparities among racial and ethnic groups in six priority areas: (1) infant mortality, (2) cancer screening and management, (3) cardiovascular disease, (4) diabetes, (5) HIV/AIDS, and (6) adult and child immunization. The Race and Health Initiative reaffirms the government's extensive focus on minority health issues by emphasizing these six health issues account for a substantial burden of disease that is highly modifiable if appropriate interventions are applied. Thus, the Race and Health Initiative is intertwined with *Healthy People 2020*'s national health promotion and disease prevention objectives.[7]

Infant Mortality

Infant mortality, defined as the death of an infant before his or her first birthday, is highly correlated to the general health and well-being of the nation. The United States made significant improvement in the twentieth century regarding infant health. However, whereas the vast majority of infants born in the United States today are healthy at birth, many are not. Additionally, infant mortality data within the United States are characterized by a longstanding and serious disparity among racial and ethnic minorities (see **Figure 8.6**). The greatest disparity exists for black

Americans, whose infant death rate is more than two times that of white American infants.

There are many reasons associated with higher infant mortality rates among black Americans. Two of the more important explanations include lack of prenatal care and giving birth to low-birth-weight (LBW) babies. Women who receive early and continuous prenatal health care have better pregnancy outcomes than women who do not. Black American, Native American, and Hispanic American women are less likely to receive early and comprehensive prenatal care.[42] In the same manner, black Americans and Native Americans are more likely to give birth to LBW babies.

Cancer Screening and Management

Cancer is the second leading cause of death in the United States, accounting for more than 550,000 deaths and some 1.4 million new cases of invasive cancer annually.[43] Nearly one-third of those who develop cancer will die from it.

More than half of all new cancer cases annually are cancers of the lung, colon and rectum, breast, and prostate. From 2002 to 2006, cancer incidence rates per 100,000 population were highest among black Americans for lung, colon and rectum, and prostate cancers compared to white Americans, Asian/Pacific Islanders, American Indian/Alaska Natives, and Hispanics (see **Figure 8.7**). During the same period of time, cancer death rates per 100,000 people were highest among black Americans for lung, colon and rectum, and prostate cancers compared to white Americans, Asian/Pacific Islanders, American Indian/Alaska Natives, and Hispanics. A number of these disparities in cancer incidence and death rates among minorities are attributed to lifestyle factors, late diagnosis, and access to health care.[44]

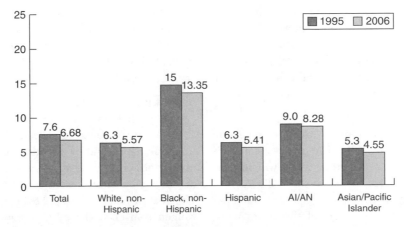

Figure 8.6 Infant mortality rates by race and Hispanic origin of mother: 1995 and 2006.
Centers for Disease Control and Prevention, National Center for Health Statistics. VitalStats. "Linked Birth and Infant Death Data." Available at: http://www.cdc.gov/nchs/vitalstats.htm.

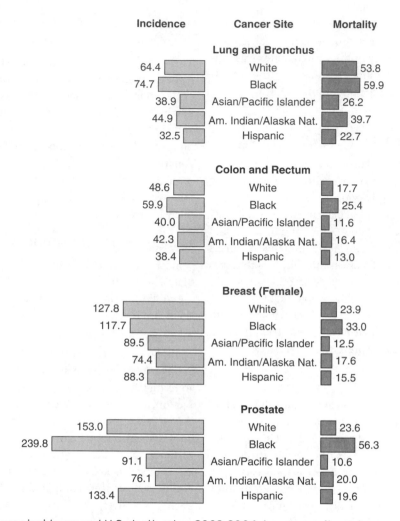

Incidence	Cancer Site	Mortality

Lung and Bronchus

64.4	White	53.8
74.7	Black	59.9
38.9	Asian/Pacific Islander	26.2
44.9	Am. Indian/Alaska Nat.	39.7
32.5	Hispanic	22.7

Colon and Rectum

48.6	White	17.7
59.9	Black	25.4
40.0	Asian/Pacific Islander	11.6
42.3	Am. Indian/Alaska Nat.	16.4
38.4	Hispanic	13.0

Breast (Female)

127.8	White	23.9
117.7	Black	33.0
89.5	Asian/Pacific Islander	12.5
74.4	Am. Indian/Alaska Nat.	17.6
88.3	Hispanic	15.5

Prostate

153.0	White	23.6
239.8	Black	56.3
91.1	Asian/Pacific Islander	10.6
76.1	Am. Indian/Alaska Nat.	20.0
133.4	Hispanic	19.6

Figure 8.7 SEER cancer incidence and U.S. death rates, 2002-2006, by cancer site and race.

Horner, M. J., L. A. G. Ries, M. Krapcho, et al. (eds.). *SEER Cancer Statistics Review, 1975-2006, based on November 2008 SEER data submission, posted to the SEER web site, 2009.* Bethesda, MD: National Cancer Institute. Available at http://seer.cancer.gov/csr/1975_2006/.

Primary cancer prevention refers to preventing the occurrence of cancer.[43] Smoking is the most preventable cause of lung cancer death in our society. The death rate for lung cancer is 20% higher in black Americans than in white Americans. Paralleling this death rate is the fact that black Americans have a higher incidence of smoking than do white Americans.

Secondary cancer prevention refers to early detection of cancer through screening tests. The earlier a cancer is detected, the greater the chances the patient will survive. The racial/ethnic disparities in lower survival rates can be attributed partially to lower cancer screening rates among specific groups. Two cancers of significant interest are colorectal and breast. Colorectal cancer remains the second leading cause of cancer deaths in the United States and the leading cause of cancer deaths among nonsmokers. According to the Centers for Disease Control and Prevention (CDC), 1,900 deaths could be prevented each year for every 10% increase in colonoscopy screening.

Breast cancer is the second leading cause of cancer death among women. Breast cancer survival rates are significantly increased if the cancer is detected early through monthly self-examination and/or periodic breast X-rays. Despite the importance of mammography, it is underutilized as an early detection procedure by many minority women (see Box 8.1). The goal of *Healthy People 2020* is to have at least 81% of women from all racial or ethnic groups age 50 or older receiving a mammogram within the preceding 2 years.[7]

Box 8.1 *Healthy People 2020:* Objective

Objective C.17: Increase the proportion of women who receive a breast cancer screening based on the most recent guidelines.

For Further Thought
Research indicates that mortality resulting from breast cancer can be reduced through the use of mammography. Data for 2008 show that 68% of white and black women received mammograms, whereas American Indian/Alaska Native, Asian/Pacific Islander, and Hispanic women were less likely to have had a mammogram. What type of program could be implemented to further increase the percentage of these minority women who participate in mammograms?

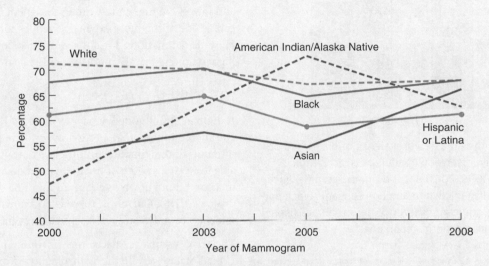

Percentage of U.S. women age 40 years and older who have had a mammogram in the last 2 years by race and ethnicity.

National Center for Health Statistics (2010). *Health, United States, 2009 with Special Feature on Medical Technology.* (DHHS pub. no. 2010-1232). Hyattsville, MD: Author. Available at http://www.cdc.gov /nchs/hus.htm.

Source: U.S. Department of Health and Human Services, Office of Disease Prevention and Health Promotion (2010). *Healthy People 2020.* Available at http://www.healthypeople.gov/2020/default.aspx.

Cardiovascular Diseases

Cardiovascular disease (CVD), especially coronary heart disease and stroke, kills more Americans annually than any other disease. In fact, CVD claims more lives each year than the next five leading causes of death combined. Death rates from coronary heart disease and stroke vary widely among racial and ethnic groups.

One of the major modifiable risk factors for coronary artery disease and stroke is hypertension. One in three adult Americans suffers from hypertension; however, rates are not evenly distributed among racial and ethnic groups,

with the highest prevalence among black Americans (see **Figure 8.8**).[45] In addition, black Americans tend to develop hypertension earlier in life than whites. The reasons for this are unknown. In fact, the cause of 90% to 95% of the cases of hypertension in all races and ethnic groups is unknown. Therefore, secondary prevention or screening for hypertension is essential.

Diabetes

Approximately 24 million people in the United States have diabetes (see **Figure 8.9**), with morbidity and mortality rates increasing for all groups in the last two decades.[46,47]

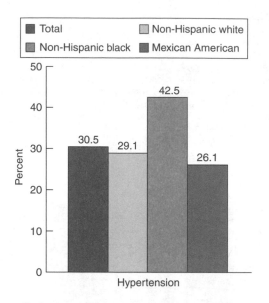

Figure 8.8 Age-adjusted prevalence of diagnosed or undiagnosed hypertension in adults, by race/ethnicity: United States, 1999–2006. 1 is the significant difference between non-Hispanic white and non-Hispanic black persons. 3 is the significant difference between non-Hispanic white and Mexican-American persons.

Note: Persons of other race/ethnicity included in total.

Centers for Disease Control and Prevention, National Center for Health Statistics. *National Health and Nutrition Examination Surveys, 1999–2006.* Available at http://www.cdc.gov/nchs/nhanes.htm.

Diabetes death rates vary considerably among racial and ethnic groups. Compared to white non-Hispanics, diabetes death rates were nearly two and a half times higher among black Americans and American Indians, and nearly two times higher among Americans of Hispanic origin.[46]

Additional serious complications from diabetes include heart disease, stroke, blindness, and kidney disease. In fact, diabetes is the leading cause of new cases of blindness in people ages 20 to 74 and the leading cause of end-stage renal disease (ESRD), accounting for nearly half of all new cases. In 2006, more than 155,000 people with ESRD resulting from diabetes were living on chronic dialysis or with a kidney transplant.[46] Between 1980 and 2006, ESRD attributable to diabetes was greatest among black men and women and lowest among white women. Inpatient hospitalization care is one of the most expensive venues for diabetes care. Hospital admissions for long-term care of diabetes are highest among black Americans and Hispanics.

HIV Infection/AIDS

A human immunodeficiency virus (HIV) infection is a chronic condition that progressively damages the body's immune system, making an otherwise healthy person less able to resist a variety of infections and disorders resulting in a condition known as acquired immune deficiency syndrome (AIDS). Currently, there is no known cure for HIV infection or AIDS and no vaccine to prevent it.

The CDC estimates that some 1.2 million people in the United States were living with diagnosed or undiagnosed HIV.[47] At the end of 2009 the CDC estimated that 878,366 people were diagnosed with AIDS in the United States. AIDS has had a disproportionate impact on racial and ethnic minority groups in the United States since the disease was first recognized, with well over half of all identified cases since 1981 being reported among racial and ethnic groups. The proportion of cases has increased among black and

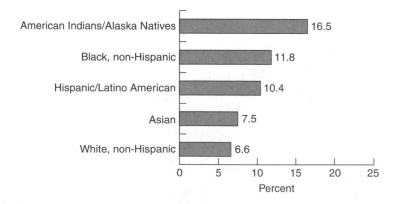

Figure 8.9 Age-adjusted percentage of civilian, noninstitionalized population with diagnosed diabetes, by race and sex, United States: 1980–2007.

Centers for Disease Control and Prevention. "National Diabetes Surveillance System." Available at http://www.cdc.gov/diabetes/statistics/prev/national/figraceethsex.htm.

Hispanic Americans and decreased among whites. In 2009, black and Hispanic Americans, who represented less than half of the population, accounted for more than one-half of the estimated number of HIV/AIDS cases diagnosed (see **Figure 8.10**). Consistent with the AIDS case rates are higher AIDS death rates for black and Hispanic Americans.[48]

Part of the reason for the disproportionate numbers of HIV and AIDS cases in black and Hispanic Americans has been attributed to a higher prevalence of unsafe or risky health behaviors (e.g., unprotected sexual intercourse and intravenous drug use), existing co-conditions (e.g., genital ulcer disease), and the lack of access to health care that would provide early diagnosis and treatment. A prevailing barrier to HIV/AIDS prevention may be that this condition is not being viewed as among the highest priorities in some minority communities when compared with other life survival problems.[49] With no cure for HIV/AIDS in sight, better health education to reduce and eliminate unsafe behaviors and increased access to medical resources for existing cases are essential to prevention.

Child and Adult Immunization Rates

As a result of widespread immunization practices, many infectious diseases that were once common have been significantly reduced. Childhood immunization rates provide one measure of the extent to which children are protected from dangerous vaccine-preventable illnesses. An important immunization rate for children ages 19 months to 35 months is the 4:3:1:3:3:1 vaccine series that includes DTP/DT/DTaP; poliovirus vaccine; measles, mumps, and rubella vaccine (MMR); *Haemophilus influenzae* type b vaccine; hepatitis B vaccine; and varicella vaccine. In 2008, coverage estimates for the 4:3:1:3:3:1 vaccine series did not vary significantly by race or ethnicity among children ages 19 months to 35 months, ranging from 76% for children of multiple races to 82% for Asians/Pacific Islanders, 78% for blacks, 76% for whites, and 78% for Hispanics.[50]

It is important for adults, especially those 65 years or older, to become immunized against certain infectious diseases that can cause illness, disability, or death (see **Figure 8.11**). Two important adult immunizations included in the 2010 adult immunization schedule, as well as among the infectious disease objectives stated in *Healthy People 2020*, are immunizations for influenza and pneumococcal diseases.[7] The goal is to increase the number of noninstitutionalized adults 65 or older who are immunized annually against influenza and who have ever received an immunization against pneumococcal disease to 90%. Immunization rates among nonminorities for influenza and pneumococcal infections are substantially lower than for white Americans.[51] Therefore, even though these two immunization rates among all adults have shown a significant increase since 1990, to reach the goal of 90% by 2020, increased efforts must be focused on minority populations.[7]

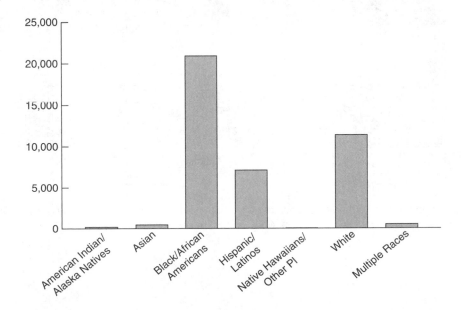

Figure 8.10 Estimated number of HIV infection diagnoses: 2009.
Data from Centers for Disease Control and Prevention (2011). *HIV Surveillance Report, 2009*, vol. 21. Available at http://www.cdc.gov/hiv/topics/surveillance/resources/reports/.

VACCINE ▼ AGE GROUP ►	19–26 years	27–49 years	50–59 years	60–64 years	≥ 65 years
Tetanus, diphtheria, pertussis (Td/Tdap)*	Substitute one-time dose of Tdap for Td booster; then boost with Td every 10 years				Td booster every 10 years
Human papillomavirus*	3 doses (females)				
Varicella*	2 doses				
Zoster				1 dose	
Measles, mumps, rubella*	1 or 2 doses		1 dose		
Influenza*	1 dose annually				
Pneumococcal (polysaccharide)	1 or 2 doses				1 dose
Hepatitis A*	2 doses				
Hepatitis B*	3 doses				
Meningococcal*	1 or more doses				

*Covered by the Vaccine Injury Compensation Program.

For all persons in this category who meet the age requirements and who lack evidence of immunity (e.g., lack documentation of vaccination or have no evidence of prior infection)

Recommended if some other risk factor is present (e.g., based on medical, occupational, lifestyle, or other indications)

No recommendation

INDICATION ► VACCINE ▼	Pregnancy	Immunocompromising conditions (excluding human immunodeficiency virus [HIV])	HIV infection CD4+ T lymphocyte count < 200 cells/μL	HIV infection CD4+ T lymphocyte count ≥ 200 cells/μL	Diabetes, heart disease, chronic lung disease, chronic alcoholism	Asplenia (including elective splenectomy and persistent complement component deficiencies)	Chronic liver disease	Kidney failure, end-stage renal disease, receipt of hemodialysis	Healthcare personnel
Tetanus, diphtheria, pertussis (Td/Tdap)*	Td	Substitute one-time dose of Tdap for Td booster; then boost with Td every 10 years							
Human papillomavirus*	3 doses for females through age 26 years								
Varicella*	Contraindicated			2 doses					
Zoster	Contraindicated			1 dose					
Measles, mumps, rubella*	Contraindicated			1 or 2 doses					
Influenza*	1 dose TIV annually								1 dose TIV or LAIV annually
Pneumococcal (polysaccharide)	1 or 2 doses								
Hepatitis A*	2 doses								
Hepatitis B*	3 doses								
Meningococcal*	1 or more doses								

*Covered by the Vaccine Injury Compensation Program.

For all persons in this category who meet the age requirements and who lack evidence of immunity (e.g., lack documentation of vaccination or have no evidence of prior infection)

Recommended if some other risk factor is present (e.g., based on medical, occupational, lifestyle, or other indications)

No recommendation

Figure 8.11 Recommended adult immunization schedule, United States, 2010, by age group and medical condition.

Centers for Disease Control and Prevention. "Recommended adult immunication schedule—United States, 2010." *Morbidity and Mortality Weekly Report,* 58(1): 1–4.

Socioeconomic Status and Racial and Ethnic Disparities in Health

The literature suggest multiple causes for health disparities in the United States including economics, education, and behavioral factors—such as lifestyle and health practices—as well as cultural, legal, and political factors (see **Figure 8.12**). We focus our discussion on **socioeconomic status (SES)**, which has been considered the single most influential contributor to premature morbidity and mortality by many public health researchers.[52–54] Furthermore, many of these factors are not always direct in nature—they are what are referred to as indirect causal associations or intermediary factors. For example, poverty by itself may not cause disease and death; however, by precluding adequate nutrition, preventive medical care, and housing, it leads to increased morbidity and premature mortality.

As we stated earlier, the categories of race are more of a social category than a biological one. In fact, biological differences between racial groups are small compared with biological differences within groups.[52] More than 90% of the differences in genetic makeup occur within racial and ethnic groups rather than between the groups. Such disparities in health status among minority groups are much better understood in terms of the groups' living circumstances.[53] A group's living circumstances may be referred to as its socioeconomic status. Common SES factors studied include level of education, level of income, and poverty.

Public health research has long studied SES factors and their relationship

socioeconomic status relating to a combination of social and economic factors

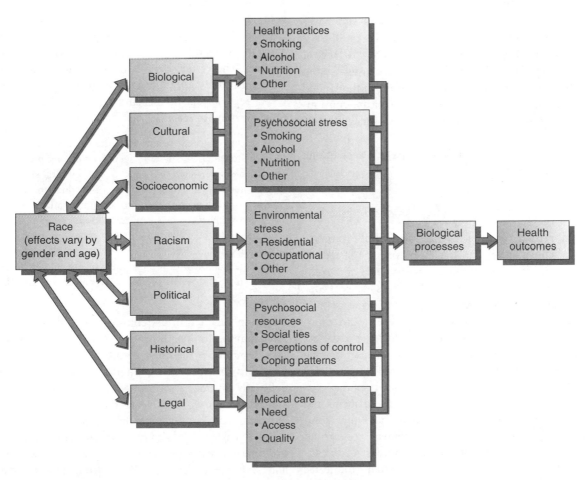

Figure 8.12 A framework for understanding the relationship between race and health.

Centers for Disease Control and Prevention (1993). "Use of Race and Ethnicity in Public Health Surveillance. Summary of CDC/ASTDR Workshop." *Morbidity and Mortality Weekly Report*, 42(RR-10).

to health. These studies have shown that better health is associated with more years of education, having more income and a more prestigious job, and living in superior neighborhoods. Similarly, elevated levels of morbidity, disability, and mortality are associated with less education, lower income, poverty, unemployment, and poor housing. An extensive amount of research shows that SES factors play a significant role in the association of race and ethnicity with health.[7] Furthermore, research in the last couple of decades indicates that the relationship between SES and health occurs at every socioeconomic level and for a broad range of SES indicators.[54] This relationship between SES and health can be described as a gradient. For example, research has documented that the more family income increases above the poverty threshold, the more health improves, and that the greater the gap in income, the greater the gap in health.

This gradient effect between SES and health has important implications that are related to the gap between the privileged and nonprivileged, or the "haves and have-nots." In the United States, many inequalities still exist between all racial and ethnic groups related to level of education, income, and poverty. Minority groups often occupy the lowest socioeconomic rankings in the United States. These low rankings become a significant community health concern when one recognizes that progress toward the *Healthy People 2020* objectives was found to be greatest among the higher SES groups and least among the lower SES groups.

Equity in Minority Health

One of the primary aims of the Race and Health Initiative consists of consultation and collaboration among federal agencies; state, local, and tribal governments; and community professionals to research and address issues of education, income, environment, and other socioeconomic factors that affect health outcomes. These health problems are inseparable from a variety of other social problems, making simple solutions unlikely. We also know that multiple resources are required to resolve these social and economic problems, and that solutions to these problems for one group may not work for another. Americans of Hispanic origin, Asian Americans, Pacific Islanders, black Americans, and Native Americans each have unique cultural traditions that must be respected if the solutions are to be successful.

cultural and linguistic competence a set of congruent behaviors, attitudes, and policies that come together in a system, agency, or among professionals, that enables effective work in cross-cultural situations

Cultural Competence

Cultural differences can and do present major obstacles to implementing effective community health programs and services. The demographic shifts in minority populations and the resulting diversity in healthcare providers treating more patients have increased interest among health professionals to increase culturally appropriate services that lead to improved outcomes, efficiency, and satisfaction for their clients.[55,56] This increased interest is not only being found among healthcare providers, but also among patients, policymakers, educators, and accreditation and credentialing agencies. In March 2001, the HHS and the Office of Minority Health published standards for culturally and linguistically appropriate services (CLAS) in health care (see **Box 8.2**).[57] These criteria are the first comprehensive and nationally recognized standards of cultural and linguistic competence in healthcare service delivery that have been developed. In the past, national organizations and federal agencies independently developed their own standards and policies. The result was a wide spectrum of ideas about what constitutes culturally appropriate health services. The CLAS report went further and defined **cultural and linguistic competence** as

> A set of congruent behaviors, attitudes, and policies that come together in a system, agency, or among professionals that enables effective work in cross cultural situations. Culture refers to integrated patterns of human behavior that include language, thoughts, communications, actions, customs, beliefs, values, and institutions of racial, ethnic, religious or social groups. Competence implies having the capacity to function effectively as an individual and an organization within the context of the cultural beliefs, behaviors, and needs presented by consumers and their communities.[57]

Based on this definition, culture is a vital factor in both how community health professionals deliver services and how community members respond to community health programs and preventive interventions. In a society as culturally diverse as the United States, community health educators need to be able to communicate with different communities and understand how culture influences health behaviors.[58,59] It is important that community health promotion/disease prevention programs be understandable and acceptable within the cultural framework of the population to be reached.

Box 8.2   National Standards for Culturally and Linguistically Appropriate Services in Health Care

1. Health care organizations should ensure that patients/consumers receive from all staff members effective, understandable, and respectful care that is provided in a manner compatible with their cultural health beliefs and practices and preferred language.

2. Health care organizations should implement strategies to recruit, retain, and promote at all levels of the organization a diverse staff and leadership that are representative of the demographic characteristics of the service area.

3. Health care organizations should ensure that staff at all levels and across all disciplines receive ongoing education and training in culturally and linguistically appropriate service delivery.

4. Health care organizations must offer and provide language assistance services, including bilingual staff and interpreter services, at no cost to each patient/consumer with limited English proficiency at all points of contact, in a timely manner during all hours of operation.

5. Health care organizations must provide to patients/consumers in their preferred language both verbal offers and written notices informing them of their right to receive language assistance services.

6. Health care organizations must assure the competence of language assistance provided to limited English proficient patients/consumers by interpreters and bilingual staff. Family and friends should not be used to provide interpretation services (except on request by the patient/consumer).

7. Health care organizations must make available easily understood patient-related materials and post signage in the languages of the commonly encountered groups and/or groups represented in the service area.

8. Health care organizations should develop, implement, and promote a written strategic plan that outlines clear goals, policies, operational plans, and management accountability/oversight mechanisms to provide culturally and linguistically appropriate services.

9. Health care organizations should conduct initial and ongoing organizational self-assessments of CLAS-related activities and are encouraged to integrate cultural and linguistic competence-related measures into their internal audits, performance improvement programs, patient satisfaction assessments, and outcomes-based evaluations.

10. Health care organizations should ensure that data on the individual patient's/consumer's race, ethnicity, and spoken and written language are collected in health records, integrated into the organization's management information systems, and periodically updated.

11. Health care organizations should maintain a current demographic, cultural, and epidemiological profile of the community as well as a needs assessment to accurately plan for and implement services that respond to the cultural and linguistic characteristics of the service area.

12. Health care organizations should develop participatory, collaborative partnerships with communities and utilize a variety of formal and informal mechanisms to facilitate community and patient/consumer involvement in designing and implementing CLAS-related activities.

13. Health care organizations should ensure that conflict and grievance resolution processes are culturally and linguistically sensitive and capable of identifying, preventing, and resolving cross-cultural conflicts or complaints by patients/consumers.

14. Health care organizations are encouraged to regularly make available to the public information about their progress and successful innovations in implementing the CLAS standards and to provide public notice in their communities about the availability of this information.

Note: The standards are organized by three themes.

1. Culturally competent care (Standards 1–3)
2. Language access services (Standards 4–7)
3. Organizational supports for cultural competence (Standards 8–14)

Source: U.S. Department of Health and Human Services, Office of Minority Health (2001). *National Standards for Culturally and Linguistically Appropriate Services in Health Care: Final Report.* Washington, DC: Author.

For community health educators whose role is to educate groups and communities of diverse cultural backgrounds, cultural competence is critical.[59] Additionally, successful community health intervention and educational activities should be firmly grounded in an understanding and appreciation of the cultural characteristics of the target group. *Healthy People 2020* is firmly devoted to the principle that "every person in every community across the Nation deserves equal access to comprehensive, culturally competent, community-based health care systems that are committed to serving the needs of the individual and promoting community health."[7]

Empowering the Self and the Community

A principle deeply etched in *Healthy People 2020* with respect to achieving equity is the ideal that the "greatest opportunities for reducing health disparities are in empowering individuals to make informed health care decisions and in promoting community-wide safety, education, and access to health care."[7] Not surprisingly, this same principle is the foundation of the eight United Nations (UN) Millennium Development Goals.[60]

A strategy to achieve the goals set forth in *Healthy People 2020* and the UN Millennium Development Goals is to promote empowerment of marginalized groups. Friedmann identifies three kinds of power associated with empowerment—social, political, and psychological.[61] An increase in social power brings with it access to bases of production, such as information, knowledge and skills, participation in social organizations, and financial resources. Increased productivity enables greater influence on markets, which in turn can influence change. Psychological power is best described as an individual sense of potency demonstrated in self-confident behavior. It is often the result of successful action in the social and political domains. With the investiture of all three types of power, empowerment can take place. Empowerment replaces hopelessness with a sense of being in control and a sense that one can make a difference.

Once people are empowered, the power then needs to be transferred to the communities. When communities are empowered, they can cause change and solve problems. Under-represented groups have the potential to have a loud voice if united. Once united, they are in a position to influence decision makers at various governmental levels. In the specific case in which the goal is greater access to health care, this could mean getting the local health department to expand the types and numbers of available clinics, to increase education opportunities, to request culturally competent health services, and to be equal partners in addressing environmental issues, among others.

The 1985 *Secretary's Task Force Report on Black and Minority Health* laid the foundation for the next three decades of *Healthy People* initiatives designed to decrease health disparities and to provide culturally competent healthcare services as well as health promotion and disease prevention programs. Although progress has been made, significant work remains to be done in achieving the goals embodied in *Healthy People 2020* and the UN Millennium Development Goals.

Chapter Summary

- One of the great strengths of the United States has been, and remains, the ethnic and racial diversity of its people. The federal government has categorized the U.S. population into five racial groups (American Indian or Alaska Native, Asian, black or African American, Native Hawaiian or Other Pacific Islander, and white) and two ethnic groups (Hispanic or Latino and non-Hispanic).
- The reporting of accurate and complete race and ethnicity data provides essential information to target and evaluate public health inventions aimed at minority populations.
- All cultural and ethnic groups hold concepts related to health and illness and associated practices for maintaining well-being or providing treatment when it is indicated.
- The Race and Health Initiative includes six priority areas: (1) infant mortality, (2) cancer screening and management, (3) cardiovascular disease, (4) diabetes, (5) HIV/AIDS, and (6) adult and child immunization. These key areas are representative of the larger minority health picture and account for a substantial burden of disease that is highly modifiable if the appropriate interventions are applied.
- Socioeconomic status (SES) has been considered the most influential single contributor to premature morbidity and mortality by many public health researchers. Research in the last couple of decades indicates that the relationship between SES and health occurs at every socioeconomic level and for a broad range of SES indicators. This relationship between SES and health can be described as a gradient.
- Significant strides in the improvement of health in minority groups can be achieved if community health professionals become more culturally sensitive and competent.
- Minority groups must be empowered to solve their own problems through the processes of social, political, and psychological empowerment.

Review Questions

1. Why is it said that the United States was built on diversity?
2. What is the Office of Management and Budget's Directive 15?
3. Why is it important for community health workers to be aware of the significant health disparities among various minority groups in the United States?

4. What were the significant findings of the 1985 landmark report *The Secretary's Task Force Report on Black and Minority Health*?
5. List and explain the six priority areas in the Race and Health Initiative.
6. What role does socioeconomic status play in health disparities among racial and ethnic minority groups?

7. Why is it important for community health professionals and workers to be culturally sensitive and competent?
8. List each of the three kinds of power associated with empowerment. What is the importance of each in empowering individuals and communities?

Activities

1. Using the most recent census report (www.census.gov), create a demographic profile of the state and county in which you live. Locate the following information—population; racial/ethnic composition; percentage of people represented by the different age groups, gender breakdown, and marital status; and percentage of people living in poverty.
2. Make an appointment with an employee of the health department in your hometown. You could conversely review published reports from your local county health department. Find out the differences in health status between the racial/ethnic groups in the community among the race/ethnicity-specific morbidity and mortality data. Discuss these differences, and then summarize your findings in a one-page paper.

3. In a two- to three-page paper, present the proposal you would recommend to the President of the United States for closing the health status gap between the races and ethnic groups.
4. Identify a specific racial/ethnic minority group and select a health problem. Study the topic, and in a three-page paper discuss the present status of the problem, the future outlook for the problem, and what could be done to reduce or eliminate the problem.
5. Write a two-page position paper on why racial/ethnic minority groups have a lower health status than the majority of white Americans.

Community Health on the Web

The Internet contains a wealth of information about community and public health. Increase your knowledge of some of the topics presented in this chapter by accessing the Jones & Bartlett Learning website at **go.jblearning.com/McKenzieBrief** and follow the links to complete the following Web activities:

- Office of Minority Health
- Eliminating Racial and Ethnic Disparities in Health
- Indian Health Service

References

1. U.S. Census Bureau (2011). "State and County Quick Facts." Available at http://quickfacts.census.gov/qfd/states/00000.html.
2. Passel, J. S., and D. Cohn (2008, February). *U.S. Population Projections: 2005-2050*. Washington, DC: Pew Hispanic Center. Available at http://pewhispanic.org/files/reports/85.pdf.
3. Centers for Disease Control and Prevention (1997). *Minority Health Is the Health of the Nation*. Washington, DC: U.S. Government Printing Office.
4. U.S. Department of Health and Human Services (1988). *Report of the Secretary's Task Force on Black and Minority Health*. Washington, DC: Author.

5. U.S. Department of Health and Human Services (1990). *Healthy People 2000: National Health Promotion and Disease Prevention Objectives* (HHS pub. no. PHS 90-50212). Washington, DC: U.S. Government Printing Office.

6. U.S. Department of Health and Human Services (2000). *Testimony of David Satcher, Assistant Secretary for Health and Surgeon General Before the House Commerce Committee, Subcommittee on Health and Environment.* Available at http://www.hhs.gov/asl/testify/t000511a.html.

7. U.S. Department of Health and Human Services, Office of Disease Prevention and Health Promotion (2010). *Healthy People 2020.* Available at http://healthypeople.gov/2020/default.aspx.

8. Office of Management and Budget (1978). "Directive 15: Race and Ethnic Standards for Federal Statistics and Administrative Reporting." In *U.S. Department of Commerce, Office of Federal Statistical Policy and Standards, Statistical Policy Handbook.* Washington, DC: Author, 37-38.

9. Office of Management and Budget (1997). "Revisions to the Standards for the Classification of Federal Data on Race and Ethnicity." Available at http://nces.ed.gov/programs/handbook/data/pdf/Appendix_A.pdf.

10. Nelson, H., and R. Jurmain (1998). *Introduction to Physical Anthropology*, 4th ed. St. Paul, MN: West Publishing.

11. Williams, D. R., R. Lavizzo-Mourey, and R. C. Warren (1994). "The Concept of Race and Health Status in America." *Public Health Reports*, 109: 26-41.

12. Senior, P. A., and R. Bhopa (1994). "Ethnicity as a Variable in Epidemiological Research." *British Medical Journal*, 309: 327-330.

13. Centers for Disease Control and Prevention (1999). "Reporting Race and Ethnicity Data—National Electronic Telecommunications System for Surveillance, 1994-1997." *Morbidity and Mortality Weekly Report*, 48(15): 305-312.

14. Cooper, R. (1994). "A Case Study in the Use of Race and Ethnicity." *Public Health Reports*, 109(1): 46-52.

15. Rosenberg, H. M., J. D. Maurer, and P. D. Sorlie (1999). "Quality of Death Rates by Race and Hispanic Origin: A Summary of Current Research." *Vital Statistics Reports*, 2: 128.

16. Ennis, S., M. Rios-Vargas, and N. Albert (May 2011). *The Hispanic Population: 2010.* Available at http://www.census.gov/prod/cen2010/briefs/c2010br-04.pdf.

17. U.S. Census Bureau (2010). *Current Population Survey, October Supplement.* Washington, DC: U.S. Department of Education, National Center for Education Statistics.

18. DeNavas-Walt, C., B. D. Proctor, and J. C. Smith (2009). *Income, Poverty, and Health Insurance Coverage in the United States: 2008.* Washington, DC: U.S. Government Printing Office.

19. Lopez, M., and D. Cohn (November 2011). "Hispanic Poverty Rate Highest in New Supplemental Census Measure." Available at http://www.pewhispanic.org/2011/11/08/hispanic-poverty-rate-highest-in-new-supplemental-census-measure.

20. Fishman, B., L. Bobo, K. Kosub, and R. Womeodu (1993). "Cultural Issues in Serving Minority Populations: Emphasis on Mexican Americans and African Americans." *American Journal of the Medical Sciences*, 306: 160-166.

21. U.S. Department of Health and Human Services (1993). "Advance Report of Final Mortality Statistics, 1990." *Monthly Vital Statistics Report*, 41(9): 42.

22. Satcher, D., and D. J. Thomas (1990). "Dimensions of Minority Aging: Implications for Curriculum Development for Selected Health Professions." In M. S. Harper, ed., *Minority Aging: Essential Curricula Content for Selected Health and Allied Health Professions* (HHS pub. no. HRS-P-DV-90-4). Washington, DC: U.S. Government Printing Office, 23-32.

23. Airhihenbuwa, C. O., and I. E. Harrison (1993). "Traditional Medicine in Africa: Past, Present and Future." In P. Conrad and E. Gallagher, eds., *Healing and Health Care in Developing Countries* (pp. 122-134). Philadelphia, PA: Temple University Press.

24. President's Advisory Commission on Asian Americans and Pacific Islanders (2001). *A People Looking Forward: Action for Access and Partnerships in the 21st Century. Interim Report to the President.* Available at http://www.scribd.com/doc/38932921/AAPI-Interim-Report.

25. President's Advisory Commission on Asian Americans and Pacific Islanders (2003). *Asian Americans and Pacific Islanders Addressing Health Disparities: Opportunities for Building a Healthier America.* Available at http://www.health.gov/communication/db/report_detail.asp?ID=160&page=2&z_8=on&sp=1.

26. Ghosh, C. (2003). "Healthy People 2010 and Asian Americans/Pacific Islanders: Defining a Baseline of Information." *American Journal of Public Health*, 93: 2093-2098.

27. Mayeno, L., and S. M. Hirota (1994). "Access to Health Care." In N. W. S. Zane, D. T. Takeuchi, and K. N. J. Young, eds., *Confronting Critical Health Issues of Asian and Pacific Islander Americans.* Thousand Oaks, CA: Sage Publications.

28. Yoon, E., and E. Chien (1996). "Asian American and Pacific Islander Health: A Paradigm for Minority Health." *Journal of the American Medical Association*, 275: 736-737.

29. Humes, K., and J. McKinnon (2000). "The Asian and Pacific Islander Population in the United States." In U.S. Census Bureau, *Current Population Reports* (Series P20-529). Washington, DC: U.S. Government Printing Office.

30. Kitano, H. H. L. (1990). "Values, Beliefs, and Practices of Asian-American Elderly: Implications for Geriatric Education." In M. S. Harper, ed., *Minority Aging: Essential Curricula Content for Selected Health and Allied Health Professions* (HHS pub. no. HRS-P-DV-90-4). Washington, DC: U.S. Government Printing Office, 341-348.

31. Frye, B. A. (1995). "Use of Cultural Themes in Promoting Health Among Southeast Asian Refugees." *American Journal of Health Promotion*, 9: 269-280.

32. Aiu, P. (June/July 2000). "Comparing Native Hawaiians' Health to the Nation." *Closing the Gap*, 8-9.

33. Hixon, A. L. and L. E. Buenconsejo-Lum (2010). "Developing the rural primary care workforce in Hawaii: A 10-Point Plan." *Hawaii Medical Journal*, 69(Suppl. 3): 53-55.

34. Blaisdell, R. K. (1989). "Historical and Cultural Aspects of Native Hawaiian Health." In E. Wegner, ed., *Social Process in Hawai'i.* Honolulu: University of Hawai'i Press, 32.

35. Garrett, J. T. (1990). "Indian Health: Values, Beliefs and Practices." In M. S. Harper, ed., *Minority Aging: Essential Curricula Content for Selected Health and Allied Health Professionals* (HHS pub. no. HRS-P-DV-90-4). Washington, DC: U.S. Government Printing Office, 179-191.

36. U.S. Department of Health and Human Services, Indian Health Services, Program Statistics Team (2000). "Regional Differences in Indian Health 1998-99." Available at http://www.ihs.gov/publicinfo/publications/trends98/region98.asp.

37. DeNavas-Walk, C., B. Proctor, and J. Smith (2011). "Income, Poverty, and Health Insurance Coverage in the United States:

2010." Available at http://www.census.gov/prod/2011pubs/p60-239.pdf.

38. Edwards, E. D., and M. Egbert-Edwards (1990). "Family Care and Native American Elderly." In M. S. Harper, ed., *Minority Aging: Essential Curricula Content for Selected Health and Allied Health Professions* (HHS pub. no. HRS-P-DV-90-4). Washington, DC: U.S. Government Printing Office, 145-163.

39. Hoffer, M., N. Rytina, & B. Baker (2010). "Estimates of the Unauthorized Immigrant Population Residing in the United States: January 2009." Available at http://www.dhs.gov/xlibrary/assets/statistics/publications/ois_ill_pe_2009.pdf.

40. Uba, L. (1992). "Cultural Barriers to Health Care for Southeast Asian Refugees." *Public Health Reports*, 107(5): 544-548.

41. Sotomayor, M. (1990). "The New Immigrants: The Undocumented and Refugees." In M. S. Harper, ed., *Minority Aging: Essential Curricula Content for Selected Health and Allied Health Professions* (HHS pub. no. HRS-P-DV-90-4). Washington, DC: U.S. Government Printing Office, 627-637.

42. Kaiser Family Foundation (n.d.). "Percentage of Mothers Beginning Prenatal Care in the First Trimester by Race/Ethnicity, 2006." Available at http://www.statehealthfacts.org/comparemaptable.jsp?cat=2&ind=45.

43. National Cancer Institute (2010). "SEER Cancer Incidence and US Death Rates, 2002-2006 by Cancer Site and Race." Available at http://seer.cancer.gov/csr/1975_2006/results_merged/topic_graph_rate_comparison.pdf.

44. Freeman, H. P. (2004). "Poverty, Culture, and Social Injustice: Determinants of Cancer Disparities." *CA: A Cancer Journal for Clinicians*, 54(2): 72-77.

45. Fryer, C. D., R. Hirsch, M. S. Eberhardt, S. S. Yoon, and J. D. Wright (2010). *Hypertension, High Serum Total Cholesterol, and Diabetes: Racial and Ethnic Prevalence Differences in U.S. Adults, 1999-2006* (NCHS Data Brief no. 36). Hyattsville, MD: National Center for Health Statistics.

46. Centers for Disease Control and Prevention (2010). "Diabetes Data and Trends." Available at http://www.cdc.gov/diabetes/statistics/index.htm.

47. Centers for Disease Control and Prevention (2011). "HIV in the United States: At a Glance." Available at http://www.cdc.gov/hiv/resources/factsheets/us.htm.

48. Centers for Disease Control and Prevention (2011). "Basic Statistics." Available at http://www.cdc.gov/hiv/topics/surveillance/basic.htm#aidsdiagnoses.

49. Barrow, R. Y., L. M. Newman, and J. M. Douglas, Jr. (2008). "Taking Positive Steps to Address STD Disparities for African-American Communities." *Sexually Transmitted Diseases*, 35(12 Suppl.) S1-S3.

50. Centers for Disease Control and Prevention (2010). "National Immunization Survey (NIS): Children (19-35 months)." Available at http://www.cdc.gov/vaccines/stats-surv/nis/default.htm#nis.

51. Centers for Disease Control and Prevention (2012). "Vaccination Coverage Among U.S. Adults National Immunization Survey: Adult, 2007." Available at http://www.cdc.gov/vaccines/stats-surv/nis/downloads/nis-adult-summer-2007.pdf.

52. Shiver, M. D. (1997). "Ethnic Variation as a Key to the Biology of Human Disease." *Annals of Internal Medicine*, 127: 401-403.

53. Navarro, V. (1990). "Race or Class Versus Race and Class: Mortality Differentials in the United States." *Lancet*, 336: 1238-1240.

54. Adler, N., and J. Ostrove (2000) "Socioeconomic Status and Health: What We Know and What We Don't." *Annals of the New York Academy of Sciences*, 896: 3-15.

55. Luquis, R. R., & M. A. Pérez (2008). "Cultural Competence and Health Education: Challenges and Opportunities for the Twenty-First Century." In M. A. Pérez and R. R. Luquis, eds., *Cultural Competence in Health Education and Health Promotion*. San Francisco, CA: Jossey Bass, 231-242.

56. Pérez, M. A. (2008). "Strategies, Practices, and Models for Delivering Culturally Competent Health Education Programs." In M. A. Pérez and R. R. Luquis, eds., *Cultural Competence in Health Education and Health Promotion*. San Francisco, CA: Jossey Bass, 183-197.

57. U.S. Department of Health and Human Services, Office of Minority Health (2001). "National Standards for Culturally and Linguistically Appropriate Services in Health Care—Final Report." Available at http://minorityhealth.hhs.gov/assets/pdf/checked/finalreport.pdf.

58. Loustaunau, M. (2000). "Becoming Culturally Sensitive: Preparing for Service as a Health Educator in a Multicultural World." In S. Smith, ed., *Community Health Perspectives*. Madison, WI: Coursewise Publishing, 33-37.

59. Luquis, R., & M. A. Pérez (2005). "Health Educators and Cultural Competence: Implications for the Profession." *American Journal of Health Studies*, 20(3): 156-163.

60. United Nations (2011). *Millennium Development Goals Reports*. Available at http://www.un.org/millenniumgoals/reports.shtml.

61. Friedmann, J. (1992). *Empowerment: The Politics of Alternative Development*. Cambridge, MA: Blackwell.

Chapter **9**

Community Mental Health

David V. Perkins, PhD

Chapter Objectives

After studying this chapter, you will be able to:

1 Define *mental health* and *mental disorders*.

2 Explain what is meant by the *DSM-IV-TR*.

3 Identify the major causes of mental disorders.

4 Define *stress*, and explain its relationship to physical and mental health.

5 Briefly trace the history of mental health care in the United States, highlighting the major changes both before and after World War II.

6 Describe the forces that brought about deinstitutionalization and the movement toward community mental health centers.

7 Identify the major problems of people who are homeless.

8 Define *primary*, *secondary*, and *tertiary prevention* as they relate to mental healthcare services, and give an example of each.

9 List and briefly describe basic approaches that provide treatment and ongoing support to people with mental disorders.

10 Describe what *recovery* means for people with mental illness.

11 Identify key challenges presently facing the mental healthcare system.

12 Describe current federal policies regarding the funding of services for people with mental illness.

Introduction

Mental illness is one of the major health issues facing every community. It is the leading cause of disability in North America and Europe and costs the United States more than half a trillion dollars per year in treatment and other expenses (see **Figure 9.1**).[1] In a given year, about 46 million people (20% of U.S. adults) have a diagnosable mental or addictive disorder, and 17.9 million of them (39.2%) receive mental health services. About 11.4 million adults (5%) have a severe mental illness, that is, one that seriously interferes with some aspect of social functioning, and 6.9 million (60.8%) of them receive treatment.[2]

The tragic shootings at Virginia Tech and Northern Illinois Universities brought the issue of mental disorder in college students to national attention. Almost half of college students show a 12-month prevalence of some form of mental disorder (most often alcohol use disorder, at 20.4%), and less than 25% receive treatment (see **Table 9.1**).[3] In 2010, 2.9 million youths (12.2% of those ages 12 to 17) received treatment or counseling for problems with emotions or behavior in a specialty mental health setting (inpatient or outpatient care).[2]

Because the needs of people with mental illness are many and diverse, the services required to meet these needs are

Table 9.1   12-Month Prevalence of Mental Disorders in College Students and Non-College-Attending Peers, in Percentage, Ages 18–25

Diagnostic Characteristic	In College	Not in College
Any psychiatric diagnosis	45.79	47.74
Any alcohol use disorder*	20.37	16.98
Any drug disorder*	5.08	6.85
Major depression	7.04	6.67
Bipolar disorder	3.24	4.62
Any anxiety disorder	11.94	12.66
Pathological gambling	0.35	0.23
Any personality disorder*	17.68	21.55

*Difference is statistically significant (p < .05).
Source: Adapted from Blanco, C., O. Mayumi, C. Wright, et al. (2008). "Mental Health of College Students and Their Non-College-Attending Peers." *Archives of General Psychiatry*, 65(12): 1429–1437.

likewise diverse and include not only therapeutic services, but also social services requiring significant community resources. As we explain, mental disorders and mental health care also occur in a diverse social, cultural, and economic context that has important ethical implications for proper diagnosis, treatment, and recovery.

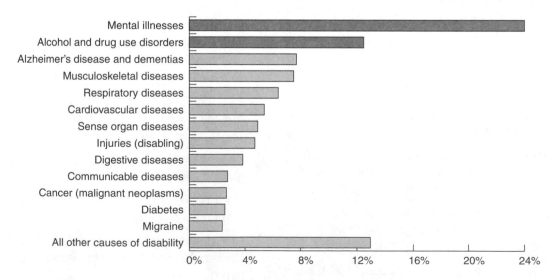

Figure 9.1 Causes of disability for all ages combined: United States, Canada, and western Europe, 2000.

Note: Measures of disability are based on the number of years of "healthy" life lost with less than full health (i.e., YLD: years lost due to disability) for each incidence of disease, illness, or condition.

President's New Freedom Commission on Mental Health (2003). *Achieving the Promise: Transforming Mental Health Care in America.* Rockville, MD: Author, 20.

Definitions

Mental health is the "state of successful performance of mental function, resulting in productive activities, fulfilling relationships with other people, and the ability to adapt to change and to cope with adversity."[4] Characteristics of people with good mental health include possessing a good self-image, valuing other people, and being able to meet the demands of everyday life.

Good mental health can be expressed as emotional maturity. In this regard, adults who have good mental health are able to do the following:

- Function under adversity
- Change or adapt to changes around them
- Manage their tension and anxiety
- Find more satisfaction in giving than receiving
- Show consideration for others
- Curb hate and guilt
- Love others

"**Mental illness** is a term that refers collectively to all diagnosable mental disorders. **Mental disorders** are health conditions that are characterized by alterations in thinking, mood, or behavior (or some combination thereof) associated with distress and/or impaired functioning."[4] People with mental illness have organic or metabolic (biochemical) disorders that prevent them from functioning effectively and happily in society. Many people with mental illness can be treated with medications and are thus able to adapt successfully to community life.

Classification of Mental Disorders

For the most part, mental disorders are diagnosed on the basis of behavioral signs and symptoms rather than definitive measurements involving the brain or another body system. The single most influential book in mental health is probably the *Diagnostic and Statistical Manual of Mental Disorders*, 4th edition, text revision (*DSM-IV-TR*), published by the American Psychiatric Association.[5] (A new edition, *DSM-5*, is expected in 2013.) It identifies the various mental disorders, provides descriptive information and diagnostic instructions for each, and has significant implications for who merits a diagnosis, whether a treatment should be reimbursed by insurance, what school and social services a person is entitled to, the top priorities for mental health research, and what kinds of new therapeutic medications should be developed.

Disorders classified in the *DSM-IV-TR* are listed in Table 9.2. Most mental disorders result from the interaction of biology and environment, so

mental disorders health conditions characterized by alterations in thinking, mood, or behavior (or some combination thereof) associated with distress and/or impaired functioning

mental health emotional and social well-being, including one's psychological resources for dealing with the day-to-day problems of life

mental illness a collective term for all mental disorders

Table 9.2 Diagnostic Categories of Mental Disorders

Category	Examples
Disorders usually first evident in infancy, childhood, or adolescence	Mental retardation; attention-deficit hyperactivity disorder
Delirium, dementia, other cognitive disorders	Alzheimer's disease; dementia associated with alcoholism or chronic drug use
Psychoactive substance use disorders	Alcohol, nicotine, cocaine, or other drug dependence
Schizophrenia	Paranoid schizophrenia
Delusional (paranoid) disorder	Persecutory delusional (paranoid) disorder
Miscellaneous psychotic disorders	Brief reactive psychosis
Mood disorders	Major depression; bipolar disorder
Anxiety disorders	Panic disorder; obsessive compulsive disorder; post-traumatic stress disorder
Somatoform disorders	Conversion disorder; hypochondriasis
Dissociative disorders	Dissociative identity disorder
Sexual disorders	Paraphilias (exhibitionism, fetishisms); sexual dysfunctions
Sleep disorders	Insomnia disorder; dream anxiety disorder
Impulse control disorders	Kleptomania; pathological gambling
Adjustment disorders	Anxious mood; withdrawal
Personality disorders	Avoidant; dependent; obsessive

one challenge in using the *DSM* is recognizing the boundary between normal reactions to life (e.g., severe grief following the death of a loved one) and a diagnosable disorder (e.g., **major depression**; see Box 9.1). Another challenge in making these diagnoses is that nearly half of people with mental illness (46.4%) have more than one disorder,[6] a problem known as comorbidity. Depression and anxiety are separate categories in the *DSM-IV-TR*, for example, yet are found together in many individuals[7] and have similar genetic risk factors.[8] Cultural differences and a lack of **cultural competence** (familiarity with language and cultural idioms of distress or body language) on the part of the clinician also complicate the application of *DSM* criteria. Worldwide, for example, women are diagnosed with mood disorders more often than are men, but this difference is smaller in countries that have less traditional gender-role differences

in employment opportunities, educational attainment, and control of fertility.[9] A further concern is that diagnosis with a mental disorder can stigmatize a person by imposing negative stereotypes, prejudice, and discrimination that the person often internalizes, reducing hope and self-esteem and hindering the person's efforts to recover.[10]

Causes of Mental Disorders

Symptoms of mental illness can arise from many causes, and the comorbidity that exists among disorders suggests they are not discrete conditions, each with a unique cause. Instead, mental disorders are understood to result from genetic influences on complex brain functions that control a person's thoughts and emotions,[11] physiologic disruptions in hormones such as testosterone and vasopressin,[12] intrauterine infections and malnutrition, maladaptive family functioning, and stress.

Two-thirds of mental retardation cases are traceable to environmental factors such as poor prenatal care, poor maternal nutrition, or maternal exposure to alcohol, tobacco, or other drugs; as such, they are preventable. For example, fetal alcohol spectrum disorder, a condition that includes mental deficiency, is the result of maternal (and fetal)

cultural competence a service provider's degree of compatibility with the specific culture of the population served, for example, proficiency in language(s) other than English, familiarity with cultural idioms of distress or body language, folk beliefs, and expectations regarding treatment procedures (such as medication or psychotherapy) and likely outcomes

major depression an affective disorder characterized by a dysphoric mood, usually depression, or loss of interest or pleasure in almost all usual activities or pastimes

---

Box 9.1 Criteria for Major Depressive Episode

A. Five (or more) of the following symptoms have been present during the same two-week period and represent a change from previous functioning. At least one of the symptoms is either (1) depressed mood or (2) loss of interest or pleasure.

Note: Do not include symptoms that are clearly due to a general medical condition, or mood-incongruent delusions or hallucinations.

- Depressed mood most of the day, nearly every day, as indicated by either subjective report (e.g., feels sad or empty) or observation made by others (e.g., appears tearful). Note: In children and adolescents, can be irritable mood
- Markedly diminished interest or pleasure in all, or almost all, activities most of the day, nearly every day (as indicated by either subjective account or observation made by others)
- Significant weight loss when not dieting or weight gain (e.g., a change of more than 5% of body weight in a month), or decrease or increase in appetite nearly every day. Note: In children, consider failure to make expected weight gains
- Insomnia or hypersomnia nearly every day
- Psychomotor agitation or retardation nearly every day (observable by others, not merely subjective feelings of restlessness or being slowed down)

- Fatigue or loss of energy nearly every day
- Feelings of worthlessness or excessive or inappropriate guilt (which may be delusional) nearly every day (not merely self-reproach or guilt about being sick)
- Diminished ability to think or concentrate, or indecisiveness, nearly every day (either by subjective account or as observed by others)
- Recurrent thoughts of death (not just fear of dying), recurrent suicidal ideation without a specific plan, or a suicide attempt or a specific plan for committing suicide

B. The symptoms do not meet criteria for a Mixed Episode.

C. The symptoms cause clinically significant distress or impairment in social, occupational, or other important areas of functioning.

D. The symptoms are not due to the direct physiological effects of a substance (e.g., a drug of abuse, a medication) or a general medical condition (e.g., hypothyroidism).

E. The symptoms are not better accounted for by bereavement, that is, after the loss of a loved one, the symptoms persist for longer than two months or are characterized by marked functional impairment, morbid preoccupation with worthlessness, suicidal ideation, psychotic symptoms, or psychomotor retardation.

Source: Adapted from American Psychiatric Association (2000). *Diagnostic and Statistical Manual of Mental Disorders*, 4th ed., text revision. Washington, DC: Author.

exposure to excessive amounts of alcohol during gestation. Mental disorders can also occur from postnatal exposure to physical, chemical, and biological agents, including secondhand cigarette smoke.[13] Brain function impairment can be caused by trauma, such as a car crash or bullet wound, or by disease, such as syphilis, cancer, or stroke. Mental impairment can also be caused by such environmental factors as chronic nutritional deficiency or lead poisoning.[14]

The brain is very sensitive to stress and other environmental influences as it develops during childhood and adolescence. Thus, other sources of mental disorders include maladaptive family functioning (such as having a parent with mental illness, or who is involved with substance abuse or criminality), poverty,[15] and experiencing violence, physical or sexual abuse, or neglect.[16] Growing up in neighborhoods marked by social fragmentation (e.g., residential instability, belonging to an "out-group" different than most other people living in the neighborhood) can lead to experiences of discrimination, isolation, and social adversity that add to the risk of mental disorder.[17]

In general, stress is a significant cause of mental illness (see Box 9.2). For example, people who survive disasters and soldiers returning from combat face increased risk of mental illness. Twenty percent of Manhattan residents living near the World Trade

diseases of adaptation diseases that result from chronic exposure to excess levels of stressors that elicit the General Adaptation Syndrome

fight or flight reaction an alarm reaction that prepares one physiologically for sudden action

General Adaptation Syndrome (GAS) the complex physiological responses resulting from exposure to stressors

---

Box 9.2   Stress: A Contemporary Mental Health Problem

Stress can be defined as one's psychologic and physiologic response to stressors–stimuli in the physical and social environment that produce feelings of tension and strain. Even Americans who believe they have good mental health carry out their everyday activities under considerable stress. Stressors can be subtle–such as having to wait in line, getting stuck in traffic, or having to keep an appointment–or they can be major life events such as getting married or divorced or losing a loved one. Although some exposure to stressors is good, perhaps even essential to a satisfying life, chronic exposure to stressors that exceed one's biological, psychological, and social coping resources can undermine one's health. Holmes and Rahe classified and ranked various stressors and found a relationship between these stressors and physical health.[19]

The process through which exposure to stressors results in health deficits has been described by Selye.[20] According to Selye's model, which he called the **General Adaptation Syndrome (GAS)**, responding to a stressor occurs in three stages: (1) an alarm reaction, (2) a stage of resistance, and finally (3) exhaustion (see **Figure 1**). In the alarm reaction stage, various hormonal changes in the body increase the individual's heart rate, respiration, and blood pressure. This is the **fight or flight reaction**, a response that the body cannot maintain for very long. Continued challenge by the stressor leads to resistance, in which the body tries to adapt to the stressor. Physiologic arousal declines and the body begins to replenish the hormones released in the alarm reaction stage, but the ability to cope with new stressors is impaired. As a result, the person is vulnerable to certain health problems that are referred to as **diseases of adaptation**, including ulcers, high blood pressure, coronary heart disease, asthma, and impaired immune function.[21] In the third stage of Selye's GAS, prolonged physiologic arousal produced by continual or repeated stress depletes energy stores to the point of exhaustion. During this stage, physiologic damage, physical diseases, mental health problems, and even death can occur.

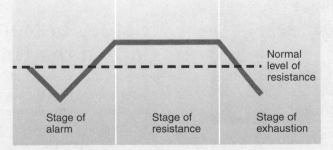

Figure 1 General adaptation syndrome.

(continues)

Box 9.2   Stress: A Contemporary Mental Health Problem (*continued*)

Evidence suggests that stress can affect health both directly, by way of physiologic changes in the body, and indirectly through changes in behavior. The release of hormones by the endocrine system during the alarm reaction affects both the cardiovascular and immune systems.[22] Hormones can produce fast or erratic beating of the heart, which can be fatal, and also increases in levels of blood lipids causing a buildup of plaque on the blood vessel walls and increasing the likelihood of hypertension, stroke, and heart attack. In terms of indirect effects, individuals under stress drink more alcohol and smoke more cigarettes,[23,24] behaviors that are associated with higher risks for heart disease and cancer, as well as injury and death from accidents.

Relationships and other social resources can mediate the effects of stress. People lacking support (in the form of marriage, church membership, social organization membership, and contacts with friends and relatives) face a greater risk than do others of experiencing mental illness, alcohol and drug abuse, suicide, illness, and mortality, independent of their overall health, socioeconomic status, smoking, drinking, obesity, and utilization of health care.[25] Effective time management, goal setting, and prioritizing tasks help reduce stress, as does being realistic about one's abilities and expectations. Experts recommend a combination of physical, social, environmental, and psychological approaches to managing stress.[26] Physical approaches to stress reduction include good nutrition and adequate sleep and aerobic exercise. Healthy social interaction and optimizing environmental factors such as noise, lighting, and living space can also reduce one's stress (see the American Institute of Stress website at www.stress.org).

Center at the time of the attacks of September 11, 2001, had symptoms consistent with post-traumatic stress disorder (PTSD) 5 to 8 weeks after the attack, and nearly 10% suffered from major depression, which occurred most often in those who had suffered losses as a result of the attack.[18]

Military service in a combat zone increases one's risk of experiencing PTSD, major depression, or other mental health problems (see **Figure 9.2**). Prevalence rates of mental health problems were especially high among veterans of Operation Iraqi Freedom (19%) and those deployed to Afghanistan (11%). Thirty-five percent of veterans returning from Iraq accessed mental health services in the year after returning home.[27]

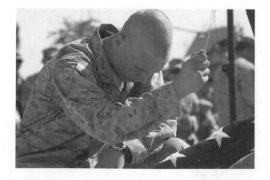

Figure 9.2 Military troops returning from duty in combat zones can be heavy users of mental health services when these services are accessible.

Courtesy of Cpl. Brian Reimers/U.S. Marines

Mental Illness in the United States

Health and social statistics clearly indicate that mental illness constitutes one of our nation's most pervasive public health problems. In 2001, for example, the second and third leading causes of death in youth ages 15 to 24 were homicide (including legal intervention) and suicide, respectively.[28] In 2010, an estimated 8.7 million adults (3.8%) had serious thoughts of suicide in the preceding year, 2.5 million (1.1%) made suicide plans, and 1.1 million (0.5%) attempted suicide.[2] However, preventing suicide is difficult because the base rate of completed suicide is only 10.9 per 100,000 people.[29] Community-wide education campaigns have shown no effects on help-seeking by people struggling with a life-ending crisis or on suicidal behavior.[30] The prevalence of alcohol, tobacco, and other drug abuse in this country is yet another social indicator of the mental illness problem.

History of Mental Health Care in the United States

The response to mental illness in the United States has a history older than the country itself, and is marked by enthusiastic reform movements followed by periods of widespread ambivalence toward people with mental disorders. Cyclical periods of reform often began when existing approaches to caring for those with mental illness became intolerable for society, and ended when their economic burden became unbearable.

In Colonial America, when communities were sparsely populated, "distracted" persons or "lunatics," as they were called, were generally cared for by their families or private caretakers, and only as a last resort became the responsibility of the local community. Institutionalization did not begin until the eighteenth century, when people with mental disorders were placed in undifferentiated poorhouses or almshouses alongside people with mental retardation, physical disabilities, and the otherwise deviant.[31]

By the early nineteenth century the situation in the poorhouses and almshouses worsened and the first efforts were made to separate people by their type of disability. In 1751 Thomas Bond opened Pennsylvania Hospital, the first institution in America specifically designed to care for those with mental illness.[32] Conditions in the hospital were harsh (see **Figure 9.3**), and treatments, which consisted of "blood letting, blistering, emetics, and warm and cold baths," were unpleasant.[33]

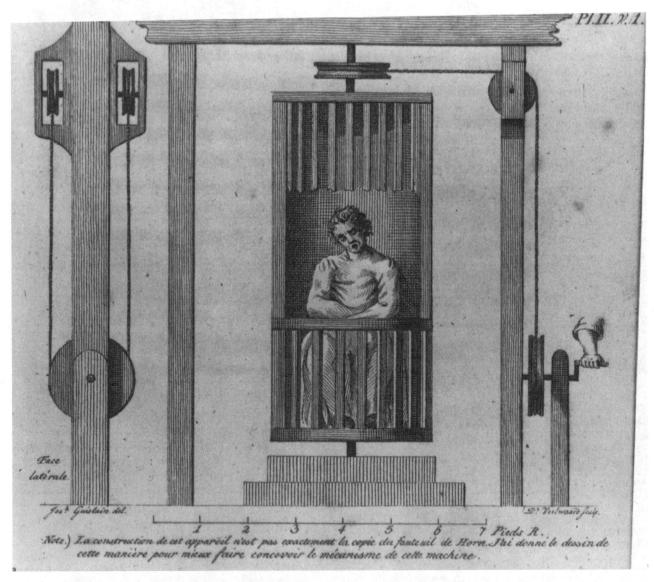

Figure 9.3 Treatment for mental illness in the eighteenth and nineteenth centuries was often inhumane and unsuccessful.

Moral Treatment

Philippe Pinel of France developed a more humane approach that he called *traitement moral*, or in English, **moral treatment**, based on the assumption that environmental changes could affect an individual's mind and thus alter behavior.[31] In the United States, William Tuke put moral treatment into practice beginning in 1792.

People with mental illness were removed from the everyday life stressors of their home environments and given "asylum" in a quiet country environment, where they received a regimen of rest, light food, exercise, fresh air, and amusements. Moral treatment was initially deemed successful and soon spread,[34] but with rising immigration and urbanization these asylums became overcrowded, and indigent patients again ended up in poorhouses. At this point, noted reformer Dorothea Lynde Dix (1802–1897) (see **Figure 9.4**) began a tireless campaign to establish public hospitals providing decent care to indigents with mental illness. When her lobbying for a federal law failed, Dix lobbied on a state-by-state basis; Dix was personally involved in the founding of 32 public mental hospitals funded by individual states.[35]

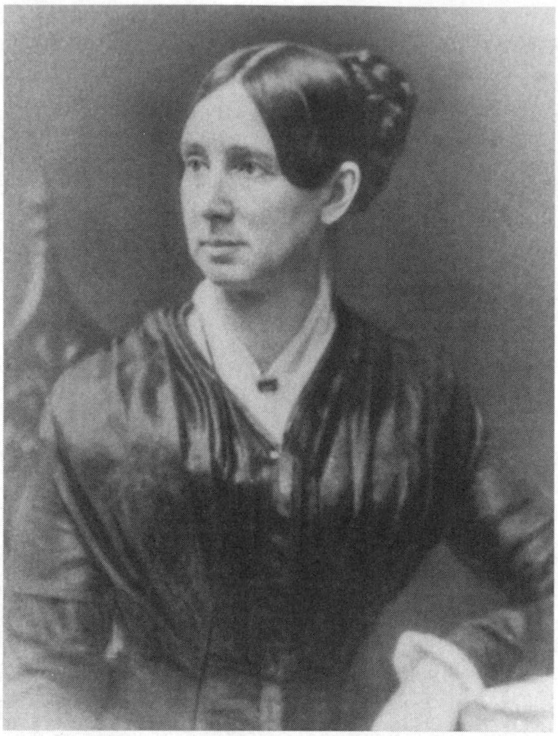

State Hospitals

The state mental hospitals were supposed to supply an environment in which therapeutic care was based on close personal relationships between patients and well-trained staff members, as prescribed in the methods of moral treatment (see **Figure 9.5**). Unfortunately, the chronic nature of mental illness made long-term or even lifetime stays increasingly the norm.[35] "Maximum capacities" were quickly reached, exceeded, and repeatedly revised upward. Personalized care became impractical and physical restraints provided the most efficient way to manage patients on large wards.[32] States repeatedly cut funding for these institutions until all that remained was custodial care by an overworked staff that turned over frequently.

By 1940 the population in state mental institutions was nearly one-half million, and staff caseloads became so large that only subsistence care was possible. In response to this situation, dramatic new approaches to treatment were developed, including

Figure 9.4 Dorothea Dix helped to establish public mental hospitals in many states.
© National Library of Medicine

electroconvulsive therapy (ECT) and **lobotomy**. ECT, which remains a treatment for severe depression, uses electric current to produce convulsions (**Figure 9.6**). The lobotomy, in which nerve fibers of the brain are severed by surgical incision, was popularized by Portuguese neuropsychiatrist Antônio Egas Moniz, and by U.S. neurologist Walter

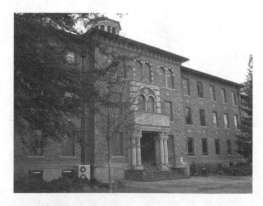

Figure 9.5 The state mental hospital was at one time viewed as the appropriate public response to the needs of people with mental illness.
Courtesy of Department of Social and Health Services, Washington State

---

electroconvulsive therapy (ECT) a method of treatment for mental disorders involving the administration of electric current to induce convulsions and unconsciousness

lobotomy surgical severance of nerve fibers of the brain by incision

moral treatment a nineteenth-century treatment in which people with mental illness were removed from the everyday life stressors of their home environments and given "asylum" in a rural setting, including rest, exercise, fresh air, and amusements

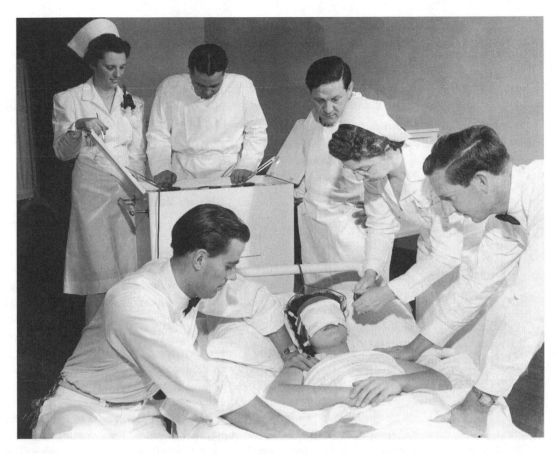

Figure 9.6 A team of doctors and nurses prepares to demonstrate procedures involved in electroconvulsive therapy (shock treatment), 1942.
© AP Photos

Freeman. Freeman streamlined the procedure with his invention of the so-called ice-pick lobotomy, enabling him and other physicians to perform tens of thousands of lobotomies between 1939 and 1967.[36] However, later research found that following this irreversible operation, only one-third of patients showed stable improvement and another one-third became worse off. The appearance of new antipsychotic and antidepressive drugs in the 1950s made the widespread use of lobotomies unnecessary.[36]

Mental Health Care After World War II

In the postwar 1940s, a number of factors brought about greater federal involvement in mental health care. New feelings of optimism in the country, together with testimony before Congress by both military and civilian experts, soon resulted in the passage of the National Mental Health Act of 1946, which established the **National Institute of Mental Health (NIMH)**. Modeled after the National Cancer Institute, NIMH came under the umbrella of the National Institutes of Health. The purposes of the NIMH were (1) to foster and aid research related to the cause, diagnosis, and treatment of neuropsychiatric disorders; (2) to provide training and award fellowships and grants for work in mental health; and (3) to aid the states in the prevention, diagnosis, and treatment of neuropsychiatric disorders.[35]

Deinstitutionalization

During the early 1950s, public distress about the conditions in state mental hospitals grew until the need to find a new approach for caring for those with mental illness was clear and inescapable. The term **deinstitutionalization** refers to the discharging of thousands of patients from state-owned mental

deinstitutionalization the process of discharging, on a large scale, patients from state mental hospitals to less restrictive community settings

National Institute of Mental Health (NIMH) the nation's leading mental health research agency, housed in the National Institutes of Health

hospitals and the resettling and maintaining of these persons in less restrictive community settings. To demonstrate the magnitude of deinstitutionalization, in 1955, 322 state psychiatric hospitals served 558,922 resident patients.[37] By 1990, the number of patients had dropped to less than 120,000 (**Figure 9.7**), and by 2004 to less than 30,000.[37,38]

Deinstitutionalization was not a preplanned policy. Rather, it was propelled by four forces that had been building up for more than half a century: (1) economics, (2) idealism, (3) legal considerations, and (4) the development and marketing of antipsychotic drugs.[31] Economically, the states needed to reduce expenditures for mental hospitals so that more money was available for the other three major state budgetary items—education, roads, and welfare. Meanwhile, Medicare and Medicaid legislation provided federal funds to reimburse the costs of outpatient and inpatient services for eligible people with mental illness.

By the early 1960s, questions arose about the legality of institutionalizing people against their will who had not been convicted of any crime, but simply because they had mental illness. The American Bar Association pointed out that people with mental disorders, even when institutionalized, had certain rights, including the right to treatment.[37] Over the ensuing decade, courts began to show more concern for the rights of individuals with mental illness—who were viewed as needing the courts' protection from inappropriate involuntary commitment—and less concern for society's right to be protected from these individuals.[33] Eventually, the test for involuntary civil commitment became one of whether these individuals could be considered dangerous to themselves or others.

Although economics, idealism, and legal considerations all helped to launch deinstitutionalization, new medications expedited it. One of the first was **chlorpromazine**, introduced as Thorazine in 1954 and characterized as a **neuroleptic** drug because it appeared to reduce nervous activity. Used first in hospitals, Thorazine and the other phenothiazines introduced later produced a remarkably calming effect in psychotic patients, and in many cases became the only form of treatment provided. In these situations, a **chemical straitjacket** was said to have been substituted for a physical one, and unfortunately some of the drugs' acute and chronic side effects were overlooked. Acute side effects (such as blurred vision, weight gain, and constipation) can cause compliance failures resulting in relapses or in attempts to self-medicate with other drugs, including drugs of abuse. Long-term use of chlorpromazine can impair the central nervous system and produce **tardive dyskinesia**, the irreversible, involuntary, and abnormal movements of the tongue, mouth, arms, and legs.[32] Despite these deleterious effects, phenothiazines are still used extensively to treat psychotic patients.

chemical straitjacket a drug that subdues a mental patient's behavior

chlorpromazine the first and most famous antipsychotic drug, introduced in 1954 under the brand name Thorazine

neuroleptic drugs drugs that reduce nervous activity; another term for antipsychotic drugs

tardive dyskinesia an irreversible condition of involuntary and abnormal movements of the tongue, mouth, arms, and legs, which can result from long-term use of certain antipsychotic drugs (such as chlorpromazine)

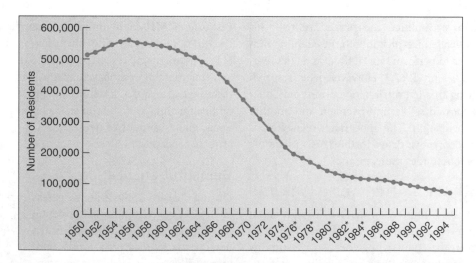

Figure 9.7 Number of resident patients in state and county mental hospitals at the end of the year, 1950–1994.

Note: Asterisk indicates linear interpolation.

Frank, Richard G., and Sherry A. Glied. Foreword by Rosalynn Carter. *Better But Not Well: Mental Health Policy in the United States Since 1950.* p. 55, figure 4.1. © 2006 The Johns Hopkins University Press. Reprinted with permission of The Johns Hopkins University Press.

Community Mental Health Centers

In 1963, mental illness and its treatment gained national attention when President John F. Kennedy addressed Congress on the subject of mental health care.[31] The resulting **Mental Retardation Facilities and Community Mental Health Centers (CMHC) Act** promised funding to establish one fully staffed, full-time **community mental health center (CMHC)** in each of 1,499 designated catchment areas covering the entire United States. These centers were to provide four core services: (1) outpatient services to older adults, children, and people with serious mental illness; (2) 24-hour-a-day emergency care; (3) day treatment or other partial hospitalization services; and (4) screenings to determine whether to admit patients to state mental facilities.[39] Hundreds of CMHCs were established in the 1960s and 1970s, but for a number of years after that they fell short of the lofty expectations outlined in Kennedy's speech. One problem was that many older patients with chronic mental illness never returned to the community and instead were simply **transinstitutionalized** to nursing homes. CMHCs also struggled to serve deinstitutionalized persons living in the community, because other than medications, no effective services to treat this population had been developed.

The federal government responded to the problems of deinstitutionalization and transinstitutionalization in 1977 by creating the Community Support Program, which was the first recognition that the problems of people with chronic mental illness are—first and foremost—social welfare problems. This program offered grants to communities to help people with chronic mental illness find the resources necessary for successful independent living, namely, income, housing, food, medical care, transportation, vocational training, and opportunities for recreation.[40] Despite the many problems resulting from deinstitutionalization, surveys indicate that most people with chronic mental illness prefer life in the community over life in an institution. Many communities now have appropriate services in place, and inpatient care is more effective and requires less time when community support is available following discharge.

Mental Healthcare Concerns in the United States Today

Today nearly everyone with serious mental illness lives in the community, receives at least some treatment, has disability income, and enjoys civil liberties; some of them also lead productive lives.[38] However, specific challenges remain, including (1) how to provide services to homeless people with serious mental illness and/or co-occurring substance use disorders, and (2) resolving the problem of the more than 1 million people with mental illness incarcerated in U.S. jails and prisons.

Serious Mental Illness in People Who Are Homeless

More than 637,000 people are homeless during any given week in the United States, and 2.1 million adults experience homelessness over the course of a year.[41] It is estimated that 80% of these homeless individuals are temporarily homeless, 10% are episodically homeless, and 10% are chronically homeless (see **Figure 9.8**).

Homeless people are more exposed to environmental stresses and threats than are people with homes, and about half of all adults who are homeless have substance use disorders, major depression, and other co-occurring mental illness.[42] Homeless people with mental illness generally have the same needs as other homeless people, and their most pressing need is safe, affordable housing. Successful interventions for homelessness require the provision of housing that these individuals choose and actually want to live in, and services they need.[43] If available at all, services to people who are homeless are often fragmented, although integration of medical, mental health, substance abuse, and housing services is possible.[44]

The New Asylums: Mental Health Care in Our Jails and Prisons

Cognitive and emotional deficits imposed by serious mental illness, coupled with homelessness and other intense stressors, increase the risk that people with serious mental illness will commit criminal acts, including violence. However, this isn't necessarily because of their mental illness, because people with psychiatric disorders are also more likely to abuse substances and be poor, unemployed, uneducated, victimized, single or divorced, and have parents who themselves have arrest records. Controlling for these social context factors shows that having severe mental illness increases the risk of future violence only when accompanied by a history of past violence.[45]

community mental health center (CMHC) a fully staffed center originally funded by the federal government that provides comprehensive mental health services to local populations

Mental Retardation Facilities and Community Mental Health Centers (CMHC) Act a law that made the federal government responsible for assisting in the funding of mental health facilities and services

transinstitutionalization transferring patients from one type of public institution to another, usually as a result of policy change

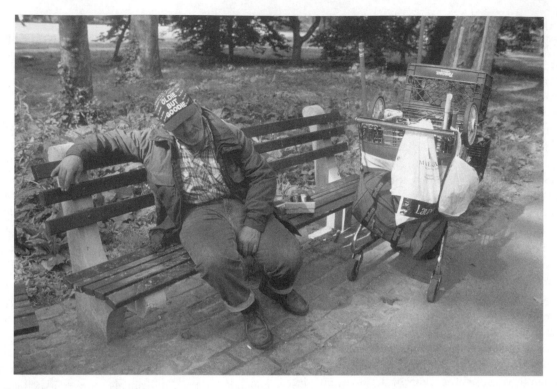

Figure 9.8 As many as two-thirds of all people with serious mental illness have experienced homelessness or been at risk for homelessness at some point in their lives.
© Photos.com

The United States imprisons a larger percentage of its citizens than any other country,[46] and approximately 15% of inmates in state and federal prisons and 24% of those in local jails have a serious mental illness[47] (see **Figure 9.9**). Incarceration is itself stressful and countertherapeutic,[48] and courts have interpreted the U.S. Constitution as ensuring a right to treatment to protect prisoners with medical and psychiatric needs against cruel and unusual punishment. However, U.S. prisons are seriously overcrowded, and effective treatment requires adequate space, a sufficient number of qualified treatment personnel, and timely access to services.[49] Some of the worst conditions are in juvenile justice centers, where adolescents from diverse cultural backgrounds and with a variety of disorders, criminal convictions, and family problems receive little or no treatment, and sometimes only multiple forms of medication.[50] Furthermore, even when treatment is available, severe mental illness (paranoid schizophrenia, **bipolar disorder**, or other serious mental disorders)

bipolar disorder an affective disorder characterized by distinct periods of elevated mood alternating with periods of depression

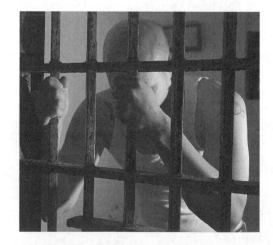

Figure 9.9 Many prison inmates with mental illness remain in prison years beyond their original sentence because they are unable to conform to good conduct requirements of the prison system.
© Tim Harman/ShutterStock, Inc.

may preclude inmates' cooperation with their prescribed medication schedules; without medication these inmates may be incapable of "good behavior," a prerequisite for parole or release.

Moreover, once released back into the community, people with serious mental illness who do not receive treatment are more likely to commit another offense than are inmates without mental disorders, leading to practices such as "legal leverage" to compel treatment and special mental health courts.[51] Legal leverage applied to the patient to accept treatment may involve service providers taking control of the patient's disability income and/or suspending the patient's eligibility for subsidized housing.[52] Such practices are controversial, but with an increased risk of violence there is an attempt to balance the values of civil rights and normalization with public safety. Mental health courts use judges who have special training and nonadversarial procedures that mandate treatment and rehabilitation if the individual is found guilty, rather than incarceration. Studies find increased amounts of treatment received by individuals diverted from criminal courts to mental health courts, improved functioning (e.g., less illicit drug use), less criminal recidivism even after court supervision ends,[53] and significant cost savings in comparison with criminal prosecution and incarceration.[54]

Meeting the Needs of Those with Mental Illness: Prevention and Treatment

Many communities find it very challenging to provide effective and economical prevention and treatment services to people with mental illness.

Prevention

The concepts of primary, secondary, and tertiary prevention can be applied to community mental health. Primary prevention in community mental health reduces the incidence (rate of new cases) of mental illness and related problems. For example, research has shown that providing high quality early education to economically disadvantaged preschool children (plus support to their families) helps the children achieve higher educational attainment and income and lower rates of justice-system involvement and substance abuse over the next 25 years.[55]

Secondary prevention, although not reducing the incidence of mental illness, can reduce its prevalence by shortening the duration of episodes through prompt intervention. For example, soldiers exposed to high levels of combat who receive intensive cognitive skills training within a few days of returning home are significantly less likely to experience symptoms of PTSD and depression later on.[56] Other examples of secondary prevention include employee assistance programs, juvenile delinquency diversion programs, and crisis intervention, which can be provided by licensed professionals in private clinics, CMHCs, hospital emergency rooms, and other social service agencies.

Tertiary prevention, treatment, and rehabilitation ameliorate the symptoms of illness and prevent further problems for the individual and the community. Intensive community treatment programs, discussed later in connection with psychiatric rehabilitation, are examples of tertiary prevention.[57]

Treatment Approaches

Treatment goals for mental disorders are to (1) reduce symptoms, (2) improve personal and social functioning, (3) develop and strengthen coping skills, and (4) promote behaviors that make a person's life better. The basic approaches to treating mental disorders include psychopharmacology, psychotherapy, and psychiatric rehabilitation.[4]

Psychopharmacology

Psychopharmacological therapy involves treatment with medications, a biological approach that is more "user friendly" than lobotomy or ECT. This treatment recognizes that mental illnesses are medical illnesses just like hypothyroidism or diabetes, and as such are treatable with drugs. Since the introduction of chlorpromazine in 1954, there has been a significant increase in the number and types of approved medications for the treatment of mental disorders. Conditions for which medications exist include schizophrenia, bipolar disorder, major depression, anxiety, panic disorder, and obsessive-compulsive disorder, although not everyone who has these disorders responds to medication.[58] Furthermore, because some of these drugs have serious side effects, and because of the nature of mental illness itself, almost half of patients may not cooperate fully in taking their medications.[59]

Another form of biomedical therapy is ECT, which was discussed earlier in this chapter. In ECT, alternating electric current passes through the brain to produce unconsciousness and a convulsive seizure. ECT is used for severe depression, selected cases of schizophrenia, or overwhelming suicide ideation, especially when the need for

psychopharmacological therapy
treatment for mental illness that involves medications

treatment is seen as urgent. Contemporary ECT methods use low doses of electric shock to the brain along with general anesthetics to reduce the unpleasant side effects.

Psychotherapy

Psychotherapy, or psychosocial therapy, involves treatment through verbal communication (see **Figure 9.10**). There are numerous approaches to psychotherapy, including interpersonal, couple, group, and family formats. Psychodynamic psychotherapy examines current problems as they relate to earlier experiences, even from childhood, whereas cognitive psychotherapy focuses on current thinking patterns that are faulty or distorted. **Cognitive-behavioral therapy** focuses on how maladaptive feelings and behaviors are the result of distorted thinking, and it uses structured procedures to promote new thought patterns and regular homework between sessions to practice more effective coping responses. In

cognitive-behavioral therapy treatment based on learning new thought patterns and adaptive skills, with regular practice between therapy sessions

psychotherapy a treatment that involves verbal communication between the patient and a trained clinician

general, psychotherapy is most likely to be successful in less severe cases of emotional distress or when used in conjunction with other approaches (such as psychopharmacological therapy).

Psychiatric Rehabilitation

One of the objectives of *Healthy People 2020* is to increase the proportion of adults with mental disorders who are receiving treatment (see **Box 9.3**). With financial considerations influencing most healthcare decisions today, the treatment of mental disorders is driven more and more by considerations of cost-effectiveness.

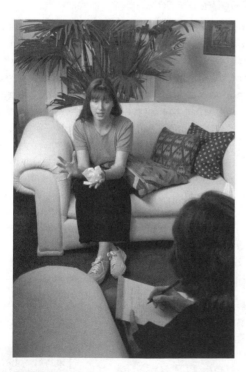

Figure 9.10 Psychotherapy is usually only one of the services needed by persons who are suffering from a mental illness.
© David Buffington/Photodisc/Getty Images

Box 9.3 *Healthy People 2020:* Objective

Mental Health and Mental Disorder Objectives
Objective MHMD-9: Increase the proportion of adults with mental disorders who receive treatment.
Targets and baselines:

Objective		2008 Baseline	2020 Target
MHMD-9.1	Adults aged 18 years and older with serious mental illness	58.7%	64.6%
MHMD-9.2	Adults aged 18 years and older with major depressive episode	68.3%	75.1%

Target setting method: 10% improvement.
Data source: National Survey on Drug Use and Health (NSDUH), SAMHSA.

For Further Thought

Just over half of adults with serious mental illness received treatment in 2008. What reasons do you think contribute to this statistic? Do you think the Affordable Care Act of 2010 will help to increase the proportion of those who receive treatment so that the *Healthy People 2020* target (10% increase) can be met? One-third of adults with major depressive episodes do not receive treatment. How would reaching the *Healthy People 2020* target (10% increase in the proportion of adults with major depression who receive treatment) affect the overall adult suicide rate?

Source: U.S. Department of Health and Human Services, Office of Disease Prevention and Health Promotion (2010). *Healthy People 2020.* Available at http://www.healthypeople.gov/2020/default.aspx.

We have seen that mental disorders are widely prevalent and can begin in adolescence, or even earlier. They entail not only neurobiological lesions that produce distortions in thinking and feeling, but also deficits in coping skills that damage relationships and stigma that interferes with social acceptance and inclusion. Mental disorders can last a lifetime, and most who have them simply live with their symptoms (e.g., people with schizophrenia learn to tolerate voices in their head), just as people with chronic arthritis or diabetes live with their disabilities. Thus, today the goal of treating mental disorders is most often one of "recovery" instead of cure. **Recovery** means progress toward financial and residential independence, managing symptoms effectively, satisfaction with life, and basic "personhood"—that is, mental and physical well-being, supportive relationships, opportunities to spend time productively, and self-determination in exercising the rights and privileges that come with community life.[60]

Recovery requires change, such as community participation in the form of work, volunteer activities, the forming of new relationships, and sometimes parenthood. Change is difficult and brings added stress, making daily pursuit of recovery a challenge to persons with mental illness and the providers who work with them. The current recovery-oriented services are collectively known as **psychiatric rehabilitation**.[61] Psychiatric rehabilitation is modeled on rehabilitation practices for people with physical and developmental disabilities (e.g., independent living, gainful employment), and its services often carry the modifier *support* (as in supported employment, supported housing, supported education) in keeping with patient self-determination. Services include medication and therapy as needed, but also changing the environment through accommodations at work or school (e.g., extended time to complete tests and other assignments, use of aids such as tape recorders, and frequent breaks), and practices must be **evidence-based**, which means there is consistent evidence showing that they improve patient outcomes. The providers of psychiatric rehabilitation services typically represent diverse professional backgrounds (psychiatry, nursing, addictions, social work, and vocational services) and work collaboratively as an integrated team. Sometimes some of these team members are themselves recovering from mental illness, which brings a different perspective to the team's efforts.[62]

One of the best-known and most successful models of psychiatric rehabilitation is Assertive Community Treatment (ACT), also called the Madison (Wisconsin) Model. ACT delivers intensive, individualized services encompassing treatment, rehabilitation, and support over an indefinite period. Active outreach is extended to individuals with severe mental disorders to help them maintain stable lives in the community (e.g., finding a place to live, learning self-care skills needed for independence, using public transportation).[40] ACT is labor-intensive, but its emphasis on community integration reduces both hospital use and costs for people with chronic and severe disorders. The cost-effectiveness of ACT for people whose needs are less severe and persistent is not as clear.[63]

Interestingly, recovery from disorders such as schizophrenia tends to be better (with longer remissions and fewer relapses) in the developing world than in developed countries such as the United States.[64] Rather than being socially isolated, homeless, or in jail, for example, people in India who have schizophrenia are usually married and living with their families.[65] Non-Western cultures use less stigmatizing explanations for mental illness and prescribe a recovery process that includes collaborative roles for everyone—patient, family, and community. In Tanzania, for example, a person with mental illness is not a source of embarrassment needing coercion but a family member or neighbor whose odd behavior is dealt with gently and, if possible, without confrontation.[66] The lesson in recovery provided by these "less developed" parts of the world is that mental disorders such as schizophrenia are not just "broken brains" but also culturally determined social and moral phenomena that involve all of us.

Self-Help Groups

Another aid to treatment and recovery is **self-help groups**, which are composed of concerned members of the community who are united by a disability or predicament not shared by other members of the community. The shared characteristic is often stigmatizing or isolating and viewed as abnormal by the rest of the community.[57] These groups meet regularly, members often share leadership responsibilities, and the roles of help-giver

evidence-based practices ways of delivering services to people using scientific evidence that shows that the services actually work

psychiatric rehabilitation intensive, individualized services encompassing treatment, rehabilitation, and support delivered by a team of providers over an indefinite period to individuals with severe mental disorder to help them maintain stable lives in the community

recovery outcome sought by most people with mental illness; includes increased independence, effective coping, supportive relationships, community participation, and sometimes gainful employment

self-help groups groups of concerned members of the community who are united by a shared interest, concern, or deficit not shared by other members of the community (Alcoholics Anonymous, for example)

and help-receiver are entirely interchangeable. These groups replace the community that was "lost" through stigmatization or isolation. Self-help groups supply feedback and guidance to their members based on unique insights gained from their own recovery, and provide their members with adaptive attitudes and expectations about the future.[57] Examples of self-help groups are the **National Alliance on Mental Illness (NAMI)**, Recovery, Inc., and Alcoholics Anonymous (AA).

Mental health care in the United States faces a variety of challenges. Multiple services are needed by people with severe or comorbid disorders, and lack of some services (such as for addictions) limits the effectiveness of other services (e.g., ACT). People with serious mental illness still face high rates of poverty, social disadvantage, and stigma, and substantial recovery (e.g., stable, gainful employment) is achieved by relatively few of them.[38] Finally, family members of people with mental illness face stigma and may need information, financial help, and therapeutic support for themselves.[67]

The mental healthcare system is very decentralized and fragmented, with many different kinds of providers[38] but few resources for rural and low-income counties.[68] Furthermore, about one-fifth of persons receiving treatment for mental disorders drop out prematurely, most after only one or two sessions. Those more likely to drop out have low incomes, lack of health insurance, and multiple (comorbid) disorders and are often ethnic minorities.[69]

General medical practitioners treat the largest number of people with mental disorders, with specialty mental health providers, human services, self-help groups, and various combinations serving the rest.[70] Patient sex, ethnicity, geography, immigration status, sexual orientation, and income are all related to the likelihood of receiving help. African Americans and Latinos, for example, consistently receive less mental health treatment than do whites.[71] The problem here may not be overt discrimination, but a lack of cultural competence[72] on the part of providers regarding their multicultural patients' attitudes toward medications and medication side effects (such as weight gain), and patients' misguided expectations of treatment in the context of particular religious, spiritual, or folk beliefs. Some of these problems are starting to be addressed using computers and other forms of technology (see Box 9.4).

Finally, in addition to their often pronounced deficits in thinking and coping, people with serious mental

National Alliance on Mental Illness (NAMI) a national grassroots mental health organization dedicated to support, education, advocacy, and research for people living with mental illness

---

Box 9.4   Psychotherapy and Technology

Psychotherapy is declining in use compared with medication. Language barriers may impair communication between therapists and clients, and the availability of psychotherapy is uneven across geographic and socioeconomic boundaries. However, technology in the form of telephone, video conferencing, Internet, e-mail, and computer software can increase the availability and flexibility of psychotherapy and also lower its cost. For example, clients may use software to complete standard steps in treatment (e.g., daily homework), contacting their therapists by telephone or e-mail only when necessary. Moving the locus of treatment from therapists and their offices to settings more comfortable and familiar to clients may reduce the feelings of coerciveness some clients experience. For certain individuals, who may have severe cognitive or language impairments or social anxiety, communicating with a therapist using a visual display of words on a screen can be more effective than face-to-face conversation.[73] Computer therapy and in-person therapy are about the same in overall effectiveness and, with greater convenience and more flexible use of client and therapist time, drop-out from computer treatments may occur less often than in face to face therapy.[74]

---

disorders tend to be among the poorest members of society and typically live in neighborhoods where crime, illicit drugs, victimization, homelessness, unemployment, and social disorganization are rampant. It may be too much to expect that medications, psychotherapy, psychosocial rehabilitation, self-help, and other circumscribed help is enough to overcome these systemic problems. From this vantage point, it is not the people with mental disorders who fail, but rather the communities and social systems they live in that have failed.

Government Policies and Mental Health Care

In recent decades the federal government's role in mental health funding and policy has been substantial. The federal Medicaid program pays more than half of publicly funded mental health care, and its policies and regulations, which vary from state to state, impact what services are covered. In addition, the Mental Health Parity and Addiction Act of 2008 requires that if healthcare coverage includes mental health or substance abuse disorders there must be parity with physical disorders in any limitations or restrictions (i.e., any limits on the number of visits per year, annual or lifetime dollars spent, and deductibles or copayments must be the same for both mental and physical disorders).[75]

The Affordable Care Act of 2010

In 2010, Medicaid's important role in covering individuals with mental disorders grew even larger with the passage of the federal Affordable Care Act (ACA). This act further extends the reach of federal parity by expanding eligibility for public programs like Medicaid and increasing the availability of private insurance. The ACA requires that individuals whose income is less than 133% of the federal poverty line be eligible for Medicaid, with all plans covering mental health and substance use disorder services at parity with medical–surgical benefits. Because individuals with mental disorders tend to have lower incomes and are more likely to be uninsured, they will disproportionately benefit from these coverage expansions.

Under the ACA, the proportion of nonelderly adults with severe mental disorders covered by Medicaid is expected to double,[76] and this group is more likely to use services once it is covered by insurance, which could exacerbate the limitations of mental health services and the shortage of professionals. States also have some control over what kinds of services are covered, and given the critical role played by intensive, team-delivered, and highly individualized services such as ACT and supported employment, the consequences of the ACA for improvements in the rate of recovery from serious mental illness remain to be seen.

These and other recent changes make it difficult to determine how the nation, states, and local communities will respond to the needs of those with mental illness in the future. The response will depend on economics, the degree to which taxpayers have been personally touched by mental illness, and the degree to which they are willing to tolerate the spectacle of homeless people with mental illness in their communities and in their jails and prisons. A key task facing communities is to find ways to unite formal services and informal supports to promote social inclusion and recovery by people who are coping with mental disorders.

Chapter Summary

- Mental illness constitutes a major community health concern because of its prevalence and chronicity and because of the social, cultural, and economic attention and resources it demands from all of us.
- Americans are afflicted with a variety of mental disorders, caused by genetic factors, environmental factors, or a combination of both. These disorders, which can range from mild to severe, are often chronic and may limit the ability of some of those afflicted to live independently.
- Over the years, society's response to the needs of those with mental illness has been characterized by long periods of apathy interrupted by enthusiastic movements for new and well-meaning approaches to care.
- Deinstitutionalization, in which hundreds of thousands of people with mental illness living in state and county hospitals were discharged and returned to their communities, was the most prominent mental health movement of the twentieth century. The origins of many of the current problems in community mental health care, such as a large number of homeless people and of prison inmates with mental illness, can be traced to this movement.

- The basic concepts of prevention in community health (primary, secondary, and tertiary prevention) can be applied to the prevention and treatment of mental disorders.
- Common treatment approaches are psychotherapy, including cognitive-behavioral therapy, and psychopharmacology, which is based on the use of medications. Self-help groups assist people at risk for relapse, and psychiatric rehabilitation programs provide ongoing support to people with severe mental disorder living in the community.
- People with severe mental illness generally pursue recovery rather than cure. Recovery entails adaptive change, including increased independence, effective coping, supportive relationships, community participation, and sometimes gainful employment.
- Important issues face those concerned with providing services for people with mental disorders. One is finding ways to provide a variety of easily accessible preventive, treatment, and rehabilitative services to people from culturally diverse backgrounds, with multiple problems and few resources, in a climate of tight funding governed by complex local, state, and federal policies.

Review Questions

1. What is meant by the term *mental health*?
2. What is a mental disorder?
3. What is the *Diagnostic and Statistical Manual of Mental Disorders*, 4th edition, text revision (*DSM-IV-TR*)?
4. Name and give examples of the different causes of mental disorders.
5. What is the relationship between stress and mental health?
6. What was included in the therapy known as "moral treatment"?
7. What role did Dorothea Dix play in the treatment of indigent people with mental illness?
8. How would you characterize the treatment of those with mental illness in state hospitals prior to World War II?
9. Define the word *deinstitutionalization*. When did it start in the United States? What caused it?
10. Why was there a movement toward community mental health centers in the early 1960s?
11. What services are provided by community mental health centers?
12. Why was the Community Support Program considered a novel approach?
13. Approximately what percentage of homeless people are living with mental illness? What percentage of state prison inmates have mental health problems?
14. How are legal leverage and mental health courts used to reduce the problem of people with mental illness ending up in jail or prison?
15. Describe primary, secondary, and tertiary prevention of mental illness and give an example of a service for each level of prevention.
16. What is involved in psychotherapy for mental illness? In cognitive-behavioral therapy? In psychopharmacological therapy?
17. What is meant by "recovery" from serious mental illness? How do psychiatric rehabilitation services such as Assertive Community Treatment promote recovery?
18. What are self-help groups? How do they increase treatment effectiveness?
19. What kinds of challenges do mental healthcare efforts face early in the twenty-first century?

Activities

1. Make a list of all the stressors you have experienced in the last 2 weeks. Select two of the items on the list and answer the following questions about them:
   - Did you realize the stressor was a stressor when you first confronted it? Explain.
   - What physiologic responses did you notice that you had when confronted with the stressor?
   - Have you confronted the stressor before? Explain your answer.
   - What stress mediators (coping responses) do you have to deal with each of the stressors?
   - Do you feel you will someday fall victim to a disease of adaptation?

2. Using a local telephone book or one from your hometown, identify the organizations in the community that you believe would provide mental health services. Then, create a list of the agencies/organizations. Divide the list into three sections based on the type of service offered (primary, secondary, or tertiary prevention). If you are not sure what types of services are offered, call the agency/organization to find out. After you have completed your list, write a paragraph or two about what you feel to be the status of mental health care in your community.

Community Health on the Web

The Internet contains a wealth of information about community and public health. Increase your knowledge of some of the topics presented in this chapter by accessing the Jones & Bartlett Learning website at **go.jblearning.com/McKenzieBrief** and follow the links to complete the following Web activities:

- Center for Mental Health Services
- National Institute of Mental Health
- National Alliance on Mental Illness

References

1. Eaton, W., S. Martins, G. Nestadt, O. Bienvenu, D. Clarke, and P. Alexandre (2008). "The Burden of Mental Disorders." *Epidemiologic Reviews*, 30: 1-14.
2. Substance Abuse and Mental Health Services Administration (2012). *Results from the 2010 National Survey on Drug Use and Health: Mental Health Findings* (NSDUH Series H-42, HHS Publication No. (SMA) 11-4667). Rockville, MD: Substance Abuse and Mental Health Services Administration.
3. Blanco, C., O. Mayumi, C. Wright, et al. (2008). "Mental Health of College Students and Their Non-College-Attending Peers." *Archives of General Psychiatry*, 65(12): 1429-1437.
4. U.S. Department of Health and Human Services (1999). *Mental Health: A Report of the Surgeon General*. Rockville, MD: Substance Abuse and Mental Health Services Administration.
5. American Psychiatric Association (2000). *Diagnostic and Statistical Manual of Mental Disorders*, 4th ed., text revision. Washington, DC: Author.
6. Kessler, R. C., W. T. Chiu, O. Demler, and E. E. Walters (2005). "Prevalence, Severity, and Comorbidity of Twelve-Month DSM-IV Disorders in the National Comorbidity Survey Replication (NCS-R)." *Archives of General Psychiatry*, 62(6): 617-627.
7. Moffit, T., H. Harrington, A. Caspi, et al. (2007). "Depression and Generalized Anxiety Disorder." *Archives of General Psychiatry*, 64: 651-660.
8. Holden, C. (2010). "Experts Map the Terrain of Mood Disorders." *Science*, 327: 1068.
9. Seedat, S., K. Scott, M. Angermeyer, et al. (2009). "Cross-National Associations Between Gender and Mental Disorders in the World Health Organization World Mental Health Surveys." *Archives of General Psychiatry*, 66(7): 785-795.
10. Yanos, P., D. Rowe, K. Markus, and P. Lysaker (2008). "Pathways Between Internalized Stigma and Outcomes Related to Recovery in Schizophrenia Spectrum Disorders." *Psychiatric Services*, 59: 1437-1442.
11. Akil, H., S. Brenner, E. Kandel, et al. (2010). "The Future of Psychiatric Research: Genomes and Neural Circuits." *Science*, 327: 1580-1581.
12. Miller, G. (2010). "Beyond DSM: Seeking a Brain-Based Classification of Mental Illness." *Science*, 327: 1437.
13. Hamer, M., E. Stamatakis, and G. Batty (2010). "Objectively Assessed Secondhand Smoke Exposure and Mental Health in Adults." *Archives of General Psychiatry*, 67(8): 850-855.
14. Bouchard, M. F., D. C. Bellinger, J. Weuve, J. Matthews-Bellinger, S. E. Gilman, et al. (2009). "Blood Lead Levels and Major Depressive Disorder, Panic Disorder, and Generalized Anxiety Disorder in US Young Adults." *Archives of General Psychiatry*, 66: 1313-1319.
15. Sareen, J., T. O. Afifi, J. Weuve, K. A. McMillan, and G. J. G. Asmundson (2011). "Relationship Between Household Income and Mental Disorders." *Archives of General Psychiatry*, 68: 419-427.
16. Green, J., K. McLaughlin, P. Berglund, et al. (2010). "Childhood Adversities and Adult Psychiatric Disorders in the National Comorbidity Survey Replication I." *Archives of General Psychiatry*, 67: 113-123.
17. van Os, J., G. Kenis, and B. P. F. Rutten (2010). "The Environment and Schizophrenia." *Nature*, 468: 203-212.
18. Galea, S., J. Ahern, H. Resnick, D. Kilpatrick, M. Bucuvalas, J. Gold, and D. Vlahov (2002). "Psychological Sequelae of the September 11 Terrorist Attacks in New York City." *New England Journal of Medicine*, 346(13): 982-1087.
19. Holmes, T. H., and R. H. Rahe (1967). "The Social Readjustment Rating Scale." *Journal of Psychosomatic Research*, 11: 213-218.
20. Selye, H. (1946). "The General Adaptation Syndrome and Disease of Adaptation." *Journal of Clinical Endocrinology and Metabolism*, 6: 117-130.
21. Sarafino, E. P. (1990). *Health Psychology: Biopsychological Interactions*. New York, NY: John Wiley & Sons.
22. Schneiderman, N., G. Ironson, and S. D. Siegel (2005). "Stress and Health: Psychological, Behavioral, and Biological Determinants." *Annual Review of Clinical Psychology*, 1: 607-628.
23. Baer, P. E., L. B. Garmezy, R. J. McLaughlin, A. D. Pokorny, and M. J. Wernick (1987). "Stress, Coping, Family Conflict, and Adolescent Alcohol Use." *Journal of Behavioral Medicine*, 10: 449-466.
24. Conway, T. L., R. R. Vickers, H. W. Ward, and R. H. Rahe (1981). "Occupational Stress and Variation in Cigarette, Coffee, and Alcohol Consumption." *Journal of Health and Social Behavior*, 22: 155-165.

25. House, J. S., K. R. Landis, and D. Umberson (1988). "Social Relationships and Health." *Science*, 241: 540–545.

26. Payne, W. A., D. B. Hahn, and E. B. Lucas (2006). *Understanding Your Health*, 9th ed. New York, NY: McGraw-Hill Higher Education.

27. Hoge, C., J. Auchterlonie, and C. Milliken (2006). "Mental Health Problems, Use of Mental Health Services, and Attrition from Military Service After Returning from Deployment to Iraq and Afghanistan." *Journal of the American Medical Association*, 295(9): 1023–1032.

28. Miniño, A. M., M. Heron, and B. L. Smith (2006). "Deaths: Preliminary Data for 2004." *National Vital Statistics Report*, 54(19): 1–52.

29. Centers for Disease Control and Prevention (2009). "National Suicide Statistics at a Glance." Available at http://www.cdc.gov/violenceprevention/suicide/statistics/trends01.html.

30. Dumesnil, H., and P. Verger (2009). "Public Awareness Campaigns about Depression and Suicide: A Review." *Psychiatric Services*, 60(9): 1203–1213.

31. Grob, G. N. (1994). *The Mad Among Us: A History of the Care of America's Mentally Ill*. New York, NY: The Free Press.

32. Johnson, A. B. (1990). *Out of Bedlam: The Truth about Deinstitutionalization*. New York, NY: Basic Books, 306.

33. Gerhart, U. C. (1990). *Caring for the Chronic Mentally Ill*. Itasca, IL: F. E. Peacock, 5.

34. Mosher, L. R., and L. Burti (1989). *Community Mental Health*. New York, NY: W. W. Norton.

35. Foley, H. A., and S. S. Sharfstein (1983). *Madness and Government*. Washington, DC: American Psychiatric Press.

36. El Hai, J. (2005). *The Lobotomist*. New York, NY: John Wiley & Sons.

37. Grob, G. N. (1991). *From Asylum to Community*. Princeton, NJ: Princeton University Press.

38. Frank, R. G., and S. A. Glied (2006). *Better But Not Well*. Baltimore, MD: Johns Hopkins University Press.

39. Centers for Medicare and Medicaid Services (2002). "Medicare Expands Crackdown on Waste, Fraud and Abuse in Community Mental Health Centers" [Press release]. Available at http://archive.hhs.gov/news/press/1998pres/980929.html.

40. Levine, M., P. A. Toro, and D. V. Perkins (1993). "Social and Community Interventions." *Annual Review of Psychology*, 44: 525–558.

41. U.S. Department of Health and Human Services, Substance Abuse and Mental Health Services Administration (2003). *Blueprint for Change: Ending Chronic Homelessness for Persons with Serious Mental Illnesses and/or Co-occurring Substance Use Disorders* (DHHS pub. no. SMA-04-3870). Rockville, MD: Author.

42. Schanzer, B., D. Boanerges, P. E. Shrout, and L. M. Caton (2007). "Homelessness, Health Status, and Health Care Use." *American Journal of Public Health*, 97(3): 464–469.

43. Gulcer, L., S. Tsemberis, A. Stefancic, and R. M. Greenwood (2007). "Community Integration of Adults with Psychiatric Disabilities and Histories of Homelessness." *Community Mental Health Journal*, 43(3): 211–228.

44. Gilmer, T., A. Stefancic, S. Ettner, W. Manning, and S. Tsemberis (2010). "Effect of Full-Service Partnerships on Homelessness, Use and Costs of Mental Health Services, and Quality of Life Among Adults with Serious Mental Illness." *Archives of General Psychiatry*, 67(6): 645–652.

45. Elbogen, E., and S. Johnson (2009). "The Intricate Link Between Violence and Mental Disorder." *Archives of General Psychiatry*, 66(2): 152–161.

46. Rich, J. D., S. E. Wakeman, and S. L. Dickman (2011). "Medicine and the Epidemic of Incarceration in the United States." *New England Journal of Medicine*, 364: 2081–2083.

47. James, D. J., and L. E. Glaze (2006). *Mental Health Problems of Prison and Jail Inmates* (NCJ pub. no. 213600). Available at http://bjs.ojp.usdoj.gov/content/pub/pdf/mhppji.pdf.

48. Wolf, N., C. Blitz, and J. Shi (2007). "Rates of Sexual Victimization in Prison for Inmates with and Without Mental Disorders." *Psychiatric Services*, 58: 1087–1094.

49. Metzner, J. L. (2012). "Treatment for Prisoners: A U.S. Perspective." *Psychiatric Services*, 63: 276.

50. Moore, S. (10 August 2009). "Mentally Ill Offenders Strain Juvenile System." *New York Times*, A1.

51. Baillargeon, J., I. Binswanger, J. Penn, B. Williams, and O. Murray (2009). "Psychiatric Disorders and Repeat Incarcerations: The Revolving Prison Door." *American Journal of Psychiatry*, 166: 103–109.

52. Swanson, J., R. Van Dorn, J. Monahan, and R. Swartz (2006). "Violence and Leveraged Treatment for Persons with Mental Disorders." *American Journal of Psychiatry*, 163: 1404–1411.

53. Steadman, H. J., A. Redlich, L. Callahan, P. C. Robbins, and R. Vesselinov (2011). "Effects of Mental Health Court on Arrests and Jail Days." *Archives of General Psychiatry*, 68: 167–172.

54. Kuehn, B. (2007). "Mental Health Courts Show Promise." *Journal of the American Medical Association*, 297(15): 1641–1643.

55. Reynolds, A. J., J. A. Temple, S. Ou, I. A. Arteaga, and B. A. B. White (2011). "School-Based Early Childhood Education and Age-28 Well-Being: Effects by Timing, Dosage, and Subgroups." *Science*, 333: 360–364.

56. Adler, A. B., R. D. Bliese, D. McGurk, S. W. Hoge, and C. A. Castro (2009). "Battlemind Debriefing and Battlemind Training as Early Interventions with Soldiers Returning from Iraq: Randomization by Platoon." *Journal of Consulting and Clinical Psychology*, 77: 928–940.

57. Levine, M., D. D. Perkins, and D. V. Perkins (2004). *Principles of Community Psychology: Perspectives and Applications*, 3rd ed. New York, NY: Oxford University Press.

58. Gaynes, B., D. Warden, M. Trivedi, et al. (2009). "What did STAR*D Teach Us? Results from a Large-Scale, Practical, Clinical Trial for Patients with Depression." *Psychiatric Services*, 60: 1439–1445.

59. Sajatovic, M., M. Valenstein, F. Blow, D. Ganoczy, and R. Ignacio (2007). "Treatment Adherence with Lithium and Anticonvulsant Medications Among Patients with Bipolar Disorder." *Psychiatric Services*, 58: 855–863.

60. Ware, N., K. Hopper, T. Tugenberg, et al. (2007). "Connectedness and Citizenship: Redefining Social Integration." *Psychiatric Services*, 58: 469–474.

61. Corrigan, P., K. Mueser, G. Bond, R. Drake, and P. Solomon (2008). *Principles and Practice of Psychiatric Rehabilitation: An Empirical Approach*. New York, NY: Guilford.

62. van Vugt, M. D., H. Droon, P. A. Delespaul, and C. L. Mulder (2012). "Consumer-Providers in Assertive Community Treatment Programs: Associations with Client Outcomes." *Psychiatric Services*, 63: 477–481.

63. Padgett, D. K., and B. F. Henwood (2011). "Moving into the Fourth Decade of ACT." *Psychiatric Services*, 62: 605.

64. Hopper, K. (2004). "Interrogating the Meaning of 'Culture' in the WHO International Studies of Schizophrenia." In J. Jenkins and R. Barrett, eds., *Schizophrenia, Culture, and Subjectivity: The Edge of Experience*. Cambridge, UK: Cambridge University Press, 62-86.

65. Miller, G. (2006). "A Spoonful of Medicine—and a Steady Diet of Normality." *Science*, 311: 464-465.

66. McGruder, J. (2004). "Madness in Zanzibar: An Exploration of Lived Experience." In J. Jenkins and R. Barrett, eds., *Schizophrenia, Culture, and Subjectivity: The Edge of Experience*. Cambridge, UK: Cambridge University Press, 255-281.

67. Drapalski, A. L., T. Marshall, D. Seybolt, et al. (2008). "Unmet Needs of Families of Adults with Mental Illness and Preferences Regarding Family Services." *Psychiatric Services*, 59: 655-662.

68. Ellis, A., T. Konrad, K. Thomas, and J. Morrissey (2009). "County-Level Estimates of Mental Health Professional Supply in the United States." *Psychiatric Services*, 60: 1315-1322.

69. Olfson, M., R. Mojtabai, N. Sampson, et al. (2009). "Dropout from Outpatient Mental Health Care in the United States." *Psychiatric Services*, 60: 898-907.

70. Wang, P., O. Demler, M. Olfson, et al. (2006). "Changing Profiles of Service Sectors Used for Mental Health Care in the United States." *American Journal of Psychiatry*, 163: 1187-1198.

71. Ault-Brutus, A. A. (2012). "Changes in Racial-Ethnic Disparities in Use and Adequacy of Mental Health Care in the United States, 1990-2003." *Psychiatric Services*, 63: 531-540.

72. Hernandez, N., T. Nesman, D. Mowery, et al. (2009). "Cultural Competence: A Literature Review and Conceptual Model for Mental Health Services." *Psychiatric Services*, 60: 1046-1050.

73. Rotondi, A. J., C. M. Anderson, G. L Haas, S. M. Eack, M. B. Spring, et al. (2010). "Web-Based Psychoeducational Intervention for Persons with Schizophrenia and Their Supporters: One-Year Outcomes." *Psychiatric Services*, 61:1099-1105.

74. Simon, G. E., and E. J. Ludman (2009). "It's Time for Disruptive Innovation in Psychotherapy." *Lancet*, 374: 594-595.

75. Centers for Medicare and Medicaid Services (2010). "The Mental Health Parity and Addiction Equity Act." Available at https://www.cms.gov/HealthInsReformforConsume/04_TheMentalHealthParityAct.asp.

76. Garfield, R. L., S. H. Zuvekas, J. R. Lave, and J. M. Donohue (2011). "The Impact of National Health Care Reform on Adults with Severe Mental Disorders." *American Journal of Psychiatry*, 168: 486-494.

Chapter 10

Alcohol, Tobacco, and Other Drugs: A Community Concern

Robert R. Pinger, PhD

Chapter Objectives

After studying this chapter, you will be able to:

1. Describe the personal and community consequences of alcohol, tobacco, and other drug abuse.

2. Define the terms *drug use*, *drug misuse*, *drug abuse*, *physical dependence*, *psychological dependence*, *psychoactive drug*, *problem drinking*, and *alcoholism*.

3. Discuss the factors that contribute to the abuse of alcohol, tobacco, and other drugs.

4. Define the terms *over-the-counter* and *prescription drugs*, explain the purposes of these categories of drugs, and describe how they are regulated.

5. Define the term *controlled substances* and provide examples.

6. Characterize recent trends in the prevalence of alcohol, tobacco, and other drug use among U.S. high school seniors.

7. Give an example of primary, secondary, and tertiary prevention activities in drug abuse prevention and control programs.

8. Explain how each of the four elements of drug abuse prevention and control—education, treatment, public policy development, and law enforcement—mitigate the damage of drug abuse in our communities.

9. Summarize governmental and nongovernmental efforts to prevent and control the misuse and abuse of alcohol, tobacco, and other drugs.

Introduction

More deaths, illnesses, and disabilities can be attributed to the abuse of alcohol, tobacco, and other drugs than to any other preventable health condition.[1,2] In this chapter, we discuss the scope of the drug problem in the United States, factors that contribute to it, and society's efforts to prevent and control further abuse.

Scope of the Current Drug Problem in the United States

Drug abuse and dependence are costly to society in terms of both lives and dollars. The deaths of more than half a million people (nearly one-fourth of all deaths) each year can be attributed to alcohol, tobacco, or illicit drug use (see Table 10.1). Estimates of the annual economic cost of substance abuse in the United States fall between $414 billion[1] and $487 billion.[1-3] These estimates include direct costs (such as healthcare expenditures, premature death, and impaired productivity) and indirect costs, which include the costs of crime and law enforcement, courts, jails, and social work. Of the $487 billion annual drug bill, the cost of alcohol abuse and alcoholism is estimated at $223 billion, drug abuse at $110 billion, and smoking at $157 billion (see Table 10.1). Another study estimates that federal, state, and local governments spend $467.7 billion as a result of substance abuse and addiction: $238.2 billion by federal governments, $135.8 billion by states, and $93.8 billion by local governments. This spending amounted to 10.7% of their entire $4.4 trillion budgets.[3] Clearly, the abuse of alcohol and other drugs is one of the United States' most expensive community health problems.

Those abusing alcohol, tobacco, and other drugs represent serious health threats to themselves, their families, and their communities because they put themselves and their families at risk for physical, mental, and financial ruin. The habitual drug user who becomes dependent on the drug will experience great difficulty in discontinuing use, even in the face of deteriorating physical and mental health and erosion of financial resources. If the drug is an illegal one, its use constitutes criminal activity, and carries the added risks of arrest, prosecution, and incarceration.

Those who abuse alcohol, tobacco, and other drugs negatively affect the community because they suffer more injuries, require more health care, and are less productive than those who do not. Community consequences range from lower productivity and loss of revenue to greater demand for social services (see Table 10.2). Additionally, those who abuse drugs may perpetrate more interpersonal violence (see Figure 10.1) and property crimes, increase the cost of insurance, and place an added burden on our legal system.

The Monitoring the Future surveys on drug use among high school and college students have been carried out annually since 1975.[4-6] Survey results for the year 1992 were remarkable because use of almost all drugs reached their lowest levels since the first survey. Since 1992, use levels for various drugs have trended up and down. The most

Table 10.1 The Annual Cost in Lives and Dollars Attributable to Alcohol, Tobacco, and Illicit Drug Abuse in the United States

Type of Drug	Estimated Number of Deaths Each Year	Economic Cost to Society (in Billions)
Alcohol	100,000	$223
Tobacco	443,000	$157
Illicit drugs	16,000	$110
Opioid pain relievers	36,450	(no estimate available)
Total	595,450	$490

Sources: Data from Horgan, C., K. C. Skwara, and G. Strickler (2001). *Substance Abuse: The Nation's Number One Health Problem.* Princeton, NJ: Robert Wood Johnson Foundation; National Center on Addiction and Substance Abuse at Columbia University (2006). *The Commercial Value of Underage and Pathological Drinking to the Alcohol Industry: A CASA White Paper.* Available at http://www.casacolumbia.org/templates/Publications_Reports.aspx#r16 ; Bouchery, E., E. H. J. Harwwod, J. J. Sacks, C. J. Simon, and R. D. Brewer (2011). "Economic Costs of Excessive Alcohol Consumption in the U.S., 2006." *American Journal of Preventative Medicine,* 41(5): 516–524; American Cancer Society (2012). *Cancer Facts and Figure—2010.* Atlanta, GA: Author; Centers for Disease Control and Prevention (2011). "Vital Signs: Overdoses of Prescription Pain Relievers—United States, 1999–2008." *Morbidity and Mortality Weekly Report,* 60(43):1487–1492. Available at http://www.cdc.gov/mmwr/PDF/wk/mm6043.pdf.

Table 10.2   Personal and Community Consequences of Drug Abuse

Personal Consequences	Community Consequences
Absenteeism from school or work	Loss of productivity and revenue
Underachievement at school or work	Lower average SAT scores
Scholastic failure/interruption of education	Loss of economic opportunity
Loss of employment	Increase in public welfare load
Marital instability/family problems	Increase in number of broken homes
Risk of infectious diseases	Epidemics of sexually transmitted infections
Risk of chronic or degenerative diseases	Unnecessary burden on healthcare system
Increased risk of accidents	Unnecessary deaths and economic losses
Financial problems	Defaults on mortgages, loans/bankruptcies
Criminal activity	Increased cost of insurance and security
Arrest and incarceration	Increased cost for police/courts/prisons
Risk of adulterated drugs	Increased burden on medical care system
Adverse drug reactions or "bad trips"	Greater need for emergency medical services
Drug-induced psychoses	Unnecessary drain on mental health services
Drug overdose	Unnecessary demand for medical services
Injury to fetus or newborn baby	Unnecessary use of expensive neonatal care
Loss of self-esteem	Increase in mental illness, underachievement
Suicide	Damaged and destroyed families
Death	

recent results (for 2011) reveal that the use of many drugs among high school seniors is now lower than it was in 1992. Most remarkable are the declines in alcohol consumption and cigarette smoking (see Table 10.3).[4,5] Marijuana use,

however, increased in 2011. Among high school seniors, 22.6% reported marijuana use in the past 30 days, compared with only 11.9% in 1992.

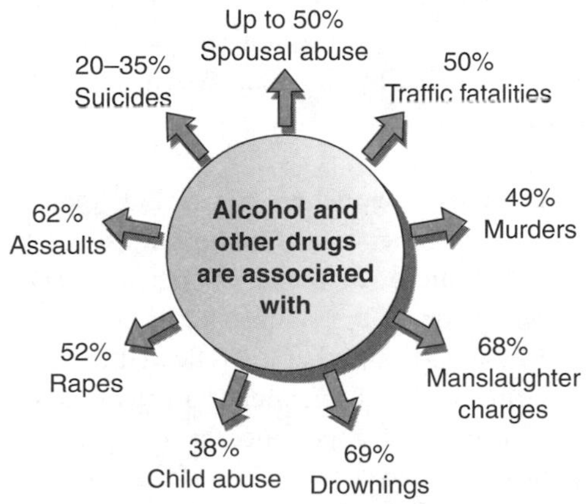

Definitions

We begin this discussion of alcohol, tobacco, and other drugs as a community health problem by defining some terms. A **drug** is a substance, other than food or vitamins, that upon entering the body in small amounts alters one's physical, mental, or emotional state. **Psychoactive drugs** are drugs that alter sensory perceptions, mood, thought processes, or behavior.

In this chapter, the term **drug use** is a nonevaluative term referring to drug-taking behavior in general, regardless of whether the behavior is appropriate. **Drug misuse** refers primarily to the inappropriate use of

Figure 10.1 Violence associated with the use of alcohol and other drugs.

National Clearinghouse for Alcohol and Drug Information (1995). *Making the Link* [fact sheets]. Rockville, MD: Author.

drug a substance other than food that when taken in small quantities alters one's physical, mental, or emotional state
drug misuse inappropriate use of prescription or nonprescription drugs
drug use a nonevaluative term referring to drug-taking behavior in general; any drug-taking behavior
psychoactive drugs drugs that alter sensory perceptions, mood, thought processes, or behavior

Table 10.3 Percentage of High School Seniors Who Have Used Drugs

	Class of 1992			Class of 2008		
	Ever Used	**Past Month**	**Daily Use**	**Ever Used**	**Past Month**	**Daily Use**
Alcohol*	87.5%	51.3%	3.4%	70.0%	40.0%	2.1%
Cigarettes	61.8	27.8	17.2	40.0	18.7	10.3
Marijuana	32.6	11.9	1.9	45.5	22.6	6.6
Amphetamines	13.9	2.8	0.2	12.2	3.7	†
Methamphetamine	–	–	–	2.1	0.6	†
Inhalants	16.6	2.3	0.1	8.1	1.0	†
Cocaine	6.1	1.3	0.1	5.2	1.1	†
Tranquilizers	6.0	1.0	†	8.7	2.3	†
LSD	8.6	2.1	0.1	4.0	0.8	†
MDMA	–	–	–	8.0	2.3	†
Crack	2.6	0.6	0.1	1.9	0.5	†
PCP	2.4	0.6	0.1	2.3	0.8	†
Heroin	1.2	0.3	†	1.4	0.4	†

*More than just a few sips.
†Less than 0.05%.
–No data.
Sources: Data from Johnston, L. D., P. M. O'Malley, and J. G. Bachman (1993). *National Survey Results from the Monitoring the Future Study, 1975–1992. Volume I: Secondary School Students* (NIH pub. no. 93-3597). Rockville, MD: National Institute on Drug Abuse; and Johnston, L. D., P. M. O'Malley, J. G. Bachman, and J. E. Schulenbert (2009). *Monitoring the Future National Survey Results on Drug Use 1975–2008, Volume I, Secondary School Students* (NIH pub. no. 09-7402). Bethesda, MD: National Institute on Drug Abuse. Available at http://www.monitoringthefuture.org/pubs.html.

drug abuse use of a drug when it is detrimental to one's health or well-being

drug (chemical) dependence a psychological and sometimes physical state characterized by a craving for a drug

physical dependence a physiological state in which discontinued drug use results in clinical illness

psychological dependence a psychological state characterized by an overwhelming desire to continue use of a drug

tolerance physiological and enzymatic adjustments that occur in response to the chronic presence of drugs, which are reflected in the need for ever-increasing doses

legally purchased prescription or nonprescription drugs. For example, drug misuse occurs when one discontinues the use of a prescribed antibiotic before the entire prescribed dose is completed or when one takes four aspirin rather than two as specified on the label. **Drug abuse** can be defined in several ways depending upon the drug and the situation. Drug abuse occurs when one takes a prescription or nonprescription drug for a purpose other than that for which it is medically approved, for example, taking a prescription diet pill for its mood altering effects (stimulation). The abuse of legal drugs such as nicotine or alcohol is said to occur when one is aware that continued use is detrimental to one's health. Because illicit drugs have no approved medical uses, any illicit drug use is considered drug abuse. Likewise, the use of alcohol and nicotine by those under legal age is considered drug abuse.

Drug (chemical) dependence, the feeling that a certain drug is necessary for normal functioning, stems from the development of **tolerance**, the physiological and enzymatic adjustments that occur in response to the chronic presence of a drug in the body and that are reflected in the need for ever-increasing doses. Dependence may be **psychological**, such that the user experiences a strong emotional or psychological desire to continue use of the drug even without clinical signs of illness, or it can be **physical**, in which case discontinuation of drug use results in clinical illness. Usually, both psychological and physical dependence are present at the same time, making abstinence from use very difficult. Abstinence in these cases is accompanied by unpleasant, or painful, clinically recognized symptoms known as **withdrawal illness (abstinence syndrome)**. Even mild withdrawal illness can make it difficult to maintain abstinence from a drug, as is frequently the case with nicotine dependence associated with cigarette smoking.

Factors That Contribute to Alcohol, Tobacco, and Other Drug Abuse

Many factors contribute to the abuse of alcohol, tobacco, and other drugs. Those that increase the probability of drug use are called *risk factors*; those that lower the probability of drug use are called *protective factors*. Individuals are differentially at risk for initiating and maintaining drug-taking behavior.[7] People with a high number of risk factors are said to be vulnerable to drug abuse or dependence, whereas those who have few risk factors and more protective factors are said to be resistant to drug abuse.

Risk and protective factors can be either genetic (inherited) or environmental. Numerous studies have concluded that inherited traits can increase one's risk of developing dependence on alcohol, and it is logical to assume that susceptibility to other drugs might also be inherited. Environmental risk factors, such as one's home and family life, school and peer groups, and society and culture, have also been identified.

Inherited Risk Factors

Evidence for the heritability of risk for alcoholism is provided by numerous studies,[8-10] which were reviewed by Tabakoff and Hoffman[11] in the *Seventh Special Report to the U.S. Congress on Alcohol and Health*, from the Secretary of Health and Human Services.[12] At least two types of inherited alcoholism exist,[9] referred to as Type I (or milieu-limited) and Type II (or male-limited) alcoholism.[12] These observational studies of alcoholics' families are supported by genetic research. Some genes predispose an individual to developing alcohol-related problems, whereas others may actually be protective in nature. Another study has provided evidence that genes may also influence cigarette smoking.[13] The heritability of susceptibility to other drugs is still under investigation.

Environmental Risk Factors

Environmental factors, both psychological and social, can influence the use and abuse of alcohol and other drugs.

Among these are personal factors, and those associated with home and family life, school and peer groups, and other components of the social and cultural environment.

Personal Factors

Personal factors include personality traits, such as impulsiveness, depressive mood, susceptibility to stress, or possibly personality disturbances. Some of these factors have been reviewed by Needle and colleagues.[14] It is difficult to determine the degree to which these factors are inherited or are simply the product of the family environment. For example, one's choice to use alcohol or drugs in response to a stressful situation (and the outcome of that decision) could be the result of either inherited characteristics, learned behavior, or a combination of these factors.

Home and Family Life

The importance of home and family life on alcohol and drug abuse has been the subject of numerous studies.[14,15] Not all family-associated risk is genetic in origin. Family structure, family dynamics, quality of parenting, and family problems can be either risk or protective factors for children and adolescents. Family turmoil (deaths and divorces) have been associated with the initiation of alcohol and other drug use.[14] In this sense, alcohol or other drug use is a symptom of personal and/or family problems, not a cause.[16]

The development of interpersonal skills, such as communication skills, independent living skills, and learning to get along with others, nurtured in the home, are viewed as protective factors. The failure of parents to provide an environment conducive to the development of these skills can result in the loss of self-esteem and an increase in delinquency, nonconformity, and sociopathic behavior, all personal risk factors for alcohol and drug abuse.[12] Finally, family attitudes toward alcohol and drug use influence adolescents' beliefs and expectations about the effects of drugs, which in turn influence decisions to initiate and continue alcohol use.[12] The age of first use of alcohol, tobacco, and illicit drugs is correlated to later development of alcohol and drug problems, especially if use begins before age 15.[1]

School and Peer Groups

Perceived support of drinking by peers is the single most important

withdrawal illness (abstinence syndrome) the unpleasant feelings or painful, clinically recognized symptoms that arise when one abstains from a dependence-producing drug after tolerance develops

factor in an adolescent's choice to drink (see Figure 10.2).[12] Peers can also influence expectations for a drug. Alcohol may be perceived as "a 'magic elixir' that can enhance social and physical pleasure, sexual performance and responsiveness, power and aggression and social competence."[12] It is interesting to note that these are precisely the mythical qualities about alcohol portrayed in advertisements for beer and other alcoholic beverages. The decision to experiment with cigarettes also often is influenced by one's peers.

Sociocultural Environment

The notion of environmental risk includes the effects of sociocultural and physical settings on drug-taking behavior. Environmental risk for drug taking can stem from one's immediate neighborhood or from society at large. For example, living in the inner city—with its sordidness, physical decay, and threats to personal safety—could set into motion a variety of changes in values and behaviors, including some related to alcohol or drug use.[17]

Opportunities for community interventions exist, though. Increasing taxes on tobacco products and alcoholic beverages and developing zoning ordinances that limit the number of bars, liquor stores, and billboards advertising tobacco and alcohol in certain neighborhoods can be effective in reducing the alcohol, tobacco, and other drug problems in a community.

Types of Drugs Abused and Resulting Problems

There are many classification systems of drugs of abuse, but none of them is perfect. In this chapter, our classification system includes legal drugs and illegal drugs. Legal (licit) drugs include alcohol, nicotine, and nonprescription and prescription drugs. Illegal (illicit) drugs are those that cannot be manufactured or grown within the confines of the law. Some prescription drugs and all of the illegal drugs are regulated under the Controlled Substance Act of 1970 and come under the purview of the Drug Enforcement Administration (DEA).

Legal Drugs

Legal drugs are drugs that can be legally bought and sold in the marketplace, including those that are closely regulated, like morphine; those that are lightly regulated, like alcohol and tobacco; and those that are unregulated, like caffeine.

Alcohol

Alcohol is the number 1 problem drug in the United States by almost any standard of measurement—the number of those who abuse it, the number of injuries and injury deaths that result from its use, the amount of money spent on it, and its social and economic costs to society in terms of broken homes and lost wages. Alcohol is consumed in a

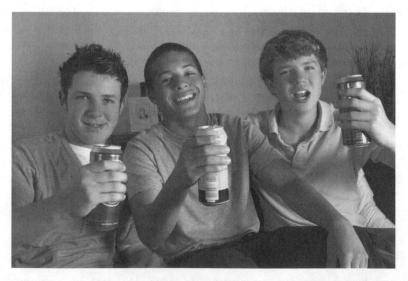

Figure 10.2 Perceived support of drinking by peers is the single most important factor in an adolescent's choice to drink.
© Monkey Business/Fotolia.com

variety of forms, including beer, wine, fortified wines and brandies, and distilled spirits. Although distilled spirits are the most concentrated form of alcoholic beverage, the form consumed most often in high risk, episodic drinking is beer. Much of this beer is drunk by young persons in the 18- to 24-year age group. **Binge drinking** (consuming five or more drinks on a single occasion for males and four or more drinks for females) "accounts for more than half of the estimated 80,000 annual deaths and three-quarters of the $223.5 billion in economic costs resulting from excessive alcohol consumption in the United States," according to a recent report from the Centers for Disease Control and Prevention (CDC).[18] In 2010, the average frequency of episodes among binge drinkers was 4.4 per month and the average number of drinks consumed on these occasions was 7.9, far above the 4–5 drinks cited in the binge drinking definition.[18]

A major community health concern is underage drinking, that is, drinking by those younger than 21 years. An analysis has revealed that nearly 26% of underage drinkers meet clinical criteria for alcohol abuse or dependence, compared with 9.6% of adult drinkers.[19] Underage drinkers, nearly all of them children and teenagers, can destroy their own lives and the lives of others through reckless driving, risky sexual behavior resulting in disease transmission and unintentional pregnancies, and acts of interpersonal violence. At issue is the fact that an estimated $22.5 billion, or 17% of all money spent on alcohol, can be accounted for by underage drinking.[19,20] The alcohol industry would take a huge hit if underage drinking were to stop. The industry relies on underage drinkers for two reasons: the amount of alcohol consumed by them and the fact that many pathological underage drinkers will become pathological adult drinkers, a group that accounts for $25.8 billion, or 20.1%, of the consumer expenditures for alcohol.[19,20]

Drinking by high school and college students is widespread despite the fact that it is illegal for virtually all high school students and for most college students to purchase these beverages. In 2011, 70% of high school seniors reported having drunk alcohol (more than a few sips) at least once in their lifetime, with 63.5% in the past year, and 40% in the past 30 days. One in four high school seniors (25%) reported having been drunk in the past 30 days.[5] Binge drinking at least once in the prior 2-week period was reported by 21.6% of high school seniors. College students reported an even higher prevalence of binge drinking; 37% stated that they had consumed five or more drinks in a row in the past 2-week period.[6]

Most of those who experiment with alcohol begin their use in a social context and become light or moderate drinkers.

Alcohol use is reinforcing in two ways: It lowers anxieties and produces a mild euphoria. For many people, alcohol use does not become a significant problem, but for about 10% of those who drink, it does. Some of these people become **problem drinkers**; that is, they begin to experience personal, interpersonal, legal, or financial problems because of their alcohol consumption. Still others lose control of their drinking and develop a dependence upon alcohol. Physical dependence on alcohol and the loss of control over one's drinking are two important characteristics of **alcoholism**. According to the *Journal of the American Medical Association*:

> Alcoholism is a primary, chronic disease with genetic, psychosocial, and environmental factors influencing its development and manifestations. The disease is often progressive and fatal. It is characterized by impaired control over drinking, preoccupation with the drug alcohol, use of alcohol despite adverse consequences, and distortions in thinking, most notably denial. Each of these symptoms may be continuous or periodic.[21]

The cost of alcohol abuse and alcoholism in the United States was estimated for 2005 to be $220 billion.[19] That is $740 for every man, woman, and child. To put it another way, it costs the United States $25 million every hour for alcohol-related problems. More than 60% of the cost is due to lost employment or reduced productivity, and 13% of the cost is due to medical and treatment costs. Healthcare costs for alcoholics are about twice those for nonalcoholics.[12]

Alcohol and other drugs are contributing factors to a variety of unintentional injuries and injury deaths; chief among these are motor vehicle–related deaths. The risk of a motor vehicle crash increases progressively with alcohol consumption and **blood alcohol concentration (BAC)**.

> Compared with drivers who have not consumed alcohol, the risk of a single-vehicle fatal crash for drivers with BAC's between 0.02 and 0.04 percent is estimated to be 1.4 times higher; for those with BAC's between 0.05 and 0.09 percent, 11.1 times higher; for drivers with BAC's between 0.10 and 0.14 percent, 48 times higher; and for those with BAC's at or above 0.15 percent, the risk is estimated to be 380 times higher.[22]

alcoholism a disease characterized by impaired control over drinking, preoccupation with drinking, and continued use of alcohol despite adverse consequences

binge drinking consuming five or more drinks in a row for males and four or more drinks in a row for females

blood alcohol concentration (BAC) the percentage of concentration of alcohol in the blood

problem drinker one for whom alcohol consumption results in a medical, social, or other type of problem

Alcohol-impaired driving is widespread in the United States. Results of a recent national survey indicate that an estimated 112,166,000 episodes of alcohol-impaired driving occurred in 2010.[23] Men accounted for 81% of these episodes; young men ages 21–34 years, who represented 11% of the U.S. adult population, reported 32% of all 2010 episodes. Binge drinking was strongly linked to impaired driving episodes; 85% of these episodes were by those who reported binge drinking. Furthermore, 4.5% of the adult population who reported binge drinking four or more times per month accounted for 55% of all alcohol-impaired driving episodes. Finally, persons reporting not always using seat belts had alcohol-impaired driving rates four times those who reported always using seat belts.[23]

The youngest drivers are particularly at risk because they are inexperienced drivers and inexperienced drinkers. This combination can be deadly. One study found that 23% of drivers 16 to 20 years old who were involved in fatal motor vehicle crashes, and for whom any alcohol consumption is illegal, had alcohol in their blood.[22]

Despite these grim figures, significant progress has been made in reducing the overall rate of alcohol-related vehicle deaths. Between 1987 and 2007 this rate declined from 9.8 to 4.0 deaths per 100,000 people, exceeding the *Healthy People 2010* objective. The *Healthy People 2020* objective, based on number of miles traveled, is to decrease the rate of alcohol-impaired driving (0.08 or greater blood-alcohol content) fatalities to 0.38 per 100 million miles traveled (see **Box 10.1**).[24]

Past success and the promise of future achievement of the target came through public policy changes—raising the minimum legal drinking age, strengthening and enforcing state license revocation laws, and lowering the BAC tolerance levels from 0.10% to 0.08% in all states—stricter law enforcement, and better education for those cited for driving while intoxicated.[25]

Alcohol consumption increases one's risk for other types of unintentional injuries, such as drowning, falls, fires, and burns and for becoming a victim or perpetrator of domestic violence, assault, rape, or murder (see Figure 10.1).

"Alcohol is the number 1 rape drug."[26] The incidence of rape on college campuses is estimated at 35 per 1,000 female students, making rape the most common violent crime on U.S. campuses. Yet, less than 5% of these rapes are reported to police. About half of the perpetrators and rape survivors on college campuses were drinking alcohol at the time of the assault. Ninety percent of college women who are raped

know their assailants. A new law in Wisconsin was designed to protect women at risk of sexual assault by acquaintances at social gatherings where alcohol is served. A person convicted under the new law can be fined up to $100,000 and sentenced to up to 25 years in prison. Wisconsin is the 50th state to enact such a law.[26]

Alcohol consumption can increase a person's risk of contracting an infectious disease. Overall, alcohol accounts for 13.5% of global mortality from infectious diseases.[27] The behavioral and physiological effects of alcohol intoxication increase the risk of contracting an infection and reduce the effectiveness of treatment should a person become infected. In one study, 35% of HIV patients were classified as currently or previously alcohol dependent.[27]

Another community health problem resulting from pathological drinking is fetal alcohol spectrum disorder (FASD). FASD includes such diagnoses as fetal alcohol syndrome (FAS), partial FAS, alcohol-related birth defects (ARBD), and alcohol-related neurodevelopmental disorders (ARND). "Every year, about 40,000 babies are born with symptoms

---

Box 10.1 *Healthy People 2020:* Objectives

Objective: SA-17 Decrease the rate of alcohol-impaired driving fatalities.

Target setting method: 5% improvement.

Data source: Analysis Reporting System (FARS), U.S. Department of Transportation.

Target and baseline:

Objective	2008 Baseline	2020 Target
SA-17 Decrease the rate of alcohol-impaired driving (0.08% or greater blood alcohol content) fatalities	Per 100 million vehicle miles traveled	
	0.40	0.38

For Further Thought

The reduction in the rate of alcohol-related vehicle deaths is one of the greatest success stories of public health during the twentieth century. What are some factors that have contributed to decreasing alcohol-related vehicle deaths? Similar success has not been achieved for substance abuse-related deaths or drug abuse-related emergency department visits overall. What explanation can you offer for this difference?

Source: U.S. Department of Health and Human Services, Office of Disease Prevention and Health Promotion (2010). *Healthy People 2020.* Available at http://www.healthypeople.gov/2020/default.aspx.

of prenatal alcohol exposure," according to the Substance Abuse and Mental Health Services Administration.[28] Estimated prevalence rates for FASD range from 0.33 to 2.0 cases of FASD per 1,000 live births. These babies cost society thousands of dollars over their lifetimes. Costs can be attributed to medical treatment for pre- and postnatal growth defects requiring surgery; services for developmentally disabled children; home health care, special education, social services, training and supervision, and institutional care for affected individuals with mental retardation to age 65 years; and lost productivity. Estimates of the annual cost of FASD in the United States range from $0.5 million to $6 billion. Likewise, estimates for the lifetime costs for a specific individual with FASD range from $1 million to $5 million.[28] Clearly, women who could become pregnant should exercise caution in their alcohol use.

Nicotine

Nicotine is the psychoactive and addictive drug present in tobacco products such as cigarettes, cigars, smokeless or "spit" tobacco (chewing tobacco and snuff), and pipe tobacco. The problem of uneven state tobacco laws regarding sales to minors and the lack of enforcement of these laws was remedied in 1992 by the **Synar Amendment**, a federal law that requires all states to adopt legislation that prohibits the sale and distribution of tobacco products to people under age 18. States that do not comply with this regulation lose federal dollars for alcohol, tobacco, and other drug prevention and treatment programs.[29] An agreement between Reynolds Tobacco and the attorneys general of 38 states to end the sale of candy-, fruit-, and liquor-flavored cigarettes popular with youth was announced October 10, 2006.[30]

On June 22, 2009, President Obama signed the Family Smoking Prevention and Tobacco Control Act into law, giving the Food and Drug Administration (FDA) oversight over tobacco products. Beginning June 22, 2010, the tobacco industry had to "halt the manufacture of its deceptively labeled 'light,' 'mild,' and 'low-tar' cigarettes."[31] It remains to be seen how effective this law will be in lowering smoking rates among young Americans.

One proven way to reduce smoking rates is to increase taxes on cigarettes, thereby increasing the financial cost of smoking. The New York State legislature added another $1.60 in state taxes to every cigarette pack sold beginning July 1, 2010, raising the average price per pack in the state of New York to $9.20. The price per pack in New York City is about $11.[32] Raising the cost of cigarettes in this manner has been shown to reduce smoking rates among young people.

The prevalence of daily smoking among high school seniors also declined in 2011, to 10.3%.[5] Although it is true that some of these students are light smokers (less than half a pack a day), studies show that many light smokers become heavy smokers (more than half a pack a day) as they become older. The prevalence of cigarette smoking in young adults (ages 19–28) in 2011 seems to be related to college attendance. For full-time college students (ages 19–22), the 30-day prevalence of daily use of cigarettes was 7.3%; among respondents 1–4 years beyond high school it was 14.8%.[6]

The health consequences of tobacco use are familiar to all, even smokers. They include increased risk for heart disease, lung cancer, chronic obstructive lung disease, stroke, emphysema, and other conditions. Smoking accounts for an estimated 443,000 premature deaths per year in the United States and 5.4 million premature deaths per year worldwide.[33] The economic costs of tobacco smoking in the United States are estimated at $193 billion, of which more than half are due to lost productivity; the remainder are attributable to medical costs.[30] A significant portion of the medical costs attributed to smoking (43%) are paid with government funds, including Medicaid and Medicare.[1] Inasmuch as tobacco use and nicotine addiction increase the cost of these programs, they clearly add to the economic burden on society.

Well-established research findings have demonstrated that one does not have to use tobacco products to be adversely affected. The 1986 Surgeon General's report on the effects of **environmental tobacco smoke (ETS) or secondhand smoke** indicated that adults and children who inhale the tobacco smoke of others (passive smoking) are also at increased risk for cardiac and respiratory illnesses.[34,35] These findings resulted in new smoking regulations in many indoor environments. Then, in December 1992, the Environmental Protection Agency (EPA) released the report *Respiratory Health Effects of Passive Smoking: Lung Cancer and Other Disorders*.[36] This report stated that ETS is a human class A carcinogen (the same class that contains asbestos) and that it is responsible for 3,000 lung cancer deaths annually among nonsmoking Americans. Further, it stated that ETS exposure is causally associated with as many as 150,000 to 300,000 cases of lower respiratory infections (such as bronchitis and pneumonia) in

environmental tobacco smoke (ETS) (secondhand smoke) tobacco smoke in the ambient air

Synar Amendment a federal law that requires states to set the minimum legal age for purchasing tobacco products at 18 years and requires states to enforce this law

infants and young children up to 18 months of age. The EPA study also found that ETS aggravates asthma in children and is a risk factor for new cases of childhood asthma. During 2007–2008, approximately 88 million nonsmokers 3 years old or older were exposed to secondhand smoke.[37]

The use of smokeless (spit) tobacco also carries with it serious health risks, including addiction, periodontal disease, and oral cancer. In high schools in 2011, 3.5% of eighth-grade males, 6.6% of tenth-grade males, and 8.3% of twelfth-grade males reported using smokeless tobacco in the past 30 days.[5]

Over-the-Counter (Nonprescription) Drugs

Over-the-counter (OTC) drugs are those legal drugs, other than tobacco and alcohol, that can be purchased without a physician's prescription. Included in this category are internal analgesics such as aspirin, acetaminophen (Tylenol), and ibuprofen (Advil); cough and cold remedies (Robitussin, Contac); emetics; laxatives; mouthwashes; vitamins; and many others.[38] Thousands of different OTC products are sold by pharmacies, supermarkets, and convenience stores, and in vending machines to those who self-diagnose and self-medicate their own illnesses. Most OTC drugs provide only symptomatic relief and do not provide a cure. For example, cough and cold remedies relieve the discomfort that accompanies a cold but do not control the cold virus that is causing these symptoms.

Food and Drug Administration (FDA) a federal agency in the Department of Health and Human Services charged with ensuring the safety and efficacy of all prescription and nonprescription drugs

over-the-counter (OTC) drugs (nonprescription drugs) drugs (except tobacco and alcohol) that can be legally purchased without a physician's prescription

prescription drugs drugs that can be purchased only with written instructions from a physician, dentist, or other licensed independent healthcare provider (a prescription)

The **Food and Drug Administration (FDA)**, in the Department of Health and Human Services, ensures the safety and effectiveness of these drugs as long as they are used according to their label directions. Misuse and abuse occur, however. Common forms of misuse are not following the dosage directions or using the drugs after their expiration date. An example of OTC drug abuse is the taking of laxatives or emetics to lose weight or to avoid gaining weight. Another form of abuse is the use of pseudoephedrine, an ingredient in common cold remedies, to manufacture the illegal drug methamphetamine. Most OTC drugs are intended for temporary use. Overuse of these drugs to relieve symptoms can cause one to delay medical treatment and may lead to dependence.

Prescription Drugs

Because all **prescription drugs** can have serious side effects, they can be purchased only with a prescription (written instructions from a physician, dentist,, or other licensed independent healthcare provider). Like OTC drugs, prescription drugs are regulated by the FDA. More than 4,000 prescription drugs are listed in each annual edition of the *Physician's Desk Reference*.[39] The written prescription connotes that the prescribed drugs are being taken by the patient under the prescribing physician's supervision.

Misuse and abuse are all-too-common occurrences. Misuse occurs whenever a prescription drug is used in a manner other than that prescribed. Examples include taking the wrong dose, giving of one person's prescription drug to another, and discontinuing an antibiotic medication before the entire dose is taken. This latter misuse can result in the development of drug-resistant strains of pathogens, such as multidrug-resistant tuberculosis (MDR-TB) and extensively drug-resistant tuberculosis (EDR-TB). Two other examples are the growing number of reports of community-associated methicillin-resistant *Staphylococcus aureus* (CA-MRSA) and multidrug-resistant *Clostridium difficile* infections. These bacterial infections are difficult to cure because they are resistant to some of our most dependable antibiotics.[40] The growing prevalence of these conditions both point to the dangers of drug misuse and necessitate the constant development of new antibiotics.

Prescription drug abuse, although not new, has become "the Nation's fastest growing drug problem."[41] Commonly abused prescription drugs are stimulants such as amphetamines, depressants such as Valium and others, and opioid pain relievers (OPRs) such as morphine and codeine, and their derivatives such as oxycodone, hydrocodone, fentanyl, propoxyphene, and methadone. These drugs rapidly induce tolerance and dependence, so that patients crave higher and higher doses. People may try to obtain these drugs from family members or friends, through duplicate prescriptions from multiple physicians, or by stealing them from hospital dispensaries or pharmacies.

In recent years, the number of deaths from unintentional drug overdoses has risen to unprecedented levels.[42] During 1999–2008, the overdose death rate for OPRs increased four-fold. In 2008, poisoning became the leading cause of injury death in the United States, exceeding motor vehicle–related deaths (see **Figure 10.3**). Nearly nine out of 10 of these deaths were caused by drugs.[43] More than 40% of the drug poisoning deaths in 2008 were caused by OPRs.[43]

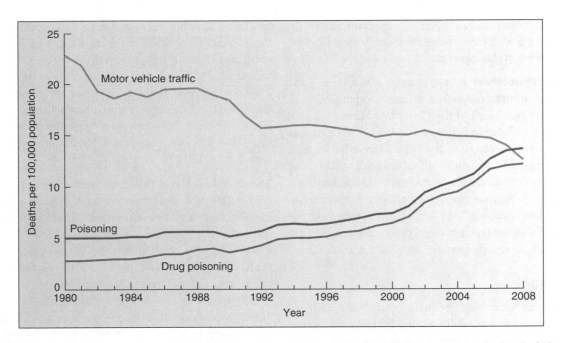

Figure 10.3 Poisoning is now the leading cause of death from injuries in the United States, and nearly 9 out of 10 poisoning deaths are caused by drugs.

Reproduced from Warner, M., L. J. Chen, D. M. Makuc, R. N. Anderson, and A. M. Miniño (2011). *Drug Poisoning Deaths in the United States, 1980–2008* (NCHS data brief no. 81). Hyattsville, MD: National Center for Health Statistics. Available at http://www.cdc.gov/nchs/data/databriefs/db81.pdf.

Sales of OPRs in 2010 were four times those for 1999, and the OPR abuse treatment admission rate in 2009 was almost six times the rate in 1999.[42] Although some of these deaths can be attributed to drugs prescribed for the decedent, at least some of these deaths occurred in people who obtained the opioid analgesics illegally. Prescription drug abuse puts an additional strain on our already overburdened emergency departments (EDs). About half of the 2 million ED visits involving drugs in 2008 were for legal drugs used nonmedically and for illegal drugs.[44] Finally, babies born to OPR-addicted mothers suffer from neonatal abstinence syndrome (NAS). Between 2000 and 2009, the percentage of newborns with NAS nearly tripled, from 1.20 to 3.39 per 1,000 live births; this amounts to 13,539 infants a year. The cost of treating these babies in 2009 was about $720 million, most of which was financed by Medicaid.[45]

Controlled Substances and Illicit (Illegal) Drugs

Controlled substances are those regulated by the **Controlled Substances Act of 1970** (CSA), officially known as the Comprehensive Drug Abuse Control Act of 1970. According to this act, drugs are listed in one of five levels according to their potential for abuse. Schedule I drugs have a high potential for abuse and have no accepted medical use. Schedule I drugs are **illicit (illegal) drugs** and cannot be legally cultivated, manufactured, bought, sold, or used in the United States. Well over 100 drugs are listed in this category, including marijuana, LSD, psilocybin, and mescaline; certain depressants such as methaqualone and Rohypnol; and other synthetic drugs such as MDMA (3,4-methylenedioxymethamphetamine) and DMT (N,N-dimethyltryptamine).[46]

Drugs that do have medical uses are placed in Schedules II to V of the act, depending on their potential for abuse and risk of causing dependence. Included in Schedule II are compounds that carry the highest risk of being abused or causing dependence. Examples are morphine, fentanyl, methadone, amobarbital, pentobarbital,

controlled substances drugs regulated by the Comprehensive Drug Abuse Control Act of 1970, including all illegal drugs and prescription drugs that are subject to abuse and can produce dependence

Controlled Substances Act of 1970 (Comprehensive Drug Abuse Control Act of 1970) the central piece of federal drug legislation that regulates illegal drugs and legal drugs that have a high potential for abuse

illicit (illegal) drugs drugs that cannot be legally manufactured, distributed, or sold, and that usually lack recognized medicinal value. Drugs that have been placed under Schedule I of the Controlled Substances Act of 1970

secobarbital, phencyclidine (PCP), amphetamine, methamphetamine, and cocaine. Schedule III to V drugs exhibit decreasing levels of abuse potential.[46]

The **Drug Enforcement Administration (DEA)**, under the Department of Justice, has the primary responsibility of enforcing the provisions of the Controlled Substances Act. Once a drug is placed in Schedule I of the CSA, it becomes the primary responsibility of the DEA to interdict its trafficking (manufacturing, distribution, and sales). The only sources of these drugs are illegal growers and manufacturers. (Marijuana represents a particular problem in this regard, as noted below.) Schedule II to V substances often reach the street illegally, either through illegal production (in clandestine labs) or by diversion from the legitimate market.

Marijuana

Marijuana and its derived products, hashish and hash oil, are the most widely abused illicit drugs in the United States. Derived from the hemp plant, *Cannabis sativa*, the products are most commonly used by smoking, although they are sometimes ingested. Marijuana use has increased in recent years. It is a community concern because (1) it is illegal (and therefore brings the user into contact with those involved in illegal activities), (2) its use is detrimental to one's health, and (3) marijuana smoking is often combined with alcohol or other drug use—**polydrug use.** The combined effects of more than one drug can be unpredictable. Finally, adolescents who smoke marijuana regularly delay completion of their personal growth and development.

In a 2011 survey, 22.6% of high school seniors reported having smoked marijuana in the past 30 days.[5] As with many other drugs, the prevalence of marijuana use has waxed and waned over the past 40 years, but the 2011 prevalence is the fifth consecutive year of increase in use. The perceived risk of harm is one of the factors correlated to the level of use. In 1992, when 76.5% of high school seniors felt there was risk of harming themselves associated with regular marijuana use, the 30-day use prevalence was 11.9%. In 2011, when only 45.7% of seniors felt there was risk of self-harm associated with regular marijuana use, the 30-day use prevalence nearly doubled

to 22.6%.[5] Another measurement of students' attitudes is the percentage of students who disapprove of smoking marijuana. The 2011 disapproval rates were the lowest on record since 1981.[5] One of the objectives of *Healthy People 2020* is to increase the proportion of adolescents (eighth, tenth, and twelfth graders) who disapprove of trying marijuana or hashish once or twice. Unfortunately, the disapproval rate for eighth, tenth, and twelfth graders decreased from 2009 to 2011.[5]

The acute health effects of marijuana use include reduced concentration, slowed reaction time, impaired short-term memory, and impaired judgment. Naturally, these effects can have serious consequences for someone operating a motor vehicle or other machinery or can even result in a medical emergency. Marijuana use in combination with other drugs can be especially dangerous because drugs in combination may affect the brain differently. In 2009, marijuana, used alone or with one or more other drugs, was involved in an estimated 376,467 emergency department visits, 38.7% of all ED visits for illicit drug use.[47]

The chronic effects of smoking marijuana, beyond damage to the lungs, include the controversial condition known as **amotivational syndrome**. Amotivational syndrome has been described as a chronic apathy toward maturation and the achievement of the developmental tasks (e.g., developing skills for independent living, setting and achieving goals, and developing an adult self-identity). There is also evidence now that long-term marijuana users experience physiological and psychological withdrawal symptoms. Although these "unpleasant behavioral symptoms are less obvious than those for heroin or alcohol, they are significant and do perhaps contribute to continued drug use."[48] Further evidence of the dependence-producing nature of marijuana is the number of persons seeking admission to treatment programs. Between 1999 and 2009, the proportion of admissions to treatment programs for marijuana abuse rose from 13% to 18% of all admissions to treatment programs nationally, ahead of admissions for cocaine and heroin addiction and trailing only alcohol and combined opiates.[49] Finally, one of the chief concerns with marijuana is that those who smoke marijuana are more likely to eventually use other, more addictive drugs. One study reported that 89% of those who use cocaine first used cigarettes, alcohol, and marijuana.[50]

As a Schedule I drug, marijuana is considered by the DEA to be an illegal drug with a high potential for abuse and without accepted medical use. However, increasingly, individual states are decriminalizing possession of small amounts

amotivational syndrome a pattern of behavior characterized by apathy, loss of effectiveness, and a more passive, introverted personality

Drug Enforcement Administration (DEA) the federal government's lead agency with the primary responsibility for enforcing the nation's drug laws, including the Controlled Substances Act of 1970

marijuana dried plant parts of the hemp plant, *Cannabis sativa*

polydrug use concurrent use of multiple drugs

of the drug, permitting its sale for medical use, and/or most recently, legalizing possession of small amounts by those over the age of 21. The enforcement of federal statutes is the duty of the executive branch of the government and President Barack Obama has suggested that enforcing the prohibition on marijuana use by adults in states where citizens have voted to legalize its use is not his top priority.

Narcotics: Opium, Morphine, Heroin, and Others

Opium and its derivatives, morphine and codeine, come from the Asian poppy plant, *Papaver somniferum*. **Narcotics** numb the senses, reduce pain, and produce drowsiness and euphoria. As such, they have a high potential for abuse. The illicit narcotic that is most widely abused is heroin. In 2010, about 0.2% of the noninstitutionalized population reported use in the past month.[51] This estimate is low because this survey undoubtedly missed a great many addicts who may be homeless and living in shelters. About 0.4% of high school seniors reported use in the past month in 2011.[5]

Opium poppies do not grow in the continental United States. They grow in Southeast and Southwest Asia (where they are native), and now, in Mexico and South America. Most of the heroin comes across our southwestern border with Mexico. Although significant amounts of heroin reaching the United States originate in South America, most of it originates in Mexico.[52]

Tolerance develops over weeks to months of use such that larger and larger doses are required to achieve the same euphoric effects as the initial dose. One of the numbing effects of opiates is to reduce the body's sensitivity to the build-up of carbon dioxide, which stimulates breathing. Although tolerance develops rapidly to a narcotic's euphoric effects, the narcotic's depression of respiration continues to increase with dose level, sometimes resulting in a fatal overdose.

The costs to the community are many, and include the death of a community member or a drug-addicted community member who is unproductive. A wealthy addict simply wastes money that could have strengthened the community. More likely, the addict is poor and must obtain money to support the addiction illegally through burglaries, thefts, robberies, muggings, prostitution (male and female), and/or selling drugs—all illegal activities deleterious to the community. Prostitution and injection drug use spread infectious diseases—gonorrhea, syphilis, *Chlamydia*, *Herpes*, hepatitis, and acquired immune deficiency syndrome (AIDS)—to other community members.

Cocaine and Crack Cocaine

Cocaine is extracted and refined from the leaves of the coca plant, *Erythroxolyn coca*, which grows in the Andes Mountains of South America. Cocaine is a **stimulant** that increases the activity of the central nervous system and produces euphoria by increasing the presence of dopamine in the brain. It produces rapid tolerance and strong psychological dependence. Cocaine use among high school seniors peaked in 1985, when 6.7% reported use within the past 30 days. By 1992 this figure had dropped to only 1.3%; in 2011, just 1.1% of high school seniors reported use in the past 30 days.[4,5]

Hallucinogens

Hallucinogens are drugs that produce illusions, hallucinations, and other changes in one's perceptions of the environment. These effects are due to the phenomenon known as **synesthesia**, a mixing of the senses. Hallucinogens include naturally derived drugs such as mescaline, from the peyote cactus, and psilocybin and psilocin, from the *Psilocybe* mushroom, as well as synthetic drugs, such as lysergic acid diethylamide (LSD). Although physical dependence has not been demonstrated with the hallucinogens, tolerance does occur. Although overdose deaths are rare, "bad trips" (unpleasant experiences) do occur, and a few people have experienced permanent visual disturbances. Because no legal sources for these Schedule I drugs exists, users have no way of knowing exactly what it is they have purchased.

Stimulants

Stimulants include the **amphetamines**, such as amphetamine itself (bennies), dextroamphetamine (dexies), methamphetamine (meth), dextromethamphetamine (ice), methylphenidate (Ritalin), and methcathinone (cat). Like cocaine, these drugs increase the activity of the central nervous system and produce euphoria by increasing the presence of the neurotransmitter dopamine in the brain. Tolerance builds quickly, resulting in the necessity of ever-increasing doses. Chronic abusers can develop tremors and confusion, aggressiveness, and paranoia. The long-term effects include permanent brain damage and Parkinson's disease–like symptoms.[53]

amphetamines a group of synthetic drugs that act as stimulants

cocaine the psychoactive ingredient in the leaves of the coca plant, *Erythroxolyn coca*, which, when refined, is a powerful stimulant/euphoriant

hallucinogens drugs that produce profound distortions of the senses

narcotics drugs derived from or chemically related to opium that reduce pain and induce stupor, such as morphine

stimulant a drug that increases the activity of the central nervous system

synesthesia impairment of mind characterized by a sensation that senses are mixed

Amphetamines are Schedule II prescription drugs that have been widely abused for many years, to stay awake and to lose weight. **Methamphetamine**, also known as "crystal," "crank," "speed," "go fast," or just "meth," produced in clandestine labs, became the fastest growing drug threat in the United States in the 1990s. The popularity of amphetamines has declined since its peak in 2001. In 2011, 0.6% of high school seniors reported abusing methamphetamine in the past 30 days.[5] Local, state, and federal agencies are tasked with finding and dismantling illegal meth labs and disposing of their hazardous materials (see **Figure 10.4**). In 2010, the DEA recorded 11,239 clandestine lab seizures in 49 states (see **Figure 10.5**).[54]

Methylphenidate (Ritalin) is a Schedule II drug used to treat attention-deficit hyperactivity disorder. Although not produced in clandestine labs, the drug is often diverted from its intended use and abused by those for whom it was not prescribed.

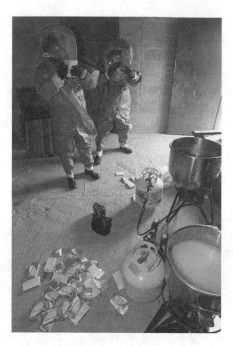

Figure 10.4 Dismantling a clandestine methamphetamine lab is hazardous work.
© Kyle Carter/The Meridian Star/AP Photos

Depressants

Barbiturates, benzodiazepines, methaqualone, and other **depressants** slow activity in the central nervous system. They are abused because, at first, like alcohol, they relieve anxiety and lower inhibitions. The result is an apparent elevation of mood. As one's dose increases, though, drowsiness, sleep, and loss of consciousness can occur. Long-term use results in tolerance and physical dependence. Abrupt withdrawal of the drug from someone who has become dependent can result in severe clinical illness and death. Medical assistance is usually required during detoxification from these depressants.

Club Drugs and Designer Drugs

Club drugs is a term for a group of illicit, synthetic drugs that are most commonly abused by teens and young adults at bars, nightclubs, concerts, raves (all-night dance parties), and other parties. These drugs include MDMA, Ketamine, GHB (gamma-hydroxybutyric acid), Rohypnol, LSD,

PCP, methamphetamine, and others.[55] Because these drugs are illegal, the user has no way of knowing the identity or purity of the drug taken.

MDMA, also known as Ecstasy, is the most popular of the club drugs. MDMA is a stimulant, and as such it can cause muscle tension, involuntary teeth clenching, nausea, blurred vision, faintness, and chills or sweating. In high doses, it can interfere with the body's ability to regulate temperature, and can cause overheating and dehydration.[56] Use of MDMA peaked in 2001 and then declined, but rose sharply again in 2011 when 5.3% of high school seniors reported use within the past year, and 2.3% within the past month.[5]

Rohypnol (flunitrazepam), another club drug, is also known as a "date-rape" or "predatory" drug. Rohypnol is a depressant that remains a legal prescription drug in more than 50 countries. In the United States, where a variety of safer depressants can be prescribed, Rohypnol is regarded as too dangerous for medical use and has been placed in Schedule I.

Anabolic Drugs

Anabolic drugs are protein-building drugs. Included are the **anabolic/androgenic steroids (AASs)** and human growth hormone (HGH). Both of these drugs have legitimate medical uses. AASs, which mimic the male hormone testosterone,

anabolic/androgenic drugs compounds, structurally similar to the male hormone testosterone, that increase protein synthesis and thus muscle building

barbiturates depressant drugs based on the structure of barbituric acid

benzodiazepines nonbarbiturate depressant drugs

club drugs a general term for those illicit drugs, primarily synthetic, that are most commonly encountered at nightclubs and "raves" (examples include MDMA, GHB, GBL, LSD, PCP, ketamine, Rohypnol, and methamphetamine)

depressants drugs that slow central nervous system activity, for example, alcohol, barbiturates, and benzodiazepines

methamphetamine the amphetamine most widely abused

methaqualone an illicit depressant drug

Rohypnol (flunitrazepam) a depressant in the benzodiazepine group that has achieved notoriety as a date-rape drug

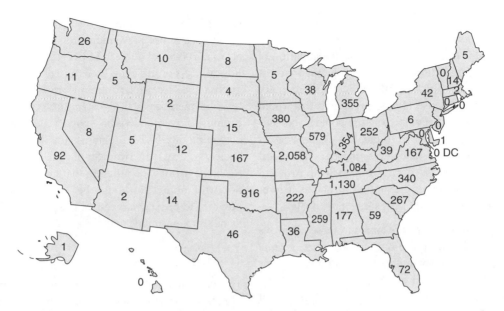

Figure 10.5 Total of all clandestine laboratory incidents involving methamphetamine (including labs, dump sites, and chemicals, glassware, or equipment), calendar year 2010.

Reproduced from Drug Enforcement Administration, Department of Justice (2011). "Methamphetamine Lab Incidents, 2004–2011." Available at http://www.justice.gov/dea/resource-center/meth_lab_maps/2011.jpg.

are used to rebuild muscles lost to starvation or disease. Human growth hormone can be used to treat clinical growth deficiencies and dwarfism. But they are sometimes abused by athletes and body builders as a shortcut to increasing muscle mass, strength, and endurance. Abuse of AASs is accompanied by numerous physiological and psychological side effects. For men, these include acne, gynecomastia (the development of breasts), baldness, reduced fertility, reduction in testicular size, and an increase in the level of "bad" cholesterol in the blood. Side effects for women are masculinizing: development of a male physique, increased body hair, failure to ovulate (menstrual irregularities), and a deepening of the voice (permanent). Long-term abuse of anabolic steroids can result in dependence, such that withdrawal causes cravings, mood swings, and, sometimes, attempted suicide.[57]

AASs are Schedule III drugs. Abuse of steroids increased during the 1990s but has since declined. About 1% of high school seniors reported using one of these drugs in the past 30 days in 2011.[5]

A brief Internet search reveals a vast marketplace for these and other psychoactive drugs. However, without any regulation, this is a clearly a case of "Buyer, beware!"

Inhalants

Inhalants are psychoactive, breathable chemicals. They include paint solvents, motor fuels, cleaners, glues, aerosol sprays, cosmetics, and other types of vapor. Because of their easy availability and low cost, they are often the drug of choice for middle school children. The primary effect of most of the inhalants is depression. As with alcohol, the user may at first experience a reduction of anxieties and inhibitions, making the user feel high. Continued use can result in hallucinations, loss of consciousness, and even death. Many inhalants are extremely toxic to the kidneys, liver, and nervous system. Boredom and peer pressure often lead to experimentation with inhalants. Parents are often unaware that their child has been abusing inhalants.

Prevention and Control of Drug Abuse

The prevention and control of alcohol and other drug abuse require the efforts of the entire community—parents, teachers, school administrators, merchants, state and local officials including law enforcement, and clergy. Also required are community organizing skills, cooperation among community leaders, and finally, persistence. The target population (innocent and curious youth) is constantly being renewed.

Levels of Prevention

Drug abuse prevention activities can be viewed as primary, secondary, or

inhalants breathable substances that produce mind-altering effects

tertiary depending on the point of intervention. The goal of *primary prevention* programs, aimed at those who have never used drugs, is to prevent or forestall the initiation of drug use. Primary prevention education programs are most appropriate and successful for children at the elementary school age. In a broader sense, almost any activity that would reduce the likelihood of primary drug use could be considered primary prevention. For example, raising the price of alcohol, increasing cigarette taxes, arresting a neighborhood drug pusher, or destroying a cocaine crop in South America could be considered primary prevention insofar as it forestalled first time drug use in at least some individuals.

Secondary prevention programs are aimed at those who have begun alcohol or other drug use but who have not become chronic abusers and have not suffered significant physical or mental impairment from their alcohol or other drug abuse. These efforts are often appropriate for those in high school or college, or in workplace settings. Intervention at this point might prevent chronic, or even fatal, drug dependence.

Tertiary prevention programs are designed to provide rehabilitation and aftercare, and prevent relapse. As such, they are usually designed for adults. Tertiary prevention programs for teenagers are far too uncommon. Clients of tertiary prevention programs may enter these programs voluntarily or by court referral.

Elements of Prevention

aftercare the continuing care provided to the recovering former drug abuser

drug abuse education providing information about drugs and the dangers of drug abuse, changing attitudes and beliefs about drugs, providing the skills necessary to abstain from drugs, and ultimately changing drug abuse behavior

treatment (for drug abuse and dependence) care that removes the physical, emotional, and environmental conditions that have contributed to drug abuse and/or dependence

Four basic elements play a role in drug abuse prevention and control. These are (1) education, (2) treatment, (3) public policy development and implementation, and (4) law enforcement. The goals of education and treatment are to reduce the demand for drugs, whereas the goals of public policy development and implementation and law enforcement are to reduce their supply and availability.

Education

Drug abuse education aims to limit the demand for drugs by providing information about drugs and the dangers of drug abuse, changing attitudes and beliefs about drugs, providing the skills necessary to abstain from drugs, and ultimately changing drug abuse behavior. Education, principally a primary prevention activity, can be school-based or community-based. Examples of school-based drug abuse prevention programs are Here's Looking at You, 2000 and Project DARE (Drug Abuse Resistance Education). For these programs and other school-based programs to be successful, community members such as parents, teachers, members of the local business community, and others must actively and visibly support the program. Examples of community-based programs are the American Cancer Society's Great American Smokeout; Race Against Drugs (RAD), a nationwide program that links drug abuse prevention with motor sports; and the Reality Check Campaign, a program to boost awareness of the harmful effects of marijuana smoking among youth.

Treatment

The goal of **treatment** is to remove the physical, emotional, and environmental conditions that have contributed to drug dependency. Successful treatment programs reduce the overall demand for drugs and save the community money. It is estimated that for every $1 invested in addiction treatment, between $4 and $7 are saved because of reduced drug-related crime, criminal justice costs, and theft. Furthermore, when healthcare savings are included, savings can be $12 for each $1 spent on treatment.[58]

Treatment for drug abuse occurs in a variety of settings and involves a variety of approaches. Treatment can be residential (inpatient) or nonresidential (outpatient). Inpatient care is normally limited to 28 days by most insurance coverage, after which the care can continue on an outpatient basis. In drug abuse treatment, **aftercare**, the continuing care provided to the recovering former drug abuser, is critical. This usually involves regular meetings with a trained counselor and/or peer group or self-help support group meetings, such as those provided by Alcoholics Anonymous (AA) or Narcotics Anonymous (NA). Despite frequent relapses, treatment for drug dependence is viewed as an important component of a community's comprehensive drug abuse prevention and control strategy.

> On January 1, 2010, the Mental Health Parity and Addiction Equity Act of 2008 (MHPAEA) took effect. This law requires group health plans and health insurance issuers to ensure that financial requirements (such as co-pays, deductibles) and treatment limitations (such as visit limits) applicable to mental health or substance use disorder are no more restrictive than the predominant requirements or limitations applied to substantially all medical/surgical benefits.[59]

Implementation of the provisions of this law should improve substance abuse treatment options for many people.

Public Policy

Public policy embodies the guiding principles and courses of action pursued by governments to solve practical problems affecting society. Examples include drunk-driving laws, zoning ordinances limiting the number of bars in a neighborhood, and smoking restrictions in public buildings. Public policy should guide budget discussions about how a community funds drug prevention education, drug treatment programs, and law enforcement.

Law Enforcement

Law enforcement is the application of federal, state, and local laws to arrest, jail, bring to trial, and sentence those who break drug laws. The primary roles of law enforcement are to (1) control drug use; (2) control crime, especially crime related to drug use and drug trafficking—the buying, selling, manufacturing, or transporting of illegal drugs; (3) prevent the establishment of crime organizations; and (4) protect neighborhoods.[60] Law enforcement is concerned with limiting the supply of drugs in the community by interrupting the source, transit, and distribution of drugs.

Governmental Drug Prevention and Control Agencies and Programs

Governmental agencies involved in drug abuse prevention, control, and treatment include a multitude of federal, state, and local agencies. At each of these levels of government, numerous offices and programs aim to reduce either the supply of or the demand for drugs.

Federal Agencies and Programs

Our nation's anti-drug efforts are headed up by the White House **Office of National Drug Control Policy (ONDCP)**, which annually publishes a report detailing the nation's drug control strategy and budget.[60,61] The goals of the current National Drug Control Strategy (to be achieved by 2015) are shown in Box 10.2.[61] In the 2011–2013 fiscal years' budget, approximately 59% of the National Drug Control budget is aimed at reducing the supply of drugs; 41% is aimed at reducing the demand for drugs. Domestic law enforcement and treatment will each receive 36–37% of the budget; 14% will be spent on interdiction, 8% on international support, and 5–6% on prevention.

The National Drug Control Strategy budget request for the fiscal year (FY) 2013 is $25.6 billion.[62] The department scheduled to receive the largest portion of funds in FY 2013 is the Department of Health and Human Services (which contains the National Institute on Drug Abuse and the Substance Abuse and Mental Health Services Administration). The Department of Justice is slated for the second-largest portion, followed by the Department of Homeland Security. The remainder of the funding is spread over the Departments

law enforcement the application of federal, state, and local laws to arrest, jail, bring to trial, and sentence those who break drug laws or break laws because of drug use

Office of National Drug Control Policy (ONDCP) the headquarters of the United States' drug control effort, located in the executive branch of the U.S. government, headed by a director appointed by the president

public policy the guiding principles and courses of action pursued by governments to solve practical problems affecting society

---

Box 10.2   National Drug Control Strategy Goals to Be Attained by 2015

Goal 1:   Curtail illicit drug consumption in America

    1a. Decrease the 30-day prevalence of drug use among 12- to 17-year-olds by 15 percent

    1b. Decrease the lifetime prevalence of 8th graders who have used drugs, alcohol, or tobacco by 15 percent

    1c. Decrease the 30-day prevalence of drug use among young adults aged 18–25 by 10 percent

    1d. Reduce the number of chronic drug users by 15 percent

Goal 2:   Improve the public health and public safety of the American people by reducing the consequences of drug abuse

    2a. Reduce drug-induced deaths by 15 percent

    2b. Reduce drug-related morbidity by 15 percent

    2c. Reduce the prevalence of drugged driving by 10 percent

Data Sources: SAMHSA's National Survey on Drug Use and Health (1a, 1c); Monitoring the Future (1b); What Americans Spend on Illegal Drugs (1d); Centers for Disease Control and Prevention (CDC) National Vital Statistics System (2a); SAMHSA's Drug Abuse Warning Network drug-related emergency room visits, and CDC data on HIV infections attributable to drug use (2b); National Survey on Drug Use and Health and National Highway Traffic Safety Administration (NHTSA) roadside survey (2c).

Source: Reproduced from Office of National Drug Control Policy, The White House (2012). *National Drug Control Strategy 2012.* Washington, DC: The White House. Available at http://www.whitehouse.gov/sites/default/files/ondcp/2012_ndcs.pdf.

of Defense, State, Veterans Affairs, Education, Treasury, and Transportation, and the Office of National Drug Control Policy.

Department of Health and Human Services

The Department of Health and Human Services (HHS) will spend its $8.4 billion on drug prevention education, treatment programs, and research into the causes and physiology of drug abuse. The preponderance of these funds is spent to reduce the demand for drugs. The approach of HHS to the drug problem is broad and includes research, treatment, and educational activities.

The HHS has published health status, risk reduction, and service and protection objectives on the use of tobacco, alcohol, and other drugs in *Healthy People 2020* (see Box 10.1). The objective in Box 10.1 is but one example of the objectives that set the direction and standards for success of all our national drug control efforts.

Several HHS agencies have as part or all of their mission the prevention or treatment of substance abuse. The **Substance Abuse and Mental Health Services Administration (SAMHSA)** and its Centers for Substance Abuse Prevention (CSAP) and for Substance Abuse Treatment (CSAT) provide leadership and guidance for the prevention and treatment of substance abuse.

The **National Institute on Drug Abuse (NIDA)** is the largest institution in the world devoted to drug abuse research. Research is aimed at understanding the causes and consequences of drug abuse and at evaluating prevention and treatment programs. Scientists conduct research and publish articles on the causes, prevention, and treatment of tobacco, alcohol, and other drug abuse.

As mentioned earlier, the Food and Drug Administration (FDA), in the Centers for Disease Control and Prevention, is charged with ensuring the safety and efficacy of all prescription and nonprescription drugs. The FDA dictates which drugs reach the market and how they must be labeled, packaged, and sold. As of June 21, 2009, the FDA also regulates the advertising, packaging, and sales of tobacco products in the United States with the goal of protecting public health.

Department of Justice

With its $7.8 billion budget, the Department of Justice (DOJ) addresses the supply side of the drug trade most directly by identifying, arresting, and prosecuting those who break drug laws. By incarcerating the most serious offenders, it hopes to deter others from becoming involved in the drug trade and provide a clear picture to all of the cost of drug trade and abuse. The DOJ also maintains prisons and prisoners, and employs marshals, attorneys, and judges. The single largest portion of the DOJ's budget goes to the Bureau of Prisons. Within these prisons, the DOJ operates treatment, education, and rehabilitation programs; this contributes to reducing the demand for drugs.

The lead agency in the DOJ is the Drug Enforcement Agency (DEA), which investigates and assists in the prosecution of drug traffickers and their accomplices in the United States and abroad and seizes the drugs as well as the assets on which traffickers depend. The DEA employs nearly 5,000 special agents and has a budget of more than $2 billion.

Three other drug fighting agencies in the DOJ are the Federal Bureau of Investigation (FBI), the Office of Justice Programs (OJP), and the **Bureau of Alcohol, Tobacco, Firearms, and Explosives (ATF)**. The FBI investigates multinational organized-crime networks that control the illegal drug market. The OJP provides leadership to federal, state, local, and tribal justice systems by disseminating knowledge and practices and providing grants for the implementation of these crime-fighting strategies. The OJP provides information, training, and coordination to state and local agencies.[63] The ATF protects our communities from the illegal diversion of alcohol and tobacco products by partnering with community institutions, industries, law enforcement, and public safety agencies to safeguard the public through information sharing, training, research, and use of technology.[64]

Department of Homeland Security

The Department of Homeland Security (DHS) will divide its $3.9 billion allotment among several agencies, namely, Immigration and Customs Enforcement (ICE), Customs and Border Protection (CBP), Counternarcotics Enforcement (CNE), and the U.S. Coast Guard (USCG). Although protection from terrorist acts is DHS's primary concern, the prevention and control of drug trafficking is

Bureau of Alcohol, Tobacco, Firearms, and Explosives (ATF) the federal agency in the Department of Justice that regulates alcohol and tobacco

National Institute on Drug Abuse (NIDA) the federal government's lead agency for drug abuse research; one of the National Institutes of Health

Substance Abuse and Mental Health Services Administration (SAMHSA) the agency within the Department of Health and Human Services that provides leadership in drug abuse prevention and treatment; houses the Center for Substance Abuse Prevention and the Center for Substance Abuse Treatment

also part of its mission. For example, ICE works to prevent the immigration to this country of criminals, including those involved in drug trafficking. Customs and Border Protection works with ICE to protect our borders from external threats, including illegal drugs (see Figure 10.6). The U.S. Coast Guard interdicts illegal drug trafficking in our coastal waters.

Other Federal Agencies

The Department of State aims to achieve reductions in the production and shipment of illicit drugs into this country through diplomacy. The Department of Defense provides military assistance to foreign allies working to eliminate the cultivation of illegal drug crops and the production of illegal drugs. The Department of Veterans Affairs expends most of its funds on the treatment of military veterans with drug dependency.

The Department of Education continues to participate in the federal drug prevention effort, although its funding is limited ($108 million for 2013).[62] Virtually all schools now have a clear no drug use policy, stemming from the "drug-free schools" initiative in the 1980s and the publication of the handbook titled *What Works: Schools Without Drugs*.[65] Funds will support the Successful, Safe, and Healthy Students state and local grants program; the Safe and Supportive Schools grants; and the Safe Students/ Healthy Schools initiative.[62]

State and Local Agencies and Programs

State support for drug abuse prevention and control is usually in the form of public policy initiatives, law enforcement expertise, the coordination of local and regional programs, and sometimes funding initiatives. It is usually up to local

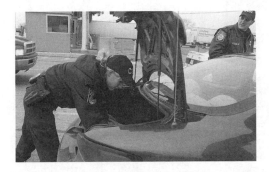

Figure 10.6 Customs agents assist in the arrest and prosecution of those involved in drug trafficking.

Courtesy of Gerald L. Nino/U.S. Customs and Border Protection

citizens to put these state initiatives into action or to begin initiatives of their own.

State Agencies

State agencies that address drug abuse prevention and control issues include the office of the governor, as well as state departments of health, education, mental health, justice, and law enforcement. To review the agencies in your state, visit your state government's home page and search using the terms "drug abuse prevention agencies" or "drug abuse prevention programs." (You can usually find your state government's home page by typing "www.*nameof yourstate*.gov". For example, www.texas.gov will take you to the Texas government's homepage.) Searching these sites in this way will reveal the agencies involved in drug abuse prevention at the state level. The role of these state-level agencies ranges from merely providing statistics and information to providing actual services and expertise. Many of these agencies serve as a conduit for federal funding that supports local initiatives.

The role of state government is to promote, protect, and maintain the health and welfare of its citizens. For example, it is the state that licenses doctors, dentists, and pharmacists; liquor stores; and taverns. Each state has its own laws regulating the sale of tobacco, alcohol, and prescription drugs. Prescription drug monitoring programs (PDMPs) are state programs that detect and prevent the diversion and abuse of prescription drugs at the retail level. The PDMPs, which are operational in 35 states, track controlled substances prescribed by authorized practitioners and dispensed by pharmacies.[41]

Each state also passes laws and sets the penalties for the manufacture, sale, and possession of illicit drugs such as marijuana. These laws vary greatly from state to state.[66] For example, some states have decriminalized possession of small amounts, others have legalized marijuana cultivation and/or sales for medical use, and more recently some have legalized possession of small amounts by those over the age of 21. The result is that those participating in marijuana-related activities deemed legal in their state could, nonetheless, be arrested by the DEA agents and prosecuted under federal law.

Local Agencies

Whereas considerable economic resources can be brought to bear on the drug problem at the federal level, and to a lesser extent from state governments, it is becoming increasingly clear that to achieve success, the drug war in the

United States must be fought at the local level—in homes, neighborhoods, and schools. Local governmental agencies involved in drug abuse prevention and control include mayors' offices, police and sheriffs' departments, schools, corporations, health departments, family services offices, mental health services, prosecutors' offices, the juvenile justice system, judges, and courts. In some communities, there is a community drug task force or coordinating council that meets to prioritize problems faced by the community and decide on approaches to solving them. The goal is to develop a coordinated and effective effort to resolve drug-related problems in the community as they arise.

Nongovernmental Drug Prevention and Control Agencies and Programs

Many nongovernmental programs and agencies make valuable contributions to the prevention and control of drug abuse in the United States. Among these are community and school-based programs, workplace programs, and voluntary agencies.

Community-Based Drug Education Programs

Community-based drug education can occur in a variety of settings, such as child care facilities, public housing, religious institutions, youth organizations, businesses, and healthcare facilities. Information about these programs can be disseminated through television and radio programs, movies, newspapers, and magazines.

Community-based drug education programs are most likely to be successful when they include six key features[67]:

1. A comprehensive strategy
2. An indirect approach to drug abuse prevention
3. The goal of empowering youth
4. A participatory approach
5. A culturally sensitive orientation
6. Highly structured activities

Community-based drug education programs that address broader issues (e.g., coping and learning skills) are most effective, as are those embedded in other existing community activities. Participation can be increased by planning drug education programs around sporting or cultural events. Culturally sensitive programs are crucial for reaching minorities in the community. Use of the appropriate language, reading level, and spokespersons can mean the difference between the success or failure of a program (see **Figure 10.7**).

In the past 30 years, a great many drug abuse prevention education programs have been conceived and tested. Some of these have been scientifically proven to be effective. The Substance Abuse and Mental Health Services Administration has a searchable database of successful programs at its National Registry of Evidence-Based Programs and Practices (NREPP).[68]

School-Based Drug Education Programs

Most health educators believe that a strong, comprehensive school health education program—one that occupies a permanent and prominent place in the school curriculum—is the best defense against all health problems, including drug abuse. However, many schools lack these strong programs

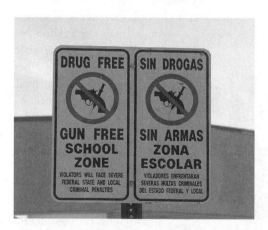

Figure 10.7 Use of appropriate language can be the difference between success and failure of a community drug prevention program.
© Lisa C. McDonald/ShutterStock, Inc.

and, in their absence, substitute drug education programs developed specifically for school use.

An example of a program from the CSAP list that has been scientifically proven to be effective is Project ALERT. Project ALERT reduced students' initiation of marijuana use by 30%, decreased current marijuana use by 60%, reduced past-month cigarette use by 20% to 25%, decreased regular and heavy smoking by 33% to 55%, and substantially reduced students' pro-drug-use attitudes and beliefs. Information about this and other programs is available on the NREPP website.[67]

One popular program, Drug Abuse Resistance Education (DARE), involves local police visiting classrooms to teach grade-school children about drugs. Although this popular program has been successful in improving children's images of the police themselves, it has been unable to demonstrate measurable success in reducing actual drug use.[69]

Student assistance programs (SAPs), modeled after employee assistance programs in the workplace, are school-based programs aimed at identifying and intervening in drug abuse cases. In **peer counseling programs,** students share personal problems, receive support, and, perhaps, learn coping skills from peers who have been trained in this intervention activity and do not use drugs.

Workplace-Based Drug Education Programs

In September 1986, concern about widespread drug use in the workplace led then-President Ronald Reagan to sign Executive Order 12564, proclaiming a Drug-Free Federal Workplace.[70] The rationale for the order was cited in the document itself: the desire and need for the well-being of employees, the loss of productivity caused by drug use, the illegal profits of organized crime, the illegality of the behavior itself, the undermining of public confidence, and the role of the federal government as the largest employer in the nation to set a standard for other employers to follow in these matters. It had also become apparent to all that drug abuse was not just a personal health problem and a law enforcement problem, but also a behavior that affected the safety and productivity of others, especially at work. Studies have shown that substance abusers (1) are less productive, (2) miss more work days, (3) are more likely to injure themselves, and (4) file more workers' compensation claims than their non–substance-abusing counterparts.

The Drug Free Federal Workplace order required federal employees to refrain from using illegal drugs, and it required agency heads to develop plans for achieving drug-free workplaces for employees in their agencies. The order further required the setting up of drug testing programs and procedures and employee assistance programs that would include provisions for rehabilitation.[70] Similar workplace substance abuse programs, which include drug testing, soon spread to the private sector so that today, such programs are in place in virtually all U.S. companies.[71]

A typical workplace substance abuse prevention program has five facets: (1) a formal written substance abuse policy that reflects the employer's commitment to a drug-free workplace, (2) an employee drug education and awareness program, (3) a supervisor training program, (4) an **employee assistance program (EAP)** to help those who need counseling and rehabilitation, and (5) a drug testing program.[72] Large companies are more likely than small companies to have the major components of a drug-free workplace program.

Although a substantial part of the problem can be attributed to alcohol consumption, illicit drug use remains a problem in many workplaces. It is true that the prevalence of illegal drug abuse in the unemployed adult population is nearly twice that of the employed adult population, but nearly 65.9% of all illegal users are employed.[51] Fortunately, the prevalence of workplace drug use has declined significantly, in part because of the proliferation of workplace drug abuse and prevention programs that include drug testing. In 1987, the first year of workplace drug testing, 18.1% of all tests were positive[73]; by 1998, this figure had dropped below 5%, where it has remained. In 2010 the general workforce positivity rate was 3.5%.[74]

Voluntary Health Agencies

A large number of voluntary health agencies have been founded to prevent or control the social and personal consequences of alcohol, tobacco, and other drug abuse. Among these are such agencies as Mothers Against Drunk Driving (MADD), Students Against Destructive Decisions (SADD), Alcoholics Anonymous (AA), Narcotics Anonymous (NA), the American Cancer Society (ACS), the American Lung Association, and many others. Each of these organizations is active locally, statewide, and nationally.

employee assistance program (EAP) a workplace drug program designed to assist employees whose work performance is suffering because of a personal problem such as alcohol or other drug problems

peer counseling programs school-based programs in which students discuss alcohol and other drug-related problems with peers

student assistance programs (SAPs) school-based drug education programs to assist students who have alcohol or other drug problems

An important function of community leaders is to encourage parents, school officials, members of law enforcement, businesses, social groups, community health workers, and the media to work together in an effort to reduce the abuse of alcohol, tobacco, and other drugs. Only through citizen support and vigilance can there be a reduction in the threat that alcohol and other drugs pose to our communities.

Chapter Summary

- The consequences of alcohol, tobacco, and other drug abuse constitute major personal and community health problems in the United States.
- Both inherited and environmental factors are associated with tendencies toward drug experimentation, drug abuse, and drug dependence.
- Chronic alcohol and tobacco use results in the loss of billions of dollars and thousands of lives in the United States each year.
- The misuse and abuse of over-the-counter and prescription drugs remain a concern.
- Education, treatment, public policy development, and law enforcement are principal elements of drug abuse prevention and control.
- Prevention activities can be categorized as primary, secondary, and tertiary prevention.
- Efforts to reduce the use, misuse, and abuse of drugs in the United States can be identified at the federal, state, and local levels of government.
- Federal agencies include the White House; the Departments of Health and Human Services, Justice, and Homeland Security; and many others.
- Efforts at the state level vary from state to state and usually include public policy development and coordination between federal and local drug programs.
- Rates of illicit drug abuse in the general workforce have declined significantly since workplace drug testing began in 1987.
- A large number of voluntary health agencies are involved in drug abuse prevention and control activities.

Review Questions

1. List the personal and community consequences of drug and alcohol abuse.
2. What are the recent trends in drug use by high school seniors?
3. Explain the differences among drug use, misuse, and abuse.
4. How do physical and psychological dependence differ? How are they related to tolerance?
5. What are the two sources of risk factors that contribute to substance abuse? Which do you feel is the more important, and why?
6. Why is alcohol abuse considered the number one problem drug in the United States?
7. In what forms do Americans consume nicotine, and in what groups of people do we see the heaviest users?
8. What agency regulates over-the-counter and prescription drugs? What two characteristics must a drug have to be approved for sale?
9. How can misuse of prescription antibiotics cause a health risk?
10. How have prescription drugs become the leading cause of poisoning deaths?
11. What is the most commonly abused illicit drug? Why is this drug a concern?
12. What are controlled substances? Give some examples.
13. List the side effects of anabolic/androgenic steroid use for men and women.
14. What are the four elements of drug prevention and control?
15. Give examples of primary, secondary, and tertiary drug abuse prevention strategies.
16. Describe the roles of the federal government in controlling drug abuse.
17. Describe the roles of state and local governments in preventing and controlling drug abuse.
18. True or false: "Most drug abusers are unemployed." Explain you answer.
19. Name four voluntary agencies and self-help groups involved in the prevention, control, and treatment of alcohol, tobacco, and other drugs of abuse.

Activities

1. Schedule an appointment with the vice president of student affairs, the dean of students, or the alcohol and drug abuse prevention educator on your campus to find out more about drug (including alcohol) problems. Find out what the greatest concerns are and how the administration is trying to deal with the issues.

2. Attend a meeting of a community group that is involved in the prevention and control of drug abuse (e.g., local drug task force, AA, a smoking cessation group, MADD, or SADD). In a two-page paper, summarize the meeting and share your reaction to it.

Community Health on the Web

The Internet contains a wealth of information about community and public health. Increase your knowledge of some of the topics presented in this chapter by accessing the Jones & Bartlett Learning website at **go.jblearning.com/McKenzieBrief** and follow the links to complete the following Web activities:

- National Clearinghouse for Alcohol and Drug Information
- MADD
- Office on Smoking and Health

References

1. Horgan, C., K. C. Skwara, and G. Strickler (2001). *Substance Abuse: The Nation's Number One Health Problem*. Princeton, NJ: Robert Wood Johnson Foundation.
2. National Center on Addiction and Substance Abuse at Columbia University (2011). *Adolescent Substance Use: America's #1 Public Health Problem*. Available at http://www.casacolumbia.org/templates/Publications_Reports.aspx.
3. National Center on Addiction and Substance Abuse at Columbia University (2009). *Shoveling Up II: The Impact of Substance Abuse on Federal, State and Local Budgets*. Available at http://www.casacolumbia.org/templates/Publications_Reports.aspx.
4. Johnston, L. D., P. M. O'Malley, and J. G. Bachman (1993). *Monitoring the Future: National Survey Results on Drug Use, 1975-1992. Volume I: Secondary School Students* (NIH pub no. 93-3597). Bethesda, MD: National Institute on Drug Abuse.
5. Johnston, L. D., P. M. O'Malley, J. G. Bachman, and J. E. Schulenberg (2012). *Monitoring the Future: National Results on Adolescent Drug Use: Overview of the Key Findings, 2011*. Ann Arbor, MD: Institute for Social Research, the University of Michigan. Available at http://www.monitoringthefuture.org/pubs/monographs/mtf-overview2011.pdf.
6. Johnston, L. D., P. M. O'Malley, J. G. Bachman, and J. E. Schulenberg (2012). *Monitoring the Future: National Survey Results on Drug Use, 1975-2011. Volume II, College Students and Adults Ages 19-50*. Ann Arbor, MD: Institute for Social Research, The University of Michigan. Available at http://www.monitoringthefuture.org/pubs/monographs/mtf-vol2_2011.pdf.
7. Glantz, M., and R. Pickens (1992). "Vulnerability to Drug Abuse: Introduction and Overview." In M. Glantz and R. Pickens, eds., *Vulnerability to Drug Abuse* (pp. 1-14). Washington, DC: American Psychological Association.
8. Cotton, N. S. (1979). "The Familial Incidence of Alcoholism: A Review." *Journal of Studies on Alcohol*, 40: 89-116.
9. Cloninger, C. R., M. Bohman, and S. Sigvardsson (1981). "Inheritance of Alcohol Abuse." *Archives of General Psychiatry*, 38: 861-868.
10. Schuckit, M. A., S. C. Risch, and E. O. Gold (1988). "Alcohol Consumption, ACTH Level, and Family History of Alcoholism." *American Journal of Psychiatry*, 145(11): 1391-1395.
11. Tabakoff, B., and P. L. Hoffman (1988). "Genetics and Biological Markers of Risk for Alcoholism." *Public Health Report*, 103(6): 690-698.
12. U.S. Department of Health and Human Services (1990). *Seventh Special Report to the U.S. Congress* (DHHS pub. no. ADM-90-1656). Washington, DC: U.S. Government Printing Office.
13. Zickler, P. (2000). "Evidence Builds That Genes Influence Cigarette Smoking." *NIDA Notes*, 15(2): 1-2.
14. Needle, R., Y. Lavee, S. Su, et al. (1988). "Familial, Interpersonal, and Intrapersonal Correlates of Drug Use: A Longitudinal Comparison of Adolescents in Treatment, Drug-Using Adolescents Not in Treatment, and Non-Drug-Using Adolescents." *International Journal of Addictions*, 239(12): 1211-1240.
15. Meller, W. H., R. Rinehart, R. J. Cadoret, and E. Troughton (1988). "Specific Familial Transmission in Substance Abuse." *International Journal of Addictions*, 23(10): 1029-1039.

16. Shedler, J., and J. Block (1990). "Adolescent Drug Use and Psychological Health: A Longitudinal Inquiry." *American Psychologist*, 45(5): 612-630.

17. Dembo, R., W. R. Blount, J. Schmeidler, and W. Burgos (1986). "Perceived Environmental Drug Use Risk and the Correlates of Early Drug Use or Nonuse Among Inner-City Youths: The Motivated Actor." *International Journal of Addictions*, 21(9-10): 977-1000.

18. Centers for Disease Control and Prevention (2012). "Vital Signs: Binge Drinking Prevalence, Frequency, and Intensity Among Adults—United States, 2010." *Morbidity and Mortality Weekly Report*, 61(1):14-19. Available at http://www.cdc.gov /mmwr/PDF/wk/mm6101.pdf.

19. National Center on Addiction and Substance Abuse at Columbia University (2006). *The Commercial Value of Underage and Pathological Drinking to the Alcohol Industry: A CASA White Paper*. Available at http://www.casacolumbia.org /templates/Publications_Reports.aspx.

20. Foster, S. E., R. D. Vaughan, W. H. Foster, and J. A. Califano (2006). "Estimate of the Commercial Value of Underage Drinking and Adult Abusive and Dependent Drinking to the Alcohol Industry." *Archives of Pediatrics and Adolescent Medicine*, 160(5): 473-478.

21. Morse, R. M., and D. K. Flavin (1992). "The Definition of Alcoholism." *Journal of the American Medical Association*, 268(8): 1012-1014.

22. National Institute on Alcohol Abuse and Alcoholism (January 1996). "Drinking and Driving." *Alcohol Alert*, 31(362): 1-4.

23. Centers for Disease Control and Prevention (2011). "Vital Signs: Alcohol-Impaired Driving Among Adults—United States, 2010." *Morbidity and Mortality Weekly Report*, 60(39): 1351-1356. Available at http://www.cdc.gov/mmwr/PDF/wk /mm6039.pdf.

24. U.S. Department of Health and Human Services, Public Health Service (2012). *Healthy People 2020*. Available at http://www .healthypeople.gov/2020/default.aspx.

25. Insurance Institute for Highway Safety, Highway Loss Data Institute (2012). "DUI/DWI Laws." Available at http://www.iihs .org/laws/state_laws/dui.htm.

26. Cole, T. B. (2006). "Rape at U.S. Colleges Often Fueled by Alcohol." *Journal of the American Medical Association*, 296(5): 504-505.

27. Bryant, K. J., S. Nelson, R. S. Braithwaite, and D. Roach. (2010). "Integrating HIV/AIDS and Alcohol Research." *Alcohol Research and Health*, 33(3): 167-178.

28. Lupton, C. (2003). "The Financial Impact of Fetal Alcohol Syndrome." Substance Abuse and Mental Health Services Administration, FASD Center for Excellence. Available at http://fasdcenter.samhsa.gov/publications/cost .cfm?&print=y.

29. Department of Health and Human Services (August 1993). "Substance Abuse Prevention and Treatment Block Grants: Sale or Distribution of Tobacco Products to Individuals Under 18 Years of Age: Proposed Rule." *Federal Register*, Part II, 45: 96.

30. Office of New York Attorney General Eliot Spitzer (11 October 2006). "Attorneys General and R. J. Reynolds Reach Historic Settlement to End the Sale of Flavored Cigarettes." Available at http://www.ag.ny.gov/press-release/ attorneys-general-and-rj-reynolds-reach.

31. American Lung Association (2009). "President Obama Signs Bill Granting the U.S. FDA Regulatory Control over Tobacco Products." Available at http://www.lungusa.org/press-room /press-releases/pres-obama-signs-bill-for-fda-tobacco-control .html.

32. Confessore, N. (21 June 2010). "Cigarette Tax Increased to Keep State Running." *New York Times*. Available at http://www .nytimes.com/2010/06/22/nyregion/22budget.html.

33. American Cancer Society (2012). *Cancer Facts and Figure–2010*. Atlanta, GA: Author.

34. U.S. Department of Health and Human Services, Public Health Service, Centers for Disease Control (1986). *The Health Consequence of Involuntary Smoking. A Report of the Surgeon General* (DHHS pub. no. CDC-87-8398). Washington, DC: U.S. Government Printing Office.

35. Byrd, J. C., R. S. Shapiro, and D. L. Schiedermayer (1989). "Passive Smoking: A Review of Medical and Legal Issues." *American Journal of Public Health*, 79(2): 209-215.

36. Environmental Protection Agency (1991). *Respiratory Health Effects of Passive Smoking: Lung Cancer and Other Disorders* (EPA/600/6-90/006F). Washington, DC: Indoor Air Quality Clearinghouse.

37. Centers for Disease Control and Prevention (2010). "Vital Signs: Nonsmokers' Exposure to Secondhand Smoke—United States, 1999-2008." *Morbidity and Mortality Weekly Report*, 59(35): 1141-1146. Available at http://www.cdc.gov/mmwr/PDF /wk/mm5935.pdf.

38. *PDR for Nonprescription Drugs*, 33rd ed. (2011). Montvale, NJ: PDR Network.

39. *Physicians' Desk Reference*, 66th ed. (2011). Montvale, NJ: PDR Network.

40. Centers for Disease Control and Prevention (2006). "MRSA (Methicillin-Resistant *Staphylococcus aureus*)." Available at http://www.cdc.gov/ncidod/diseases/submenus/sub_mrsa.htm.

41. Office of National Drug Control Policy, The White House (2011). *Epidemic: Responding to America's Prescription Drug Abuse Crisis*. Available at http://www.whitehouse.gov /sites/default/files/ondcp/issues-content/prescription-drugs /rx_abuse_plan.pdf.

42. Centers for Disease Control and Prevention (2011). "Vital Signs: Overdoses of Prescription Pain Relievers—United States, 1999-2008." *Morbidity and Mortality Weekly Report*, 60(43): 1487-1492. Available at http://www.cdc.gov/mmwr /PDF/wk/mm6043.pdf.

43. Warner, M., L. J. Chen, D. M. Makuc, R. N. Anderson, and A. M. Miniño (2011). *Drug Poisoning Deaths in the United States, 1980-2008* (NCHS data brief no. 81). Hyattsville, MD: National Center for Health Statistics. Available at http://www.cdc.gov /nchs/data/databriefs/db81.pdf.

44. Centers for Disease Control and Prevention (2010). "Emergency Department Visits Involving Nonmedical Use of Selected Prescription Drugs—United States, 2004-2008." *Morbidity and Mortality Weekly Report*, 59(23): 705-709.

45. Patrick, S. W., R. E. Schumacher, B. D. Benneyworth, E. E. Krans, J. M. McAllister, and M. M. Davis (2012). "Neonatal Abstinence Syndrome and Associated Health Care Expenditures, United States, 2000-2009." *Journal of the American Medical Association,* 307(18): 1934-1940.

46. "Schedules of Controlled Substances." (1 April 1998). *Federal Register*, Code of Federal Regulations, Food and Drugs, Part 1308. Washington, DC: Author.

47. Substance Abuse and Mental Health Services Administration (2011). *Drug Abuse Warning Network, 2009: National Estimates of Drug-Related Emergency Department Visits* (HHS pub. no. (SMA) 11-4659), DAWN Series D-35. Rockville, MD: Substance Abuse and Mental Health Services Administration. Available at http://www.samhsa.gov/data/DAWN.aspx.

48. Zickler, P. (2000). "Evidence Accumulates That Long-Term Marijuana Users Experience Withdrawal." *NIDA Notes*, 15(1).

49. Substance Abuse and Mental Health Services Administration (2011). *Treatment Episode Data Set (TEDS). 1999-2009. National Admissions to Substance Abuse Treatment Services* (DASIS Series: S-56, HHS pub no. (SMA) 11-4646). Rockville, MD: Author. Available at http://www.samhsa.gov/data/DASIS/teds09/teds2k9nweb.pdf.

50. Center for Addiction and Substance Abuse at Columbia University (1994). *Cigarettes, Alcohol, Marijuana: Gateways to Illicit Drug Use*. New York: Author.

51. Substance Abuse and Mental Health Services Administration (2011). *Results from the 2010 National Survey on Drug Use and Health: Summary of National Findings* (NSDUH Series H-41, HHS pub. no. (SMA) 11-4658). Rockville, MD: Author. Available at http://oas.samhsa.gov/NSDUH/2k10NSDUH/2k10Results.pdf.

52. Department of Justice, National Drug Intelligence Center (2011). *National Drug Threat Assessment 2011* (Product no. 2011-Q0317-001). Johnstown, PA: Author. Available at http://www.justice.gov/archive/ndic/about.htm.

53. Volkow, N. D. (2005). "Message from the Director: Communities Across the Country Are Trying to Respond to Increased Abuse of Methamphetamine, a Powerfully Addictive Stimulant." Available at http://www.drugabuse.gov/about/welcome/messagemeth405.html.

54. Drug Enforcement Administration, Department of Justice (2011). "Methamphetamine Lab Incidents, 2004-2011." Available at http://www.justice.gov/dea/resource-center/meth-lab-maps.shtml.

55. National Institute on Drug Abuse, National Institutes of Health (2010). *InfoFacts: Club Drugs (GHB, Ketamine, and Rohypnol)*. Available at http://www.drugabuse.gov/publications/drugfacts/club-drugs-ghb-ketamine-rohypnol.

56. National Institute on Drug Abuse, National Institutes of Health (2010). *InfoFacts: MDMA (Ecstasy)*. Available at http://www.drugabuse.gov/drugs-abuse/mdma-ecstasy.

57. National Institute on Drug Abuse, National Institutes of Health (2009). *InfoFacts: Steroids (Anabolic-Androgenic)*. Available at http://www.drugabuse.gov/drugs-abuse/mdma-ecstasy.

58. National Institute on Drug Abuse, National Institutes of Health (2009). *Principles of Drug Addiction Treatment: A Research-Based Guide*, 2nd ed. Available at http://www.drugabuse.gov/publications/principles-drug-addiction-treatment/frequently-asked-questions/drug-addiction-treatment-worth-its-cost.

59. Centers for Medicare and Medicaid Services (2011). "The Mental Health Parity and Addiction Equity Act." Available at http://www.samhsa.gov/healthreform/parity/.

60. Bureau of Justice Statistics (1992). *Drugs, Crime and the Justice System 1992*. Washington, DC: U.S. Government Printing Office.

61. Office of National Drug Control Policy, The White House (2012). *National Drug Control Strategy 2012*. Washington, DC: The White House. Available at http://www.whitehouse.gov/ondcp/2012-national-drug-control-strategy.

62. Office of National Drug Control Policy, The White House (2012). *The National Drug Control Budget: FY 2013 Funding Highlights*. Available at http://www.whitehouse.gov/ondcp/the-national-drug-control-budget-fy-2013-funding-highlights.

63. U.S. Department of Justice, Office of Justice Programs (n.d.). "About Us." Available at http://www.ojp.usdoj.gov/about/about.htm.

64. U.S. Department of Justice, Bureau of Alcohol, Tobacco, Firearms, and Explosives (n.d.). "ATF's Mission." Available at http://www.atf.gov/about/mission/.

65. U.S. Department of Education (1987). *What Works: Schools Without Drugs*. Washington, DC: U.S. Government Printing Office.

66. NORML (National Organization for the Reform of Marijuana Laws) (n.d.). Home page. Available at http://www.norml.org.

67. Brown, M. E. (1993). "Successful Components of Community and School Prevention Programs." *National Prevention Evaluation Report: Research Collection*, 1(1): 4-5.

68. Substance Abuse and Mental Health Services Administration (2012). "NREPP: SAMHSA's National Registry of Evidence-Based Programs and Practices." Available at http://www.nrepp.samhsa.gov.

69. Lynam, D. R., R. Milich, R. Zimmerman, S. P. Novak, T. K. Logan, C. Martin, C. Leukefeld, and R. Clayton (1999). "Project DARE: No Effects at 10-Year Follow-up." *Journal of Consulting and Clinical Psychology*, 67(4): 590-593.

70. Drug-Free Federal Workplace (Executive Order 12564) (17 September 1986). *Federal Register*, 51(180): 32889-32893.

71. American Management Associates (1996). *AMA Survey: Workplace Drug Testing and Drug Abuse Policy*. New York: Author.

72. U.S. Department of Labor (1991). *What Works: Workplaces Without Alcohol or Other Drugs* (Pub. no. 282-148/54629). Washington, DC: U.S. Government Printing Office.

73. SmithKline Beecham Clinical Laboratories (29 February 1996). "Drug Detection in the Workplace in 1995 Declines for the Eighth Straight Year." [Press release]. Collegeville, PA: Author.

74. Quest Diagnostics (2010). *Hawaii, Arkansas and Oklahoma Lead the Nation for Methamphetamine Use in the Workforce, Reveals Quest Diagnostics Drug Testing Index*. Available at http://www.questdiagnostics.com/home/physicians/health-trends/drug-testing/archives.html.

Chapter 11

Healthcare Delivery in the United States

James F. McKenzie, PhD, MPH, MCHES

Chapter Objectives

After studying this chapter, you will be able to:

1. Define the term *healthcare system*.

2. Trace the history of healthcare delivery in the United States from colonial times to the present.

3. Discuss and explain the concept of the spectrum of healthcare delivery.

4. Distinguish among the different kinds of health care, including population-based public health practice, medical practice, long-term practice, and end-of-life practice.

5. List and describe the different levels of medical practice.

6. List and characterize the various groups of healthcare providers.

7. Explain the differences among allopathic, osteopathic, and nonallopathic providers.

8. Define the term *complementary and alternative medicine*.

9. Explain why there is a need for healthcare providers.

10. Prepare a list of the different types of facilities in which health care is delivered.

11. Explain the differences among private, public, and voluntary hospitals.

12. Explain the difference between inpatient and outpatient care facilities.

13. Briefly discuss the options for long-term care.

14. Identify the major concerns with the healthcare system in the United States.

15. Explain the various means of reimbursing healthcare providers.

16. Briefly describe the purpose and concept of insurance.

17. Define the term *insurance policy*.

18. Explain the insurance policy terms *deductible*, *co-insurance*, *copayment*, *fixed indemnity*, *exclusion*, and *preexisting condition*.

19. Explain what is meant when a company or business is said to be self-insured.

20. List the different types of medical care usually covered in a health insurance policy.

21. Briefly describe Medicare, Medicaid, and Medigap insurance.

22. Briefly describe the Children's Health Insurance Program (CHIP).

23. Briefly explain long-term care health insurance.

24. Define the term *managed care*.

25. Define the terms *health maintenance organization (HMO), preferred provider organization (PPO),* and *point-of-service option*.

26. Identify the advantages and disadvantages of managed care.

27. Define the term *consumer-directed health plans* and give several examples.

28. Provide a brief overview of the Affordable Care Act passed in 2010.

Introduction

The process by which health care is delivered in the United States is unlike the processes used in other countries of the world. Other developed countries have national health insurance run or organized by the government and paid for, in large part, by general taxes. Also, in these countries almost all citizens are entitled to receive healthcare services, including routine and basic health care.[1] Health care in the United States is delivered by an array of **providers**, in a variety of settings, under the watchful eye of regulators, and paid for in a variety of ways. Because of this process, many question the notion that the United States has a healthcare delivery system (see **Figure 11.1**). That is, "[a]lthough these various individuals and organizations are generally referred to collectively as 'the health care delivery system,' the phrase suggests order, integration, and accountability that do not exist. Communication, collaboration, or systems planning among these various entities is limited and is almost incidental to their operations."[2] Whether or not healthcare delivery in the United States should be called a "system," there is a process in place in which healthcare professionals, located in a variety of facilities, provide services to deal with disease and injury for the purpose of promoting, maintaining, and restoring health to the citizens. In this chapter, we outline the history of healthcare delivery in the United States, examine the structure of

providers healthcare facilities or health professionals that provide healthcare services

third-party payment system a health insurance term indicating that bills will be paid by the insurer and not the patient or the healthcare provider

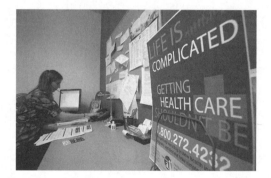

Figure 11.1 Do we really have a healthcare system?
© Brian Snyder/Reuters/Landov

health care, and describe how our unique system functions. Finally, we discuss healthcare reform in the United States.

History of Healthcare Delivery in the United States

Healthcare delivery in the United States has evolved much differently than in other developed countries of the world. It is unique because it is based upon U.S. values and beliefs and has been greatly influenced by the social, political, and economic environments in which it has matured.[1] As such, initiatives toward a national healthcare program have failed to make significant inroads[1] (see **Figure 11.2**). However, over the years, a **third-party payment system** was created and compromises have led to providing government

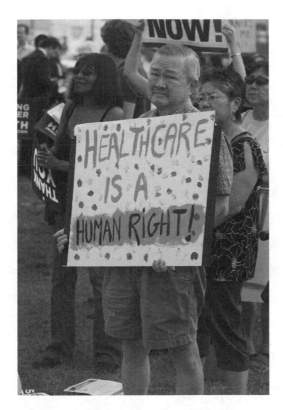

Figure 11.2 Health benefits have become an important part of the total compensation package for workers.
© Gerry Boughan/ShutterStock, Inc.

healthcare insurance (i.e., Medicare, Medicaid, Children's Health Insurance Program [CHIP]) and consequently access to health care, for certain defined groups of people in the United States.[1] Box 11.1 provides a listing of some of the history and major events that have helped to shape healthcare delivery in the United States.

Healthcare System: Structure

The structure of the healthcare system of the United States is unique in the world. In the sections that follow, we examine the spectrum of healthcare delivery and describe the various types of healthcare providers and the facilities in which health care is delivered.

The Spectrum of Healthcare Delivery

Because health care in the United States is delivered by an array of providers in a variety of settings, reference is sometimes made to the spectrum of healthcare delivery (see Table 11.1). The spectrum of healthcare delivery refers to the various types of care. Within this spectrum, four levels of practice have emerged: population-based public health practice, medical practice, long-term practice, and end-of-life practice.

Box 11.1   Timeline and Highlights of the History of Healthcare Delivery in the United States

A. Colonial Times Through the Nineteenth Century

1. U.S. health care and medical practice lagged behind Great Britain and Europe.
2. Much of early health care was provided by family members and neighbors based on home and folk remedies.
3. Medical education was not grounded in science but rather based on experience via an apprenticeship with a practicing physician.[1,3]
4. Much health care was provided in patients' homes, not in clinics or offices.
5. Hospitals called almshouses (or poorhouses) were used primarily to provide food, shelter, and basic care for the indigent; some local governments operated pesthouses as places to isolate those with infectious diseases.[1]
6. In the last third of the nineteenth century, medicine began to be based on science; the scientific method was used, germ theory was accepted, and infectious agents were identified.
7. In the late nineteenth century health care moved from patient homes to physician offices and hospitals.[4]

B. First Half of Twentieth Century

1. As the century began, the leading causes of death were communicable diseases.
2. In 1911, Montgomery Ward and Company sold health insurance based on many of the principles still used today; however, very few people had insurance.
3. From 1918-1919, the influenza pandemic occurred. It was the deadliest in history, killing 100 million people worldwide.
4. In the 1920s, noncommunicable diseases surpassed communicable diseases as the leading cause of death.
5. The 1920s saw new medical procedures (e.g., X-rays, specialized surgical procedures, chemotherapy), group medical practices, and new medical equipment (e.g., electrocardiograph).
6. In 1929, the United States spent 3.9% of its gross domestic product (GDP) on health care.
7. Through the 1930s, most health care was delivered through a two-party system—patients and physicians.
8. In the 1940s, World War II led to huge technical strides in medical procedures. Employer-provided health insurance was used to lure workers to companies because recruitment

(continues)

Box 11.1 Timeline and Highlights of the History of Healthcare Delivery in the United States (*Continued*)

of soldiers to the armed services left many shortages back home.

9. The **Hospital Survey and Construction Act of 1946** (i.e., Hill-Burton Act), a federal-state partnership, provided substantial funds for hospital construction.

C. Second Half of Twentieth Century

1. In the 1950s, healthcare costs rose and were too expensive for some; the debates about whether health care was a right or privilege and who should pay for it began in earnest.

2. At the end of the 1950s there was a shortage of quality health care in the United States.

3. In the 1960s, healthcare costs continued to rise, and the third-party payment system became solidified with the help of unions negotiating with employers for employees.

4. In 1965, Medicare and Medicaid were authorized by Titles XVIII and XIX, respectively, of the Social Security Act.

5. The Health Maintenance Organization (HMO) Act of 1973 was passed.[4]

6. The National Health Planning and Resources Development Act of 1974 (P.L. 93-641) was passed, aimed at comprehensive planning for health care.[5]

7. In 1980, P.L. 93-641 was eliminated.

8. In 1981, then-President Reagan announced he would let the competitive market, not governmental regulation, shape healthcare delivery.[6]

9. The 1980s saw a proliferation of medical technology.

10. In 1994, Congress discussed the **American Health Care Security Act of 1993**, proposed by then-President Clinton, but never acted on it.

11. In the 1990s, managed care became the dominant form of healthcare financing and delivery.[7]

12. In 1996, for the first time the healthcare bill in the United States topped $1 trillion—13.6% of GDP.[8]

13. The State Children's Health Insurance Program (SCHIP), now known as just CHIP, was created by the Balanced Budget Act of 1997.[9]

D. Twenty-First Century

1. The Medicare Prescription Drug, Improvement, and Modernization Act of 2003 (MMA) passed, creating Medicare Part D (prescription drugs) and health savings accounts (HSAs).[10]

2. In 2006, Massachusetts mandated that all residents have health insurance by 2009.

3. The CHIP Reauthorization Act of 2009 passed and was paid for by new tax on cigarettes.

4. In 2010, the healthcare bill in the United States was $2.6 trillion—17.9% of GDP.[11]

5. The Patient Protection and Affordability Care Act (PPACA) (P.L. 111-148) and Health Care and Education Reconciliation Act of 2010 (HCERA) (P.L. 111-152) were passed; the two acts were consolidated and called the Affordable Care Act.

6. In 2012, the U.S. Supreme Court ruled to uphold the Affordable Care Act.

7. In 2013, the healthcare bill was projected to be $2.9 trillion—17.6% of GDP.[11]

American Health Security Act of 1993 the comprehensive healthcare reform introduced by then-President Clinton, but never enacted

Hospital Survey and Construction Act of 1946 (Hill-Burton Act) federal legislation that provided substantial funds for hospital construction

population-based public health practice incorporates interventions aimed at disease prevention and health promotion, specific protection, and a good share of case findings

Population-Based Public Health Practice

Population-based public health practice incorporates interventions aimed at disease prevention and health promotion, specific protection, and a good share of case findings.[12,13] A primary component of population-based public health practice is education. If people are going to behave in a way that will promote their health and the health of their community, they first must know how to do so. Health education not only provides such information, but also attempts to empower and motivate people to put this information to use by discontinuing unhealthy behaviors and adopting healthy ones. Although much of public health practice takes place in governmental health agencies, it also takes place in a variety of other settings (such as voluntary health agencies, social service agencies, schools, businesses and industry, and even in some traditional medical care settings).[12]

Medical Practice

Medical practice means "those services usually provided by or under the supervision of a physician or other traditional health care provider."[12] Such services are offered at several different levels—primary, secondary, and tertiary.

Table 11.1 The Spectrum of Healthcare Delivery

Level of Practice	Description	Examples of Delivery Settings
Population-Based Public Health Practice	Practice aimed at disease prevention and health promotion that shapes a community's overall health; emphasizes education and prevention	Public, community, and school health programs; public health clinics
Medical Practice		
Primary care	Clinical preventive services, first-contact treatment services, and ongoing care for commonly encountered medical conditions; emphasizes prevention, early detection, and routine care	Primary care provider offices; public clinics; managed care organizations; community mental health centers
Secondary care	Specialized attention and ongoing management for common and less frequently encountered medical conditions, including support services for people with special challenges due to chronic or long-term conditions	Physician offices, hospitals
Acute care	Short-term, intense medical care that may require hospitalization	Emergency rooms; urgent/emergency care centers; outpatient/inpatient surgical centers; hospitals
Subacute care	After acute care, need for more nursing intervention	Special subacute units in hospitals (e.g., transitional care units); skilled nursing facilities; home health care
Tertiary care	Subspecialty referral care requiring highly specialized personnel and facilities	Specialty hospitals (e.g., psychiatric, chronic disease) and general hospitals with highly specialized facilities
Long-Term Practice		
Restorative care	Intermediate follow-up care such as surgical postoperative care	Home health; progressive and extended care facilities; rehabilitation facilities that specialize in therapeutic services; halfway houses
Long-term care	Care for chronic conditions; personal care	Nursing homes; facilities for the mentally retarded or emotionally disturbed; geriatric day care centers
End-of-Life Practice	Care provided to those who have less than 6 months to live	Hospice services provided in a variety of settings

Sources: Cambridge Research Institute (1976). *Trends Affecting the U.S. Health Care System*. Washington, DC: U.S. Government Printing Office; U.S. Public Health Service (1994). *For a Healthy Nation: Return on Investments in Public Health*. Washington, DC: Author; Turnock, B. J. (2012). *Public Health: What It Is and How It Works*, 5th ed. Burlington, MA: Jones & Bartlett Learning; and Shi, L., and D. A. Singh (2012). *Delivering Health Care in America: A Systems Approach*, 5th ed. Burlington, MA: Jones & Bartlett Learning.

Primary Medical Care

Primary care is "front-line" or "first-contact" care. "The unique characteristic of primary care is the role it plays as a regular or usual source of care for patients and their families."[2] Formally, primary care has been defined as "clinical preventive services, first-contact treatment services, and ongoing care for commonly encountered medical conditions."[12] Eighty percent of medical care is primary care.[12] Primary care includes routine medical care to treat common illnesses or to detect health problems in their early stages, and thus includes such things as semiannual dental checkups; annual physical exams; health screenings for hypertension, high blood cholesterol, and breast or testicular cancer; and sore throat cultures. Primary care usually is provided in practitioners' offices, clinics, and other outpatient facilities by physicians, nurse practitioners, physician assistants, and an array of other individuals on the primary care team. Primary care is the most difficult for the poor and uninsured to obtain (see **Box 11.2**).

Secondary Medical Care

Secondary medical care is "specialized attention and ongoing management for common and less frequently encountered medical conditions, including support services for people

> **primary care** "clinical preventive services, first-contact treatment services, and ongoing care for commonly encountered medical conditions"[12]
>
> **secondary medical care** "specialized attention and ongoing management for common and less frequently encountered medical conditions, including support services for people with special challenges due to chronic or long-term conditions"[12]

Such facilities are equipped and staffed to provide advanced care for people with illnesses such as cancer and heart disease, and procedures such as heart bypass surgery.

Long-Term Practice

Long-term practice can be divided into two subcategories—restorative care and long-term care.

Restorative Care

Restorative care is the health care provided to patients after surgery or other successful treatment, during remission in cases of an oncogenic (cancerous) disease, or when the progression of an incurable disease has been arrested. This level of care includes follow-up to secondary and tertiary care, rehabilitative care, therapy, and home care (see **Figure 11.3**). Typical settings for this type of care include both inpatient and outpatient rehabilitation units, nursing homes, assisted-living facilities, halfway houses, and private homes.

Long-Term Care

Long-term care includes the different kinds of help that people with chronic illnesses, disabilities, or other conditions that limit them physically or mentally need. In some situations, time-intensive skilled nursing care is needed, whereas some people just need help with basic daily tasks like bathing, dressing, and preparing meals. This type of care is provided in various settings such as nursing homes, with special challenges due to chronic or long-term conditions."[12] This type of care is usually provided by physicians, ideally upon referral from a primary care source.[12]

long-term care different kinds of help that people with chronic illnesses, disabilities, or other conditions that limit them physically or mentally need

restorative care care provided after successful treatment or when the progress of an incurable disease has been arrested

tertiary medical care "specialized and technologically sophisticated medical and surgical care for those with unusual or complex conditions (generally no more than a few percent of the need in any service category)"[12]

Tertiary Medical Care

Tertiary medical care "is even more highly specialized and technologically sophisticated medical and surgical care than secondary medical care for those with unusual or complex conditions (generally no more than a few percent of the need in any service category)."[12] This care is not usually performed in smaller hospitals; however, it is provided in specialty hospitals, academic health centers, or on specialized floors of general hospitals.

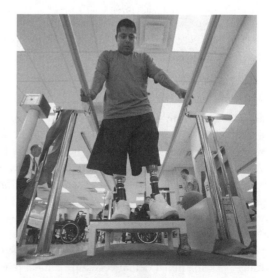

Figure 11.3 Restorative care can follow either secondary or tertiary care.
© Jason Reed/Reuters/Landov

facilities for the mentally and emotionally disturbed, assisted-living facilities, and adult and senior day care centers, but often long-term care is used to help people live at home rather than in institutions.

End-of-Life Practice

The final level of practice in the healthcare delivery spectrum is end-of-life practice. **End-of-life practice** is usually thought of as those healthcare services provided to individuals shortly before death. The primary form of end-of-life practice is hospice care. **Hospice care** "is a cluster of special services for the dying, which blends medical, spiritual, legal, financial, and family-support services. The venue can vary from a specialized facility to a nursing home to the patient's own home."[1] The most common criterion for admission to hospice care is being terminally ill with a life expectancy of less than 6 months. The first hospice program in the United States was established in 1974[14]; by 2009 there were 3,405 Medicare-certified providers and suppliers of hospice services.[15]

Types of Healthcare Providers

To offer comprehensive health care that includes services at each of the levels just mentioned, a great number of healthcare workers are needed. In 2009, almost 15.5 million civilians were employed in the health service industry, representing approximately 1 of every 10 (11.1%) employed civilians in the United States.[16]

Despite the large number of healthcare workers, the demand for more is expected to continue to grow. "Employment growth is expected to be driven by technological advances in patient care, which permit a greater number of health problems to be treated, and by an increasing emphasis on preventive care. In addition, the number of older people, who are much more likely than younger people to need nursing care, is projected to grow rapidly."[17] Due to the continuing geographic maldistribution of healthcare workers, the need will be greater in rural and inner-city areas (see Box 11.3).

In 2009, just more than two-fifths (40.5%) of all healthcare workers were employed in hospitals, just more than one-fourth (25.4%) worked in outpatient healthcare settings (i.e., offices and clinics of physicians, dentists, chiropractors, optometrists, and other health practitioners, and outpatient care centers), about one-sixth (16.6%) worked in nursing and residential care facilities, and the remaining one-sixth (17.5%) worked in home health care or other settings.[16] As changes have come to the way health care is offered, the proportions of healthcare workers by setting

have also changed, with fewer persons working in hospitals (in 1970, 63% worked in hospitals), and more employed in nursing homes and ambulatory care settings (such as surgical and emergency centers). This trend is expected to continue in the future, with special needs in the area of long-term care workers to meet the needs of the aging baby boom generation.

There are well over 200 different careers in the healthcare industry. To help simplify the discussion of the different types of healthcare workers, they have been categorized into six different groups—independent providers, limited care providers, nurses, nonphysician practitioners, allied healthcare professionals, and public health professionals.

Independent Providers

Independent providers are those healthcare workers who have the

> **Box 11.3** *Healthy People 2020*: Objectives
>
> ***Access to Health Services***
> **Goal:** Improve access to comprehensive, quality health care services.
> **Objective:** AHS-4 (Developmental), Increase the number of practicing primary care providers.
> **Objective:** AHS-4.1 (Developmental), medical doctors
> **Target:** TBD
> **Baseline:** TBD
> **Target setting method:** TBD
> **Potential data source:** American Medical Association (AMA), Masterfile, AMA.
> **Objective:** AHS-4.2 (Developmental), doctors of osteopathy
> **Target:** TBD
> **Baseline:** TBD
> **Target setting method:** TBD
> **Potential data source:** American Osteopathic Association (AMA), Masterfile, AOA.
> ***For Further Thought***
> What impact would reaching these objectives have on access to health care in the United States, especially in rural and inner-city areas? Provide a rationale for your response.
> TBD = To be determined
> *Source:* Reproduced from U.S. Department of Health and Human Services, Office of Disease Prevention and Health Promotion (2010). *Healthy People 2020.* Available at http://www.healthypeople.gov/2020/topicsobjectives2020/pdfs/HP2020objectives.pdf.

end-of-life practice healthcare services provided to individuals shortly before death

hospice care "a cluster of special services for the dying, which blends medical, spiritual, legal, financial, and family-support services"[1]

independent providers healthcare professionals with the education and legal authority to treat any health problem

specialized education and legal authority to treat any health problem or disease that an individual has. This group of workers can be further divided into allopathic, osteopathic, and nonallopathic providers.

Allopathic and Osteopathic Providers

Allopathic providers are those who use a system of medical practice in which specific remedies for illnesses, often in the form of drugs or medication, are used to produce effects different from those of diseases. The practitioners who fall into this category are those who are referred to as Doctors of Medicine (MDs). The usual method of practice for MDs includes the taking of a health history, a physical examination—perhaps with special attention to one area of the complaint—and the provision of specific treatment, such as antibiotics for a bacterial infection or a tetanus injection and sutures for a laceration.

> **allopathic providers** independent providers whose remedies for illnesses produce effects different from those of the disease
>
> **chiropractor** a nonallopathic, independent healthcare provider who treats health problems by adjusting the spinal column
>
> **complementary/ alternative medicine (CAM)** "a group of diverse medical and health care systems, practices, and products that are not presently considered to be a part of conventional medicine"[4]
>
> **nonallopathic providers** independent providers who provide nontraditional forms of health care
>
> **osteopathic providers** independent healthcare providers whose remedies emphasize the interrelationships of the body's systems in prevention, diagnosis, and treatment

Another group of physicians that provides services similar to those of MDs are **osteopathic providers**—Doctors of Osteopathic Medicine (DOs). At one time, MDs and DOs would not have been grouped together because of differences in their formal education, methods, and philosophy of care. Although the educational requirements and methods of treatment used by MDs have remained essentially consistent over the years, those of DOs have not. The practice of osteopathy was started in 1874 by Andrew Taylor Still, MD, DO, who was dissatisfied with the effectiveness of nineteenth-century medicine.[18] The distinctive feature of osteopathic medicine is the recognition of the reciprocal interrelationship between the structure and function of the body. The actual work of DOs and MDs is very similar today. Both types of physicians use all available scientific modalities, including drugs and surgery, in providing care to their patients. Both can also serve as primary care physicians (a little over one-third of MDs[15] and more than three-fifths of DOs are primary care physicians)[19] or as board-certified specialists. Their differences

are most notably the DOs' greater tendency to use more physical manipulation in treating health problems and the DOs' perception of themselves as being more holistically oriented than MDs. Few, if any, patients today would be able to tell the difference between the care given by a DO and an MD.

The educational requirements for MD and DO degrees are very similar. Both complete a bachelor's degree, 4 years of medical education, and 3 to 7 years of medical specialty training known as a *residency*. By completing a residency, physicians are eligible to sit for the board specialty examinations. Passing this examination makes them "board certified" in their specialty.

Nonallopathic Providers

Nonallopathic providers are identified by their nontraditional means of providing health care. Some have referred to much of the care provided by these providers as **complementary/alternative medicine (CAM)** or complementary/integrative medicine. Included in this group of providers are **chiropractors**, acupuncturists (see **Figure 11.4**), naturopaths (those who use natural therapies), herbalists (those who use plant-based medicines to treat their patients), and

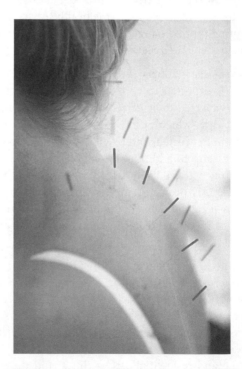

Figure 11.4 Many people seek out nontraditional means of health care, such as acupuncture.
© Stuart Pearce/Pixtal/age fotostock

homeopaths (those who use small doses of herbs, minerals, and even poisons for therapy).

CAM has been defined as "a group of diverse medical and health care systems, practices, and products that are not presently considered to be a part of conventional medicine."[20] When used together with conventional medicine, a therapy is identified as *complementary*. An example of a complementary medicine is using acupuncture in addition to usual care to help lessen pain. When a therapy is used in place of a conventional medicine, it is labeled as *alternative*. An example of an alternative therapy is using a special diet to treat cancer instead of undergoing surgery, radiation, or chemotherapy that has been recommended by a conventional doctor.[20] When mainstream medical therapies are combined with CAM therapies for which there is some high-quality scientific evidence of safety and effectiveness, it is referred to as *integrative medicine*.[20] CAM is one of the fastest growing areas of health care today.

> Private health insurance plans may offer coverage of certain CAM therapies, such as chiropractic and massage. Overall, however, coverage of CAM therapies is relatively limited—compared with coverage of conventional therapies. One factor is a lack of scientific evidence regarding the cost-effectiveness of CAM therapies. As consumer interest in CAM grows, more insurance companies and managed care organizations may consider offering coverage of CAM therapies shown to be safe and effective.[20]

There are literally hundreds of systems, approaches, and techniques that fall within the CAM rubric. CAM practices are often grouped into broad categories, such as natural products (e.g., herbal medicines, also known as botanicals), mind–body medicine (e.g., meditation, yoga, acupuncture, hypnotherapy, tai chi), manipulative and body-based practices (e.g., spinal manipulation and massage therapy), and other CAM practices (e.g., movement therapies [e.g., Pilates], traditional healers, manipulation of energy fields [e.g., magnet therapy], and whole medical systems [e.g., Ayurvedic medicine, homeopathy, naturopathy]).[20]

Limited (or Restricted) Care Providers

Much health care is provided by **limited (or restricted) care providers** who have advanced training, usually a doctoral degree, in a healthcare specialty. Their specialty enables them to provide care for a specific part of the body. This group of providers includes, but is not limited to, dentists (teeth and oral cavity), optometrists (eyes, specifically refractory errors), podiatrists (feet and ankles), audiologists (hearing), and psychologists (mental health).

Nurses

We have categorized nurses into a group of their own because of their unique degree programs, the long-standing tradition of nursing as a profession, and their overall importance in the healthcare industry. It has been estimated that between 4 and 5 million individuals work in the nursing profession. These include registered nurses, licensed practical nurses, and ancillary nursing personnel such as nurses' aides.[15] Nurses outnumber physicians, dentists, and every single other group of healthcare workers in the United States.[15] Even with such numbers, the need for more nurses will continue[21] (see **Figure 11.5**).

Training and Education of Nurses

Nurses can be divided into subcategories based on their level of education and type of preparation. The first are those who complete 1 to 2 years of education in a vocational, hospital, or associate degree program and pass a licensure examination. These nurses are then referred to as **licensed practical nurses (LPNs)**, or licensed vocational nurses (LVNs) in some states. LPNs "care for people who are sick, injured, convalescent, or disabled under the supervision of physicians or registered nurses."[22] "The nature of the direction and supervision required varies by state and job setting."[22] In 2010, there were 752,300 LPNs or LVNs working

> **licensed practical nurse (LPN)** those prepared in 1- to 2-year programs to provide nontechnical bedside nursing care under the supervision of physicians or registered nurses
>
> **limited (or restricted) care providers** healthcare providers who provide care for a specific part of the body

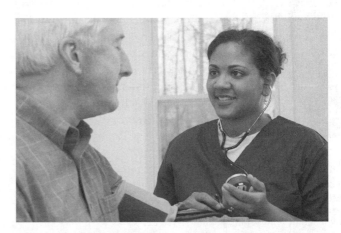

Figure 11.5 There is still a need for more nurses.
© Rob Marmion/ShutterStock, Inc.

in the United States, and that number was projected to grow by 22% to 920,800 by 2020.[23]

A second group of nurses is registered nurses. **Registered nurses (RNs)** are those who have successfully completed an accredited academic program and a state licensing (registration) examination. The three typical educational paths to registered nursing are a bachelor's degree (BSN), an associate degree (ADN), or a diploma from an approved nursing program.[24] ADN programs take about 2 to 3 years to complete and are typically offered by community or junior colleges. Diploma programs are offered by hospitals and last about 3 years. RNs holding BSN degrees are referred to as **professional nurses** and are considered to have been more thoroughly prepared for additional activities involving independent judgment. Of the employed registered nurses, 54% worked in hospitals, about 8% in offices of physicians, 5% in home healthcare services, and 5% in nursing care facilities. The remainder worked mostly in government agencies, social assistance agencies, and educational services.[24] In 2008, there were more than 2.7 million RNs working in the United States, and that number was projected to grow by 26% to more than 3.4 million by 2020.[24]

Advanced Practice Nurses

With advances in technology and the development of new areas of medical specialization, there is a growing need for specialty-prepared **advanced practice registered nurses (APRNs)**. Many professional nurses continue their education and earn master's and doctoral degrees in nursing. The master's degree programs are aimed primarily at specialties such as nurse practitioners (NPs) (e.g., pediatric nurse practitioners and school nurse practitioners), clinical nurse specialists (CNSs), certified registered nurse anesthetists (CRNAs), and certified nurse midwives (CNMs). These APRNs are qualified to conduct health assessments, diagnose and treat a range of common acute and chronic illnesses, and manage normal maternity care. They not only provide high-quality care in a cost-effective manner, but also are considered primary care

providers in chronically medically underserved inner-city and rural areas. Like other nurses, the demand for APRNs is also expected to increase, especially as a greater portion of the population gains access to health care and more of the population becomes enrolled in managed care. In 2008, the number of RNs prepared to practice in at least one advanced practice role was estimated to be 250,527, or 8.2% of the total RN population.[25] The largest portion of these APRNs were nurse practitioners.

The relatively few nurses who hold doctorate degrees in nursing are highly sought after as university faculty. Nurses with doctorates teach, conduct research, and otherwise prepare other nurses or hold administrative (leadership) positions in healthcare institutions.

Nonphysician Practitioners

Nonphysician practitioners (NPPs) (also known as nonphysician clinicians [NPCs], midlevel providers, or physician extenders) constitute a relatively new classification of healthcare workers. This group is composed of those "clinical professionals who practice in many of the areas in which physicians practice, but do not have an MD or a DO degree."[1] NPPs are mid-level health workers with training and skills beyond those of RNs and less than those of physicians.[22] This group typically includes the just discussed nurse practitioners and certified nurse midwives as well as physician assistants (PAs).[1] Because the former two were just presented as part of the section on advanced practice nurses, we discuss only PAs here.

Physician assistant programs began in response to the shortage of primary care physicians. PAs' academic programs usually last 2 years and are offered in a variety of formats, including diploma and certificate programs, or as associate, bachelor's, or master's degrees. After completion of the program or degree, PAs must pass a national certifying examination. PAs always work under the direct supervision of a licensed physician (thus the name *physician extenders*). They carry out many of the same duties that are thought of as the responsibilities of physicians, such as taking medical histories, examining patients, ordering and interpreting laboratory tests and X-rays, counseling patients, making preliminary diagnoses, treating minor injuries, and, in most states, prescribing medications.[22]

Allied Healthcare Professionals

Allied health describes a large group of health-related professions that fulfill necessary roles in the healthcare

advanced practice registered nurse (APRN) registered nurse who has completed graduate training as a clinical nurse specialist, nurse anesthetist, nurse-midwife, or nurse practitioner
nonphysician practitioners (NPPs) "clinical professionals who practice in many of the areas similar to those in which physicians practice, but who do not have an MD or DO degree"[1]
professional nurse a registered nurse holding a bachelor of science degree in nursing (BSN)
registered nurse (RN) one who has successfully completed an accredited academic program and a state licensing examination

delivery system. These **allied healthcare professionals** assist, facilitate, and complement the work of physicians, dentists, and other healthcare specialists. These healthcare workers provide a variety of services that are essential to patient care. Often they are responsible for highly technical services and procedures. Allied healthcare professionals can be categorized into several groups,[4] including (1) laboratory technologists and technicians (e.g., medical technologists, emergency medical technicians, nuclear medicine technicians, operating room technicians, dental technicians and hygienists, and radiographers [X-ray technicians]); (2) therapeutic science practitioners (e.g., physical and respiratory therapists); (3) behavioral scientists (e.g., health education specialists and social workers); and (4) support services (e.g., medical record keepers and medical secretaries). The educational backgrounds of allied health workers range from vocational training to master's degrees. Many of these professionals also must pass a state or national licensing examination before they can practice. The demand for allied healthcare workers in all of the areas previously noted is expected to continue well into the twenty-first century.

Public Health Professionals

A discussion about healthcare providers would be incomplete without the mention of a group of health workers who provide unique healthcare services to the community— **public health professionals**. They support the delivery of health care by such hands-on providers as public health physicians, dentists, nurses, and dieticians who work in public health clinics sponsored by federal, state, local, and voluntary health agencies (see **Figure 11.6**). Examples of other public health professionals are environmental health workers, public health administrators, epidemiologists, health education specialists, public health nurses and physicians, biostatisticians, the

allied healthcare professionals healthcare workers who provide services that assist, facilitate, and complement the work of physicians and other healthcare specialists

public health professional a healthcare worker who works in a public health organization

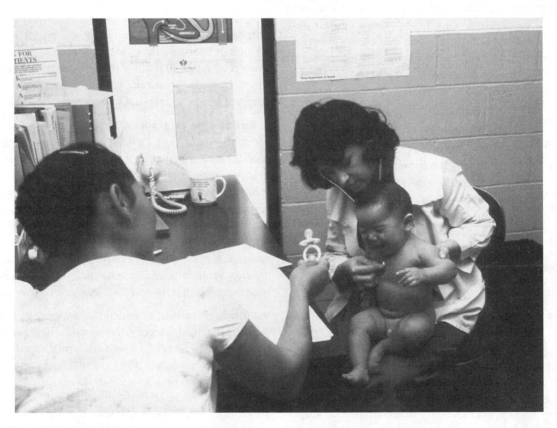

Figure 11.6 Public health professionals make up a key component of the healthcare system.
© Susan Van Etten/PhotoEdit, Inc.

Surgeon General, and the research scientists at the Centers for Disease Control and Prevention. Public health professionals often make possible the care that is practiced in immunization clinics; nutritional programs for women, infants, and children (WIC); dental health clinics; and sexually transmitted infection clinics. School nurses are also considered public health professionals. Public health services are usually financed by tax dollars and, although available to most taxpayers, serve primarily the economically disadvantaged.

Healthcare Facilities

Healthcare facilities are the physical settings in which health care is actually provided. They include a wide variety of settings but can be divided into two large categories of inpatient and outpatient care facilities. Inpatient care facilities include any in which a patient stays overnight, such as a hospital. Outpatient care facilities refer to any facility in which the patient receives care and does not stay overnight.

Inpatient Care Facilities

The primary inpatient care facilities are hospitals, nursing homes, and assisted-living facilities; we will discuss only hospitals here. In 2009, there were 5,795 hospitals in the United States,[16] varying in size, mission, and organizational structure. The major purpose of hospitals is to provide secondary and tertiary care.

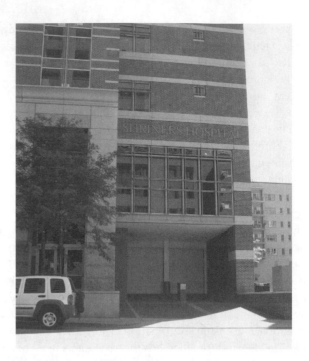

Figure 11.7 Hospitals are often categorized by ownership.

private (proprietary) or investor-owned hospitals for-profit hospitals

public hospitals hospitals that are supported and managed by governmental jurisdictions

specialty hospital a hospital that provides mainly one type of medical service, is for-profit, and is owned at least in part by the physicians who practice in it

voluntary hospitals nonprofit hospitals administered by not-for-profit corporations or charitable community organizations

Hospitals can be categorized in several different ways; one way is by hospital ownership (see **Figure 11.7**). A **private (proprietary or investor-owned) hospital**, of which there were 989 in 2009,[16] is one that is owned as a business for the purpose of making a profit. "Most for-profit hospitals belong to one of the large hospital management companies that dominate the for-profit hospital network."[4] A subset of the private hospitals is **specialty hospitals**. These are hospitals that provide mainly one type of medicine—usually surgery, either cardiac or orthopedic; most are owned, at least in part, by the physicians who practice in them.[4] A lot of controversy surrounds these hospitals. Larger general hospitals, which are losing patients and revenue to the specialty

hospitals, say that these specialty hospitals are just a "grab for money" by the physicians who own them. Physicians say specialty hospitals allow them to practice medicine the way it should be practiced, without answering to a hospital administrator who is trying to cut corners to make a profit.

A second type is a **public hospital**. These hospitals, of which there were 1,303 in 2009,[16] are supported and managed by governmental jurisdictions and are usually found in larger cities. Public hospitals can be operated by agencies at all levels of government. Hospitals operated by the federal government include military hospitals (e.g., Bethesda Naval Hospital) and the many hospitals run by the Veterans Administration and Indian Health Service. There are also hospitals that are owned or partially financed by states and local governments. Examples include university hospitals, state mental hospitals, and local city and county hospitals.

Voluntary hospitals, of which there were 2,918 in 2009,[16] make up the third category of hospitals. These are nonprofit hospitals administered by not-for-profit corporations or religious, fraternal, and other charitable community organizations. These hospitals make up about one-half of all hospitals in the United States. Examples of this latter group are the Southern Baptist hospitals, the many Shriners' hospitals, and many community hospitals. In recent years, voluntary hospitals have been expanding their scope of services and many now include wellness centers, stress centers, chemical dependency programs, and a variety of satellite centers.

A second way of classifying hospitals is by dividing them into teaching and nonteaching hospitals. Teaching hospitals have, as a part of their mission, the responsibility to prepare new healthcare providers. These hospitals are typically aligned with medical schools, universities, and medical residency programs. However, a number of hospitals not affiliated with medical schools provide medical residency programs, and clinical education for nurses, allied health personnel, and a wide variety of technical specialties.

A third means of categorizing hospitals is by the services offered. **Full-service hospitals**, or general hospitals, are those that offer care at all or most of the levels of care discussed earlier in the chapter. These are the most expensive hospitals to run and are usually found in metropolitan areas. **Limited-service hospitals** offer the specific services needed by the population served, such as emergency, maternity, general surgery, and so on, but they lack much of the sophisticated technology available at full-service hospitals. This type of hospital is more common in rural areas. Many limited-service hospitals were once full-service hospitals but have become limited-service hospitals because of the low volume of patients, a shortage of healthcare personnel, and financial distress.

Outpatient Care Facilities

An outpatient care facility is one where a patient receives ambulatory care (i.e., patients voluntarily leave their home to seek care) without being admitted as an inpatient.[1,26] Because of the variety of outpatient care services offered throughout the United States and the variety of arrangements for ownership of the services (i.e., hospitals, hospital systems, physician groups, and for-profit or not-for-profit chains), it is difficult to identify all possible outpatient care facilities.

What is known is that today, care and procedures that once were performed only on an inpatient basis are increasingly being performed in a variety of outpatient settings.[14] In fact, today the majority of all surgical procedures are performed on an outpatient basis.[4] The growth and movement of services to outpatient care facilities have resulted from a combination of new medical and diagnostic procedures, technological advances, consumer demand for user-friendly environments, the reimbursement process, and financial mandates from insurance companies and government.[4] The types of outpatient care facilities found in communities are healthcare practitioners' offices, clinics, primary care centers, retail clinics, urgent/emergent care centers, ambulatory surgery centers, and freestanding service facilities (see Figure 11.8).

Probably the outpatient care facilities with which people have the most familiarity are healthcare practitioners' offices that house private practices. Because it is very expensive to set up a private practice, it is increasingly common to see more than one practitioner sharing both an office and staff. These practices are often referred to as group practices to distinguish them from solo (single practitioner) practices.

Primary care centers present another way to offer primary care in addition to the more traditional physician office mode. Although they may appear to be just another physician's office or group practice, many of these facilities are owned by hospitals and also include laboratory, radiology, and pharmacy services. "In hospital-operated facilities, staff physicians are commonly employees of the owner hospital, or, in the case of a teaching facility, physicians may be jointly compensated through a medical school–affiliated faculty practice group and the hospital."[4] In some parts of the country, depending on licensing procedures, it may be common to see nurse practitioners and physician assistants, under physician supervision, as the primary care practitioners in these facilities.[4]

Some of the most recent additions to outpatient care facilities are retail clinics found in pharmacies (e.g., Walgreens), supermarkets, and retail stores (e.g., Walmart). The services offered are limited, but they "represent an entrepreneurial response to consumer demand for fast, affordable treatment of easy-to-diagnose, acute conditions."[4] The facilities are often operated by an outside company, maybe even a hospital, and are generally staffed by nurses, nurse practitioners, and physician assistants. Initially, payment at these clinics was out of the pocket of the consumer, but the concept has caught the eye of insurers as a lower cost way of providing acute care, and thus many insurers now have contracts with the clinics.[4] Employers like the idea too, and waive the copay when employees use them,[4] and some employers have even set up similar "quick clinics" within their own facility. Response to these clinics has been good from the insurers and consumers, but some in the medical community question the quality of care received.

full-service hospitals hospitals that offer services in all or most of the levels of care defined by the spectrum of healthcare delivery

limited-service hospitals hospitals that offer only the specific services needed by the population served

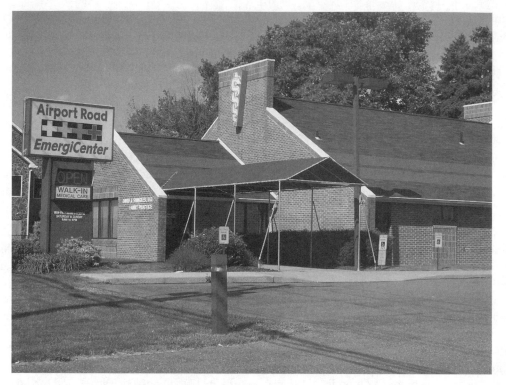

Figure 11.8 Many outpatient care facilities provide medical services safely and efficiently without the overhead of a hospital.

Urgent/emergent care centers have been around in the United States since the early 1970s. They "fill gaps in the delivery system created by the rigidity of private physician appointment and unavailability during nonbusiness hours. The centers also can provide a much more convenient and user friendly alternative to a hospital emergency department during hours when private physicians are not available."[4] Urgent/emergent care centers often provide quicker service with less paperwork, particularly for those with cash or credit cards. These facilities are not appropriate for all emergency cases. A majority of patients with life-threatening conditions are still taken to hospital emergency rooms, where top-of-the-line, advanced life support equipment and emergency physicians are on staff. Although emergency rooms are expensive for hospitals to maintain, they obviously perform a needed service.

Ambulatory surgery centers do not perform major surgery, such as heart transplants, but perform same-day surgeries where a hospital stay following the surgery is not needed. As noted earlier, today the majority of all surgical procedures are performed in these types of facilities.[4] The factors that have promoted the increase in ambulatory surgical procedures as alternatives to inpatient surgery include the development of new, safe, and faster-acting general anesthetics; advances in surgical equipment and materials; development of noninvasive or minimally invasive surgical and nonsurgical procedures; and reduced coverage by insurance companies for hospital stays.

One area of tremendous growth in outpatient care facilities in recent years has been in the development of freestanding, non–hospital-based, specialty facilities. Often, these facilities offer a single service, such as dialysis for individuals with kidney failure, or several similar services, such as those found in a diagnostic imaging center (e.g., X-rays, CT, and MRI). These technologies are ideal for outpatient facilities because of their noninvasive nature and profitability.

Clinics

When two or more physicians practice as a group, the facility in which they provide medical services is called a *clinic*. Some clinics are small, with just a few providers, whereas others are very large with many providers, such as the Mayo

Clinic in Rochester, Minnesota, or the Cleveland Clinic in Cleveland, Ohio. Some clinics provide care only for individuals with special health needs, such as treatment of cancer or diabetes or assistance in family planning; others accept patients with a wide range of problems. A misconception held by many is that clinics are not much different from hospitals, but clinics do not have inpatient beds.

Although many of the clinics are run as either for-profit or not-for-profit facilities, some are also funded by tax dollars. These clinics have been created primarily to meet the needs of the **medically indigent**—those lacking the financial ability to pay for their own medical care. Most of these clinics are located in large urban areas or rural areas that are underserved by the private sector. Two examples of this type of clinic are public health clinics and community health centers (CHCs). The former are usually a part of a local health department (LHD). The scope of healthcare services offered by LHDs varies greatly. These services can range from prevention-oriented programs, such as immunizations and well-baby care, to complete personal health services such as those offered at private-sector clinics. CHCs have been around since the late 1960s, and were known initially as neighborhood health centers. Today, the 1,200 CHCs with over 20 million patients operate under the auspices of the Bureau of Primary Health Care, which is part of the U.S. Department of Health and Human Services.[27] The importance of CHCs to the primary care and behavioral and mental health needs of the medically underserved populations in the United States is huge.[4]

Rehabilitation Centers

Rehabilitation centers are healthcare facilities in which patients work with healthcare providers to restore functions lost because of injury, disease, or surgery. These centers are sometimes part of a clinic or hospital but may also be freestanding facilities. Rehabilitation centers may operate on both an outpatient and an inpatient basis. Those providers who commonly work in a rehabilitation center include physical, occupational, and respiratory therapists as well as exercise physiologists.

Long-Term Care Options

Not too many years ago, when the topic of long-term care was mentioned, most people thought of nursing homes and state hospitals for the mentally ill and emotionally disabled. Today, however, the term *long-term care* includes not only the traditional institutional residential care, but also special units within these residential facilities (such as for Alzheimer

patients), halfway houses, group homes, assisted-living facilities, transitional (step-down) care in a hospital, day care facilities for patients of all ages with health problems that require special care, and personal home health care.

One area of long-term care that has received special attention in recent years is **home health care**. The demand for home health care has been driven by the restructuring of the healthcare delivery system, technological advances that enable people to be treated outside a hospital and to recover more quickly, and the cost containment pressures that have shortened hospital stays. Home health care should not be confused with home care. *Home care* is a more inclusive term and "denotes a range of services provided in the home, including skilled nursing and therapies, personal care, and even social services, such as meals, and home modifications."[28] Home health care involves providing health care via health personnel and medical equipment to individuals and families in their places of residence, for the purpose of promoting, maintaining, or restoring health or to maximize the level of independence while minimizing the effects of disability and illness, including terminal disease. Home health care can be either long term, to help a chronically ill patient avoid institutionalization, or short term to assist a patient following an acute illness and hospitalization until the patient is able to return to independent functioning. Home health care can be provided either through a formal system of paid professional health caregivers (e.g., home healthcare agency) or through an informal system where the care is provided by family, friends, and neighbors.[4] Medicare is the largest single payer for home health care, accounting for about one-third of the total annual expenditures.[4]

The need for professional home health caregivers will continue into the future because of the "increase in the number of older persons and their expressed desire to remain in their homes for care whenever possible."[4] In 2009, there were 10,184 Medicare-certified home health agencies in the United States. That number is more than three times as many as existed in 1980.[15] Even though Medicare and Medicaid are the largest payers for home healthcare services, the amounts spent are relatively small in comparison to the total dollars spent on the Medicare and Medicaid programs.

home health care care provided in the patient's residence for the purpose of promoting, maintaining, or restoring health

rehabilitation center a facility in which restorative care is provided following injury, disease, or surgery

medically indigent those lacking the financial ability to pay for their own medical care

Healthcare System: Function

Like the structure of the healthcare system, the function of the U.S. healthcare system is also unique compared to the healthcare systems of other developed countries of the world. However, with the passage of the Patient Protection and Affordable Care Act (PPACA; Public Law 111-148) and the Health Care and Education Reconciliation Act of 2010 (HCERA; Public Law 111-152) in 2010, changes have occurred and more will come in the next few years. (Note: Because these two laws were consolidated with each other and some other legislation, we refer to them collectively from here on as the "Affordable Care Act.") After the Affordable Care Act (ACA) was approved, a number of states felt the law was unconstitutional. Mixed rulings of cases in lower courts led the U.S. Supreme Court to hear the case and rule on the constitutionality of the law. In June 2012 the U.S. Supreme Court largely upheld the constitutionality of the ACA. The bulk of the ACA goes into effect in 2014, but some aspects became effective in mid-2010, and the final portions will be implemented in 2020.

Understanding the Structure of the Healthcare System

To begin, it must be understood that the U.S. healthcare system is big and complicated.[29] It is big from the standpoint of cost—it is very expensive (see **Figure 11.9**)—and because of the many stakeholders that include, but are not limited to, healthcare consumers, healthcare providers, healthcare administrators, politicians, policymakers, government regulators, insurance companies, and professional and trade associations. It is complicated because healthcare policy is intertwined with other policies (e.g., the U.S. tax code; for example, credits for employers who provide health insurance for employees and healthcare consumers who get deductions on their income taxes if their healthcare spending reaches certain levels in a year) and because of the politics and ideological viewpoints of the decision makers.

The major issues of the U.S. healthcare system can be represented by the cost containment, access, and quality triangle noted by Kissick[30] (see **Figure 11.10**). In Kissick's equilateral triangle, the equal 60-degree angles represent equal priorities; that is, access is just as important as quality and cost containment. However, an expansion of any one of the angles compromises one or both of the other two. For example, if we were interested in increasing the quality of our already good services, it would also increase the costs and decrease access. Or, some feel, if we increase access, costs will go up, and the quality will decrease. Or, if we concentrate on containing costs, both quality of care and access will decrease. With such dilemmas, the United States continues to struggle to find the right combination of policy and accountability to deal with these shortcomings.

Access to Health Care

Even with several different means of gaining access to healthcare services, access has been and continues to be a major health policy issue in the United States. Health

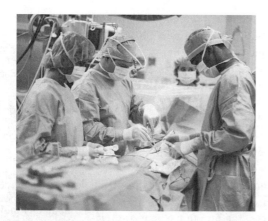

Figure 11.9 Healthcare services offered by U.S. providers are perhaps the best in the world, but at what cost?
© Photos.com

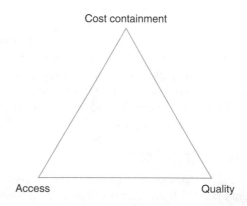

Figure 11.10 The cost containment, access, and quality triangle of health care.

Kissick, W. L. (1994). *Medicine's Dilemmas: Infinite Needs Versus Finite Resources.* New Haven, CT: Yale University Press. Copyright © 1994. Reprinted by permission of Yale University Press.

insurance coverage and the generosity of coverage are major determinants of access to health care.[31] In 2010, 48.6 million persons of all ages (16%) were uninsured, 60.3 million (19.8%) had been uninsured for at least part of the year, and 35.7 million (11.7%) had been uninsured for more than a year[32] (see **Box 11.4**). The likelihood of being uninsured is greater for younger persons, those with less education, those with lower incomes, nonwhites, those who are not U.S. citizens, and males.[32] The greatest reason for lack of insurance coverage is cost of insurance followed by lost job or change in employment.[33]

Box 11.4 *Healthy People 2020:* Objectives

Access to Health Services

Goal: Improve access to comprehensive, quality health care services.

Objective: AHS-1, Increase the proportions of persons with health insurance.

Objective: AHS-1.1, Medical insurance

Target: 100 percent.

Baseline: 83.2 percent of persons had medical insurance in 2008.

Target setting method: Total coverage.

Data source: National Health Interview Survey (NHIS), CDC, NCHS.

Objective: AHS-1.2 (Developmental), Dental insurance

Target: TBD

Baseline: TBD

Target setting method: TBD

Potential data source: National Health Interview Survey (NHIS), CDC, NCHS.

Objective: AHS-1.3 (Developmental), Prescription drug insurance

Target: TBD

Baseline: TBD

Target setting method: TBD

Potential data source: National Health Interview Survey (NHIS), CDC, NCHS.

For Further Thought

Do you think the Affordable Care Act was the best way to go about reaching these objectives? Defend your response. Do you think the United States should adopt a national health insurance plan like the other developed countries of the world to make sure all persons have health insurance? Why or why not?

TBD = To be determined

Source: Reproduced from U.S. Department of Health and Human Services, Office of Disease Prevention and Health Promotion (2010). *Healthy People 2020.* Available at http://www.healthypeople .gov/2020/topicsobjectives2020/pdfs/HP2020objectives.pdf.

Interestingly enough, the uninsured do not lack emergency or urgent care because no one needing such care and willing to go to a hospital emergency room will be turned away. However, the uninsured usually do not have access to primary care, such as checkups, screenings for chronic illnesses, and prenatal care. Without adequate primary care, many patients eventually find themselves in need of more costly and often less effective medical treatment. The primary factors that limit access to this type of care are total lack of health insurance, inadequate insurance, and poverty. Those who are unable to receive medical care because they cannot afford it are referred to as "medically indigent."[34] The medically indigent in the United States include people and families with income above the poverty level who are thus ineligible for Medicaid, or government health insurance for the poor, but who are unable to afford health care or health insurance. "Eight out of ten uninsured persons are members of working families. In most of these cases, the worker holds a job that does not offer health insurance. In others, subsidized coverage may be offered, but the employee turns it down because of the cost or because they do not perceive the need for coverage."[31] Those who have a job but are unable to afford health insurance are referred to as the working poor. It has been estimated that there are 30 million working poor in the United States.[35] Others may be uninsured because individual health policies are quite expensive and may be unavailable for those who have a preexisting health problem. Young adults often lose their eligibility under their parents' policy. In summary, in the United States, access to a regular source of health care is closely tied to having health insurance.

To deal with the problem of lack of access to health care, a major component of the Affordable Care Act passed in 2010 was aimed at increasing the number of Americans with health insurance. **Box 11.5** provides a brief summary of some of the steps that were included in the Affordable Care Act to increase access to care. The Congressional Budget Office has estimated that by taking all these steps, the number of uninsured could be reduced by 32 million by 2019.[36] The majority of those who will be uninsured in 2019 will be those who have entered the country illegally.

Quality of Health Care

All people are entitled to and should receive quality health care. Yet several different reports indicate that people in the United States could be receiving better care. Quality health care has been defined as "the degree to which health

---

Box 11.5   Components of the Affordable Care Act to Increase Access to Care*

1. *Individual mandate:* Beginning in 2014, all individuals will be required to have health insurance or pay a penalty. The penalty will be phased in from 2014–2016. There are some exceptions to this requirement that include financial hardship, religious objections, and for American Indians.

2. *Expansion of public programs:* Medicaid can be expanded to cover those up to 133% of the federal poverty level. In 2012, that level would have been $14,856 for an individual and $30,657 for a family of four. This expansion will create a national uniform eligibility standard across states. The federal government will pay for much of the expansion. In June 2012 the U.S. Supreme Court ruled that states could opt out of this provision. (Note: At the time this book was written it was too soon to know how many states would opt out.)

3. *American Health Benefit Exchanges:* For people who do not receive employer-sponsored insurance and who make more than 133% of the federal poverty level, health insurance will be available through new American Health Benefit Exchanges created by states. Plans in the exchanges must provide benefits that meet a minimum set of standards. Insurers will offer four levels of coverage that vary based on premiums, out-of-pocket costs, and benefits beyond the minimum required plus a catastrophic coverage plan. Various premium subsidies will be available to those with incomes between 100% and 400% of the federal poverty level.

4. *Changes to private insurance:* New health insurance regulations will change the way insurers operate. Insurers will: (1) not be able to deny coverage to people because of health status (i.e., preexisting condition); (2) not be able to charge people more because of health status or gender; (3) for all new health plans, have to provide comprehensive coverage that includes a minimum set of services, caps out-of-pocket spending, does not impose cost-sharing for preventive services, and does not impose annual or lifetime limits on coverage; (4) have to allow young adults to remain on their parents' health insurance up until age 26; and (5) have to limit waiting periods to no longer than 90 days.

5. *Employer requirements:* There is no employer mandate to offer health insurance to employees, but employers with 50+ employees will be assessed a fee of $2,000 per full-time employee (in excess of 30 employees) if they do not offer coverage and if they have at least one employee who receives a premium credit through an exchange. Employers with 50+ employees who do offer health insurance but have at least one employee who receives a premium credit through an exchange will be required to pay the lesser of $3,000 per employee who receives a premium credit or $2,000 per employee (in excess of 30 employees). If employers offer coverage and have workers who do not sign up for the plan or do not opt out of a plan, the employer must automatically enroll employees in the lowest cost premium plan. Also, if employers offer coverage to employees with incomes less than 400% of the federal poverty level and the employees' share of the premium is between 8% and 9.8% of their income, then employers will be required to provide vouchers so that employees can enroll in a plan in an exchange

*Limited to U.S. citizens and legal immigrants.

Sources: Adapted from Henry J. Kaiser Family Foundation (2010). "Summary of Coverage Provisions in the Patient Protection and Affordable Care Act (#8023)." Available at http://www.kff.org/healthreform/8023.cfm; and data from Supreme Court of the United States (2012, June 28). "2011 Term Opinions of the Court." Available at http://www.supremecourt.gov/opinions/11pdf/11-393c3a2.pdf.

---

services for individuals and populations increase the likelihood of desired health outcomes and are consistent with current professional knowledge."[37] The Institute of Medicine (IOM) has further delineated that quality health care should be[37]:

Effective: Delivering health care based on scientific evidence to all who could benefit based on need

Safe: Delivering health care to patients that avoids injuries to patients from the care that is intended to help them

Timely: Delivering health care in a way that reduces waits and sometimes harmful delays

Patient centered: Providing health care that is respectful of and responsive to individual patient preferences, needs, and values

Equitable: Delivering health care that does not vary in quality because of personal characteristics of patients

Efficient: Delivering health care that maximizes resources and avoids waste

Although the definitions of quality health care are easily understood, operationalizing quality health care is not as easy; yet a number of groups have created measures for healthcare quality. Since 2003, the Agency for Healthcare Research and Quality (AHRQ), together with the U.S. Department of Health and Human Services (HHS) and some private-sector partners, has annually reported on progress and opportunities for improving healthcare quality, as mandated by Congress, by publishing the National Healthcare Quality Report (NHQR)[38] and the National Healthcare Disparities Report (NHDR).[39] Both the NHQR and the NHDR are built on, for the most part, the same 250 measures assembled across 7 dimensions of quality—effectiveness of care, patient safety, timeliness of care, patient centeredness, care coordination, efficiency of care, and health system infrastructure.

Another group that measures healthcare quality is the National Committee for Quality Assurance (NCQA).[40] The NCQA is a private, not-for-profit organization that has been assessing and accrediting healthcare plans since 1990.

It assesses how well a health plan manages and delivers health care in four different ways: (1) through **accreditation** (a rigorous on-site review of key clinical and administrative processes); (2) through certification (a rigorous review of certain functions—for example, credentialing or utilization management—that health plans or employers have delegated to another organization); (3) through the Health Plan Effectiveness Data and Information Set (HEDIS—a tool that consists of 76 measures across five domains that is used to measure performance in key areas such as immunization and mammography screening rates) and members' satisfaction with their care in areas such as claims processing, customer service, and getting needed care quickly; and (4) through physician recognition programs that identify physicians who provide quality care in areas such as diabetes and heart/stroke care. The data available from these assessments are available at NCQA's website. Many employers use the data as a way of selecting the best managed care programs for their employees.

Regardless of which method is used to measure the quality of health care delivered in the United States, the results have been similar. The general consensus is that the quality of health care has been getting better at a modest pace but is not as good as it could or should be.

Dealing with the problem of "less than desirable quality in health care" is not easy because it runs through every aspect of care. That is why there are not just a few items in the Affordable Care Act that deal with quality—there are many. Box 11.6 provides a sampling of some of the items of the law that address quality.

The Cost of and Paying for Health Care

The cost of health care and paying for health care continue to be burdens on both individuals and the U.S. population as a whole. In 2013, health expenditures were projected to be almost $2.9 trillion and to consume 17.6% of the gross domestic product (GDP), and they are expected to reach more than $4.6 trillion and 19.7% of the GDP by 2020.[11] The United States spends more per capita annually on health care (estimated at $9,349 in 2013[11]) than any other nation. Other developed countries in the world spend between one-third (Japan and New Zealand) and two-thirds (Switzerland and Norway) as much.[41] Under the U.S. system, the actual cost of the service is usually not known until after the service has been provided, unless the consumer is bold enough to inquire ahead of time. Most are not.

> **accreditation** the process by which an agency or organization evaluates and recognizes an institution as meeting certain predetermined standards

---

Box 11.6   Some of the Components of the Affordable Care Act That Will Affect Quality of Care

- *Wellness and preventive services:* New health plans available on or after September 23, 2010, are required to cover recommended preventive services (e.g., screenings, vaccinations, counseling) without charging a copay, co-insurance, or deductible. Similar benefits apply to Medicare. Effective January 1, 2011.

- *Center for Medicare and Medicaid Innovation:* A new center will begin testing new ways of delivering care to patients. These methods are expected to improve the quality of care and reduce the rate of growth in healthcare costs for Medicare, Medicaid, and the Children's Health Insurance Program (CHIP). Effective January 1, 2011.

- *Providing better information and accountability for nursing home care:* It will be easier to file complaints about the quality of care in a nursing home. Consumers also will have access to more information on nursing home quality and resident rights. Effective January 1, 2011.

- *Linking payment to quality outcomes:* A hospital Value-Based Purchasing program (VBP) will become a part of traditional Medicare, which will offer financial incentives to hospitals to improve the quality of care. Hospital performance is required to be publicly reported, beginning with measures relating to heart attacks, heart failure, pneumonia, surgical care,

healthcare-associated infections, and patients' perception of care. Effective September 30, 2012.

- *Encouraging integrated health systems:* Incentives will be available for physicians to join together to form accountable care organizations (ACOs). These groups allow doctors to better coordinate patient care and improve its quality, help prevent disease and illness, and reduce unnecessary hospital admissions. If ACOs provide high-quality care and reduce costs to the healthcare system, they can keep some of the money that they have helped save. Effective January 1, 2012.

- *Reducing paperwork and administrative costs:* A series of changes to be made to standardize billing that requires health plans to begin adopting and implementing rules for the secure, confidential, electronic exchange of health information. Using electronic health records will reduce paperwork and administrative burdens, cut costs, reduce medical errors, and, most important, improve the quality of care. Effective October 1, 2012.

- *Paying physicians based on value not volume:* Physician payments will be tied to the quality of care they provide. Physicians will see their payments modified so that those who provide higher value care will receive higher payments than those who provide lower quality care. Effective January 1, 2015.

Source: Modified from U.S. Department of Health and Human Services (2012). "What's Changing and When." Available at http://www.healthcare.gov/law/timeline/index.html.

Payments for the U.S. healthcare bill come from four sources. The first is the consumers themselves. In 2013, it was estimated these direct or out-of-pocket payments represented approximately one-tenth (11.2%) of all payments. The remaining portion of healthcare payments, nine-tenths, comes almost entirely from indirect, or third-party, payments. The first source of third-party payments is private insurance companies. It was estimated that private insurance companies paid 31.1% of the healthcare bill in 2013. The second source of third-party payments is governmental insurance programs (i.e., Medicare, Medicaid, Veterans Administration, Children's Health Insurance Program, Indian Health Service, or military). These government programs are funded by a combination of taxes and premiums from those insured. In 2013 it was estimated that 40.7% of the healthcare bill was paid for by governmental insurance programs. Finally, the remaining portion of healthcare bills are paid by other private funds; in 2013, it was approximately 17%.[11]

It is clear that the cost of health care is going to continue to rise. One of the major selling points of the Affordable Care Act was to try to slow down the cost of health care, thus the title "Affordable Care." The Congressional Budget Office (CBO) "estimates the cost of the coverage components of the new law to be $938 billion over ten years. These costs are financed through a combination of savings from Medicare and Medicaid and new taxes and fees."[42] Examples of new taxes include taxes on high-cost health insurance and tanning bed use; examples of new fees include those that have to be paid by pharmaceutical and insurance companies. Many feel that in addition to the cost savings from Medicare and Medicaid, healthcare costs have the potential to be lower because many people who were uninsured before the law will now be paying premiums, and many of them are young and healthy and will not use a lot of health care.

As noted earlier, *third-party payers* (i.e., insurance companies and government entities) make a majority of the payments for health services. The payments made by the third-party payers to providers are referred to as **reimbursement**.[1] The process for receiving a third-party payment usually begins when a healthcare provider or his or her staff requests information about the patient's health insurance plan. They normally request the name of the insuring company (e.g., Blue Cross/Blue Shield), the policy number, and a personal identification number (PIN).

fee-for-service a method of paying for health care in which a fee is paid after the service is rendered

reimbursement payments made by third-party payers to providers

This information is usually provided to the insured on a wallet-sized card by the insurer. The provider may then ask the patient to sign an insurance claim form in two places. The first signature indicates that the service has been provided and authorizes the provider to submit patient information with the claim for payment. The second signature instructs the insurance company to make the payment directly to the provider. Upon receiving and reviewing the completed and signed form, the insurance company then issues payments to the provider for services based on the provisions of the insurance policy. Depending on the level of reimbursement for the claim, the provider will either consider the bill paid in full or will request payment from the patient in the amount of the difference between the provider's full fee and the portion paid by the insurance company.

In recent years, the methods by which the amount of the reimbursement has been determined have changed. Traditionally, providers have favored the **fee-for-service** method, but it is not used much any more because of the cost escalation.[1] The fee-for-service method is based on the assumption that services are provided in a set of identifiable and individually distinct units such as a doctor's office visit or a specific medical procedure.[1] Under the fee-for-service format, consumers select a provider, receive care (service) from the provider, and incur expenses (a fee) for the care. The provider is then reimbursed for covered services in part by the insurer and in part by the consumer, who is responsible for the balance unpaid by the insurer. Initially, the providers set the fees and insurers would pay the claim. But because of increased costs, insurers started to limit the amount they would pay to "usual, customary, and reasonable." The biggest drawback of the fee-for-service format is that providers have a greater incentive to provide services, some of which sometimes are nonessential.[1]

Under the fee-for-service format, consumers are obligated to pay their fee at the time the service is rendered. Today, for patients to receive care via fee-for-service, they are often required to demonstrate the ability to pay (to assume financial responsibility for the fee) before the service is rendered. A provider's receptionist may ask, "How do you plan to settle your bill?" In other cases, providers have signs placed around the waiting room that state, "Payment is expected when service is rendered, unless other arrangements have been made prior to the appointment."

The more recent methods of paying for health services have included packaged pricing, resource-based relative value scale, capitation, and prospective reimbursement.

In **packaged pricing**, also referred to as bundled charges, several related services are included in one price. For example, optometrists will bundle the cost for an eye exam, frames, and lenses into a single charge.[1]

Resource-based relative value scale was created for Medicare as part of the Omnibus Budget Reconciliation Act of 1989 to reimburse physicians according to the relative value of the service provided. The relative value units (RVUs) are derived through a complex formula based on time, skill, and intensity to provide the service. Also included in the RVU is an overhead charge to run a practice.[1] Each year, Medicare publishes the Medicare Physician Fee Schedule, adjusted for geographic areas of the country, which provides the reimbursement amount for services and procedures under the Current Procedural Terminology (CPT) code.[1]

Managed care organizations (MCOs) (see information about managed care later in this chapter) use a couple different approaches for reimbursement. Preferred provider organizations (PPOs) use a variation of the fee-for-service method. The variation is that the PPOs "establish fee schedules based on discounts negotiated with providers"[1] participating in their network. Health maintenance organizations (HMOs), depending on their structure, have either paid providers a salary if they are employed by the HMO or have reimbursed using a mechanism called capitation.

Under **capitation**, insurers make arrangements with healthcare providers to provide agreed-upon covered healthcare services to a given population of consumers for a (usually discounted) set price—the per-person premium fee—over a particular time period. Often the arrangements are set up on a per-member, per-month (PMPM) rate called a *capitated fee*. The provider receives the capitated fee per enrollee regardless of whether the enrollee uses healthcare services and regardless of the quality of services provided. The provider is responsible for providing all needed services determined to be medically necessary and covered under the plan.[1] In addition to the capitated fee, consumers may pay additional fees (copayments) for office visits and other services used. The insurer organizes the delivery of care by building an infrastructure of providers and implementing the systems to monitor and influence the cost and quality of care.

Prospective reimbursement has been around since 1983, when it was first used in the form of diagnosis-related groups (DRGs) for hospital stays under Medicare Part A. It replaced retrospective reimbursement that was based on the length of stay and services provided. Thus, providers were rewarded for longer stays and more services, which increased costs. Prospective reimbursement, referred to as the prospective pricing system (PPS), "uses certain established criteria to determine the amount of reimbursement in advance, before services are delivered."[1] Because of the success of DRGs, the Balanced Budget Act of 1997 mandated implementation of a Medicare PPS for hospital outpatient services and postacute providers such as skilled nursing facilities, home health agencies, and inpatient rehabilitation facilities.[1] Thus, the four primary prospective reimbursement methods used today are DRGs (used for Medicare Part A), ambulatory payment classifications (APCs; used for payment to hospital outpatient departments), resource utilization groups (RUGs; used for payment to skilled nursing facilities), and home health resource groups (HHRGs; used for payment of home health care).[1]

Health Insurance

Health insurance, like all other types of insurance, is a risk- and cost-spreading process; that is, the cost of one person's injury or illness is shared by all in the group. Each person in the group has a different chance (or risk) of having a problem and thus needing health care. Some members of the group, for example, those who suffer from chronic and/or congenital health problems, will probably need more care whereas others in the group will need less. The concept of insurance has everyone in the group, no matter what their individual risk, helping to pay for the collective risk of the group. The risk of costly ill health is spread in a reasonably equitable fashion among all persons purchasing insurance, and everyone is protected from having to pay an insurmountable bill for a catastrophic injury or illness.

There are some exceptions to the "equitable fashion." If someone in the group knowingly engages in a behavior that increases his or her risk, such as smoking cigarettes or driving in a reckless manner, that person may have to pay more for the increased risk. In short, the greater the risk (or probability of using the insurance), the more the individual or group has to pay for insurance.

The concept of health insurance is not a new one in this country. Group

capitation a method of paying for covered healthcare services on a per-person premium basis for a specific time period prior to the service being rendered

packaged pricing several related health services are included in one price

prospective reimbursement uses preestablished criteria to determine in advance the amount of reimbursement

resource-based relative value scale reimbursement to physicians according to the relative value of the service provided

health and life insurance are considered American inventions of the early twentieth century. In 1911, Montgomery Ward and Company sold health insurance policies based on the principles still used today in the business. Currently, hundreds of companies in the United States sell health and life insurance policies.

The Health Insurance Policy

A *policy* is a written agreement between a private insurance company (or the government) and an individual or group of individuals to pay for certain healthcare costs during a certain time period in return for regular, periodic payments (a set amount of money) called *premiums*. The insurance company benefits in that it anticipates collecting more money in premiums than it has to pay out for services; hence, it anticipates a profit. The insured benefits by not being faced with medical bills he or she cannot pay, because the insurance company is obligated to pay them according to the terms of the contract. The added benefit for those insured as a group is that group premiums are less expensive than premiums for individuals.

Although the language of health insurance policies can be confusing, everyone needs to understand several key terms. One of the most important is **deductible**. The deductible is the amount of expenses (money) that the beneficiary (insured) must incur (pay out of pocket) before the insurance company begins to pay for covered services. A common yearly deductible level is $250 per individual policy holder, or a maximum of $1,000 per family. This means that the insured must pay the first $250/$1,000 of medical costs before the insurance company begins paying. The higher the deductible of a policy, the lower the premiums will be.

Usually, but not always, after the deductible has been met, most insurance companies pay a percentage of what they consider the "usual, customary, and reasonable" charge for covered services. The insurer generally pays 80% of the usual, customary, and reasonable costs, and the insured is responsible for paying

co-insurance the portion of the insurance company's approved amounts for covered services that a beneficiary is responsible for paying

copayment a negotiated set amount that a patient pays for certain services

deductible the amount of expenses that the beneficiary must incur before the insurance company begins to pay for covered services

exclusion a health condition written into the health insurance policy indicating what is not covered by the policy

fixed indemnity the maximum amount an insurer will pay for a certain service

preexisting condition a medical condition that had been diagnosed or treated usually within the 6 months before the date a health insurance policy goes into effect

the remaining 20%. This 20% is referred to as **co-insurance**. If the healthcare provider charges more than the usual, customary, and reasonable rates, the insured will have to pay both the co-insurance and the difference. A form of co-insurance, often associated with managed care programs, is **copayment** (or copay for short). A copayment is a negotiated set amount a patient pays for certain services—for example, $20 for an office visit and $15 for a prescription. Some insurance policies may have both co-insurance and copayments included. The greater the proportion of co-insurance paid by the insured, the lower the premiums.

A fourth key term, **fixed indemnity**, refers to the maximum amount an insurer will pay for a certain service. For example, a policy may state that the maximum amount of money paid for orthodontia is $2,000. Depending on the language of a policy, the fixed indemnity benefit may or may not be subject to the provisions of the deductible or co-insurance clause. Costs above the fixed indemnity amount are the responsibility of the insured.

Another key term related to health insurance is **exclusion**. When an exclusion is written into a policy, it means that a specified health condition is excluded from coverage; that is, the policy does not pay for service to treat the condition. Common exclusions include a pregnancy that began before the health insurance policy went into effect or a chronic disease or condition such as diabetes or hypertension that has been classified as a preexisting condition. A **preexisting condition** is a medical condition that had been diagnosed or treated usually within the 6 months before the date the health insurance policy went into effect. Because of such exclusions, people who have a serious condition or disease are often unable to get health insurance coverage for the condition/disease or in general. Some health insurance policies also exclude a condition/disease for a specified period of time, such as 9 months for pregnancy or 1 year for all other exclusions.

The rule that a preexisting condition could be an exclusion "trapped" many people in jobs, because the employees were afraid of losing their health insurance for the condition if they changed employers. To deal with this issue, Congress passed the Health Insurance Portability and Accountability Act of 1996 (Public Law 104-102, known as HIPAA). This law was created, in part, to ensure that people will not have to wait for health insurance to go into effect when changing jobs. More specifically, a preexisting condition had to be covered without a waiting period when a person joined a new plan if the person had been insured for the previous 12 months. If a person had a preexisting condition and it had not been covered in the previous 12 months before joining a new plan, the longest that person had to wait before being covered for that condition was 12 months.

Even with HIPAA many people, mostly older Americans, were unable to get health insurance because of preexisting conditions. Thus, preexisting conditions were addressed in the Affordable Care Act passed in 2010. Beginning 90 days after enactment of the law, older adults with preexisting conditions who had been uninsured for at least 6 months were eligible for subsidized insurance through a national high-risk pool. Then, in 2014, insurance companies will be required to cover all individuals regardless of health status and charge the same premium regardless of preexisting conditions.[43]

Types of Health Insurance Coverage

As has been noted in the previous discussions, health insurance policies cover a number of different types of services. The more common types of coverage are hospitalization, surgical, regular medical, major medical, dental, and disability. Although the types of health insurance coverage remain constant, several trends associated with health insurance plans and the products they offer are emerging. The trends that characterize health insurance plans today are (1) the plans are becoming more complex and are concentrated in a smaller number of companies; (2) there is an increase in the diversity of products, so consumers have many more options in the type of plan they select; (3) there is an increased focus on delivering care through a network of providers rather than independent providers; (4) there is a movement of shifting to financial structures and incentives among purchasers, health plans, and providers; and (5) more health insurance plans are developing clinical infrastructures to manage utilization and to improve the quality of care. Such trends will make understanding health insurance plans more challenging for consumers. These trends will require a greater investment in education and information to help consumers understand how insurance products differ, how best to navigate managed care systems, and what differences exist in structure or performance across the plans.

The Cost of Health Insurance

Over the years, the cost of health insurance has pretty much mirrored the cost of health care. From the early 1970s through the early 1990s, healthcare costs and the costs of healthcare insurance were growing in the neighborhood of 10% to 12% per year.[42] But as the increase in the cost

of health care slowed in the early to mid-1990s, so did the increase in the cost of health insurance. This deceleration in premium growth paralleled the dramatic shift in the health insurance marketplace away from traditional fee-for-service indemnity insurance to managed care. However, the managed care revolution created a one-time-only cost savings, and all the underlying cost drivers, such as an aging population, increased use of prescription drugs, and technology, have again increased costs. The burden of the cost of health insurance for those who are working falls primarily on the employer and, to a lesser extent, on the employee. Most Americans younger than 65 years of age receive their health insurance through their employer or the employer of their parent or spouse/partner. Even though the Affordable Care Act mandates that all citizens and legal immigrants have health insurance, much of the responsibility will continue to fall on employers. Because of the increasing costs of health insurance and its impact on the bottom line of companies, employers are shifting more of the cost onto their employees by (1) increasing the workers' share of the premium, (2) raising the deductibles that workers must pay, (3) increasing the copayments for prescription drugs, and (4) increasing the number of items on the exclusion list.

In the end, the actual cost of a policy is determined by two major factors—the risk of those in the group and the amount of coverage provided. An increase in either risk or coverage will result in an increase in the cost of the policy.

Self-Funded Insurance Programs

With the high cost of health care today, some employers "(or other group, such as a union or trade association)"[4] who provide health insurance for their employees are deciding to cut their costs by becoming self-insured. With such an arrangement, a **self-funded insurance program** pays the healthcare costs of its employees with the premiums collected from the employees and the contributions made by the employer instead of using a commercial carrier.[4] Self-funded insurance programs "often use the services of an actuarial firm to set premium rates and a third-party administrator to administer benefits, pay claims, and collect data on utilization. Many third-party administrators also provide case management services for potentially extraordinarily expensive cases to help coordinate care and control employee risk of catastrophic expenses."[4] There are several benefits to being self-funded. First, the organization gets to

self-funded insurance program one that pays the healthcare costs of its employees with the premiums collected from the employees and the contributions made by the employer

set most of the parameters of the policy—deductibles, co-insurance, fixed indemnities, and exclusions. If the organization wants to exclude some services and include others, it can. For example, if the organization has an older workforce, it may wish to delete obstetrics from the policy but include a number of preventive health services. Second, the organization holds on to the cash reserves in the benefits account instead of sending them to a commercial carrier, and thus gets to accrue interest on them. Third, the self-funded organizations have been exempt from the Employee Retirement and Income Security Act of 1974 (ERISA), which mandates minimum benefits under state law.[4] And fourth, generally the administrative costs of self-funded organizations have been less than those of traditional commercial carriers and, in general, health insurance costs to these groups have risen at a slower rate.[4] It appears that these benefits will not be affected by the Affordable Care Act; however, the law did include language that indicates that the Secretary of the U.S. Department of Labor is required to provide an annual report about self-funded insurance programs to the appropriate committees of Congress so that they can study their workings. In addition, the law requires the Secretary of the U.S. Department of Health and Human Services to conduct a study of self-funded insurance programs to determine if there are any adverse effects on the components of healthcare reform.[44]

For self-funded insurance to work, there must be a sizable group of employees over which to spread the risk. Larger organizations usually find it more useful than smaller ones do. However, if a small workforce is composed primarily of low-health-risk employees, say, for example, younger employees, self-funded programs make sense.

Health Insurance Provided by the Government

Although there are some in the United States who would like to see all health insurance provided by the government—a national health insurance plan—at the present time government health insurance plans are only available to select groups in the United States. The only government health insurance plans—those funded by governments at federal, state, and local levels—that exist today are Medicare, Medicaid, the Children's Health Insurance Program (CHIP), Veterans Administration (VA) benefits (see **Figure 11.11**), Indian Health Service, and healthcare

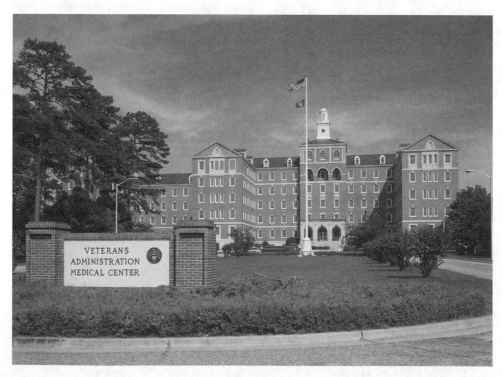

Figure 11.11 Insurance provided for veterans is one of several insurance plans paid for by the U.S. government.
© SuperStock/age fotostock

benefits for the uniformed services (military and Public Health Service) (TRICARE), federal employees (Federal Employees Health Benefits Program), and prisoners. Our discussion here is limited to Medicare, Medicaid, and CHIP. Medicare and Medicaid were created in 1965 by amendments to the Social Security Act and were implemented for the first time in 1966. CHIP was created in 1997 and codified as Title XXI of the Social Security Act.

Medicare

Medicare, which currently covers more than 47.5 million people,[15] is a federal health insurance program for people 65 years of age or older, people of any age with permanent kidney failure, and certain disabled people under 65. It is administered by the Centers for Medicare and Medicaid Services (CMS) of the U.S. Department of Health and Human Services (HHS). The Social Security Administration provides information about the program and handles enrollment. Medicare is considered a contributory program, in that employers and employees are required to contribute a percentage of each employee's wages/salaries through Social Security (FICA) tax to the Medicare fund. Medicare has four parts: hospital insurance (Part A), medical insurance (Part B), managed care plans (Part C), and prescription drug plans (Part D).

The Medicare hospital insurance (Part A) portion is mandatory and is provided for those eligible without further cost. Some seniors who are not eligible for premium-free Part A because they or their spouses did not pay into Social Security at all, or paid only a limited amount, may be able to purchase Part A coverage. In 2013, those premiums were $441 per month.[45] Although Medicare Part A has deductible ($1,184 in 2013) and co-insurance provisions, it helps pay for inpatient care in a hospital and in a skilled nursing facility after a hospital stay, hospice care, and some home health care.[45] Those who are enrolled in Part A of Medicare are automatically enrolled in Part B unless they decline. In 2013, the premium for Part B was $104.90 per month.[45] Most Part A enrollees are also enrolled in Part B and have their premium deducted directly from their Social Security check. Part B of Medicare helps cover physicians' and other healthcare providers' services, outpatient care, durable medical equipment, home health care, and some preventive services. Part B also has a deductible ($147 per year in 2013) and co-insurance (80/20 coverage). Whereas most Medicare beneficiaries pay the standard premium rate, a small percentage pay a higher rate based on their income. In 2013, the higher rates ranged from $146.90 to $335.70

per month depending on the extent to which an individual beneficiary's income exceeded $85,000 (or $170,000 for those filing a joint tax return), with the highest rates paid by those whose incomes were more than $214,000 (or $428,000 for those filing a joint tax return).[45]

Part C of Medicare is the managed care plans of Medicare (see the discussion of managed care later in this chapter). Formally, Part C is called Medicare Advantage (MA plans) and was added to Medicare as part of the Balanced Budget Act (BBA) of 1997. It was introduced primarily as a means to try to reduce costs compared with the original fee-for-service Medicare plan. Medicare Advantage plans provide all of the coverage provided in Parts A and B and must cover medically necessary services except for hospice care. They generally offer extra benefits; thus, there is no need to purchase a separate supplemental Medigap policy (see the discussion of Medigap later in this chapter), and many include Part D prescription drug coverage. Part C plans are offered by private insurance companies and are not available in all parts of the country. Because private companies offer them, the specifics of the plans are not consistent from plan to plan. Some are set up on a fee-for-service arrangement whereas others are offered as managed care plans (i.e., PPOs, HMOs, and medical savings accounts). Most have an annual deductible and require a monthly premium in addition to premiums paid for Part B.[45] In 2010, 11.4 million people were enrolled in Part C plans.[46]

Medicare Part D is the prescription drug program and currently has 34.5 million enrollees.[15] Part D is optional and run by insurance companies and other private companies approved by Medicare. To use it, those eligible must sign up for it and pay a monthly premium (most range from $20 to $40 per month). The premium varies based on the plan selected (most states offer approximately 50 different plans). Like Part A, there is an additional fee for those with higher incomes. A special provision in Part D—"Extra Help"— offers drug coverage at low cost for qualified people with limited incomes and resources. Although Part D has provided welcome help with the cost of prescription drugs to those who are eligible, the process of using Part D has been hard for many seniors to understand. It is complicated for several reasons. The first is the large number of plans available. The plans vary in drugs covered and costs. For example, one drug may be on the list of drugs covered (called the formulary) for one plan but not another. Many plans cover

Medicare a national health insurance program for people 65 years of age or older, certain younger disabled people, and people with permanent kidney failure

only generic drugs, whereas others cover both generic and brand-name drugs. Most plans have copayments or co-insurance. And then there is the coverage gap, or what has become known as the donut hole. In 2012, all plans (with the exception of the Extra Help plan) had a $320 deductible. Once the deductible was met, the plans covered the cost of drugs (minus copayment/co-insurance) between $321 and $2,930. Then, at $2,930, the enrollees had to pay out of pocket (in 2012, 50% of the cost of covered brand-name drugs and 86% of the cost of covered generic drugs) for drugs while in the coverage gap until they had spent $4,700. (This includes yearly deductible, copayment/co-insurance, and costs while in the coverage gap. This does not include the plan's premium.) Once enrollees reached the plan's out-of-pocket limit, the donut hole closed and the enrollees had catastrophic coverage. This means that those covered paid a small co-insurance amount or a copayment for the rest of the calendar year.[45] Some of the complexity of Part D will be resolved with the Affordable Care Act. As part of that legislation, the confusing donut hole (i.e., coverage gap) is to be gradually reduced, and by 2020 it will be eliminated.[44]

It should be noted that when healthcare providers take assignment (are willing to accept Medicare patients) on a Medicare claim, they agree to accept the Medicare-approved amount as payment in full. These providers are paid directly by the Medicare carrier, except for the deductible and co-insurance amounts, which are the patient's responsibility. Finally, Medicare, like private health insurance programs, is affected by the high costs of health care and, therefore, the government is always looking for ways of cutting the costs of the programs. In recent years, much discussion has centered around whether there are sufficient funds in Medicare to pay for the healthcare costs of the 76 million baby boomers when they started to become eligible in 2011. Most projections about the Medicare program indicate that there is enough money to begin to cover the baby boomers, but as they age Medicare will run out of money unless changes are made. To deal in part with this problem, a number of changes were made to Medicare as part of the Affordable Care Act. Box 11.7 presents some of the components of the Affordable Care Act that will affect the way the Medicare program is delivered.

Box 11.7 Implementation Timeline for Key Medicare Provisions of the 2010 Health Care Reform Law, 2010–2015

2010	
Cost containment	• Reduce annual market basket updates for inpatient hospital, home health, skilled nursing facility, hospice, and other Medicare providers, and adjust payments for productivity • Ban new physician-owned hospitals in Medicare
Delivery system reforms	• Establish a new office within the Centers for Medicare and Medicaid Services (CMS), the Federal Coordinated Health Care Office, to improve care coordination for dual eligibles
Part D	• Provide a $250 rebate for beneficiaries who reach the Part D coverage gap
2011	
Cost containment	• Establish a new Center for Medicare and Medicaid Innovation within CMS • Freeze the income threshold for income-related Medicare Part B premiums for 2011 through 2019 at 2010 levels ($85,000/individual and $170,000/couple), and reduce the Medicare Part D premium subsidy for those with incomes above $85,000/individual and $170,000/couple • Provide Medicare payments to qualifying hospitals in counties with the lowest quartile Medicare spending for 2011 and 2012
Medicare Advantage	• Prohibit Medicare Advantage (MA) plans from imposing higher cost sharing for some Medicare covered benefits than is required under the traditional fee-for-service program • Restructure payments to MA plans by phasing payments to different percentages of Medicare fee-for-service rates; freezes payments for 2011 and 2010 levels
Physician payment	• Provide a 10 percent Medicare bonus payment to primary care physicians and general surgeons practicing in health professional shortage areas

Box 11.7 Implementation Timeline for Key Medicare Provisions of the 2010 Health Care Reform Law, 2010–2015 (*Continued*)

Part D	• Begin phasing in federal subsidies for generic drugs in the Medicare Part D coverage gap (reducing coinsurance from 100 percent in 2010 to 25 percent by 2020) • Require pharmaceutical manufacturers to provide a 50 percent discount on brand-name prescriptions filled in the coverage gap (reducing coinsurance from 100 percent in 2010 to 50 percent in 2011)
Preventive services	• Eliminate Medicare cost sharing for some preventive services • Provide Medicare beneficiaries access to a comprehensive health risk assessment and creation of a personalized prevention plan
2012	
Cost containment	• Allow providers organized as accountable care organizations (ACOs) that voluntarily meet quality thresholds to share in the savings they achieve for the Medicare program • Reduce Medicare payments that would otherwise be made to hospitals by specified percentages to account for excess (preventable) hospital readmissions
Delivery system reforms	• Create the Medicare Independence at Home demonstration program • Establish a hospital value-based purchasing program and develop plans to implement value-based purchasing for skilled nursing facilities, home health agencies, and ambulatory surgical centers
Medicare Advantage	• Reduce rebates for Medicare Advantage plans • High-quality Medicare Advantage plans begin receiving bonus payments
Part D	• Make Part D cost sharing for dual eligible beneficiaries receiving home and community-based care services equal to the cost sharing for those who receive institutional care
2013	
Delivery system reforms	• Establish a national Medicare pilot program to develop and evaluate paying a bundled payment for acute inpatient hospital services, physician services, outpatient hospital services, and postacute care services for an episode of care
Part D	• Begin phasing in federal subsidies for brand-name drugs in the Part D coverage gap (reducing coinsurance from 100 percent in 2010 to 25 percent in 2020, in addition to the 50 percent manufacturer brand discount)
Tax changes	• Increase the Medicare Part A (hospital insurance) tax rate on wages by 0.9 percent (from 1.45 percent to 2.35 percent) on earnings over $200,000 for individual taxpayers and $250,000 for married couples filing jointly • Eliminate the tax deduction for employers who receive Medicare Part D retiree drug subsidy payments
2014	
Cost containment	• Independent Payment Advisory Board composed of 15 members begins submitting legislative proposals containing recommendations to reduce Medicare spending if spending exceeds a target growth rate • Reduce disproportionate share hospital (DSH) payments initially by 75 percent and subsequently increase payments based on the percentage of the population uninsured and the amount of uncompensated care
Medicare Advantage	• Require Medicare Advantage plans to have medical loss ratios no lower than 85 percent
Part D	• Reduce the out-of-pocket amount that qualifies for Part D catastrophic coverage (through 2019)
2015	
Cost containment	• Reduce Medicare payments to certain hospitals for hospital-acquired conditions by 1 percent

Source: "Summary of Key Changes to Medicare in 2010 Health Reform Law," (#7948-02) The Henry J. Kaiser Family Foundation, May 2010. This information was reprinted with permission from the Henry J. Kaiser Family Foundation. The Kaiser Family Foundation, a leader in health policy analysis, health journalism and communication, is dedicated to filling the need for trusted, independent information on the major health issues facing our nation and its people. The Foundation is a nonprofit operating foundation, based in Menlo Park, California.

Medicaid

A second type of government health insurance is **Medicaid**, a health insurance program for low-income Americans. Currently, approximately 56 million people are covered by Medicaid (almost three-fifths of those covered are children).[15] Eligibility for enrollment in Medicaid is determined by each state. Many Medicaid recipients are also enrolled in other types of public assistance programs (welfare). Unlike Medicare, there is no age requirement for Medicaid; eligibility requirements are primarily tied to income. Also, unlike Medicare, Medicaid is a noncontributory program jointly paid for and administered through federal and state governments. Both programs cover skilled nursing care but under different conditions.

For many states, one of the more costly items appearing in the annual state budget is the Medicaid program. Thus, like the federal government, state governments are always looking for ways to reshape their programs to become more efficient. Several states have combined their Medicaid program with their Children's Health Insurance Program (CHIP) (see CHIP discussion that follows) to provide better health care for low-income Americans. In addition, the HHS has provided, on a competitive basis, some states with special grants to develop other plans for extending healthcare coverage to the uninsured.

The Affordable Care Act made some significant changes to the Medicaid program. The U.S. Supreme Court ruling in June 2012 also had an impact. The biggest change deals with eligibility for the program. Eligibility prior to the new law was determined by each state in consultation with the federal government. Under healthcare reform, eligibility will be based solely on income and will be extended to more low-income people, including both parents and adults without dependent children.[47] As a result of these changes, nearly everyone under the age of 65 years with income below 133% of the poverty level (in 2011 that was $29,700 for a family of four) could qualify for Medicaid, significantly reducing the number of uninsured and state variation in coverage.[47] In the previous sentence we used the phrase "could qualify." The reason for this deals with the 2012 Supreme Court ruling regarding the constitutionality of the ACA that allow states to opt out of this Medicaid provision. As a part of that ruling the court limited, but did not invalidate, the provision. Prior to the ruling, states had to expand Medicaid or risk losing all Medicaid funding—an option no state could afford. The Supreme Court ruled that the federal government could not force this significant change to an already-existing program on the states.[48] Thus, states could opt out of covering up to 133% of the poverty level. At the time of the writing of this book it was unclear how many states might opt out, but several governors had pledged to do so.

> Some health care experts said it was unthinkable that state leaders would really opt out, since the vast majority of the cost is covered by the federal government—taxes their citizens will pay, regardless of whether the state opts in or out. For the first two years, the federal government pays for 100 percent of the expansion. Starting in 2017, the states start chipping in, but they will never contribute more than 10 percent of the cost.[48]

Children's Health Insurance Program

The **Children's Health Insurance Program (CHIP)** was created as part of the Balanced Budget Act of 1997. It was enacted to provide coverage to eligible low-income, uninsured children who do not qualify for Medicaid. Currently, approximately 8 million children are covered by CHIP. In 2009, President Obama extended CHIP through 2013 by signing the 2009 Children's Health Insurance Program Reauthorization Act (CHIPRA, or Public Law 111-3).[49] The Affordable Care Act has provisions to increase enrollment and extend funding until 2015.[49] Like Medicaid, this is a joint state–federal funded program. To help offset the cost of the reauthorization, the new law included an increase in the federal excise tax rate on tobacco products.[49]

Problems with Medicare and Medicaid

In theory, both the Medicare and Medicaid programs seem to be sound programs that help provide health care to two segments of society who would otherwise find it difficult or impossible to obtain health insurance. In practice, there are two recurrent problems with these programs. One problem is that some physicians and hospitals do not accept Medicare and Medicaid patients because of the tedious and time-consuming paperwork, lengthy delays in reimbursement, and insufficient reimbursement. As a result, it is difficult if not impossible for many of those eligible for Medicare and Medicaid to receive health care. The second problem occurs when physicians and hospitals file Medicare and Medicaid paperwork for care or services not rendered or rendered incompletely. This is known as *Medicare/Medicaid fraud*. These problems were known to Congress, so when the Affordable Care Act passed in 2010

Children's Health Insurance Program (CHIP) a title insurance program under the Social Security Act that provides health insurance to uninsured children

Medicaid a jointly funded federal–state health insurance program for low-income Americans

it included provisions to both increase payment to physicians and hospitals and crack down on fraud.

Supplemental Health Insurance

Medigap

As noted earlier, Parts A and B of Medicare have deductibles and co-insurance stipulations. To help cover these out-of-pocket costs and some other services not covered by Medicare, people can purchase supplemental policies from private insurance companies. These policies have come to be known as **Medigap** (also called Medicare Supplement Insurance) policies because they cover the "gaps" not covered by Medicare. Federal and state laws mandate national standardization of Medigap policies. Since their inception, 14 different standardized Medigap plans (titled A through N) have been used. Currently, there are only 10 plans (A–D, F, G,

K–N) available[50] (see **Box 11.8**). All plans are required to have a core set of benefits referred to as *basic benefits*; however, some of the basic benefits of plans K through N are offered at a reduced level. By law, the letters and benefits of the individual plans cannot be changed by the insurance companies. However, they may add names or titles to the letter designations. Companies are not required to offer all the plans. "Insurance companies selling Medigap policies are required to make Plan A available. If they offer any other Medigap plan, they must also offer either Medigap Plan C or Plan F."[50] Three states—Minnesota, Massachusetts, and Wisconsin—have exceptions to the 10-plan setup because they had alternative Medigap standardization programs in effect before the federal legislation was enacted. Individuals should contact the state insurance office in these states if interested in these plans.

Medigap private health insurance that supplements Medicare benefits

---

Box 11.8   Medigap Policies

How to read the chart:

If a check mark appears in a column of this chart, the Medigap policy covers 100% of the described benefit. If a row lists a percentage, the policy covers that percentage of the described benefit. If a row is blank, the policy doesn't cover that benefit. *Note:* The Medigap policy covers coinsurance only after you have paid the deductible (unless the Medigap policy also covers the deductible).

Medigap Benefits	Medigap Plans									
	A	B	C	D	F*	G	K	L	M	N
Medicare Part A Coinsurance and hospital costs up to an additional 365 days after Medicare benefits are used up	✓	✓	✓	✓	✓	✓	✓	✓	✓	✓
Medicare Part B Coinsurance or Copayment	✓	✓	✓	✓	✓	✓	50%	75%	✓	✓***
Blood (First 3 Pints)	✓	✓	✓	✓	✓	✓	50%	75%	✓	✓
Part A Hospice Care Coinsurance or Copayment	✓	✓	✓	✓	✓	✓	50%	75%	✓	✓
Skilled Nursing Facility Care Coinsurance			✓	✓	✓	✓	50%	75%	✓	✓
Medicare Part A Deductible		✓	✓	✓	✓	✓	50%	75%	50%	✓
Medicare Part B Deductible			✓		✓					
Medicare Part B Excess Charges					✓	✓				
Foreign Travel Emergency (Up to Plan Limits)			✓	✓	✓	✓			✓	✓
							Out-of-Pocket Limit**			
							$4,660	$2,330		

*Plan F also offers a high-deductible plan. If you choose this option, this means you must pay for Medicare-covered costs up to the deductible amount of $2,070 in 2012 before your Medigap plan pays anything.

**After you meet your out-of-pocket yearly limit and your yearly Part B deductible ($140 in 2012), the Medigap plan pays 100% of covered services for the rest of the calendar year.

***Plan N pays 100% of the Part B coinsurance, except for a copayment of up to $20 for some office visits and up to a $50 copayment for emergency room visits that don't result in an inpatient admission.

Source: Reproduced from Centers for Medicare and Medicaid Services (2011). *2012 Choosing a Medigap Policy: A Guide to Health Insurance for People with Medicare.* Baltimore, MD: Author, 11. Available at http://www.medicare.gov/Pubs/pdf/02110.pdf.

Two other variances to these Medigap rules should be noted. The first deals with those individuals enrolled in the Medicare Advantage program. Because Medicare Advantage is more comprehensive in coverage than is the traditional Medicare program, Medigap policies are not needed. In fact, it is illegal for insurance companies to sell a Medigap policy if they know a person is enrolled in Medicare Advantage.[50] Another variance in Medigap policy deals with Medicare SELECT, which is a type of Medigap policy that is available in some states. This type of policy still provides one of the standardized Medigap plans (A–D, F, G, K–N), but requires policy holders to use specific hospitals and, in some cases, doctors (except in emergencies) to receive full Medigap benefits.[50]

Other Supplemental Insurance

Medigap is a supplemental insurance program specifically designed for those on Medicare. However, a number of supplemental insurance policies exist for people regardless of their age. Included are specific-disease insurance, hospital indemnity insurance, and long-term care insurance. Specific-disease insurance, though not available in some states, provides benefits for only a single disease (such as cancer) or a group of specific diseases. Many policies are written as fixed-indemnity policies. Hospital indemnity coverage is insurance that pays a fixed amount for each day a person receives inpatient hospital services, and it pays up to a designated number of days. Long-term care insurance, which pays cash amounts for each day of covered nursing home or at-home care, is of great concern to many people, and it is presented next.

Long-Term Care Insurance

With people living longer and the cost of health care on the rise, more and more individuals are considering the purchase of long-term care insurance. It has been estimated that "(a)bout 70 percent of people over age 65 will require some type of long-term care services during their lifetime. More than 40 percent will need care in a nursing home."[51] Women need care for longer than do men. Most—about 80%—of long-term care will be provided in the home by unpaid caregivers,[52] usually family and friends. "The typical caregiver is a 46-year-old woman who is married and employed, and is caring for her widowed mother who

managed care "a system of health care delivery that (1) seeks to achieve efficiency by integrating the basic functions of health care delivery, (2) employs mechanisms to control utilization of medical services, and (3) determines the price at which the services are purchased and how much the providers get paid"[54]

does not live with her."[52] Yet, planning for long-term care requires people to think about possible future healthcare needs and how they will pay for them. Obviously, the cost of long-term care varies based on the level of care, the length of time the care is provided, where the care is provided, and in what part of the country. Recent figures show that "nursing home care averages $72,000 per year, assisted living facilities average $38,000 per year, and home health services average $21 per hour."[53] This cost is something that can quickly deplete a lifetime of savings. Medicare and other health insurance do not include most long-term care services. If people have fairly low income and savings, they may qualify for Medicaid, the federal public program that pays for most long-term care services. There is a good chance that individuals will have to pay for all or some of these services out of pocket; therefore, it may be important to consider long-term care insurance.[51]

Although long-term care is expensive, not everyone needs to buy long-term care insurance. Those who do not need it are those with low incomes and few assets who could be covered by Medicaid and the very wealthy who are able to pay the cost of the care out of pocket. Those who are most likely to benefit from long-term care insurance are those in between the poor and wealthy, especially older women. However, there are several reasons why all people should consider purchasing long-term care insurance. They include the following:

- To preserve financial assets
- To prevent the need for family members or friends to provide the care
- To enable people to stay independent in their homes longer
- To make it easier to get into the nursing home or assisted-living home of their choice

Managed Care

The failed attempt to adopt universal health care in the United States during the first term of President Clinton led to the movement of **managed care**. "Managed care refers to arrangements that link health care financing and service delivery and allows payers to exercise significant economic control over how and what services are delivered."[4] The transition to managed care in the United States was largely driven by a desire of employers, insurance companies, and the public to control soaring healthcare costs. Although the exact number of individuals enrolled in managed care programs is constantly changing, it has been estimated that in 2011, more than 210 million Americans,[55] approximately two-thirds of the total population, belonged to some form of a managed healthcare plan. These numbers cover not only workers who received their healthcare coverage from employers, but also some individuals who were covered by Medicare, Medicaid, and the military. Notably, more than 90% of employees insured through employer-sponsored health insurance are enrolled in managed care programs.

Managed healthcare plans are offered by managed care organizations (MCOs). MCOs function like insurance organizations. They offer policies, collect premiums, and bear financial risk; that is, MCOs take on the financial responsibility if the costs of the services exceed the revenue from the premiums. These organizations have agreements with certain doctors, hospitals, and other healthcare providers to give a range of services to plan members at reduced cost. MCOs have been structured in a variety of ways and are similar to the other healthcare organizations with which we are familiar (such as hospitals). Some are structured as nonprofit organizations, whereas others are for-profit and owned by a group of investors. "Regardless of their structure, their goals, however, are similar: to control costs through improved efficiency and coordination, to reduce unnecessary or inappropriate utilization, to increase access to preventive care, and to maintain or improve quality of care."[56]

The managed healthcare plans offered by these organizations vary and are always evolving as managed care practices mature. The plans also differ, both in cost and ease of receiving needed services. Although no plan pays for all the costs associated with medical care, some plans cover more than others do. Common features in managed care arrangements include:

- *Provider panels, often referred to as the network*: Specific physicians and other providers who are selected to care for plan members
- *Limited choice*: Members must use the providers affiliated with the plan or pay an additional amount
- *Gatekeeping*: Members must obtain a referral from a case manager for specialty care or inpatient services
- *Risk sharing*: Providers bear some of the health plan's financial risk through capitation and withholds
- **Quality management and utilization review**: The plan monitors provider practice patterns and medical outcomes to identify deviations from quality and efficiency standards.[4]

The utilization review can take the form of prospective utilization review (as precertification), concurrent utilization review (i.e., during the course of healthcare utilization), or retrospective utilization review (completed by reviewing medical records after the care has been provided).[1]

Types of Managed Care

As noted earlier, there are several different types of managed care arrangements, and because of the increasing cost of health care and the demands of consumers for better healthcare service, these arrangements continue to be adapted and developed. Prior to 1990, the types of MCOs were quite distinct. Since then, the differences between traditional forms of health insurance and managed care have narrowed considerably.[1] The following are the most commonly available arrangements.

Preferred Provider Organizations

The **preferred provider organization (PPO)** is a form of managed care closest to a fee-for-service plan. A PPO differs from the traditional fee-for-service plan in that the fee has been fixed (at a discounted rate) through a negotiation process between a healthcare provider (e.g., physicians, dentists, hospitals) and the PPO, and the provider agrees to accept this discounted rate as payment in full. It works in the following manner: A PPO approaches a provider, such as a group dental practice, and contracts with the dentists to provide dental services to all those covered by the PPO's insurance plan at a fixed (discount) rate. To the extent that the PPO succeeds in obtaining favorable prices, it can offer lower premiums, co-insurance, and copayments, and hence can attract more patients to enroll in its insurance plan. In addition to the PPO doctors making referrals, plan members can refer themselves to other doctors, including ones outside the plan. However, if they do choose to go outside the plan, they will have to meet the deductible and pay higher co-insurance. In addition, they may have to pay the difference between what the provider charges and what the plan pays. PPOs also control costs by requiring (1) preauthorization for hospital admissions (excluding emergencies), and (2) second opinions for major procedures such as surgery.[4] Advantages for the providers are that they (1) do not share in any financial risk as a condition of participation,[4] (2) are reimbursed on a fee-for-service basis to which they are accustomed,[4] (3) are assured a certain volume of patients, and (4) are assured that the patients will pay promptly (via the PPO). Approximately 108 million people were enrolled in PPOs in 2011.[55]

preferred provider organization (PPO) an organization that buys fixed-rate health services from providers and sells them to consumers

quality management and utilization review the analysis of provided health care for its appropriateness by someone other than the patient and provider

Health Maintenance Organizations

Health maintenance organizations (HMOs) are the oldest form of managed care. In 2011, just over 68 million people were enrolled in HMOs.[55] In an HMO, the insurance coverage and the delivery of medical care are combined into a single organization. The organization hires (through salaries or contracts) an individual doctor or groups of doctors to provide care and either builds its own hospital or contracts for the services of a hospital within the community. The organization then enrolls members, usually, but not always, through the workplace. Members (or their employers or the government [in the case of HMOs for Medicare and Medicaid]) make regular payments in advance on a fixed contract fee to the HMO. This contract may also include a deductible and copayment when service is provided. In return, the HMO is contractually obligated to provide the members with a comprehensive range of outpatient and inpatient services that are spelled out in the contract for a specific time period.

When members enroll in an HMO, they are given a list (network) of specific physicians/providers from which to select their primary care doctor (usually a family physician, internist, obstetrician-gynecologist, or pediatrician) and other healthcare providers. The primary care doctor (which some have referred to as the gatekeeper) serves as the member's regular doctor and coordinates the member's care, which means the member must contact his or her primary care doctor to be referred to a specialist. In many plans, care by a specialist is only paid for if the member is referred by the primary care doctor, thus the term *gatekeeper*. Also, if patients receive care outside the network, they must pay for all the costs, except in cases of emergency when physically not near a member of the network.

How do HMOs make a profit? An HMO's focus of care is different from that of a traditional fee-for-service provider. In an HMO, ill and injured patients become a "cost." An HMO does not make money on the ill but on keeping people healthy. The less the providers of an HMO see a patient, the lower the costs and the more profitable the organization. Therefore, most HMOs emphasize health promotion activities and primary and secondary care.

There are two main organizational models of HMOs—staff models and individual practice models—and each type has spawned several hybrids. These hybrids are referred to as **mixed model HMOs**.

Staff model: In **staff model HMOs**, the healthcare providers are employed (usually salaried) by the HMO and practice in common facilities paid for by the HMO. Staff model HMOs employ providers in all common specialties to provide services to their members. Special contracts are established with subspecialties for infrequently needed services. These providers are expected to follow the practice and procedures determined by the HMO. With the exception of the special contracts, the providers work only for the HMO, and thus do not have their own private practices. In most instances, the HMO contracts with a hospital for inpatient services. Nationwide, the number of staff model HMOs has been declining.

Independent practice association model: **Independent practice associations (IPAs)** are the most common type of HMO today. IPAs are legal entities separate from the HMO[1] that are physician organizations composed of community-based independent physicians in solo or group practices who provide services to HMO members.[4] "Instead of establishing contracts with individual physicians or groups, the HMO contracts with the IPA for physician services. Physicians do not have contracts with the HMO, but with the IPA."[1] Thus, the IPA acts as an intermediary and is paid a capitation amount by the HMO.[1]

Other HMO models: Three other HMO models are the group model, the network model, and the direct contract model. A **group model HMO** contracts with a multispecialty group practice and separately with one or more hospitals to provide services, whereas a **network model HMO** contracts with more than one medical group practice.[1] A **direct contract HMO** contracts with individual physicians as opposed to group practices.[4]

Point-of-Service Option

One of the major objections to HMOs is that the patients cannot freely select their provider. They are restricted to those with whom the HMO has contracted. Some HMOs have solved this problem with the **point-of-service (POS)**

---

direct contract HMO one that contracts with individual physicians as opposed to group practices

group model HMO one that contracts with a multispecialty group practice

health maintenance organizations (HMOs) groups that supply prepaid comprehensive health care with an emphasis on prevention

independent practice associations (IPAs) legal entities separate from the HMO that are physician organizations composed of community-based independent physicians in solo or group practices who provide services to HMO members

mixed model HMO a hybrid form of health maintenance organization

network model HMO one that contracts with more than one medical group practice

point-of-service (POS) option an option of an HMO plan that enables enrollees to be at least partially reimbursed for selecting a healthcare provider outside the plan

staff model HMO a health maintenance organization that hires its own staff of healthcare providers

option, which allows for a more liberal policy of enabling patients to select providers. With this option, members may choose a provider from within or outside the HMO network. Patients who obtain services outside the network generally must pay a higher deductible and co-insurance.

Medicare Advantage

As noted earlier, in some parts of the country Medicare recipients may have an HMO option available to them through the Medicare Advantage plan. In such plans, the Medicare recipient receives all Medicare-covered services from the HMO. In addition, the HMO may charge the beneficiary a premium (in addition to the Medicare Part B premium) to cover co-insurance and deductibles of Medicare and may include items and services not covered by Medicare. If this is the case, Medigap coverage cannot be purchased. In other cases, beneficiaries may receive other services not covered by Medicare at no charge or at a much lower cost than might be expected. In 2011, a little over one-fourth of the people in Medicare were covered by managed care plans.[55]

Medicaid and Managed Care

As has been noted throughout this chapter, managed care plans are also available for those covered by Medicaid. The rationale for offering such plans is to improve access to care by the establishment of contracted provider networks, as well as by promoting greater accountability for quality and costs. Each state in the United States offers such a plan, and depending on the state requirements, enrollment may or may not be voluntary. If it is mandatory, then the state is required to offer a choice of managed care plans and make efforts to inform beneficiaries about their choices.[4] In 2011, approximately 71% of the people covered by Medicaid were enrolled in managed care plans.[55]

National Health Insurance

National health insurance, or national health care, suggests a system in which the federal government assumes the responsibility for the healthcare costs of the entire population. In such a system, the costs are primarily paid for with tax dollars. Presently among all the developed countries of the world, there is only one that does not have a national healthcare plan for its citizens: the United States.

The national healthcare systems of the developed countries of the world fall into two basic models. The first is a national health service model with universal coverage and a general tax-financed government ownership of the facilities

and doctors as public employees. Countries using this model include the United Kingdom, Spain, Italy, Greece, and Portugal. The second is a social insurance model that provides universal coverage under social security, financed in various ways including taxes or contributions paid by employers and employees. In Canada, contributions are made to a government entity. In France and Germany, contributions go to nonprofit funds with national negotiation on fees. Japan also has a compulsory system that relies heavily on employer-based coverage.

When one considers the level of satisfaction with health care, the better access to healthcare services, the lower healthcare costs, and the superior health status indicators in these other countries, one must ask why the United States has not adopted such a program. It is not because the United States has not considered such a plan—in fact, there have been seven failed attempts at addressing the issue over the past 70+ years. The first came when President Roosevelt tried to include it as part of the New Deal. President Harry Truman presented a proposal to Congress on two different occasions, only to have it defeated twice. Other unsuccessful attempts at national healthcare legislation were made during the Kennedy, Nixon, and Clinton administrations. The most recent talk about a national health insurance program in the United States came during the presidential campaign and debates of 2008.

Although the push for national health insurance has not been successful, several states—including Florida, Hawaii, Massachusetts, Minnesota, Oregon, and Vermont—prior to 2010 passed major healthcare reform packages aimed at providing increased access to health insurance and basic health services to all or most of their residents.

Healthcare Reform in the United States

Prior to the passage of the Affordable Care Act (ACA) in 2010, the healthcare reform that took place in the United States in recent times was with specific smaller, but not insignificant, portions of the healthcare system—for example, President Clinton's creation of the Children's Health Insurance Program (CHIP) in 1997 and the reauthorization of the program by President Obama in 2009. During President George W. Bush's term in office, the reform came in the form of the Medicare Prescription Drug Improvement and Modernization Act (MMA) of 2003 (Public Law 108-173). The portion of the MMA that gained the greatest publicity—that dealing with prescription drugs via Medicare

Part D—was discussed earlier in the chapter. However another significant component of the MMA was health savings accounts (HSAs). HSAs are one of several different forms of consumer-directed health plans (CDHPs). In the sections that follow, we discuss both CDHPs and the major features of the Affordable Care Act.

Consumer-Directed Health Plans

Consumer-directed health plans (CDHPs) (also called consumer-driven health plans, consumer-directed health arrangements [CDHAs], consumer choice, and self-directed health plans [SDHPs][34]) have been defined several different ways. But whichever definition is used, they are health plan options that combine more consumer responsibility for healthcare decisions with a tax-sheltered account that consumers may use to pay for out-of-pocket healthcare costs and usually a high-deductible health insurance policy. A critical part of the CDHPs is providing those enrolled in such plans with comparative information to increase their knowledge about healthcare choices and associated costs.[4] The central idea behind CDHPs is that consumers will still have catastrophic health insurance, but because they are required to use more of their own money to pay for health care they will be more careful about their use of services than they would be under a traditional health plan that provides greater coverage of their initial healthcare costs.[34] Those options usually included in CDHPs are health savings accounts (HSAs), usually coupled with high-deductible health plans (HDHPs), health reimbursement arrangements (HRAs), flexible spending accounts (FSAs), and Archer Medical Savings Accounts (MSAs).

CDHPs are not without critics. There are three major concerns about CDHPs. One, will consumers become educated enough to make good decisions? Health insurance and health care are very complicated, and will consumers take the time to become well educated? Two, is the healthcare field transparent enough to get enough information to make a good decision? When was the last time a patient received a healthcare service and knew in advance what the cost would be? Also, how do consumers know when they are receiving quality care? Who is the best physician in the community? Who is the worst? And three, will consumers seek health care in a timely manner because with CDHPs they have to use more of their own money? For example, on a traditional plan maybe annual influenza

> **consumer-directed health plans (CDHPs)** health plan options that combine more consumer responsibility for decisions with a tax-sheltered account to pay for out-of-pocket costs for health care and a high-deductible health insurance policy

vaccinations were covered with a zero deductible, but with a CDHP that has a high deductible it now costs consumers $50 out of pocket. Will they still get the vaccine or will they try to save the $50 and forgo the vaccine?

The most visible of the CDHPs is the health savings account (HSA). An HSA is a type of medical savings account that allows people to save money to pay for current and future medical expenses on a tax-free basis. To be eligible for an HSA, people must be covered by a high-deductible plan (in 2013, the deductible was $1,250 for individuals and $2,500 for families),[58] not have any other health insurance (including Medicare), and not be claimed as a dependent on someone else's tax return. Those with HSAs can use this account to pay for qualified health expenses, including expenses that the plan ordinarily does not cover, such as hearing aids. By law, there is a maximum amount that people with HSAs would have to pay out of pocket for health expenses in a year. The amount is adjusted for inflation each year, but in 2013 the amount was $6,250 for individuals and $12,500 for families.[58]

During the year, those with HSAs can make voluntary contributions to the account using before-tax dollars. In 2013, the maximum amount that could be set aside was $3,250 for an individual, $6,450 for families, or the amount of the deductible of the health insurance policy, whichever was lower.[58] People age 55 or older can make addition "catch-up" contributions (in 2013, $1,000) until they enroll in Medicare.[57] In some cases, employers may set up and help fund HSAs for their employees, but they are not required to do so. An HSA earns interest. If there is a balance in a person's HSA at the end of the year, it will roll over, allowing the person to build up a cushion against future health expenses. In addition, HSAs allow people to accumulate funds and retain them when they change plans or retire.[57] Money can be withdrawn from the account without penalty to pay for care before the deductible is met and for things not covered under the health insurance policy after the deductible is met. Money can be withdrawn and pay for anything (nonhealth expenses) after 65 years of age, but the person must pay income tax on it. The advantages of such a plan are reduced premiums and, it is hoped, more prudent use of healthcare dollars—which should be good for both employers and employees. The major disadvantage for consumers is that they might have to pay more out of pocket for health care, and therefore might skip needed care. At the present, HSAs seem best suited for the healthy and wealthy.

The Affordable Care Act made several changes to HSAs. As of January 2011, HSAs could no longer be used tax-free for over-the-counter medications unless the medications were prescribed by a doctor. In addition, if people use their HSA funds for nonmedical expenses, they must pay a 20% penalty instead of the former 10% penalty.[42]

Although HSAs must be combined with high-deductible health plans (HDHPs), HDHPs do not have to be combined with HSAs. In fact, HDHPs are expected to grow in popularity because of their lower premium costs.[1] When these plans are used they are often accompanied by health promotion and wellness, disease management, case management, and health coaching programs to help participants improve and maintain health and keep medical conditions under control.[34]

Another type of CDHP is health reimbursement arrangements (HRAs). HRAs may be established by employers to pay employees' medical expenses. Only employers can set up HRAs for employees, and only employers can contribute to them. The employer decides how much money to put in a health reimbursement arrangement, and the employee can withdraw funds from the account to cover allowed expenses. HRAs often are established in conjunction with an HDHP, but they can be paired with any type of health plan or used as a standalone account. In addition, federal law allows employers to determine whether employees can carry over all or a portion of unspent funds from year to year. Also, employers can decide whether account balances will be forfeited if an employee leaves the job or changes health plans.[59] The Affordable Care Act also affected HRAs. Like HSAs, as of January 2011, HRA funds could no longer be used tax-free for over-the-counter medications unless the medications were prescribed by a doctor.[42]

Flexible spending accounts (FSAs) are set up by employers to allow employees to set aside pre-tax money to pay for qualified medical expenses during the year. Only employers may set up an account, and employers may or may not contribute to the account. There may be a limit on the amount that employers and employees can contribute to a health flexible spending arrangement. FSAs can be offered in conjunction with any type of health insurance plan, or they can be offered on a standalone basis. The tricky part of having an FSA is trying to determine how much money to place in the account in a year to avoid losing any money at year's end because unspent money does not roll over in the account; it goes back to the employer. Just like HRAs, as of January 2011, the Affordable Care Act no longer allowed FSA funds to be used tax-free for over-the-counter medications unless the medications were prescribed by a doctor.[42]

Archer Medical Savings Accounts (MSAs), the oldest of the CDHPs in use today, are individual accounts that may be set up by self-employed individuals and those who work for small businesses (less than 50 employees). To set up an MSA, people must be covered by an HDHP. Either the employee or the employer may contribute to the account, but both cannot contribute to the account in the same year. Individuals control the use of funds in the accounts and can withdraw funds for qualified medical expenses. Funds can be rolled over from year to year, and balances in the accounts are portable when changing jobs or retiring.

The Affordable Care Act made several changes to MSAs that were much like those made to HSAs. As of January 2011, MSAs could no longer be used tax-free for over-the-counter medications unless the medications were prescribed by a doctor. In addition, if people use their MSA funds for nonmedical expenses, they must pay a 15% penalty instead of the former 10% penality.[42]

Enrollment in CDHPs has been rising in recent years for three major reasons: (1) employers trying to cut healthcare costs, (2) consumers trying to reduce the cost of health insurance premiums, and (3) the tax advantages of most of the plans. Data from the National Health Interview Study showed that those more likely to be enrolled in a CDHP were those (1) who directly purchased private health plans, (2) with more education, and (3) with higher incomes.[60] More recent data show that "25.3% of persons under age 65 years with private health insurance were enrolled in a HDHP, including 7.7% who were enrolled in a CDHP and 17.6% who were enrolled in a HDHP without a health savings account (HSA)"[61] (see **Figure 11.12**). In terms of numbers, the American Association of Preferred Provider Organizations estimated that 28 million people were enrolled in CDHPs in 2010, up from 23 million in 2009—an increase of 22%.[62]

Affordable Care Act

Throughout this chapter, we have made reference to the Affordable Care Act (ACA) passed in 2010, and upheld by the U.S. Supreme Court in 2012, when information included in the act applied to a specific topic in the chapter. Here, we will provide some background on the ACA and some of its major features. Portions of the ACA went into effect in 2010, and the final portion will go into effect in 2020. Much of the law takes effect in 2014.

At the heart of the ACA was increasing the number of Americans who had health insurance and providing consumers with some healthcare/insurance rights that they have not received in the past. This will happen because of the mandate (i.e., individual mandate) that U.S. citizens

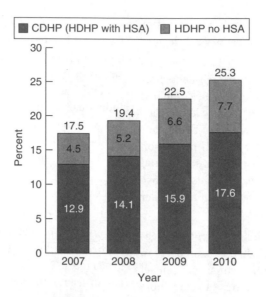

Figure 11.12 Percentage of persons under age 65 who are enrolled in a high-deductible health plan without a health savings account or in a consumer-directed health plan, among those with private health insurance: United States, 2007–2010.

Notes: HDHP no HSA is high-deductible health plan without a health savings account. CDHP is consumer-directed health plan, which is a HDHP with a HSA. The individual components of HDHPs may not add to up to the total, due to rounding.

Reproduced from Cohen, R. A., B. W. Ward, and J. S. Schiller (2012). *Health Insurance Coverage: Early Release of Estimates from the National Health Interview Survey, 2010.* Hyattsville, MD: National Center for Health Statistics. Available at http://www.cdc.gov/nchs/data/nhis/earlyrelease/insur201106.htm#fig03.

and legal residents have "'minimum essential' health insurance coverage"[63] or face a penalty up to 2.5% of income. As noted throughout this chapter, both the health care that is received and the health of people are better when people are insured. The people helped most by the ACA will be "the uninsured and intermittently insured, the underinsured, those who cannot afford their out-of-pocket costs or health insurance premiums, small businesses and their employees, young adults who will be able to stay on their parents' policies until they find a job with health benefits, and those who are denied coverage because they have preexisting conditions or major health problems."[43] Those individuals who are not covered under the ACA are the 15 million or so undocumented immigrants. In addition, it is unclear at this time what impact the "opt out" clause in the Medicaid expansion provision will have on the number of uninsured.

During his administration, President Clinton tried to pass a Patient's Bill of Rights at the national level. When those efforts fell short, many states created and passed their own Patient's Bill of Rights. The ACA included several different components that addressed patients' rights "to put

American consumers back in charge of their health coverage and care."[62] In June 2010,

> the Departments of Health and Human Services (HHS), Labor, and Treasury issued regulations to implement a new Patient's Bill of Rights under the Affordable Care Act—which will help children (and eventually all Americans) with preexisting conditions gain coverage and keep it, protect all Americans' choice of doctors and end lifetime limits on the care consumers may receive. These new protections apply to nearly all health insurance plans.[64]

Box 11.9 provides a brief summary of the major components of the ACA that address patients' rights.

As noted throughout this chapter, the ACA is not a simple piece of legislation. It included many items that changed the way health insurance is provided in the United States. Some of the changes are very obvious and easy to understand, whereas others could be skipped over by one not reading closely. Others are complicated and will take many people much time to completely understand and implement. To keep consumers up-to-date on the implementation of the ACA, the U.S. government has created an information website at www.healthcare.gov.

Box 11.9   The Affordable Care Act's New Patient's Bill of Rights

- *No pre-existing condition exclusions for children younger than age 19:* As of September 2010, the ACA prohibited insurance plans from limiting benefits for children and from refusing to sell children coverage at all based on the fact that a child had a pre-existing condition. This policy applies to all types of insurance except for individual market plans that were "grand-fathered." This critical policy will be broadened to Americans of all ages in 2014.

- *No unjustified rescissions of insurance coverage:* Prior to passage of ACA, insurance companies were able to retroactively cancel someone's policy when they became sick, or if they or their employers made an unintentional mistake on their paperwork. Under the ACA, insurers are prohibited from rescinding coverage—for individuals or groups of people—except in cases involving fraud or an intentional misrepresentation of material facts. There are no exceptions to this policy.

- *No lifetime limits on coverage:* The ACA prohibited insurance plans from stopping benefits when the cost of care for a patient reached a lifetime limit set by the insurance company. No plan issued or renewed after September 23, 2010, could use such a limit.

- *Restricted annual limits on coverage:* Even more binding than lifetime limits were annual dollar limits on what an insurance company would pay for health care. The ACA is phasing out the use of annual limits over a 3-year period for most health plans before banning such limits entirely in 2014.

- *Protecting choice of doctors:* The ACA made it clear that health plan members were free to designate any available (in the plan network) participating primary care provider as their primary care provider.

- *Removing insurance company barriers to emergency department services:* The ACA made emergency services more accessible for consumers. Health insurers are not able to charge higher cost sharing (copayments or co-insurance) for emergency services obtained outside the health plan's network.

Source: Sebelius, K. (2010). "Health Care Notes: Protecting Patients with Private Insurance." Available at http://www.healthcare.gov/blog/2010/06/patient protections.html.

Chapter Summary

- The concept of a healthcare system has been and continues to be questioned in the United States. Is it really a system or is treatment provided in an informal, cooperative manner?
- There are medical specialists and healthcare facilities for almost every type of illness and health problem.
- The spectrum of health care includes four domains of practice—population-based public health practice, medical practice, long-term practice, and end-of-life practice.
- Within the medical practice domain of health care are the following types of healthcare providers: independent providers (allopathic, osteopathic, and nonallopathic), limited (restricted) care providers, nurses, nonphysician practitioners, allied healthcare professionals, and public health professionals.
- Complementary and alternative medicine (CAM) is "a group of diverse medical and health care systems, practices, and products that are not presently considered to be a part of conventional medicine."[4]
- Healthcare providers perform services in both inpatient and outpatient care facilities.
- Inpatient care facilities include hospitals, nursing homes, and assisted living facilities.

- The types of outpatient care facilities found in communities include healthcare practitioners' offices, clinics, primary care centers, retail clinics, urgent/emergent care centers, ambulatory surgery centers, and freestanding service facilities.
- Long-term care options include traditional institutional residential care as well as special units within these residential facilities, halfway houses, group homes, assisted-living facilities, transitional (step-down) care in a hospital, day care facilities for patients, and personal home health care.
- The major issues of concern with the healthcare system in the United States can be summed up by the cost containment, access, and quality triangle.
- Some of the barriers to access to health care in the United States have been the lack of health insurance, inadequate insurance, and poverty.
- There are a number of different methods by which the amount of reimbursement to healthcare providers is determined. They include fee-for-service, packaged pricing, resource-based relative value scale, capitation, and prospective reimbursement.
- Most health care in the United States is paid for via third-party payment.

- Key health insurance terms include *deductible, co-insurance, copayment, fixed indemnity, exclusion*, and *preexisting condition.*
- The two largest government-administered health insurance programs in the United States are Medicare and Medicaid.
- The government's Children's Health Insurance Program (CHIP) is for many children who were previously uninsured.
- Two major supplemental insurance programs in the United States are Medigap and long-term care insurance.
- A significant portion of Americans today are covered by some form of managed care.
- The more common forms of managed care are health maintenance organizations (HMOs), preferred provider organizations (PPOs), and point-of-service (POS) options.
- The United States is the only developed country in the world without national health insurance.
- Consumer-directed health plans, including health savings accounts (HSAs), high-deductible health plans (HDHPs), health reimbursement arrangements (HRAs), flexible spending accounts (FSAs), and Archer Medical Savings Accounts (MSAs), are becoming more popular health plan options.
- Healthcare reform in the United States did not come easily, but the Affordable Care Act will significantly increase the number of Americans who have health insurance.

Review Questions

1. Why have some questioned whether the United States really has a healthcare system?
2. Describe some of the major changes that have taken place in healthcare delivery over the years.
3. What is meant by third-party payment?
4. Why has the cost of health care in the United States continued to grow faster than the cost of inflation?
5. What is meant by a spectrum of health care?
6. What are the domains of practice noted in the spectrum of health care?
7. Is there a demand for healthcare workers in the United States today? If so, why?
8. In what type of facility are most healthcare workers employed?
9. What is the difference between independent and limited (restricted) care providers?
10. What are the differences between allopathic and nonallopathic healthcare providers?
11. Define *complementary and alternative medicine* and give a few examples of each.
12. What kind of education do limited (restricted) care providers have?
13. What is the difference between LPNs and RNs?
14. What are advanced practice nurses (APRNs)?
15. What are nonphysician practitioners?
16. What role do public health professionals play in healthcare delivery?
17. What are the advantages of outpatient care facilities?
18. What is a long-term care facility? Give two examples.
19. Why has the number of home healthcare agencies increased in recent years?
20. What are three major problems facing the healthcare system in the United States?
21. How is the quality of healthcare services measured?
22. Explain how each of the following types of reimbursement works: fee-for-service, packaged pricing, resource-based relative value scale, capitation, and prospective reimbursement.
23. On what basic concept is insurance based?
24. Explain the following insurance policy provisions: (a) a $200 deductible, (b) 20/80 co-insurance, (c) a $4,500 fixed indemnity for a basic surgical procedure, (d) an exclusion of the preexisting condition of lung cancer, and (e) a $10 copayment.
25. What is the difference between Medicare and Medicaid?
26. What is covered in each of the four parts of Medicare—Parts A, B, C, and D?
27. What relationship does Medigap insurance have to Medicare?
28. What is the Children's Health Insurance Program (CHIP)?

29. Briefly explain the differences among health maintenance organizations (HMOs), preferred provider organizations (PPOs), and a point-of-service option.
30. What are the advantages and disadvantages of managed care?
31. What is meant by the term *consumer-directed health plans*? Give some examples.
32. What is the major result of the Affordable Care Act passed in 2010?

Activities

1. Using Table 11.1 from this chapter, identify two different healthcare facilities in your community for each of the levels of care. Briefly describe each facility and determine whether each is private, public, or voluntary.
2. Make an appointment to interview three healthcare workers in your community who have different types of jobs. Ask them what they like and dislike about their work, what kind of education they needed, whether they are happy with their work, and whether they would recommend that others seek this line of work. Summarize your findings in a written paper.
3. Make an appointment to interview an administrator in the local (city or county) health department. In the interview, find out what kind of people, by profession, work in the department. Also find out what type(s) of healthcare services and clinics are offered by the department. Summarize your findings in a two-page paper.
4. Obtain a copy of the student health insurance policy available at your school. After reading the policy, summarize in writing what you have read. In your summary, indicate what type of reimbursement system is used to pay providers, and list specifics about the premium costs, deductible, co-insurance, copayment, fixed indemnity, and any exclusions.
5. Visit an HMO in your area and find the answers to the following: (a) What type of HMO is it? (b) How does one enroll? (c) What does it cost? (d) What services are provided? and (e) Why should someone get his or her health care from an HMO instead of the more traditional private-practice physician?

Community Health on the Web

The Internet contains a wealth of information about community and public health. Increase your knowledge of some of the topics presented in this chapter by accessing the Jones & Bartlett Learning website at **go.jblearning.com /McKenzieBrief** and follow the links to complete the following Web activities:

- The Henry J. Kaiser Family Foundation, Health Reform Source
- Medicare and Medicaid
- Affordable Care Act

References

1. Shi, L., and D. A. Singh (2012). *Delivering Health Care in America: A Systems Approach*, 5th ed. Burlington, MA: Jones & Bartlett Learning.
2. Institute of Medicine (2003). *The Future of the Public's Health in the 21st Century*. Washington, DC: National Academy Press.
3. Rothstein, W. G. (1972). *American Physicians in the Nineteenth Century: From Sect to Science*. Baltimore, MD: Johns Hopkins University Press.
4. Sultz, H. A., and K. M. Young (2011). *Health Care USA: Understanding Its Organization and Delivery*, 7th ed. Burlington, MA: Jones & Bartlett Learning.

5. Koff, S. Z. (1987). *Health Systems Agencies: A Comprehensive Examination of Planning and Process*. New York, NY: Human Services Press.

6. Stockman, D. A. (1981). "Premises for a Medical Marketplace: A Neoconservative's Vision of How to Transform the Health System." *Health Affairs*, 1(1): 5–18.

7. Zatkin, S. (1997). "A Health Plan's View of Government Regulation." *Health Affairs*, 16(6): 33–35.

8. MacKay, A. P., L. A. Fingerhut, and C. R. Duran (2000). *Health, United States, 2000, with Adolescent Health Chartbook*. Hyattsville, MD: National Center for Health Statistics.

9. Dickerson, J. F. (8 December 1997). "Dr. Clinton Scrubs Up." *Time*, 48.

10. White House (5 April 2006). "Fact Sheet: Health Savings Accounts: Affordable and Accessible Health Care" [Press release]. Available at http://georgewbush-whitehouse.archives.gov/news/releases/2006/04/20060405-6.html.

11. U.S. Department of Health and Human Services, Centers for Medicare and Medicaid Services (2012). "National Health Expenditure Data." Available at http://www.cms.gov/Research-Statistics-Data-and-Systems/Statistics-Trends-and-Reports/NationalHealthExpendData/index.html.

12. Turnock, B. J. (2012). *Public Health: What It Is and How It Works,* 5th ed. Burlington, MA: Jones & Bartlett Learning.

13. U.S. Public Health Service (1994). *For a Healthy Nation: Return on Investments in Public Health*. Washington, DC: U.S. Department of Health and Human Services.

14. Bernstein, A. B., E. Hing, A. J. Moss, K. F. Allen, A. B. Siller, and R. B. Tiggle (2004). *Health Care in America: Trends in Utilization*. Hyattsville, MD: National Center for Health Statistics.

15. National Center for Health Statistics (2012). *Health, United States, 2011: With Special Feature on Socioeconomic Status and Health*. Hyattsville, MD: Author.

16. National Center for Health Statistics (2011). *Health, United States, 2010: With Special Feature on Death and Dying*. Hyattsville, MD: Author.

17. U.S. Department of Labor, Bureau of Labor Statistics (2009). "Spotlight on Statistics: Health Care." Available at http://www.bls.gov/spotlight/2009/health_care/.

18. American Osteopathic Association (2006). "The History of Osteopathic Medicine: Virtual Museum." Available at http://history.osteopathic.org.

19. American Osteopathic Association (2012). "What Is a DO?" Available at http://www.osteopathic.org/osteopathic-health/about-dos/what-is-a-do/Pages/default.aspx.

20. National Institutes of Health, National Center for Complementary and Alternative Medicine (2011). "What Is Complementary and Alternative Medicine?" Available at http://nccam.nih.gov/health/whatiscam.

21. American Association of Colleges of Nursing (2012). "Nursing Shortage." Available at http://www.aacn.nche.edu/media-relations/fact-sheets/nursing-shortage.

22. Stanfield, P. S., N. Cross, and Y. H. Hui (2012). *Introduction to the Health Professions*, 6th ed. Burlington, MA: Jones & Bartlett Learning.

23. U.S. Department of Labor, Bureau of Labor Statistics (2012). "*Occupational Outlook Handbook*: Licensed Practical and Licensed Vocational Nurses." Available at http://www.bls.gov/ooh/healthcare/licensed-practical-and-licensed-vocational-nurses.htm.

24. U.S. Department of Labor, Bureau of Labor Statistics (2012). "*Occupational Outlook Handbook*: Registered Nurses." Available at http://www.bls.gov/ooh/Healthcare/Registered-nurses.htm.

25. U.S. Department of Health and Human Services, Health Resources and Services Administration (2010). "The Registered Nurse Population: Initial Findings from the 2008 National Sample Survey of Registered Nurses." Available at http://bhpr.hrsa.gov/healthworkforce/rnsurvey2008.html.

26. Griffin, D. J. (2012). *Hospitals: What They Are and How They Work*, 4th ed. Burlington, MA: Jones & Bartlett Learning.

27. National Association of Community Health Centers (2012). "Research & Data." Available at http://www.nachc.org/Research%20Snapshots.cfm.

28. Coleman, B. (2000). *Assuring the Quality of Home Care: The Challenge of Involving the Consumer*. Washington, DC: American Association of Retired People.

29. Alliance for Health Reform (2010). *Covering Heath Issues,* 5th ed. Available at http://www.allhealth.org/covering-health-issues-5th-edition/toc.asp.

30. Kissick, W. L. (1994). *Medicine's Dilemmas: Infinite Needs Versus Finite Resources*. New Haven, CT: Yale University Press.

31. Institute of Medicine (2004). *Insuring America's Health: Principles and Recommendations*. Available at http://www.iom.edu/Reports/2004/Insuring-Americas-Health-Principles-and-Recommendations.aspx.

32. Cohen R. A., B. W. Ward, and J. S. Schiller (2011). "Health Insurance Coverage: Early Release of Estimates from the National Health Interview Survey, 2010." Available from: http://www.cdc.gov/nchs/nhis.htm.

33. Adams, P. F., and P. M. Barnes (2006). "Summary Health Statistics for U.S. Population: National Health Interview Survey, 2004." *Vital and Health Statistics*, 10(229). Available at http://www.cdc.gov/nchs/products/series/series10.htm.

34. Slee, D. A., V. N. Slee, and H. J. Schmidt (2008). *Slee's Health Care Terms*, 5th ed. Sudbury, MA: Jones & Bartlett.

35. Institute of Medicine (2002). *Care Without Coverage: Too Little, Too Late*. Washington, DC: National Academies Press.

36. Kaiser Family Foundation (2010). "Summary of Coverage Provisions in the Affordable Care Act." Available at http://www.kff.org/healthreform/8023.cfm.

37. Institute of Medicine (2001). *Crossing the Quality Chasm: A New Health System for the 21st Century*. Washington, DC: Author. Available at http://iom.edu/Reports/2001/Crossing-the-Quality-Chasm-A-New-Health-System-for-the-21st-Century.aspx.

38. U.S. Department of Health and Human Services, Agency for Healthcare Research and Quality (2012). *National Healthcare Quality Report–2011* (AHRQ pub. no. 12-0005). Rockville, MD: Author. Available at http://www.ahrq.gov/qual/qrdr11.htm.

39. U.S. Department of Health and Human Services, Agency for Healthcare Research and Quality (2012). *National Healthcare Disparities Report–2011* (AHRQ pub. no. 12-0006). Rockville, MD: Author. Available at http://www.ahrq.gov/qual/qrdr11.htm.

40. National Committee for Quality Assurance (2012). "About NCQA." Available at http://www.ncqa.org/tabid/675/Default.aspx.

41. Squires, D. A. (2012). *Explaining High Health Care Spending in the United States: An International Comparison of Supply, Utilization, Prices, and Quality*. New York, NY: Commonwealth

Fund. Available at: http://www.commonwealthfund.org/Publications/Issue-Briefs/2012/May/High-Health-Care-Spending.aspx.

42. Kaiser Family Foundation (2010). "Summary of New Health Reform Law." Available at http://www.kff.org/healthreform/8061.cfm.

43. Davis, K. (2010). *A New Era in American Health Care: Realizing the Potential of Reform.* New York, NY: Commonwealth Fund. Available at http://www.commonwealthfund.org/Content/Publications/Fund-Reports/2010/Jun/A-New-Era-in-American-Health-Care.aspx.

44. The Patient Protection and Affordable Care Act, Public Law Numbers 111-148 and 111-152, Consolidated Print.

45. Centers for Medicare and Medicaid Services (2013). *Medicare & You.* Baltimore, MD: Author. Available at http://www.medicare.gov/medicare-and-you/medicare-and-you.html.

46. Kaiser Family Foundation (2010). *Medicare: A Primer.* Menlo Park, CA: Author. Available at http://www.kff.org/medicare/7615.cfm.

47. Kaiser Family Foundation (2010). *Medicaid: A Primer.* Menlo Park, CA: Author. Available at http://www.kff.org/medicaid/7334.cfm.

48. Condon, S. (2 July 2012). "States Opting Out of Medicaid Expansion Could Leave Many Uninsured." Available from http://www.cbsnews.com/8301-503544_162-57465110-503544/states-opting-out-of-medicaid-expansion-could-leave-many-uninsured/?tag=cbsnewsMainColumnArea.

49. U.S. Department of Health and Human Services, Centers for Medicare and Medicaid Services (2012). "Children's Health Insurance Program (CHIP)." Available at http://www.medicaid.gov/Medicaid-CHIP-Program-Information/By-Topics/Childrens-Health-Insurance-Program-CHIP/Childrens-Health-Insurance-Program-CHIP.html.

50. Centers for Medicare and Medicaid Services (2011). *2012 Choosing a Medigap Policy: A Guide to Health Insurance for People with Medicare.* Baltimore, MD: Author.

51. U.S. Department of Health and Human Services (2012). "National Clearinghouse for Long Term Care Information." Available at http://www.longtermcare.gov/LTC/Main_Site/Index.aspx.

52. Kaiser Family Foundation (2009). *The Sleeper in Health Reform: Long-Term Care and the CLASS Act.* Menlo Park, CA:

Author. Available at http://www.kff.org/healthcareform/kcmv102009pkg.cfm.

53. Kaiser Family Foundation (2009). "Medicaid and the Uninsured: Fact Sheet." Menlo Park, CA: Author. Available at http://www.kff.org/medicaid/2186.cfm.

54. Shi, L., and D. A. Singh (2013). *Essentials of the U.S. Health Care System,* 3rd ed. Burlington, MA: Jones & Bartlett Learning.

55. MCOL (2011). "Managed Care Fact Sheets." Available at http://www.mcol.com/factsheetindex.

56. Institute of Medicine (1997). *Managing Managed Care: Quality Improvement in Behavioral Health.* Washington, DC: National Academy Press.

57. MCOL (2012). "Home." Available at http://www.mcol.com.

58. Internal Revenue Service (2012). *Publication 969.* Available at http://www.irs.gov/publications/p969/ar02.html#d0e710.

59. U.S. Department of Health and Human Services, Agency for Healthcare Research and Quality (2007). *What Is Consumer-Directed Coverage?* Available at http://innovations.ahrq.gov/content.aspx?id=2421.

60. Cohen, R. A., and M. E. Martinez (2009). *Consumer-Directed Health Care for Persons Under 65 Years of Age with Private Health Insurance: United States, 2007* (NCHS Data Brief no. 15). Hyattsville, MD: National Center for Health Statistics.

61. Cohen, R. A., B. W. Ward, and J. S. Schiller (2012). *Health Insurance Coverage: Early Release of Estimates from the National Health Interview Survey, 2010.* Hyattsville, MD: National Center for Health Statistics. Available at http://www.cdc.gov/nchs/data/nhis/earlyrelease/insur201106.htm.

62. American Association of Preferred Provider Organizations (2012). *2011 Study of Consumer-Directed Health Plan (CDHP) Growth.* Available at http://www.aappo.org/Newsroom.aspx.

63. Supreme Court of the United States (28 June 2012). "2011 Term Opinions of the Court." Available at http://www.supremecourt.gov/opinions/slipopinions.aspx?Term=11.

64. U.S. Department of Health and Human Services (2010). "The Affordable Care Act's New Patient's Bill of Rights." Available at http://www.healthcare.gov/news/factsheets/aca_new_patients_bill_of_rights.html.

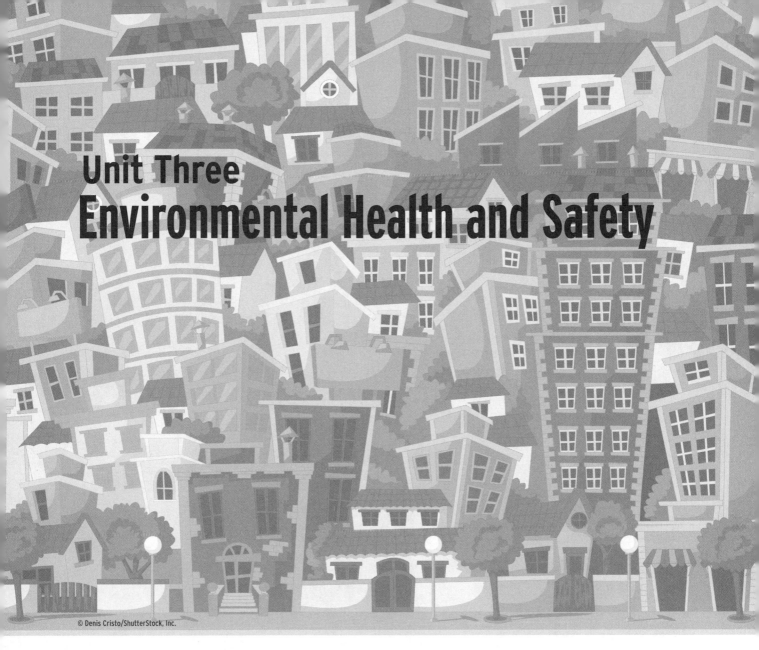

Unit Three
Environmental Health and Safety

© Denis Cristo/ShutterStock, Inc.

Chapter 12

Community Health and the Environment

Robert R. Pinger, PhD

Chapter Objectives

After studying this chapter, you will be able to:

1. List the sources and types of air pollutants, including the criteria pollutants, and explain the difference between primary and secondary pollutants.

2. Describe the role of the Environmental Protection Agency (EPA) in protecting the environment.

3. Outline the provisions of the Clean Air Act and the purposes of the National Ambient Air Quality Standards and the Air Quality Index.

4. List the major types of indoor air pollutants and describe ways to reduce exposure to them.

5. Explain the difference between point source and nonpoint source pollution.

6. Define what is meant by the term *waterborne disease outbreak* and list some of the causative agents.

7. Describe the measures communities take to ensure the quality of drinking water and the measures communities take to manage wastewater.

8. Explain the purposes of the Clean Water and the Safe Drinking Water Acts.

9. Name some of the agents associated with foodborne disease outbreaks and list some of the factors that lead to their occurrence.

10. Describe the roles of the agencies that help protect the safety of our food.

11 Explain the advantages and hazards of agricultural pesticide use.

12 Describe the composition of municipal solid waste (MSW) and outline acceptable MSW management strategies.

13 Define *hazardous waste* and give some examples.

14 Explain the purposes of the Resource Conservation and Recovery Act (RCRA) and the Comprehensive Environmental Response, Compensation, and Liability Act (CERCLA).

15 Describe the health hazards associated with lead in our environment.

16 Explain how environmental mismanagement can lead to vectorborne disease outbreaks.

17 List the kinds of environmental hazards found in our places of work and provide examples of these.

18 Define *ionizing radiation* and explain how it is deleterious to our health.

19 List the ways that natural disasters can affect the health of a community.

20 Explain how overpopulation can affect the environment and our health.

21 Define *terrorism* and explain how it can affect the environment of a community.

22 Explain the roles of the Federal Emergency Management Agency (FEMA) and the American Red Cross in disaster preparedness and relief.

Introduction

Our health is affected by the quality of our environment where we live and work, including the air we breathe, the water we drink, and the food we eat. The demands of our growing population for food, water, living space, and energy endanger the quality of our air, the purity of our water, the safety of our food, and the health of our planet. Having recognized the implications of environmental degradation on our health and the health of our communities, we have begun to accept our responsibility for the stewardship of our planet and enact regulatory measures to address some of our most egregious environmental assaults.

Environmental health is the study and management of environmental conditions that affect our health and well-being. **Environmental hazards** are those factors or conditions in the environment that increase the risk of human injury, disease, or death. The aim of this chapter is to examine common environmental hazards and describe community efforts to protect our health. We begin with a discussion of environmental concerns surrounding our air, water, and food resources. Then, we discuss solid and hazardous waste management and environmental concerns in the workplace. We conclude with a discussion of natural and sociological environmental hazards.

air pollution contamination of the air that interferes with the comfort, safety, and health of living organisms

environmental hazards factors or conditions in the environment that increase the risk of human injury, disease, or death

environmental health the study and management of environmental conditions that affect the health and well-being of humans

primary pollutants air pollutants emanating directly from transportation, power and industrial plants, and refineries

The Air We Breathe

Nothing has been more important to the development of life as we know it on earth than the composition of the air we breathe. By polluting the air, we endanger our health and risk leaving a deteriorating environment to future generations.

Outdoor Air Pollution

Air pollution is the contamination of the air by substances—gases, liquids, or solids—in amounts great enough to harm humans, other living organisms, or the ecosystem, or that alter climate. These contaminants or pollutants can arise from natural or human sources. Natural sources include dust storms, forest fires, and volcanic eruptions. Human sources can be divided into mobile sources, such as motor vehicles, and stationary sources, such as power plants and factories.

In the United States, major sources are (1) transportation, including privately owned motor vehicles; (2) electric power plants fueled by oil and coal; and (3) industry, primarily mills and refineries. In addition to these major sources, there are many smaller sources, such as wood- and coal-burning stoves, fireplaces, dry-cleaning facilities, and incinerators.

Polluting chemicals can be divided into primary and secondary pollutants. **Primary pollutants** include those emanating directly from the sources listed previously. They include carbon monoxide, carbon dioxide, sulfur dioxide, nitrogen oxides, most hydrocarbons, and most suspended particles. **Secondary pollutants** are formed when primary pollutants react with one another or with other atmospheric components to form new harmful chemicals. Secondary pollutants include nitrogen dioxide, nitric acid, nitrate salts, sulfur trioxide, sulfate salts, sulfuric acid, peroxyacyl nitrates, and ozone.[1] Because sunlight promotes the formation of these secondary pollutants, the resulting smog is referred to as **photochemical smog** (brown smog). This term is used to contrast photochemical smog with **industrial smog** (gray smog) formed primarily by sulfur dioxide and suspended solid particles.

Living in communities where air pollution reaches harmful levels can result in both acute and chronic health problems. Acute effects include burning eyes, shortness of breath, and increased incidence of colds, coughs, nose irritation, and other respiratory illness. In severe pollution episodes, deaths have been reported.[2] Chronic effects include chronic bronchitis, emphysema, increased incidence of bronchial asthma attacks, and, perhaps, lung cancer from air pollution.

Ozone represents perhaps the single most dangerous air pollutant. Breathing ozone can cause chest pain, coughing, throat irritation, congestion, bronchitis, emphysema, asthma, and reduced lung function. Repeated exposure to ground level ozone may permanently scar lung tissue. Even healthy people can experience breathing problems if exposed to ozone at high enough levels. In many urban and suburban areas throughout the United States concentrations of ground-level ozone exceed air quality standards.

One cause of excessive levels of ground-level ozone is a phenomenon referred to as a **thermal inversion**. This occurs when a layer of warm air settles above cooler air close to the earth's surface, preventing the cooler air from rising. Ozone then accumulates in the cooler air, the air we breathe. The longer a thermal inversion continues, the more likely it is that pollutants will reach dangerously high levels (see **Figure 12.1**).[2]

Regulation of Outdoor Air Quality

Steady deterioration of air quality in the 1950s and 1960s led to passage of the **Clean Air Act (CAA)** of 1963, which provided the federal government with the authority to address interstate air pollution problems. The 1970 amendments to the CAA issued emission standards for automobiles and new industries, and ambient air quality standards for urban areas.[2] The latter are known as the **National Ambient Air Quality Standards (NAAQSs)**.

The **Environmental Protection Agency (EPA)**, the federal agency primarily responsible for setting, maintaining, and enforcing environmental standards, is empowered to regulate air quality and is authorized to levy fines against those who violate the standards. The EPA sets limits on how much of a pollutant can be in the air anywhere in the United States. The air pollutants of greatest concern in the United States are called **criteria pollutants**, namely, sulfur dioxide, carbon monoxide, nitrogen oxides, ground-level ozone, respirable particulate matter, and lead (see **Table 12.1**). The EPA monitors the levels of each of these six pollutants in the ambient (outdoor) air to determine if and when they exceed the NAAQSs. Between 1990 and 2008, the United States substantially reduced the ambient air concentrations of all six of the criteria.[3] Nonetheless, in 2008, approximately 127 million people in the United States lived in counties with pollution levels above the NAAQSs.[3] To make it easier for all of us to understand daily air quality and what it means for your health, the EPA calculates the **Air Quality Index (AQI)** for five criteria air pollutants regulated by the Clean Air Act. The index tells you how clean or polluted your air is, and what associated health effects might be of concern for you or sensitive people in your community.

The value of the AQI on a particular day can range from 0 (good air quality) to 500 (hazardous air quality). AQI values below 100 are generally thought of as satisfactory, whereas values above 100 are considered to be unhealthy—at first for certain sensitive groups of people. Weather channels and websites might use a

Air Quality Index (AQI) an index that indicates the level of pollution in the air and the associated health risk

Clean Air Act (CAA) the federal law that provides the government with authority to address interstate air pollution

criteria pollutants the most pervasive air pollutants and those of greatest concern in the United States

Environmental Protection Agency (EPA) the federal agency primarily responsible for setting, maintaining, and enforcing environmental standards

industrial smog smog formed primarily by sulfur dioxide and suspended particles from the burning of coal, also known as gray smog

National Ambient Air Quality Standards (NAAQSs) standards created by the Environmental Protection Agency for allowable concentration levels of outdoor air pollutants

ozone O_3, an inorganic molecule considered to be a pollutant in the atmosphere because it harms human tissue, but considered beneficial in the stratosphere because it screens out ultraviolet radiation

photochemical smog smog formed when air pollutants interact with sunlight

secondary pollutants air pollutants formed when primary air pollutants react with sunlight and other atmospheric components to form new harmful compounds

thermal inversion a condition that occurs when warm air traps cooler air at the surface of the earth

Table 12.1 Criteria Pollutants

Pollutant (designation)	Form(s)	Major Sources (in order of percentage of contribution)
Carbon monoxide (CO)	Gas	Transportation, industrial processes, other solid waste, stationary fuel combustion
Lead (Pb)	Metal or aerosol	Transportation, industrial processes, stationary fuel combustion, solid waste
Nitrogen dioxide (NO$_2$)	Gas	Stationary fuel combustion, transportation, industrial processes, solid waste
Ground-level ozone (O$_3$)	Gas	Transportation, industrial processes, solid waste, stationary fuel combustion
Particulate matter	Solid or liquid	Industrial processes, stationary fuel combustion, transportation, solid waste
Sulfur dioxide (SO$_2$)	Gas	Stationary fuel combustion, industrial processes, transportation, other wastes

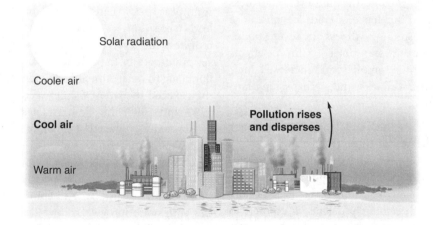

(a) Normal pattern

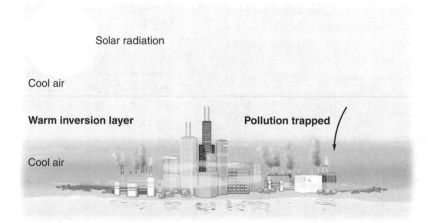

(b) Thermal inversion

Figure 12.1 A thermal inversion.

Chiras, D. D. (2010). *Environmental Science*, 8th ed. Sudbury, MA: Jones & Bartlett Learning.

color-coded AQI to make it more easily understood (see **Figure 12.2**).[4]

The 1990 amendments to the CAA set deadlines for establishing emission standards for 190 toxic chemicals that had not been previously addressed, established pollution taxes on toxic chemical emissions, and tightened emission standards for automobiles.

Although our primary focus has been on the health benefits of air quality regulation, some mention should be made of the role of air pollution in climate change. In this regard, it should be noted that reducing the level of **greenhouse gases**, such as carbon dioxide, chlorofluorocarbons, ozone, methane, water vapor, and nitrous oxide, will reduce heat retention in the atmosphere and slow global climate change.

Indoor Air Pollution

Sources of indoor air pollution include building and insulation materials, biogenic pollutants, combustion by-products, home furnishings, paint, cleaning agents, radon gas, and tobacco smoke (see **Figure 12.3**). **Asbestos** was often used in older buildings to insulate pipes, walls, and ceilings; as a component of floor and ceiling tiles; and was sprayed in structures for fireproofing. It is harmless if intact and left alone, but, when disturbed, the airborne fibers can cause serious health problems.

Biogenic pollutants are airborne materials of biological origin such as living and nonliving fungi and their toxins, bacteria, viruses, molds, pollens, insect parts and wastes, and animal dander. Inhaling these contaminants can trigger allergic reactions, including asthma; cause infectious illnesses, such as influenza and measles; or release disease-producing toxins. Symptoms of health problems include sneezing, watery eyes, coughing, shortness of breath, dizziness, lethargy, fever, and even digestive problems. Children, elderly people, and people with breathing problems, allergies, or lung diseases are particularly susceptible to airborne biogenic pollutants. People can minimize exposure to these pollutants by controlling the relative humidity level in a home or office; a relative humidity of 30% to 50% is generally recommended for homes. To reduce airborne biogenic pollutants in their homes, people should clean up standing water, remove any wet or water-damaged materials from around the home, and, if they suspect a problem, have the home inspected by someone knowledgeable about indoor air pollution problems.

Combustion by-products include gases (e.g., carbon monoxide [CO], nitrous dioxide [NO_2], and sulfur dioxide [SO_2]) and particulates

> **asbestos** a naturally occurring mineral fiber that has been identified as a Class A carcinogen by the Environmental Protection Agency
>
> **biogenic pollutants** airborne biological organisms or their particles or gases or other toxic materials that can produce illness
>
> **combustion by-products** gases and particulates generated by burning
>
> **greenhouse gases** atmospheric gases, principally carbon dioxide, chlorofluorocarbons, ozone, methane, water vapor, and nitrous oxide, that are transparent to visible light but absorb infrared radiation

Air Quality Index Levels of Health Concern	Numerical Value	Meaning
Good (green)	0–50	Air quality is considered satisfactory, and air pollution poses little or no risk.
Moderate (yellow)	51–100	Air quality is acceptable; however, for some pollutants there may be a moderate health concern for a very small number of people who are unusually sensitive to air pollution.
Unhealthy for Sensitive Groups (orange)	101–150	Members of sensitive groups may experience health effects. The general public is not likely to be affected.
Unhealthy (red)	151–200	Everyone may begin to experience health effects; members of sensitive groups may experience more serious health effects.
Very Unhealthy (purple)	201–300	Health alert: everyone may experience more serious health effects.
Hazardous (maroon)	> 300	Health warnings of emergency conditions. The entire population is more likely to be affected.

Figure 12.2 Color codes for various air quality indices.

Environmental Protection Agency (2009). "Air Quality Index (AIQ): A Guide to Air Quality and Your Health." Available at http://airnow.gov/index.cfm?action=aqibasics.aqi.

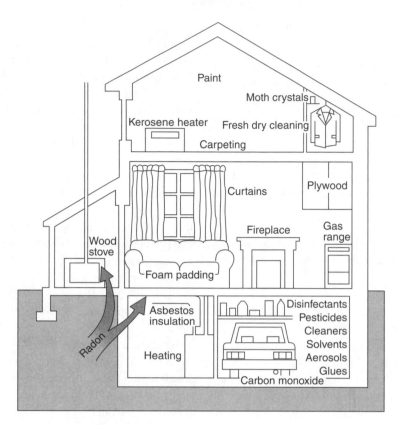

Figure 12.3 Air pollution sources in the home.

Environmental Protection Agency (1988). *The Inside Story: A Guide to Indoor Air Quality.* Washington, DC: Author, 2.

(e.g., ash and soot). The major sources of these items are fireplaces, wood stoves, kerosene heaters, gas ranges and engines, candles, incense, secondhand tobacco smoke, and improperly maintained gas furnaces. Prolonged exposure to these substances can cause serious illness and possibly death.

Volatile organic compounds (VOCs) are compounds that exist as vapors over the normal range of air pressures and temperatures. VOCs irritate the eyes and respiratory tract, and cause headaches, dizziness, memory impairment, and, sometimes, cancer. Sources of VOCs include construction materials (e.g., insulation and paint), structural components (e.g., vinyl tile and sheet rock), furnishings (e.g., drapes and upholstery fabric), cleansers and solvents (e.g., liquid detergent and furniture polish), personal care products (e.g., deodorant and eyeliner

pencils), insecticides/pesticides, electrical equipment (e.g., computers and VCRs), and combustion of wood and kerosene.[5] **Formaldehyde**, a pungent water-soluble gas, is one of the most ubiquitous VOCs. It is a widely used chemical that can be found in hundreds of products. Exposure occurs when it evaporates from wood products such as plywood and particle board, in which it is a component of the glue that binds these products together. Formaldehyde can also be found in products such as grocery bags, wallpaper, carpet, insulation, wall paneling, and wallboard.[5] Exposure to formaldehyde can cause watery eyes, burning in the eyes and throat, and difficulty in breathing, and precipitate asthma attacks in susceptible people. Formaldehyde may also be a **carcinogen**, a cancer-causing agent. When building or renovating a residence, use products that emit less formaldehyde. Increase ventilation in the home, use a dehumidifier and air conditioning to control humidity, and keep the temperature at moderate levels in the home to reduce formaldehyde emissions.

Radon is the number 1 cause of lung cancer among nonsmokers and the second leading cause of lung cancer

carcinogens agents, usually chemicals, that cause cancer

formaldehyde (CH₂O) a water-soluble gas used in aqueous solutions in hundreds of consumer products

radon a naturally occurring colorless, tasteless, odorless, radioactive gas formed during the radioactive decay of uranium-238

volatile organic compounds (VOCs) compounds that exist as vapors over the normal range of air pressures and temperatures

overall. This radioactive gas, which cannot be seen, smelled, or tasted, is responsible for about 21,000 lung cancer deaths every year.[6] It is a naturally occurring gas that seeps into a home from surrounding soil, rocks, and water and through openings such as cracks, drains, and sump pumps. However, exposure to radon is preventable, and homeowners can do something about it. Every home and office building should be tested for radon, and homeowners can administer this inexpensive and easy test. More homes with operating radon mitigation systems is one of the *Healthy People 2020* objectives (see Box 12.1).

Environmental tobacco smoke (ETS), also known as **secondhand smoke**, includes both **mainstream smoke** (the smoke inhaled and exhaled by the smoker) and **sidestream tobacco smoke** (the smoke that comes off the end of a burning tobacco product). The involuntary inhalation of ETS by nonsmokers is referred to as **passive smoking**. Hundreds of toxic agents and more than 40 carcinogens are in secondhand smoke. A few of these harmful agents are CO, NO_2, carbon dioxide (CO_2), hydrogen cyanide, formaldehyde, nicotine, and suspended particles.[7]

Twenty-three percent of adult Americans (about 58.3 million people) are current cigarette smokers,[8] so many Americans are regularly exposed to ETS. Epidemiological studies have revealed an association between exposure to ETS and cancer and heart disease.[9,10] ETS is classified as a known human (group A) carcinogen and causes approximately 3,000 lung cancer deaths annually in U.S. nonsmokers.[9] In addition, studies show that about 50% of all U.S. children 5 years of age or younger have been exposed to ETS from prenatal maternal smoking and/or sidestream smoke from household members after their birth. Such exposure has been shown to increase the risk of intrauterine growth retardation, low birth weight, preterm delivery, respiratory tract infections, and behavioral and cognitive abnormalities.[11] Furthermore, young children are especially susceptible to secondhand smoke and are likely to suffer from coughing, wheezing, phlegm production, breathlessness, and an increased risk of developing asthma.

Although indoor air is more polluted than outdoor air, identifying the source of pollution in a building can be difficult. **Sick building syndrome** refers to a situation in which the air quality in a building produces nonspecific signs and symptoms of ill health in the building occupants. Often the problem lies with the building's ventilation system.

Protecting Indoor Air

Because we spend 50% to 90% of our time indoors,[2,12] we need to take measures to protect the quality of our indoor air. In the absence of a federal indoor clean air act, some

environmental tobacco smoke (ETS) tobacco smoke in the environment that can be inhaled by nonsmokers

mainstream smoke tobacco smoke inhaled and exhaled by the smoker

passive smoking the inhalation of environmental tobacco smoke by nonsmokers

secondhand smoke environmental tobacco smoke

sick building syndrome a situation in which the air quality in a building produces generalized signs and symptoms of ill health in the building's occupants

sidestream tobacco smoke tobacco smoke that comes off the end of burning tobacco products

---

Box 12.1 *Healthy People 2020*: Objectives

Objective EH-14 Increase the number of homes with an operating radon mitigation system for persons in homes at risk for radon exposure.
Target setting method: Consistency with national programs/regulations/policies/laws
Data sources: Annual report to EPA by radon vent fan manufacturers, EPA, Indoor Environments Division

Target and baseline:		
Objective	2007 Baseline	2020 Target
EH-14 Increase the number of homes at risk (radon level of 4 Pico curies per liter of air (pCi/L or more) with an operating radon mitigation system	788,000 of 7.7 million homes (10.2%)	3.1 million of 9.2 million homes (30%)

For Further Thought
Have you tested your house for radon? What was the reading? What is the potential radon level in your area? Go to the EPA map of radon zones and search for the map of your state, where you can identify the potential by county.

Source: U.S. Department of Health and Human Services, Office of Disease Prevention and Health Promotion (2010). *Healthy People 2020.* Available at http://www.healthypeople.gov/2020/default.aspx.

states, counties, and municipalities have developed their own regulations, particularly with regard to ETS. In an attempt to protect workers and citizens from heart disease, cancer, and respiratory illness and to reduce passive smoking, many states and local jurisdictions have banned smoking in workplaces and in public buildings. In some areas, even outdoor smoking has been banned within a certain distance of exits and air intakes of public and state-owned building entrances. As of January 2012, 24 states and the District of Columbia received a grade of "A" for smoke-free air, based on their legislation prohibiting smoking in all public places and workplaces. Still, only one state, Alaska, met the Centers for Disease Control and Prevention's (CDC) guidelines for best practices in funding of comprehensive tobacco control programs.[13]

The Water We Use

Clean, uncontaminated water is essential for life and health. Consumption of polluted water can result in outbreaks of such waterborne diseases such as cholera, typhoid fever, dysentery, and other gastrointestinal diseases. One-seventh of the world's population has no access to a supply of clean drinking water.[14]

Here in the United States, virtually 100% of the population has access to a clean water supply (see **Figure 12.4**), and the **sanitation** rate, the establishment and maintenance of healthy or hygienic conditions in the environment, is the highest reported rate for any world region.[15] Nonetheless, more than 100 waterborne disease outbreaks (WBDOs) linked to drinking or recreational use water continue to occur annually. A major source of drinking water contamination is wastes produced by humans through their daily activities. Thus, both the prevention of water pollution and the treatment of polluted water are essential community activities.

Sources of Water

We acquire water for our domestic, industrial, and agricultural needs from either surface water or groundwater. Water in streams, rivers, lakes, and reservoirs is called **surface water**. The water that infiltrates into the soil is referred to as subsurface water or **groundwater**. Groundwater that is not absorbed by the roots of vegetation moves slowly downward until it reaches the zone of soil completely saturated with water, referred to as an aquifer. **Aquifers** are porous, water-saturated layers of underground bedrock, sand, and gravel that can yield economically significant amounts of water.[1]

aquifers porous, water-saturated layers of underground bedrock, sand, and gravel that can yield economically significant amounts of water

groundwater water located under the surface of the ground

sanitation the practice of establishing and maintaining healthy or hygienic conditions in the environment

surface water precipitation that does not infiltrate the ground or return to the atmosphere by evaporation; the water in streams, rivers, and lakes

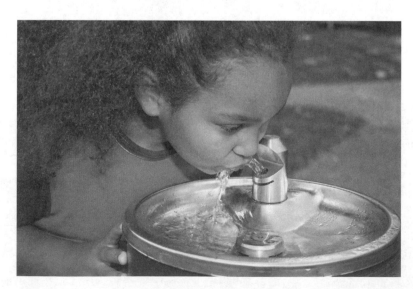

Figure 12.4 In the United States, virtually 100% of the population has access to clean, safe drinking water.
© Jaimie Duplass/ShutterStock, Inc.

Sources of Water Pollution

Water pollution includes any physical or chemical change in water that can harm living organisms or make it unfit for other uses, such as drinking, domestic use, recreation, fishing, industry, agriculture, or transportation.[1] The sources of water pollution fall into two categories—point sources and nonpoint sources[2] (see **Figure 12.5**). **Point source pollution** refers to a single identifiable source that discharges pollutants into the water, such as release of pollutants from a factory or sewage treatment plant. Point sources of pollution are relatively easy to identify, control, and treat.

Nonpoint source pollution includes all pollution that occurs through the runoff, seepage, or falling of pollutants into the water. Examples include the **runoff** of water from cities, highways, and farms resulting from rain events (called stormwater runoff); seepage of leachates from landfills; and acid rain. Nonpoint source pollution is a greater problem than point source pollution is because it is often difficult to track the actual source of pollution and, therefore, to control it.

Types of Water Pollutants

Water pollutants can be classified as biological or nonbiological. Biological pollutants include pathogens such as parasites, bacteria, viruses, and other undesirable living microorganisms. These pathogens enter the water mainly through human and other animal wastes that were disposed of improperly or without being treated before their disposal. Nonbiological pollutants include physical conditions and chemical substances neither produced by nor derived from plants or animals.

Biological Pollutants of Water

Biological pollutants are living organisms or their products that make the water unsafe for human consumption. Waterborne viral agents and the diseases they cause include poliomyelitis virus (polio), hepatitis A virus (hepatitis), and norovirus. Waterborne bacteria and the diseases they cause include *Escherichia coli* (gastroenteritis), *Legionella* species (legionellosis), *Salmonella typhi* (typhoid fever), *Shigella* species (shigellosis or bacillary dysentery), and *Vibrio cholerae* (cholera). Waterborne parasites

nonpoint source pollution all pollution that occurs through the runoff, seepage, or falling of pollutants into the water

point source pollution pollution that can be traced to a single identifiable source

runoff water that flows over land surfaces (including paved surfaces), typically from precipitation

water pollution any physical or chemical change in water that can harm living organisms or make the water unfit for other uses

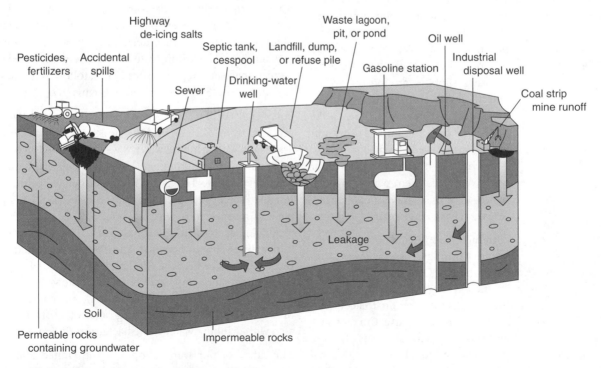

Figure 12.5 Sources of groundwater contamination.
U.S. Environmental Protection Agency.

include *Entamoeba histolytica* (amebiasis or amebic dysentery), *Giardia lamblia* (giardiasis), and *Cryptosporidium parvum* (cryptosporidiosis). Each of these diseases can be serious, and two in particular—typhoid fever and cholera—have killed thousands of people in single epidemics.

Nonbiological Pollutants of Water

Nonbiological pollutants include heat; inorganic chemicals such as lead, copper, and arsenic; organic chemicals, such as pesticides, industrial solvents, and chlorinated compounds like polychlorinated biphenyls (PCBs); and radioactive pollutants. These pollutants, present in high concentrations and known to be detrimental to human health, are relatively easy to identify. Within the past decade, however, two new types of pollutants have been detected in our waterways and are raising health concerns. These are **endocrine-disrupting chemicals (EDCs)** and **pharmaceuticals and personal care products (PPCPs)**. Endocrine disruptors include pesticides, commercial chemicals, and environmental contaminants that can disrupt, imitate, or block the body's normal hormonal activity, causing developmental or reproductive problems. Thus far, the relationship between EDCs and human diseases of the endocrine system is poorly understood and remains scientifically controversial.[16]

PPCPs are synthetic chemicals found in over-the-counter drugs; cosmetics, including soaps and shampoos; fragrances; sunscreens; diagnostic agents; biopharmaceuticals; and many other products. PPCPs have been detected in water supplies around the world, and their effects on human health are as yet unknown. PPCPs reach the waterways by being flushed down our toilets and rinsed down our drains. They are then transported to our wastewater treatment plants, through which they pass, mostly unchanged, into our rivers and streams.

Although the EPA and other researchers are working to assess the effects of EDCs and PPCPs, there are no governmental regulations or guidance for the disposal of pharmaceuticals meant for personal use. Current suggestions for safe disposal of these products are to (1) contact a local pharmacy to see if it takes expired or unwanted medicines, or (2) turn them in to a local hazardous waste collector. If neither of these options is available, disposal in household trash is a better alternative than disposal in the sewage system.[17]

Waterborne Disease Outbreaks

A **waterborne disease outbreak (WBDO)** is a water exposure in which at least two persons have been epidemiologically linked to recreational or drinking water by location, time, and illness. In the case of a recreational exposure, two or more persons must experience a similar illness after ingestion of drinking water or after exposure to water used for recreational purposes, and epidemiological evidence must implicate water as the probable source of the illness.[18]

In recent years, the number of WBDOs associated with drinking water has declined; however, the number of those associated with recreational exposure has increased. The Centers for Disease Control and Prevention issues biennial surveillance summaries based on WBDOs reported to the Waterborne Disease and Outbreak Surveillance System (WBDOSS). In the most recent biennial report, 134 WBDOs associated with recreational water were reported from 38 states and Puerto Rico. These resulted in 13,966 cases of illness.[16] Eighty-six percent of these outbreaks were traced to exposure to treated water venues (swimming pools, wading pools, spas, etc.); 14% were associated with untreated water (springs, rivers, reservoirs). In about 60% of the outbreaks, the illnesses were described as acute gastroenteritis illnesses, 18% as skin disorders, and 13% as acute respiratory illnesses. The leading cause of WBDOs associated with recreational water was parasites (65%), followed by bacteria (21%), viruses (5%), and chemicals/toxins (8%).[16]

Forty-eight WBDOs associated with drinking water were reported from 24 states and Puerto Rico. Of these, 36 were associated with drinking water, 8 were associated with water not intended for drinking, and 4 were associated with water of unknown intent. The 36 WBDOs associated with water intended for drinking caused illness in at least 4,128 people and resulted in 3 deaths. About 61% of the outbreaks resulted in acute gastrointestinal illness, 33% in acute respiratory illness, 3% in hepatitis, and 3% in skin irritation. In those outbreaks where the etiological agent was determined, the leading cause was bacteria (58%), followed by viruses (14%), parasites (8%), chemical (3%), mixed (8%), and unidentified (11%).[16] The leading cause of WBDOs associated with drinking water is the bacterium *Legionella*.

The safety of our water supply in the United States has deteriorated in many communities. This deterioration can be attributed to four causes: (1) population growth,

endocrine-disrupting chemical (EDC) a chemical that interferes in some way with the body's endocrine (hormone) system

pharmaceuticals and personal care products (PPCPs) synthetic chemicals found in everyday consumer healthcare products and cosmetics

waterborne disease outbreak (WBDO) a disease in which at least two persons experience a similar illness after the ingestion of drinking water or after exposure to water used for recreational purposes, and epidemiological evidence implicates water as the probable source of the illness

(2) chemical manufacturing, (3) reckless land use practices, and (4) mismanagement and irresponsible disposal of hazardous wastes.[19] As the public's knowledge of the endangerment of water quality in the United States grows, it is hoped that greater efforts will be made to protect our water.

Ensuring the Safety of Our Water

Ensuring the safety of our water in the United States involves the proper treatment and distribution of water intended for drinking and the proper construction and maintenance of water-associated recreation facilities. Safe water also depends on the enactment and enforcement of well-conceived water quality regulations and the proper treatment of wastewater.

Treatment of Water for Domestic Use

Water in the United States is used for many purposes, including agriculture, industry, energy generation, and domestic use. Domestic water use in the United States (6% of the total) includes water for drinking, cooking, washing dishes and laundry, bathing, flushing toilets, and outdoor use (such as watering lawns and gardens and washing cars). Each U.S. resident uses an average of 80–100 gallons of water each day, just by flushing the toilet, showering, washing laundry, and other domestic uses.[20,21]

Whereas many rural residents in the United States obtain their water from untreated private wells (groundwater), urban residents usually obtain their water from municipal water treatment plants. About two-thirds of the municipalities use surface water, and one-third use groundwater.

Virtually all surface water is polluted and needs to be treated before it can be safely consumed. The steps in the treatment of water for domestic use vary, but usually include removing solids through coagulation, flocculation, and filtration. This is followed by disinfection, during which chlorine (or sometimes ozone) is added to the water to kill remaining viruses, bacteria, algae, and fungi. Disinfection is sometimes accompanied by fluoridation, which helps prevent dental decay.[22]

The responsibility of municipal water treatment plants is to provide water that is chemically and bacteriologically safe for human consumption. It is also desirable that the water be aesthetically pleasing in regard to taste, odor, color, and clarity. Above all, the municipal water supply must be reliable. Reliability in regard to both quantity and quality has always been regarded as nonnegotiable in planning a treatment facility.

Wastewater Treatment

Wastewater is the substance that remains after humans have used water for domestic or commercial purposes. Such water, also referred to as liquid waste or sewage, consists of about 99.9% water and 0.1% suspended and dissolved solids. The solids consist of human feces, soap, paper, garbage grindings (food parts), and a variety of other items that are put into wastewater systems from homes, schools, commercial buildings, hotels/motels, hospitals, industrial plants, and other facilities connected to the sanitary sewer system. The primary purpose of **wastewater treatment** is to improve the quality of wastewater to the point that it might be released into a body of water without seriously disrupting the aquatic environment, causing health problems in humans in the form of waterborne disease, or causing nuisance conditions. Most municipalities and many large companies have wastewater treatment plants that incorporate at least primary and secondary treatment processes (see **Figure 12.6**).

Primary Wastewater Treatment

Primary wastewater treatment occurs in a sedimentation tank, also called a clarifier, where wastewater remains in a quiescent condition for about 2 to 4 hours. Here, the solids (sludge and scum) are separated from the aqueous solution. The layers of sludge and scum are removed, and the clarified

> **wastewater** the aqueous mixture that remains after water has been used or contaminated by humans
>
> **wastewater treatment** the process of improving the quality of wastewater (sewage) to the point that it can be released into a body of water without seriously disrupting the aquatic environment, causing health problems in humans, or causing nuisance conditions

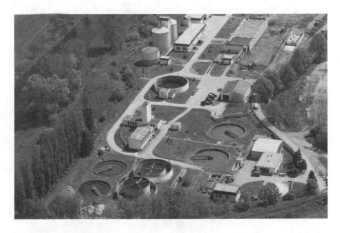

Figure 12.6 A wastewater treatment facility.
© Robert Malota/Dreamstime.com

wastewater enters the secondary stage of treatment. During secondary treatment, aerobic bacteria and oxygen are added to the wastewater to break down organic waste into carbon dioxide, water, and minerals. When this biological process is completed (after about 6 to 10 hours), the wastewater is sent to sedimentation tanks, where the water is clarified under quiescent conditions. After this process, many treatment plants disinfect and discharge the treated wastewater to surface water bodies; other wastewater plants perform tertiary treatment, involving filtration with sand and carbon filters. The treated water is finally disinfected and discharged. Discharges of treated wastewater are regulated by the EPA.

absorption field the element of a septic system in which the liquid portion of waste is distributed

septic tank a watertight concrete or fiberglass tank that holds sewage; one of two main parts of a septic system

Septic Systems

Those who live in unsewered areas (25% of Americans) dispose of their wastewater using a septic system. A septic system consists of two major components—a septic tank and a buried sand filter or absorption field (see Figure 12.7). The **septic tank**, a watertight concrete or fiberglass tank, is buried in the ground and is connected to the house by a pipe. Sewage leaves the home via the toilets or drains and goes through the pipe to the septic tank. The wastewater is retained in quiescent conditions for 1 to 2 days, during which separation of heavier solids and lighter scum from liquid wastewater occurs by sedimentation. The liquid portion of wastewater is then carried by a pipe to an **absorption field**, a system of trenches (dugout channels) where perforated pipes are surrounded by gravel. As wastewater trickles through the gravel, films of aerobic microorganisms develop and feed on this liquid wastewater, causing decomposition of organic waste. This treated wastewater then infiltrates through the soil profile into the groundwater.

Clearly, proper installation and regular maintenance of the septic system are absolutely crucial for its optimal

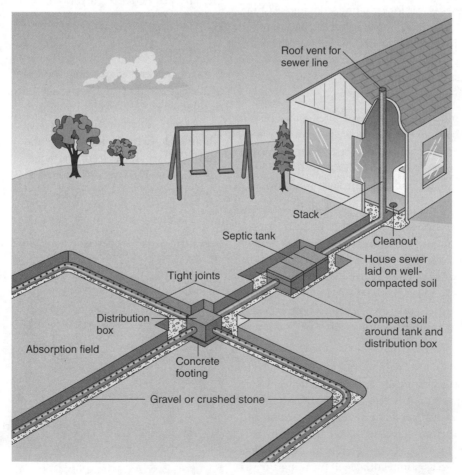

Figure 12.7 A septic system consists of a septic tank and an absorption field.

performance. Septic systems cannot be legally installed in most communities without a permit. Local health departments are responsible for issuing permits, inspecting the systems, and enforcing state and local regulations regarding them. Improperly functioning or overflowing septic systems also provide optimal breeding sites for disease-transmitting mosquitoes such as the northern house mosquito, *Culex pipiens*, the vector of West Nile fever.

Regulating Water Quality

Surface water and drinking water are regulated by two important laws, the Clean Water Act and the Safe Drinking Water Act. The goal of the 1972 **Clean Water Act (CWA)** and its 1977 amendments is to restore and maintain the chemical, physical, and biological integrity of the waters in the United States for "the protection and propagation of fish, shellfish, and wildlife and recreation in and on the water."[23] In other words, the goal is to return the quality of surface waters to swimmable and fishable status.

The CWA made it unlawful for any person or agency to discharge any pollutant from a point source into navigable waters without a permit. Since the late 1980s, the EPA has significantly increased its efforts to address polluted nonpoint source runoff. In its efforts to reduce and manage water pollution, the EPA considers land use and sources of pollution within the entire **watershed** rather than controlling and regulating only individual pollution sources or contaminants. The watershed approach emphasizes protecting healthy waters and restoring impaired ones to protect not only human health, but also environmental health.

The quality of drinking water is regulated by the **Safe Drinking Water Act (SDWA)** and its amendments. Its goal is to protect drinking water and its sources (rivers, lakes, reservoirs, springs, and groundwater). Under the SDWA, the EPA sets national standards to limit the levels of more than 90 contaminants in drinking water and oversees the states, localities, and water suppliers who implement those standards.[24] The EPA must periodically release a list of unregulated contaminants—the Contaminant Candidate List—to prioritize research and data collection that can help determine whether it should regulate a specific contaminant. The latest list included 104 chemicals and 12 microbiological agents.[25]

The Food We Eat

In a worldwide comparison, the U.S. food supply probably ranks as one of the safest, a result of a century of public health efforts. Nonetheless, we have not completely eliminated foodborne disease. "More than 200 known diseases are transmitted through food. In these cases, food is the vehicle; and the agents can be viruses, bacteria, parasites, toxins, metals, and prions."[26] Foodborne diseases cause an estimated 47.8 million cases of illness, 127,839 hospitalizations, and 3,037 deaths per year in the United States.[27-29] A majority of these cases are never reported to the CDC. The annual economic cost of foodborne illness in the United States has been estimated at $152 billion.[30] Healthy food can become contaminated at several points between the farm or factory and the consumer. When this happens, a foodborne disease outbreak can occur.

Foodborne Disease Outbreaks

The CDC defines a **foodborne disease outbreak (FBDO)** as the occurrence of two or more cases of a similar illness resulting from the ingestion of a common food.[31] Symptoms of foodborne illness range from mild to severe, and organs involved can include stomach and intestines, liver, kidneys, and brain and nervous system. During the most recent year for which data are available (2008), 1,034 FBDOs were reported from 47 states, the District of Columbia, and Puerto Rico, resulting in 23,152 cases and 22 deaths. Among the 429 outbreaks in which a single cause was confirmed, norovirus (49% of outbreaks and 46% of illnesses) was the leading cause. *Salmonella* (23% of outbreaks and 31% of illnesses) was the second leading cause, and the leading cause of FBDO-related hospitalizations. Among the 22 reported deaths, 20 were attributed to bacterial agents: *Salmonella* (13), *Listeria monocytogenes* (3), *Escherichia coli* (3), and *Staphylococcus* (1). One death was attributed to norovirus, and one to mycotoxin. Poultry (15%), beef (14%), and finfish (14%) were associated with the largest number of outbreaks, but vine-stalk vegetables (24%), fruits/nuts (23%), and beef (13%), were the commodities with the most outbreak-associated illnesses.[31]

Leading factors that contributed to FBDOs were inadequate cooking temperatures or improper holding temperatures for foods (especially for bacterial outbreaks); unsanitary

Clean Water Act (CWA) the federal law aimed at ensuring that all rivers are swimmable and fishable and that limits the discharge of pollutants in U.S. waters to zero

foodborne disease outbreak (FBDO) the occurrence of two or more cases of a similar illness resulting from the ingestion of food

Safe Drinking Water Act (SDWA) the federal law that regulates the safety of public drinking water

watershed the area of land from which all of the water that is under it or drains from it goes; for example, the Mississippi River watershed drains and collects all the water from the land extending from east of the Rocky Mountains to the Appalachian Mountains and from the upper Midwest all the way south to the Gulf of Mexico

conditions or practices at the point of service, such as failure to wash hands (norovirus outbreaks); or drinking raw milk (bacterial outbreaks).[31] Other factors that often contribute to FBDOs are contaminated equipment or obtaining food from an unsafe source (such as shellfish from polluted waters).

Protecting the public from foodborne diseases requires the coordinated efforts of federal, state, and local health agencies. At the federal level, the CDC, under its Emerging Infections Program, has established the Foodborne Diseases Active Surveillance Network (FoodNet) to provide better data on foodborne diseases.[32] The CDC coordinates these surveillance activities with officials from the U.S. Department of Agriculture's Food Safety and Inspection Service, the Food and Drug Administration's Center for Food Safety and Applied Nutrition, and state epidemiologists. The goal is to reduce the human and economic burden of FBDOs. Salmonella infections alone result in an estimated $365 million in direct medical costs each year.[32]

Growing, Processing, and Distributing Our Food Safely

In spite of the surveillance efforts described earlier, greater efforts need to be made to make sure our plants and animals are free from harmful chemical and biological agents during growing, harvesting, and processing of food products.

Pesticides

Two health concerns with the ubiquitous nature of agricultural chemicals, especially pesticides, are (1) the risk of unintentional poisonings where these chemicals are stored and used, and (2) the residues reaching food workers and consumers. **Pesticides** are natural or synthetic chemicals that have been developed and manufactured for the purpose of killing pests—organisms (plant, animal, or microbe) that have adverse effects on human interests. The EPA regulates the registration and labeling of pesticides, but individual state agencies license those who can buy, sell, or apply pesticides within their state. An estimated 18,625 products containing a total of 1,110 active ingredients have a current registration. These products are marketed by 1,720 companies.[33] Many of these pesticides are used in agriculture, where it is estimated that

pesticides synthetic chemicals developed and manufactured for the purpose of killing pests

registered environmental health specialists (REHSs) (sanitarians) environmental workers responsible for the inspection of restaurants, retail food outlets, public housing, and other sites to ensure compliance with public health codes

pests destroy about 40% of the food crop before it reaches the marketplace. Without the use of agricultural chemicals, farm production could decrease by as much as 30%.[1] Because of this, it seems certain that pesticides will be present in our environment for the foreseeable future.

The two groups at highest risk for pesticide poisoning are young children and the workers who apply the pesticides. Poisonings can be acute (single, high-level exposure) or chronic (repeated exposure over an extended period of time). Some signals of poisoning are headaches, weakness, rashes, fatigue, and dizziness. More serious effects include respiratory problems, convulsions, coma, and death. Chronic effects can include cancer, mutations, and birth defects.

Regulating Food Safety

Two other federal agencies regulate our food supply. The U.S. Department of Agriculture (USDA) inspects meat and dairy products, and the Food and Drug Administration (FDA) is charged with ensuring the safety of the remainder of our foods (see **Figure 12.8**). In recent years, several instances have occurred that call into question the quality of food processing and its inspection process. These include scares associated with fresh spinach, tomatoes, and peanut butter products.

The task of enforcing state regulations at the local level falls on **registered environmental health specialists (REHSs)**, more commonly known as sanitarians. Hired by local health departments, REHSs inspect restaurants and other food-serving establishments (such as hospitals, nursing homes, churches,

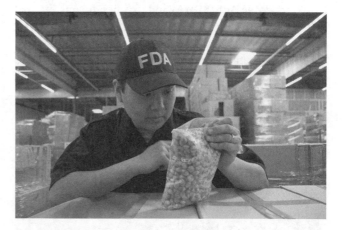

Figure 12.8 The Food and Drug Administration (FDA) is charged with ensuring the safety of our foods, except for meat and dairy products.
Courtesy of U.S. Food and Drug Administration

and schools), retail food outlets (grocery stores and super-markets), temporary and seasonal points of food service (such as those at fairs and festivals), and food vending machines to ensure that environmental conditions favorable to the growth and development of pathogens do not exist. When unsafe or unhealthy conditions are found, establishments are cited or, in cases of imminent danger to the public, closed. By enforcing food safety laws, public health officials protect the health of the community by reducing the incidence of FBDOs.

Finally, it is important to recognize that consumers, them-selves, can further reduce their risk for foodborne illness by following safe food-handling practices and by avoiding con-sumption of certain unsafe foods. Examples of foods that are often unsafe include unpasteurized milk and milk products, raw or undercooked oysters, raw or undercooked eggs, and raw or undercooked ground beef, pork, fish, and poultry. Guidelines for preventing foodborne disease transmission at home are simple and straightforward (see the text's website).

Where We Live

The production and mismanagement of our solid waste can result in a community's exposure to unsanitary and hazard-ous materials, serve as a reservoir for disease vectors, and lead to environmental degradation.

Solid and Hazardous Waste

Solid waste is garbage, refuse, sludge, and other discarded solid materials. Most solid waste, 95% to 98%, can be traced to agriculture, mining and gas and oil production, and industry.[1,2] The remaining 2% to 5%, termed **municipal solid waste (MSW)**, comprises the waste generated by households, businesses, and institutions (e.g., universities, schools, and colleges) located within municipalities. In 2010, we produced a daily average of 4.43 pounds of MSW per person, up from the 2.6 pounds of waste produced per person in 1960, but down slightly from the 4.72 pounds per person we gener-ated in 2000 (see **Figure 12.9**). There are nine major categories—paper, yard waste, food scraps, rubber and textiles, wood, metals, glass, plastics, and other. Paper makes up the largest percent-age (28.5%), followed by food scraps (13.9%), yard trimmings (13.4%), and plastics (12.4%) (see **Figure 12.10**).[34]

Hazardous waste is solid waste with properties that make it dangerous or potentially harmful to human health or the environment and, therefore,

> **hazardous waste** a solid waste or combination of solid wastes that is dangerous to human health or the environment
>
> **municipal solid waste (MSW)** waste generated by individual households, businesses, and institutions located within municipalities
>
> **solid waste** solid refuse from house-holds, agriculture, and businesses

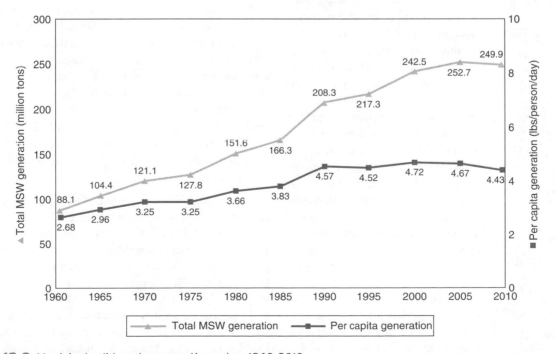

Figure 12.9 Municipal solid waste generation rates, 1960–2010.

requires special management and disposal. A waste is hazardous if it is ignitable, corrosive, reactive, or toxic, or if it is otherwise designated hazardous by the EPA. Designated hazardous wastes can be found among the by-products of manufacturing and industrial processes (e.g., solvents and cleaning fluids), and the by-products of petroleum refining operations and pesticide manufacturing. Electronic waste (e-waste), not included in the preceding total, often contains hazardous components, such as polyvinylchloride, brominated flame retardants, lead, and mercury. Each year Americans discard an estimated 48 million personal computers, 155 million cell phones, 68 million television sets, and millions of iPods and Blackberries.[1]

Managing Our Solid Waste

The **Resource Conservation and Recovery Act of 1976 (RCRA)** (pronounced *rick-rah*) was the first comprehensive law to address the collection and disposal of both solid and hazardous wastes. **Solid waste management** (integrated waste management) encompasses all of the approaches to managing all of the constantly accumulating solid waste. These approaches include source reduction, product reuse and recycling, and disposal. Of these approaches, the most desirable is **source reduction**. Examples of solid waste source reduction include not buying or using such throwaway products as paper towels and disposable diapers and minimizing packaging associated with groceries and carryout foods. The second best approach to solid waste management is to reuse or recycle the waste. **Recycling** is the collecting, sorting, and processing of materials that would otherwise be considered waste into raw materials that can be used to manufacture new products. Recycling diverts items, such as paper, glass, plastic, and metals, from the waste stream and conserves sanitary landfill space.

composting the natural, aerobic biodegradation of organic plant and animal matter to compost

leachates liquids created when water mixes with wastes and removes soluble constituents from them by percolation

recycling the collecting, sorting, and processing of materials that would otherwise be considered waste into raw materials for manufacturing new products, and the subsequent use of those new products

Resource Conservation and Recovery Act of 1976 (RCRA) the federal law that sets forth guidelines for the proper handling and disposal of hazardous wastes

sanitary landfills waste disposal sites on land suited for this purpose and on which waste is spread in thin layers, compacted, and covered with a fresh layer of clay or plastic foam each day

solid waste management (integrated waste management) the collection, transportation, and disposal of solid waste

source reduction a waste management approach involving the reduction or elimination of the use of materials that produce an accumulation of solid waste

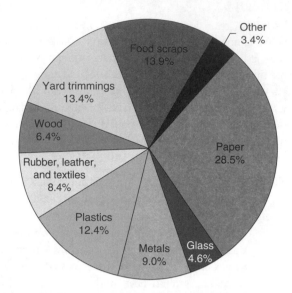

Figure 12.10 Total municipal solid waste generation (by material), 2010: 250 million tons (before recycling).

Reproduced from Environmental Protection Agency (2011). "Municipal Solid Waste Generation, Recycling, and Disposal in the United States: Facts and Figures for 2010." Available at http://www.epa.gov/osw /nonhaz/municipal/pubs/msw_2010_rev_factsheet.pdf.

The United States currently recycles about 34% of its MSW.[34] Only about 59% of our population is served by a curbside recycling program.[35] Although progress has been made, the recycling rate in the United States is far below the rates of some European countries. Austria, for example, recycles or composts 60% of its household solid waste.[36] **Composting** is a form of recycling that can be done easily at home because it doesn't require special knowledge or equipment. In composting, yard and food wastes are biodegraded naturally by microorganisms that convert organic plant and animal matter into compost that can be used as a mulch or fertilizer, thereby conserving precious landfill space.

Once created, MSW that cannot be reused or recycled must be disposed of either in a sanitary landfill or by combustion (incineration). Currently, 54.2% of municipal solid waste is placed in **sanitary landfills**, sites judged suitable for in-ground disposal of solid waste.[34] RCRA permits only state-of-the-art landfills to operate. At the end of 2008, there were 1,812 approved landfills.[35] Landfills must be located and constructed so that **leachates**, that is, liquids created when water mixes with wastes and drains from beneath a landfill, do not contaminate the groundwater beneath them (see **Figure 12.11**). Despite these precautions, according to the EPA, all landfills will eventually leak.[1]

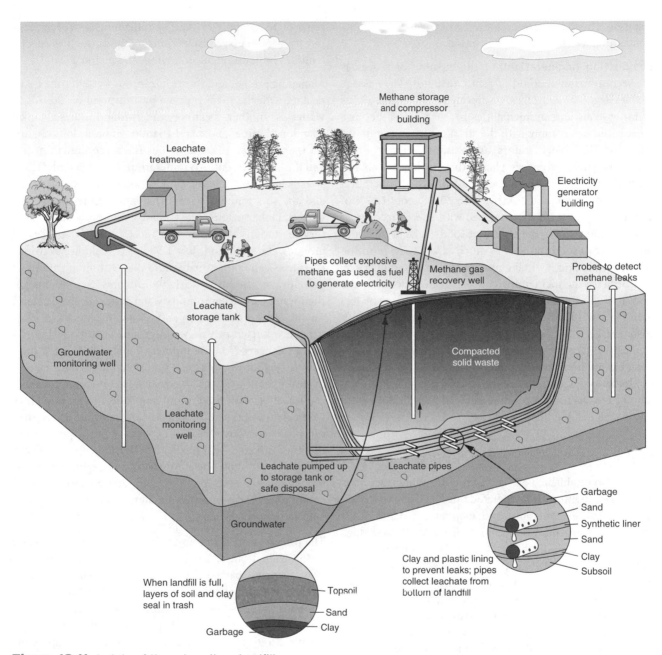

Figure 12.11 A state-of-the-art sanitary landfill.

Adapted from Miller, G. T. (2008). *Living in the Environment: Principles, Connections, and Solutions*, 16th ed. Pacific Grove, CA: Brooks/Cole; and SWACO Sanitary Landfill Poster, Solid Waste Authority of Central Ohio. Available http://www.swaco.org/SmartKids/Presentations.aspx.

Another concern with landfills is the accumulation of dangerous amounts of methane gas (a greenhouse gas) created by the anaerobic decomposition of refuse. In some cases, explosions have occurred when the methane gas was ignited. Only a small minority of communities have systems in place to harness the methane gas and use it as an energy source. It has been estimated that landfills were responsible for 17% of all methane emissions in the United States in 2009.[37]

Because nobody wants to live next to a sanitary landfill, even a properly operating one, it is exceedingly difficult to establish new landfills. As existing landfill space becomes more restricted, demand will drive up the cost of MSW disposal. This has led to an increased interest in combustion as an alternative to MSW disposal.

Combustion (incineration), or the burning of wastes, is the second major method of refuse disposal. The passage of the Clean Air Act of 1970 severely restricted the rights of individuals and municipalities to burn refuse because most could not comply with the strict emission standards. Some of these incinerators are waste-to-energy incinerators or energy recovery plants; that is, they are able to convert some of the heat generated from the incineration process into steam and electricity. In 2010, about 12.7% of all municipal waste was combusted with energy recovery.[34] Combustion reduces the weight of solid waste by 75% and the volume of solid waste by as much as 90%. The resulting waste, if nontoxic, will take up less sanitary landfill space, and because an incinerator can be located closer to the source of the solid waste, transportation costs may be less than for landfills. But there are disadvantages: (1) startup costs are high because large commercial incinerators are expensive, (2) nitrogen oxides, sulfur dioxide, and other toxic air pollutants are produced, and (3) the ash may be too toxic to place in a sanitary landfill. Regular testing is required to ensure that residual ash is nonhazardous before it is placed in a landfill.

Managing Our Hazardous Waste

RCRA also established a system for controlling hazardous waste from the time it is generated until its disposal (called cradle-to-grave regulation) and mandated strict controls over the treatment, storage, and disposal of hazardous waste. It is the responsibility of the EPA to implement the legislation created by RCRA. More than 400 substances are now listed on the EPA's hazardous waste list, which does not include radioactive wastes controlled by the Nuclear Regulatory Commission or biomedical wastes regulated by the individual states. The EPA's Office of Solid Waste has the responsibility of overseeing hazardous waste treatment, storage, and disposal. More than 35 million tons of hazardous waste were generated in the United States in 2009.[38] There are about 15 methods of hazardous waste management overseen and regulated by the EPA. The most commonly used method is deep well (underground) injection, which is used for disposal of about 50% of hazardous waste.[38] Most of these wells are found in the

states of Texas and Florida. The remaining 50% of hazardous waste is managed by various methods, such as special landfills, impoundment, recycling, and incineration.

Managing present and future hazardous wastes is one issue; dealing with the inappropriate past disposal of hazardous wastes is another. Leaking underground storage tanks, abandoned mine lands, and abandoned hazardous chemical waste sites all present serious threats to human health and the environment. An underground storage tank (UST) system includes the tank, underground connected piping, and any containment system that stores either petroleum or certain hazardous substances. Gasoline leaking from service stations is one of the most common sources of groundwater pollution. Just 1.5 cups of leaking hazardous chemicals can contaminate more than 1 million gallons of groundwater. Because nearly 90 million U.S. residents get their water from a community water system derived at least in part from groundwater, and 15 million more U.S. residents drink from private wells, groundwater pollution is a serious concern.[39] Many municipal and private wells have had to be shut down as a result of contamination caused by leaky UST systems. Additionally, fumes and vapors can travel beneath the ground and collect in areas such as basements, utility vaults, and parking garages, where they can pose a serious threat of explosion, fire, asphyxiation, or other adverse health effects. Cleaning up petroleum releases in the subsurface is difficult and expensive; therefore, the best prevention of groundwater contamination is appropriate management and maintenance of the UST systems to prevent releases.

The primary participant in the cleanup of hazardous waste in the United States has been the federal government. In 1980, Congress passed the **Comprehensive Environmental Response, Compensation, and Liability Act (CERCLA)** in response to the public's demand to clean up leaking dump sites. This law, known as the Superfund, created a tax on the chemical and petrochemical industries to clean up abandoned hazardous waste sites that might endanger human health and the environment. The guiding principle was that the government would make responsible parties pay for those cleanups whenever possible. The Superfund did not provide compensation to victims for health-related problems.

Since the inception of this program, more than 47,929 contaminated sites have been placed in the database from which the individual states and the U.S. EPA select the sites for cleanup. Of the 12,595 active, selected sites, 1,587 were listed on the National Priority List (NPL) for cleanup. Through the end of 2008, construction of the remedy was

combustion (incineration) the burning of solid wastes

Comprehensive Environmental Response, Compensation, and Liability Act (CERCLA) the federal law (known as the Superfund) created to clean up abandoned hazardous waste sites

complete at 1,060 of the 1,587 final and deleted sites from the National Priority List (NPL).[40] The Superfund is now more than 30 years old and has provided billions of dollars for the assessment and cleanup of the NPL sites.

Brownfields

Another problem is the more than 450,000 abandoned industrial plants, factories, commercial worksites, junkyards, and gas stations. These so-called **brownfields** are contaminated properties where expansion, redevelopment, or reuse may be complicated by the presence or potential presence of a hazardous substance, pollutant, or contaminant that can pose a threat to human health.[1] Cleaning up and reinvesting in these properties take development pressures off undeveloped open land, increase local tax bases, facilitate job growth, and improve and protect both the environment and human health.

Lead and Other Heavy Metals

Among the more ubiquitous and harmful environmental hazards are heavy metals, such as lead, mercury, cadmium, chromium, and arsenic. They often contaminate well water and are ingested by unsuspecting people. Heavy metals occur naturally throughout the environment, and many are also used in industrial processes or products. For example, **lead** is used in electric batteries, pipe, solder, paint and plastic pigments, and, until 1986, in leaded gasoline.[1]

Because of its past widespread use, lead can be found in soil, household dust, air, paint, old painted toys and furniture, and foods and liquids stored in lead crystal or lead-based porcelain. Those who are at greatest risk of lead poisoning are young children, who may inadvertently ingest lead paint, but adults can be poisoned too. It is estimated that as much as 50% of the lead ingested by young children is absorbed, compared with only 10% in adults.

The health problems from exposure to lead include anemia, birth defects, bone damage, depression of neurological and psychological functions, kidney damage, learning disabilities, miscarriages, and sterility.[2] Lead poisoning was once cited as the most significant and prevalent disease of environmental origin among U.S. children,[41] but the prevalence of elevated blood lead levels among U.S. children has declined significantly since widespread testing began in 1976.[42] Between 1997 and 2009 the percentage of children under 6 years of age with elevated blood lead levels declined from 7.61% to 0.64% of those tested.[43] Unfortunately, disparities remain among racial and ethnic groups. The children with the highest blood lead levels are non-Hispanic African American children,[42] many of whom live in older homes. The major source of lead exposure for these children is dust and chips of lead paint in their homes (see Figure 12.12).

The major source of lead intake for adults is occupational exposure. In this case, the method of exposure is usually inhalation. Adults may also be exposed in their homes if they have lead water pipes or have used lead to solder water pipes. The exposed lead dissolves in the flowing water and is delivered to the tap. Americans who live in homes built before 1930 (when copper began to replace lead in pipes) may be drinking water containing more than the legally permissible level of lead (15 parts per billion). Well water can also become contaminated with lead by the inappropriate disposal of lead-containing materials such as old automobile batteries or solvents containing lead.

Public health education about the dangers of lead and testing for lead levels in older homes with children present are the most effective control

> **brownfields** property where reuse is complicated by the presence of hazardous substances from prior use
>
> **lead** a naturally occurring mineral element found throughout the environment and used in large quantities for industrial products, including batteries, pipes, solder, paints, and pigments

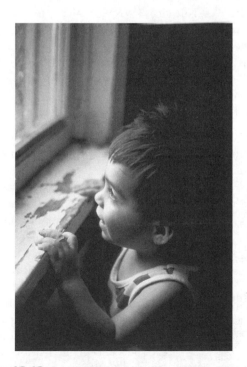

Figure 12.12 Lead poisoning from paint dust continues to be a problem in the United States.
© Tony Freeman/PhotoEdit, Inc.

measures. Educational efforts to inform people of the dangers of lead in paint in older homes have been well received. Those living in older homes with children should have their homes tested for lead. Most local health departments provide this service.

Controlling Vectorborne Diseases

Standing water, including runoff water from overflowing septic systems or overloaded sewer systems; improperly handled solid waste; and malfunctioning irrigation systems are more than unsavory sights. They provide a habitat for, and support the proliferation of, disease vectors. A **vector** is a living organism, usually an insect or other arthropod, that transmits microscopic disease agents to susceptible hosts.

Mosquitoes, perhaps the most notorious and ubiquitous vectors, require standing water in which to complete their development. The improper handling of wastewater, rainwater, or water for agricultural use can promote substantial populations of mosquitoes and put communities at risk for a **vectorborne disease outbreak (VBDO)**. Of particular concern in this regard is the northern house mosquito— *Culex pipiens* is the most important vector of St. Louis encephalitis (SLE) in the eastern United States and *Culex tarsalis* is the SLE vector in the far West. *Cx. pipiens* also transmits West Nile virus (WNV), which causes West Nile fever, West Nile encephalitis, and West Nile meningitis. The latter two are severe forms of the disease that affect the nervous system. In 2011, a relatively mild year for WNV, 690 cases were reported from 43 states and the District of Columbia.[44] However, as recently as 2006, 4,269 cases were reported from 44 states.[45]

Another species of mosquito that thrives on environmental mismanagement in the north-central and eastern United States is the eastern tree-hole mosquito, *Aedes triseriatus*. Although the natural habitat for this mosquito is tree holes, it flourishes in water held in discarded automobile and truck tires. It is estimated that there are 2 billion used tires discarded in various places in the United States today, and 2 million more discarded tires are added to the environment each year. *Ae. triseriatus* transmits LaCrosse encephalitis virus, a neuroinvasive, California serogroup virus. The disease, which is often fatal in children, occurs primarily in states east of the Great Plains. An average of 80–100 cases are reported each year.[46]

Cx. pipiens, *Cx. tarsalis*, and *Ae. triseriatus* are only three of several hundred species of mosquitoes that occur in the United States. Because we have become a global economy, new exotic pest species are continually being introduced into our country. Two of these are the Asian tiger mosquito, *Ae. albopictus*, first discovered in Texas in 1985,[47] and *Ae. japonicus*, first detected in 1998.[48] Although no human cases of disease have been traced directly to either of these vectors in the United States, laboratory studies indicate that both of them can transmit pathogenic viruses.

Federal, state, and local governments all have units whose primary responsibility is the prevention and control of vectorborne diseases. At the federal level, the lead agency is the CDC's National Center for Emerging and Zoonotic Infectious Diseases (NCEZID), located in Atlanta, Georgia. It conducts and funds research on vectorborne diseases, maintains surveillance of vectorborne diseases, assists states in investigating vectorborne disease outbreaks, and, in some cases, assists other countries with vectorborne problems. Most state departments of health have offices or labs that maintain vectorborne disease surveillance programs and provide expertise to local health departments, which have the primary task of reducing mosquito populations and preventing disease transmission. Most of us have seen county or mosquito abatement district workers inspecting or treating standing water or driving through a neighborhood with a mosquito sprayer or fogger. Proper land, solid waste, and wastewater management; mosquito control efforts; the promotion of personal protection against mosquito bites; and active surveillance for vectorborne diseases are all important defenses against mosquito-borne disease outbreaks.

The number one vectorborne disease in the United States is not a mosquito-borne disease, but a tick-borne disease, Lyme disease. In 2011, more than 33,000 confirmed and probable cases of Lyme disease were reported to the CDC (see **Figure 12.13**).[49] Lyme disease is transmitted by the blacklegged tick, *Ixodes scapularis*, a species of tick that flourishes when deer are abundant. Because there is no vaccine for Lyme disease, and community tick control is virtually nonexistent, state and local health departments promote personal protection as the best way to prevent Lyme disease. (Please see the text's website for these precautions.) They also recommend various measures for the home including landscaping techniques that discourage ticks—reduce leaf litter and tall grass, and establish a

vector a living organism, usually an insect or other arthropod (e.g., a mosquito or tick), that can transmit a communicable disease agent to a susceptible host

vectorborne disease outbreak (VBDO) an occurrence of an unexpectedly large number of cases of disease caused by an agent transmitted by insects or other arthropods

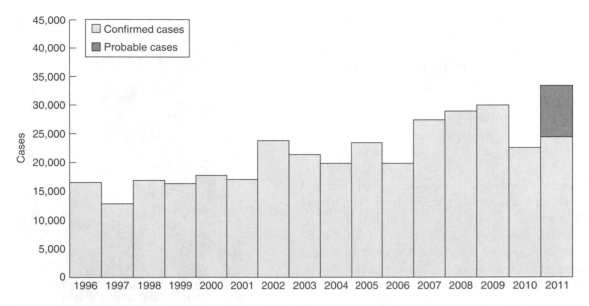

Figure 12.13 Number of reported cases of Lyme disease in the United States from 1994 to 2011.

Reproduced from Centers for Disease Control and Prevention (2012). "Reported Cases of Lyme Disease by Year, United States, 2002-2011." Available at http://www.cdc.gov/lyme/stats/chartstables/casesbyyear.html.

litter-free (and tick-free) border around the perimeter of the yard. Keep the lawn short and, if using acaricides, do so in accordance with instructions on the label. Finally, support any community efforts at tick control.

Improper management of solid waste—such as occurs at open dumps, ill-managed landfills, and urban slums—fosters the expansion of rat and mouse populations. These rodents are hosts for fleas that transmit murine typhus, a Rickettsial disease characterized by headache, fever, and rash. The closing of most of the open dumps has relegated murine typhus to the status of an uncommon disease in the United States, but improper MSW management could provide an environment conducive to murine typhus transmission.

The Place We Work

Because we spend more time at work than anywhere except home, we must be concerned about the healthiness of our workplace environments. The healthiness of our workplaces has greatly improved over the past century, but environmental hazards remain. Workers are at risk for occupational diseases and disorders caused by the inhalation of harmful airborne particles and gasses, contact with toxic chemicals and heavy metals, and exposure to infectious biological agents.

Inhalation of Airborne Particles and Gases

Among the occupational respiratory disorders attributable to workplace exposure are work-related asthma, pneumoconiosis, and several other lung diseases. Occupational lung diseases are difficult to detect in their early stages, develop slowly (the latent period for such diseases may be 15 to 30 years), and are chronic in nature.

Work-related asthma (WRA) is the most commonly reported occupational respiratory disease, even though estimates suggest that most cases are not recognized or reported as being work related. There is no estimate of how many cases of WRA occur nationwide. The highest percentage of cases occur among operators, fabricators, and laborers.[50]

Pneumoconiosis is a fibrotic lung disease caused by the inhalation of dusts, especially mineral dusts. Types of pneumoconiosis include coal workers' pneumoconiosis, asbestosis, silicosis, and byssinosis. Deaths from **coal workers' pneumoconiosis (CWP)** (also called black lung disease), an acute or chronic lung disease that is caused by inhaling coal dust, historically have

coal workers' pneumoconiosis (CWP) acute and chronic lung disease caused by the inhalation of coal dust (black lung disease)

pneumoconiosis fibrotic lung disease caused by the inhalation of dusts, especially mineral dusts

outnumbered all other types of pneumoconiosis deaths. However, deaths from CWP have declined during the last 30 years, from a high of 2,870 in 1972 to 525 (24% of all pneumoconiosis deaths) in 2007.[50,51] The human cost of CWP can be measured another way, through analysis of years of potential life lost (YPLL). During the period 1998–2006, a total of 22,625 YPLL were attributed to CWP, an average of 5.7 years per fatality.[52] Most troubling is the finding that, after a period of decline, the number of YPLL has been increasing, from an average of 5.3 during 1968–1972 to 7.8 in 2002–2006, perhaps because of inadequate enforcement of standards and unrepresentative dust sample measurements. Also, miners worked an average of 25.6% more hours underground during 2003–2007 than they did during 1978–1982, thereby increasing their exposure to coal dust.[51] No effective medical treatment is available for CWP (see **Figure 12.14**); therefore, primary prevention is essential.

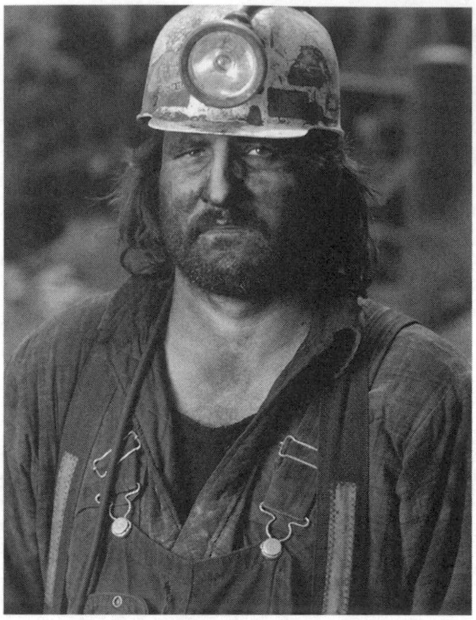

Asbestos workers suffer from diseases that include **asbestosis** (an acute or chronic lung disease caused by the deposition of asbestos fibers on their lungs), lung cancer, and mesothelioma (cancer of the epithelial linings of the heart and other internal organs). In contrast to CWP, asbestosis deaths have increased from 77 in 1968 to 1,401 in 2007, when it accounted for 63% of pneumoconiosis deaths.[50,51] A total of 2,606 work-related mesothelioma deaths also occurred in 2007.[50]

Workers in mines, stone quarries, sand and gravel operations, foundries, abrasive blasting operations, and glass manufacturing run the risk of **silicosis**, which is caused by inhaling crystalline silica. Silicosis deaths represent nearly 6% of all pneumoconiosis deaths in the United States. Mortality from silicosis has significantly declined in recent years, from 1,157 in 1968 to 123 in 2007.[50,51]

Textile factory workers who inhale dusts from cotton, flax, or hemp often acquire **byssinosis** (sometimes called brown lung disease). These days, byssinosis deaths are uncommon—10 or fewer cases were reported annually between 1996 and 2007. There were also 160 unspecified pneumoconiosis deaths in 2007.[50]

Other agents that can affect the lungs include metallic dusts, gases and fumes, and aerosols of biological agents (viruses, bacteria, and fungi). Health conditions that can result from exposure to these agents include occupational asthma, asphyxiation, pulmonary edema, histoplasmosis, and lung cancer.

asbestosis acute or chronic lung disease caused by the deposition of asbestos fibers on lungs

byssinosis acute or chronic lung disease caused by the inhalation of cotton, flax, or hemp dusts (brown lung disease)

silicosis acute or chronic lung disease caused by the inhalation of free crystalline silica

Figure 12.14 There is no effective medical treatment for CWP.
© Rubberball Productions/Creatas

Workplace Poisonings

Poisoning agents in the workplace include heavy metals (including lead), toxic gases, organic solvents, pesticides, and other substances. Pesticides represent a health risk for agricultural workers. Approximately 1 billion pounds of pesticide active ingredients are used annually in the United States, where 16,000 separate pesticide products are marketed. Each year, 10,000 to 20,000 physician-diagnosed pesticide poisonings occur among the approximately 3,380,000 agricultural workers.[53] The vast majority of these cases (71%) occurred in farm workers.[54] Insecticides are responsible for the highest percentage of occupational poisoning cases (49%).[50]

Exposure to Infectious Agents

In 2010, more than 16 million people were employed in the health service industries in the United States, making up 11% of the employed workforce.[55] More than 8 million of these workers are exposed to a variety of hazardous conditions, including infectious disease agents. Among the agents of concern are hepatitis B virus and human immunodeficiency virus (HIV). Healthcare workers are at risk if they become exposed to the blood or bodily fluids of patients or coworkers. The major route of exposure to these agents (82% of the cases) is percutaneous exposure (injuries through the skin) via contaminated sharp instruments such as needles and scalpels. Exposure also occurs through contact with the mucous membranes of the eyes, nose, or mouth (14%); exposure to broken or abraded skin (3%); and through human bites (1%). Up to 800,000 percutaneous injuries occur annually, with an average risk of infection for HIV of 0.3% (3 per 1,000) and for hepatitis B of from 6% to 30%.[50] Healthcare workers are also at increased risk for acquiring other infectious diseases such as tuberculosis (TB); the incidence for healthcare workers is 3.7 cases per 100,000 workers.[50]

Another risk in healthcare settings is occupational exposure to antineoplastic drugs (drugs used in cancer treatment) and other hazardous drugs. Exposure to these substances can cause skin rashes, infertility, miscarriage, birth defects, and possibly leukemia or other cancers.[56] Exposure can occur while crushing tablets, reconstituting powdered drugs, expelling air from syringes filled with hazardous drugs, administering these drugs, or handling contaminated clothing, dressings, or body fluids. The National Institute for Occupational Safety and Health (NIOSH) has issued an alert and guidelines for preventing exposure.[56]

Preventing and controlling exposure to environmental hazards in the workplace require the vigilance of employer and employee alike and the assistance of governmental agencies. **Industrial hygienists** are health professionals trained to identify environmental factors that might cause illness and make recommendations for their reduction or elimination.

Natural Disasters

Natural hazards are natural phenomena or events that produce/release energy in amounts that exceed human endurance, causing injury, disease, or death. Examples include high-energy radiation, geologic activity (earthquakes and volcanoes), and weather-driven events (tornados, hurricanes, and floods). When natural hazards involve human injuries and deaths, they are often termed **natural disasters**.

Radiation

Radiation is the process in which energy is emitted as particles or waves. Heat, sound, and visible light are examples of long-wavelength, low-energy radiation. High-energy (ionizing) radiation is radiation with shorter wavelengths, such as ultraviolet light, X-rays, and gamma rays, or particles, such as alpha or beta particles (see **Box 12.2**). High-energy

industrial hygienists health professionals trained to identify environmental factors in the workplace that might cause illness and make recommendations for their reduction or elimination

natural disaster a natural hazard that results in substantial loss of life or property

natural hazard naturally occurring phenomenon or event that produces or releases energy in amounts that exceed human endurance, causing injury, disease, or death (such as radiation, earthquakes, tsunamis, volcanic eruptions, hurricanes, tornados, and floods)

radiation a process in which energy is emitted as particles or waves

---

Box 12.2 About the Electromagnetic Spectrum

Electromagnetic radiation emitted from different sources has characteristic wavelengths. Taken together, these types of radiation make up the electromagnetic spectrum, which ranges from the very-long-wavelength radiation of power lines (thousands of meters) to the very-short-wavelength cosmic radiation that originates in outer space (less than one-trillionth of a meter).

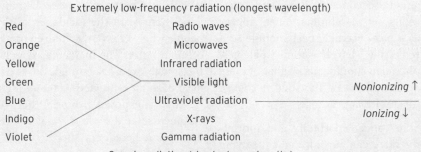

In the middle of the electromagnetic spectrum, infrared and ultraviolet radiation bracket the familiar spectrum of visible light. Sunlight is made up of infrared radiation, visible light, and ultraviolet radiation. Infrared radiation is simply heat; any object that is warmer than its surroundings gives off infrared radiation.

ionizing radiation is released when atoms are split or naturally decay from a less stable to a more stable form. This type of radiation has enough energy to knock electrons out of orbit and break chemical bonds among molecules in living cells and tissues. Mild tissue damage may be able to be repaired, but if the damage is too severe or widespread, it cannot be repaired and is manifest in radiation burns, radiation sickness, or both. Symptoms of radiation sickness include nausea, weakness, hair loss, skin burns, diminished organ function, premature aging, cancer, or even death. The amount of radiation and the duration of exposure affect the severity of the injury or illness.

Radiation from Natural Sources

Sunshine is composed of radiation in many wavelengths, including visible light, heat, and **ultraviolet (UV) radiation**. UV radiation includes energy at wavelengths between 0 and 400 nanometers (nm). UV radiation between 290 and 330 nm, called UV-B, causes most of the harm to humans.

Much of the UV radiation emanating from the sun is screened out by the layer of ozone in the stratosphere. In recent years, with the erosion of the ozone layer, the quantity of UV-B radiation reaching the earth has been increasing.[1,2] Each year, 2–3 million new cases of skin cancer are diagnosed in the United States.[57] The vast majority of these cases are the highly curable basal cell and squamous cell carcinomas, the most common forms of cancer. The most serious and least common skin cancer is malignant melanoma. More than 75,000 new cases of melanoma are diagnosed and about 12,000 patients die from this disease each year. Although malignant melanomas grow and spread quickly, they are curable if discovered and treated early.[57] Melanomas often appear first as small mole-like growths. A new mole that wasn't apparent during a previous month's self-examination should raise concern. Basal and squamous cell carcinomas often appear as a pale, waxlike, peely nodule or a red, scaly, sharply outlined patch. A physician should check either of these abnormalities or the sudden change in a mole's appearance.

Skin cancer morbidity and mortality rates can be lowered by staying out of the sun, by covering the skin with clothing when in direct sunlight, and by eschewing tanning beds. Avoiding terrestrial radiation, radiation from uranium ore, is more difficult, especially for those who live or work in buildings made of brick and stone that contain radioactive materials. Similarly, miners and bricklayers are at greater risk for terrestrial exposure, as are those who drink from wells contaminated with radioactive materials.

Radiation from Humanmade Sources

Sources of humanmade radiation are those associated with medical and dental procedures, such as X-rays, nuclear medicine diagnoses, and radiation therapy; most would agree that most of the radiation used for medical and dental purposes is justified. Some consumer products, such as smoke detectors, and television and computer screens, also emit radiation at levels generally regarded as safe. Two other humanmade sources of radiation are much more controversial—nuclear power and weaponry.

The advantages and disadvantages of nuclear power are often discussed, and have been in the news recently in the aftermath of the earthquake and tsunami in Japan, which disabled the Fukushima nuclear power plant. The 103 nuclear power stations operating in the United States currently generate about 8.5% of our nation's total energy and fit comfortably into the nation's electricity grid.[2] They do this while producing very little air pollution (carbon dioxide, sulfur oxides, nitrogen oxides) and reducing our dependence on foreign oil. However, these facilities produce large volumes of radioactive waste, pose significant environmental and human health risks should failure occur, and are costly to build, run, and decommission at the end of their expected life. The contamination of the environment caused by any accident during shipment or use of nuclear materials is long lasting because the half-life of uranium is measured in the billions of years.

In the aftermath of the 1986 meltdown of the nuclear facility at Chernobyl, in the Ukraine, there has been a large increase in the incidence of thyroid cancer among people who were young children or adolescents at the time of the disaster. The incidence of leukemia has doubled in those who experienced high doses of radiation, and there have been an estimated 4,000 additional cancer deaths in the highest exposed groups. Other concerns are cataracts, cardiovascular disease, mental health effects, and reproductive and hereditary effects.[58]

It has been more than 30 years since there has been a serious nuclear accident in the United States and global warming concerns have fostered growing interest in maintaining existing nuclear power plants and in building new ones. However, the Fukushima nuclear disaster in

ionizing radiation high-energy radiation that can knock an electron out of orbit, creating an ion, and can thereby damage living cells and tissues (e.g., ultraviolet radiation, gamma rays, X-rays, alpha and beta particles)

ultraviolet (UV) radiation radiation energy with wavelengths of 0–400 nanometers

Japan in 2011 has been a reminder of the inherent dangers of nuclear power.

Natural Environmental Events

Natural environmental events include geologic activity such as volcanic eruptions and earthquakes (and resulting tsunamis), and weather-driven events such as tornados, cyclones, hurricanes, and floods. Natural environmental hazards can result in serious physical and psychological health consequences for humans, resulting in natural disasters or catastrophic events. Examples of recent natural disasters are the tsunami in Southeast Asia (2004), Hurricane Katrina (2005), the earthquakes that struck Haiti and Chile (2010), the earthquake and tsunami in Japan (2011), and Hurricane Sandy (2012) (see **Figure 12.15**). Each of these natural disasters resulted in the immediate loss of lives and destruction of homes and businesses followed by unavailability of clean water, food, and sanitation. Survivors were in immediate need of emergency services as well as other social services.

Longer-term environmental hazards usually follow for days or months after these natural events. For example, homes flooded because of Hurricane Katrina were contaminated with high levels of mold that led to respiratory problems. Similarly, volcanic eruptions that release large quantities of ash into the atmosphere are responsible for the acute respiratory symptoms commonly reported by people during and after ash falls, including nasal irritation and discharge (runny noses), throat irritation and sore throat, coughing, and uncomfortable breathing. People with preexisting conditions can develop severe bronchitis, shortness of breath, wheezing, and coughing.[59] Flooding can result in outbreaks of cholera or other waterborne diseases and the production of prodigious numbers of mosquitoes, resulting in outbreaks of mosquito-borne diseases, such as encephalitis and malaria.

After a natural disaster, because of the remaining physical, biological, sociological, and psychological conditions, a variety of needs may exist, including clean water, food, shelter, health care, and clothing. Failure of a community, state, or nation to provide for these needs in an efficient and effective manner can exacerbate the extent of human suffering.

Psychological and Sociological Hazards

Living around other people exposes us to psychological and sociological hazards that can affect our health. Among these are overpopulation and crowding, hate crimes, wars, and acts of terrorism. Many of these hazards can be related directly or indirectly to population growth.

Population Growth

The world population now exceeds 7 billion. During the past three decades, the rate of world population growth began to decline because of worldwide efforts to curb the growth and avoid disaster caused by exceeding the earth's **carrying capacity**, the maximum population size that can be supported by available resources (air, water, shelter, etc.). Although the growth rate of the world's population will continue to decline (see **Figure 12.16**), the world population will continue to grow during the twenty-first century, but at only half the rate it grew in the recent past. At this rate, the United Nations projects that world population will reach 9 billion by the year 2043.[60]

The ramifications of overpopulation include the prospects of global warming, acid rain, bulging landfills, depletion of the ozone layer, increasing crime rates, increasing vulnerability to epidemics and pandemics, smog, exhaustion and contamination of soils and groundwater, degradation of arable land, and growing international tensions. Each year we degrade millions of acres of arable land.[61] Also, there will be a dwindling of natural resources for energy, housing, and living space—especially in large cities. Since 1950, the urban population has

carrying capacity
the maximum population of a particular species that a given habitat can support over a given period of time

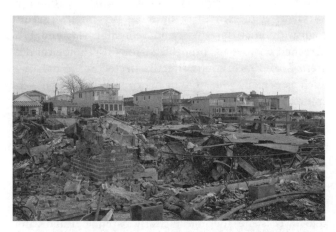

Figure 12.15 Aftermath of 2011 tsunami in Japan.
© Leonard Zhukovsky/ShutterStock, Inc.

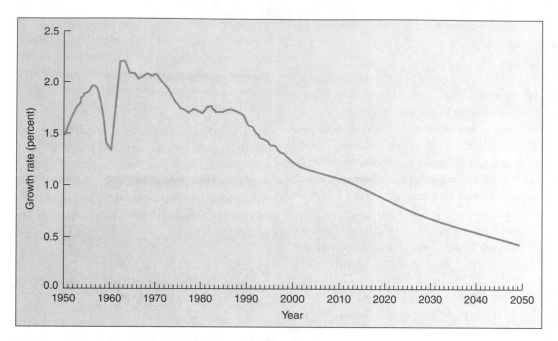

Figure 12.16 World population growth rate between 1950 and 2050.

U.S. Census Bureau (2008). International Data Base, December 2008 Update. Available at http://www.census.gov/ipc/www/img/worldgr.gif.

more than tripled. It is estimated that three-fourths of the current population growth is urban.

Most experts agree that the world population is approaching the maximum sustainable limit. However, no one knows what the ultimate population size will be, what the ultimate carrying capacity of the earth is, and how many people it can support. The world population growth rate was over 2% just 35 years ago; it is now just 1.092%.[62] Most of the population increase will be in the less developed countries, with growth rates in some of the more developed countries now falling below replacement levels.[63]

Terrorism

Terrorism is the calculated use of violence (or the threat of violence) against civilians to attain goals that are political, religious, or ideological in nature; this is done through intimidation, coercion, or instilling fear.[64] Terrorism is a sociological hazard because it affects entire societies, but it is also a psychological hazard because it produces fear, stress, and hysteria and endangers mental health.

One or more of these psychological conditions may have been experienced by those present in New York

terrorism calculated use of violence (or threat of violence) against civilians to attain goals that are political, religious, or ideological in nature

City during the terrorist attacks on the World Trade Center (WTC) on September 11, 2001. The attack not only caused 2,726 civilian deaths, but also caused an unprecedented environmental assault on Lower Manhattan that resulted in both physical and mental health problems in survivors. According to the World Trade Center Health Registry survey, the survivors caught in the dust cloud were two to five times more likely to report physical or mental health problems after September 11 than were those who were not. Based on the registry data survey, 64% of building survivors witnessed three or more potentially psychological traumatizing events on September 11, and 11% screened positive for probable serious psychological distress. Also, 15% of adults directly affected by the attacks—such as persons who were in the complex and who were injured; those who lost possessions, a job, a friend, or a relative in this event; or those who were part of the rescue effort—had probable post-traumatic stress disorder (PTSD), compared with only 7.4% of all New York City residents.[65]

A study of Manhattan residents found that 20% of those living near the WTC had symptoms consistent with PTSD 5 to 8 weeks after the attack. Clearly, psychological hazards are an important community health concern, especially during a disaster.

Responding to Environmental Hazards

The **Federal Emergency Management Agency (FEMA)**, an agency within the U.S. Department of Homeland Security, leads our nation's terrorism and natural disaster preparation and response efforts. "FEMA's mission is to support our citizens and first responders to ensure that as a nation we work together to build, sustain, and improve our capability to prepare for, protect against, respond to, recover from, and mitigate all hazards."[66]

Today, FEMA has 7,474 regular employees supplemented by nearly 4,000 stand-by, disaster assistant employees (see **Figure 12.17**).[66] The FEMA website (www.fema.gov) provides links to a vast array of information, reports, and publications that can help individuals and communities prepare for emergencies. Often FEMA works in partnership with other organizations that are part of the nation's emergency management system, including state and local emergency management agencies, 27 other federal agencies, and the American Red Cross.

In the United States, the **American Red Cross (ARC)**, a humanitarian organization led by volunteers and guided by its Congressional Charter and the Fundamental Principles of the International Red Cross Movement, provides relief to victims of disaster and helps people prevent, prepare for, and respond to emergencies.[67] The ARC works to prevent and alleviate human suffering wherever it may be found, with the purpose of protecting life and health while ensuring respect for human beings. The organization is responsible for giving aid to members of the U.S. Armed Forces and to disaster victims in the United States and abroad while staying neutral and impartial.

Each year, the ARC responds to more than 70,000 emergencies—from small emergencies such as apartment fires to large ones such as earthquakes and floods.[67] The ARC has 35,000 employees, more than 500,000 volunteers, and 700 local chapters throughout the United States.

Natural disasters can occur at any place and at any time. Although a variety of federal and state agencies and organizations have as all or part of their mission to respond to such disasters, recent experiences with disasters should have taught us that local communities, especially those located in high-risk areas, need to prepare too. Only through careful planning and preparation can communities hope to minimize loss of human health and life if a disaster should occur.

American Red Cross (ARC) a nonprofit, humanitarian organization led by volunteers and guided by its Congressional Charter that provides relief to victims of disasters

Federal Emergency Management Agency (FEMA) the nation's official emergency response agency

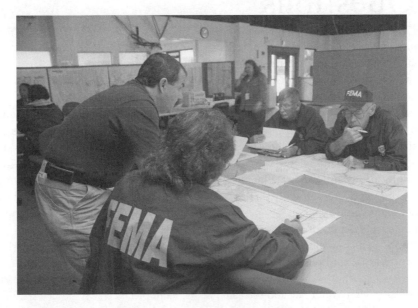

Figure 12.17 The Federal Emergency Management Agency (FEMA) helps communities prepare for disasters and manages federal response and recovery efforts following a national incident.
Courtesy of Patsy Lynch/FEMA

Chapter Summary

- Environmental health is the study and management of environmental conditions that affect our health and well-being.
- Environmental hazards increase our risk of injury, disease, or death.
- Air pollution is contamination of the air by gases, liquids, or solids in amounts that harm humans, other living organisms, or the ecosystem or that alter climate.
- Sources of primary air pollutants are stationary or mobile. Secondary air pollutants arise from the interaction of primary air pollutants and sunlight.
- Federal efforts to regulate air quality began with the Clean Air Act of 1963.
- Indoor air pollutants include asbestos, biogenic materials, combustion by-products, volatile organic compounds, and radon gas.
- The United States has the safest water in the world; nonetheless, waterborne disease outbreaks occasionally occur.
- The Clean Water Act and the Safe Drinking Water Act regulate water quality.

- Foodborne disease outbreaks, caused by unsafe food handling, are reported to and monitored by the Centers for Disease Control and Prevention.
- The U.S. Department of Agriculture and the Food and Drug Administration inspect food processing plants and enforce health and safety standards.
- Registered environmental health specialists inspect local restaurants and retail food outlets.
- The Resource Conservation and Recovery Act (RCRA) governs the management of both municipal and hazardous solid waste; the Comprehensive Environmental Response, Compensation, and Liability Act (CERCLA) governs the cleanup of existing hazardous waste sites.
- Natural hazards include high-energy radiation and natural environmental events such geologic and weather-related events.
- Uncontrolled population growth can contribute to psychological and sociological hazards.
- FEMA and the American Red Cross prepare for and respond to natural disasters.

Review Questions

1. What are the major sources of air pollutants? What are criteria pollutants? What is the difference between primary and secondary pollutants?
2. What role does the Environmental Protection Agency (EPA) play in protecting the environment?
3. What is the Clean Air Act? What are the National Ambient Air Quality Standards? What is the Air Quality Index?
4. What are some major kinds of indoor air pollutants? How can we reduce our exposure to them? What is radon, and why is it dangerous?
5. What is the difference between point source and non-point source pollution? Which is the bigger problem?
6. What is a waterborne disease outbreak? Name some causative agents.
7. List the purposes of the Clean Water Act and the Safe Drinking Water Act.
8. What is a foodborne disease outbreak? What factors contribute to foodborne disease

outbreaks? Name some common foodborne disease causative agents.
9. List the local, state, and federal agencies that help protect our food.
10. What types of refuse make up our municipal solid waste? How much MSW do we generate per person per year? How is MSW managed?
11. What is hazardous waste? Provide some examples.
12. What are the purposes of the Resource Conservation and Recovery Act (RCRA) and the Comprehensive Environmental Response, Compensation, and Liability Act (CERCLA)?
13. How does lead poisoning occur? Who is most vulnerable?
14. What is a vectorborne disease? Provide some examples.
15. What kinds of environmental hazards can be found in our places of work? List some examples.
16. What is ionizing radiation? Why is it a health issue?

17. What are natural disasters? How do they affect the health of a community?
18. How would you interpret the relationships among population growth, the environment, and human health?
19. How would you define *terrorism*? How did the World Trade Center attacks result in environmental health repercussions?

20. What role does the Federal Emergency Management Agency (FEMA) play in preparing for and responding to catastrophic events? What is the role of the American Red Cross in providing assistance to people and communities after a natural disaster?

Activities

1. In a one-page paper, identify what you feel to be the number-one waste or pollution problem faced by the United States, and then detail your rationale for feeling this way.
2. Make arrangements to interview a director of environmental health in a local health department. Find answers to the following questions and summarize these answers in a two-page paper:

a. What are all the tasks this division of the health department carries out?
b. What is the primary environmental health problem of your community? Why is it a problem? How is it being dealt with?

References

1. Miller, G. T., Jr., and S. Spoolman (2010). *Environment Science: Principles, Concepts, and Solutions*, 13th ed. Belmont, CA: Brooks/Cole, Cengage Learning.
2. Chiras, D. D. (2013). *Environmental Science*, 9th ed. Burlington, MA: Jones & Bartlett Learning.
3. U.S. Environmental Protection Agency (2012). "Air Quality Trends." Available at http://www.epa.gov/airtrends/aqtrends.html.
4. U.S. Environmental Protection Agency (2009). *Air Quality Index (AQI): A Guide to Air Quality and Your Health*. Available at http://www.epa.gov/airnow/aqi_brochure_08-09.pdf.
5. U.S. Environmental Protection Agency (2010). "Indoor Air: An Introduction to Indoor Air Quality." Available at http://www.epa.gov/iaq/ia-intro.html.
6. U.S. Environmental Protection Agency (2012). "Radon: Health Risks." Available at http://www.epa.gov/radon/healthrisks.html.
7. U.S. Department of Health and Human Services (1991). *Environmental Tobacco Smoke in the Workplace* (DHHS [NIOSH] pub. no. 91-108). Washington, DC: U.S. Government Printing Office.
8. Substance Abuse and Mental Health Services Administration, Center for Behavioral Health Statistics and Quality (2011). *Results from the 2010 National Survey on Drug Use and Health: National Findings* (Office of Applied Studies, NSDUH Series H-41, DHHS pub. no. SMA 11-4658). Rockville, MD: Author. Available at http://oas.samhsa.gov/NSDUH/2k10NSDUH/2k10Results.pdf.
9. U.S. Environmental Protection Agency (1993). *Respiratory Health Effects of Passive Smoking: Lung Cancer and Other Disorders* (EPA/600/6-90/006f). Washington, DC: U.S. Government Printing Office.
10. U.S. Department of Health and Human Services (1991). *Environmental Tobacco Smoke in the Workplace* (DHHS [NIOSH] pub. no. 91-108). Washington, DC: U.S. Government Printing Office.
11. Overpeck, M. D., and A. J. Moss (1991). *Children's Exposure to Environmental Cigarette Smoke Before and After Birth* (DHHS pub. no. PHS-91-1250). Washington, DC: U.S. Government Printing Office.
12. California Air Resources Board (2005). *Report to the California Legislature: Indoor Air Pollution in California*. Sacramento, CA: Author. Available at http://www.arb.ca.gov/research/indoor/ab1173/rpt0705.pdf.
13. American Lung Association (2006). *State of Tobacco Control: 2012*. New York: Author. Available at http://www.stateoftobaccocontrol.org/SOTC_2012.pdf.
14. World Health Organization and United Nations Children's Fund Joint Monitoring Programme for Water Supply and Sanitation (2008). *Progress on Drinking Water and Sanitation*. New York and Geneva: UNICEF and WHO.
15. World Health Organization and UNICEF (2000). *Global Water Supply and Sanitation Assessment 2000 Report*. Geneva: WHO/UNICEF Joint Monitoring Programme for Water Supply and Sanitation. Available at http://www.who.int/water_sanitation_health/monitoring/globalassess/en/index.html.
16. U.S. Environmental Protection Agency (2006). "The Endocrine Disruption Screening Program." Available at http://www.epa.gov/scipoly/oscpendo/pubs/edspoverview/primer.htm#3.
17. U.S. Environmental Protection Agency (2006). "Pharmaceuticals and Personal Care Products as Environmental Pollutants." Available at http://www.epa.gov/ppcp/.

18. Centers for Disease Control and Prevention (23 September 2011). "Surveillance for Waterborne Disease and Outbreaks and Other Health Events Associated with Recreational Water–United States, 2007-2008 and Surveillance for Waterborne Disease and Outbreaks Associated with Drinking Water–United States, 2007-2008." *Morbidity and Mortality Weekly Report, Surveillance Summaries* 60(No. SS-12).

19. Steward, J. C. (1990). *Drinking Water Hazards: How to Know If There Are Toxic Chemicals in Your Water and What to Do If There Are*. Hiram, OH: Envirographics.

20. Barber, N. L. (2009). *Summary of Estimated Water Use in the United States in 2005* (U.S. Geological Survey Fact Sheet 2009-3098). Available at http://pubs.usgs.gov/fs/2009/3098/.

21. U.S. Geological Survey (2009). "Water Questions and Answers." Available at http://ga.water.usgs.gov/edu/qahome.html.

22. Centers for Disease Control and Prevention (1999). "Achievements in Public Health, 1900-1999: Fluoridation of Drinking Water to Prevent Dental Caries." *Morbidity and Mortality Weekly Report*, 48(41): 933-940.

23. Federal Water Pollution Control Act (33 U.S.C. 1251 ed seq.) [As Amended Through P.L. 107-303, November 27, 2002]. Available at http://epw.senate.gov/water.pdf.

24. U.S. Environmental Protection Agency (2012). "Water: Contaminant Candidate List–CCL and Regulatory Determinations Home." Available at http://water.epa.gov/scitech/drinkingwater/dws/ccl/index.cfm.

25. U.S. Environmental Protection Agency (2009). "Water: Contaminant Candidate List–Basic Information on CCL and Regulatory Determinations." Available at http://water.epa.gov/scitech/drinkingwater/dws/ccl/basicinformation.cfm.

26. Centers for Disease Control and Prevention (1999). "Achievements in Public Health, 1900-1999: Safer and Healthier Foods." *Morbidity and Mortality Weekly Report*, 48(4): 905-913.

27. Morris, Jr., J. G. (2012). "How Safe Is Our Food?" *Emerging Infectious Diseases*, 17(1): 126-127.

28. Scallan, E., R. M. Hoekstra, F. J. Angulo, R. V. Tauxe, M.-A. Widdowson, S. L. Roy, J. L. Jones, and P. M. Griffin. (2012). "Foodborne Illness Acquired in the United States–Major Pathogens." *Emerging Infectious Diseases*, 17(1): 7-15.

29. Scallan, E., P. M. Griffin, F. J. Angulo, R. V. Tauxe, M.-A. Widdowson, and R. M. Hoekstra (2012). "Foodborne Illness Acquired in the United States–Unspecified Agents." *Emerging Infectious Diseases*, 17(1): 16-22.

30. Scharff, R. L. (2010). "Health-Related Costs from Foodborne Illness in the United States." Available at http://www.pewhealth.org/uploadedFiles/PHG/Content_Level_Pages/Reports/PSP-Scharff%20v9.pdf.

31. Centers for Disease Control and Prevention (2011). "Surveillance for Foodborne Disease Outbreaks–United States, 2008." *Morbidity and Mortality Weekly Report*, 60(35): 1197-1202. Available at http://www.cdc.gov/mmwr/PDF/wk/mm6035.pdf.

32. Centers for Disease Control and Prevention (2011). "Vital Signs: Incidence and Trends of Infection with Pathogens Transmitted Commonly Through Food – Foodborne Diseases Active Surveillance Network, 10 U.S. Sites, 1996-2010." *Morbidity and Mortality Weekly Report*, 60(22): 749-755. Available at http://www.cdc.gov/mmwr/pdf/wk/mm6022.pdf

33. National Pesticide Information Retrieval Systems (2012). "PPIS." Available at http://ppis.ceris.purdue.edu.

34. U.S. Environmental Protection Agency (2011). *Municipal Solid Waste Generation, Recycling, and Disposal in the United States: Facts and Figures for 2010.* Available at http://www.epa.gov/osw/nonhaz/municipal/pubs/msw_2010_rev_factsheet.pdf.

35. U.S. Environmental Protection Agency, Office of Resource Conservation and Recovery (2009). *Municipal Solid Waste Generation, Recycling, and Disposal in the United States Detailed Tables and Figures for 2008.* Available at http://www.epa.gov/epawaste/nonhaz/municipal/pubs/msw2008data.pdf.

36. BBC News (2005). "Recycling Around the World." Available at http://news.bbc.co.uk/2/hi/europe/4620041.stm.

37. U.S. Environmental Protection Agency (2011). "Methane: Sources and Emissions." Available at http://www.epa.gov/methane/sources.html.

38. U.S. Environmental Protection Agency (2010). *National Analysis: The National Biennial RCRA Hazardous Waste Report (Based on 2009 Data)* (EPA530-R-10-014A). Available at http://www.epa.gov/wastes/inforesources/data/br09/national09.pdf.

39. Centers for Disease Control and Prevention (2012). "Ground Water Awareness Week–March 11-18, 2012." Available at http://www.cdc.gov/Features/GroundWaterAwareness/.

40. U.S. Environmental Protection Agency (September 2009). *Superfund Annual Report FY 2008* (EPA 9200.2-87 5101T). Washington, DC: Author. Available at http://www.epa.gov/superfund/accomp/pdfs/sf_annual_report_2008.pdf.

41. Silbergeld, E. K. (1997). "Preventing Lead Poisoning in Children." *Annual Review of Public Health*, 18: 187-210.

42. Jones, R. L., D. M. Homa, P. A. Meyer, D. J. Brody, K. L. Caldwell, J. L. Pirkle, and M. J. Brown. (2009). "Trends in Blood Lead Levels and Blood Lead Testing Among US Children Aged 1 to 5 Years, 1988-2004." *Pediatrics*, 123: e376-e385. Available at http://www.pediatrics.org/cgi/content/full/123/3/e376.

43. Centers for Disease Control and Prevention, National Center for Environmental Health (2010). "Number of Children Tested and Confirmed EBLLs by State, Year and BLL Group, Children < 72 Months Old." Available at http://www.cdc.gov/nceh/lead/data/StateConfirmedByYear_1997_2009.htm.

44. Centers for Disease Control and Prevention, Division of Vector-Borne Infectious Diseases (2012). "Final 2011 West Nile Virus Human Infections in the United States." Available at http://www.cdc.gov/ncidod/dvbid/westnile/surv&controlCaseCount11_detailed.htm.

45. Centers for Disease Control and Prevention, Division of Vector-Borne Infectious Diseases (2011). "2006 West Nile Virus Activity in the United States." Available at http://www.cdc.gov/ncidod/dvbid/westnile/surv&controlCaseCount06_detailed.htm.

46. Centers for Disease Control and Prevention (2011). "LaCrosse Encephalitis: Epidemiology and Geographic Distribution." Available http://www.cdc.gov/lac/tech/epi.html.

47. Centers for Disease Control and Prevention, Division of Vector-Borne Diseases (2011). "Information on *Aedes albopictus*." Available at http://www.cdc.gov/ncidod/dvbid/arbor/albopic_new.htm.

48. Centers for Disease Control and Prevention, Division of Vector-Borne Diseases (2005). "Information on *Aedes japonicus*." Available at http://www.cdc.gov/ncidod/dvbid/arbor/japonicus.htm.

49. Centers for Disease Control and Prevention (2011). "Lyme Disease: Reported cases of Lyme disease by state or locality, 2002-2011." Available at http://www.cdc.gov/lyme/stats /chartstables/reportedcases_statelocality.html.

50. United States Department of Health and Human Services, Centers for Disease Control and Prevention, National Institute for Occupational Safety and Health (2004). *Worker Health Chartbook*, 2004. DHHS (NIOSH) Publication No. 2004-146. Available at http://www.cdc.gov/niosh/docs/2004-149.

51. National Institute for Occupational Safety and Health (2012). *Work-Related Lung Disease Surveillance System (eWoRLD)*. Available at http://www2a.cdc.gov/drds/WorldReportData/.

52. Centers for Disease Control and Prevention (2009). "Coal Worker's Pneumoconiosis-Related Years of Potential Life Lost Before Age 65 Years–United States, 1968-2006." *Morbidity and Mortality Weekly Report*, 58(50): 1412-1416. Available at http://www.cdc.gov/mmwr/PDF/wk/mm5850.pdf.

53. Centers for Disease Control and Prevention, National Institute for Occupational Safety and Health (2005). "Pesticide Illness and Injury Surveillance." Available at http://www.cdc.gov /niosh/topics/pesticides/.

54. Calvert, G. M., J. Karnik, L. Meler, J. Beckman, B. Morrissey, J. Sievert, R. Barrett, M. Lackovic, L. Mabee, A. Schwartz, Y. Mitchell, and S. Moraga-McHaley (2008). "Acute Pesticide Poisoning Among Agricultural Workers in the United States, 1998-2005." *American Journal of Industrial Medicine*, 2008: 883-898.

55. U.S. Bureau of the Census, Statistical Abstract of the United States (2012). "Table 16.1. Revenue for Selected Health Care Industries by Source of Revenue: 2008 and 2009." Available at http://www.census.gov/compendia/statab/2012/tables /12s0162.pdf.

56. Centers for Disease Control and Prevention, National Institute for Occupational Safety and Health (2004). *NIOSH Alert: Preventing Occupational Exposures to Antineoplastic and Other Hazardous Drugs in Health Care Settings* (DHHS [NIOSH] pub. no. 2004-165). Cincinnati, OH: Author.

57. American Cancer Society (2012). *Cancer Facts and Figure–2010*. Atlanta, GA: Author.

58. World Health Organization (n.d.). "Health Effects of the Chernobyl Accident: An Overview." Available at http://www .who.int/mediacentre/factsheets/fs303/en/index.html.

59. Centers for Disease Control and Prevention (2005). "Infectious Disease and Dermatological Conditions in Evacuees and Rescue Workers After Hurricane Katrina–Multiple States, August–September, 2005." *Morbidity and Mortality Weekly Report*, 54(Dispatch): 1-4.

60. United Nations, Department of Economic and Social Affairs, Population Division, Population Estimates and Projections Section (2011). "World Population Prospects, the 2010 Revision: Frequently Asked Questions." Available at http://esa .un.org/unpd/wpp/Other-Information/faq.htm#q3.

61. Hinrichsen, D., and B. Robey (Fall 2000). *Population and the Environment: The Global Challenge* (Population Reports, Series M, no. 15). Baltimore, MD: Johns Hopkins University School of Public Health, Population Information Program. Available at http://www.actionbioscience.org/environment /hinrichsen_robey.html.

62. Kluger, J. (2000). "The Big Crunch." *Time* (Special Edition), Earth Day 2000: 44-47.

63. Index Mundi (2011). "World Demographics Profile 2012." Available at http://www.indexmundi.com/world/demographics _profile.html.

64. WordNet Search (n.d.). "Terrorism." Available at http://wordnetweb.princeton.edu/perl/webwn?s=terrorism.

65. New York City Department of Health and Mental Hygiene (7 April 2006). "Substantial Physical and Mental Health Effects Reported by WTC Building Survivors" [Press release]. Available at http://www.nyc.gov/html/doh/html/pr2006 /pr021-06.shtml.

66. Federal Emergency Management Agency (2010). "About FEMA." Available at http://www.fema.gov/about.

67. American Red Cross (2010). "Disaster Relief." Available at http://www.redcross.org/what-we-do/disaster-relief.

Chapter 13

Injuries and Injury Prevention at Home, on the Road, at Work, and at Play

Robert R. Pinger, PhD

Chapter Objectives

After studying this chapter, you will be able to:

1. Describe the scope and importance of injuries as a health issue and an economic issue in our communities.

2. Explain the difference between intentional and unintentional injuries and provide examples of each.

3. List the four elements usually included in the definition of the term *unintentional injury*.

4. Describe the epidemiology of unintentional injuries in the United States.

5. List strategies for the prevention and control of unintentional injuries.

6. Explain how education, regulation, automatic protection, and litigation can reduce the number and seriousness of unintentional injuries.

7. Describe the scope and importance of intentional injuries as a community health problem in the United States.

8. List some factors that contribute to domestic violence and some strategies for reducing it.

9. List some factors that contribute to violence among youths and explain what communities can do to reduce this level of violence.

10. Discuss local, state, and national resources for preventing or controlling intentional injuries.

Introduction

In this chapter we first define the terms *injury, unintentional injury,* and *intentional injury.* Then we describe the scope and importance of injuries as both a health and an economic problem for communities. We describe the various types of injuries in epidemiological terms—when and where injuries occur and to whom. Then we review approaches to the prevention and control of injuries and injury deaths. We do this first for unintentional injuries, and then for intentional injuries.

Definitions

The word **injury** is derived from the Latin word for "not right."[1] Injuries result from "acute exposure to physical agents such as mechanical energy, heat, electricity, chemicals, and ionizing radiation interacting with the body in amounts or at rates that exceed the threshold of human tolerance."[2] In this chapter we first discuss **unintentional injuries**, injuries judged to have occurred without anyone intending that harm be done. These include injuries that result from motor vehicle crashes, poisonings, falls, drowning, suffocation, fires and burns, and the unintentional discharge of firearms. Then, we discuss **intentional injuries**, injuries judged to have been purposely inflicted, either by another or oneself. These include assaults, intentional shootings and stabbings, and suicides.

> **fatal injury** an injury that results in one or more deaths
>
> **injury** physical damage to the body resulting from mechanical, chemical, thermal, or other environmental energy
>
> **intentional injury** an injury that is purposely inflicted, either by the victim or by another
>
> **unintentional injury** an injury that occurred without anyone intending that harm be done

Cost of Injuries to Society

Injuries are a leading cause of death and disability in the United States. Each year more than 150,000 people die from **fatal injuries**, making this the fifth leading cause of death in this country. Specifically, in 2010, there were 176,939 injury deaths, which accounted for 7.2% of all deaths among residents of the United States.[3] Of these deaths, 118,043 (67%) were classified as unintentional injury deaths, 37,793 (21%) as suicides, and 16,065 (9%) as homicides. The remaining 5,038 (3%) deaths were either of undetermined intent (4,629 [3%]) or the result of legal intervention (409 [< 1%]) (see **Figure 13.1**).[3]

Injuries are a major cause of premature deaths (deaths that occur before reaching the age of one's life expectancy) in the United States. To simplify calculating years of potential life lost (YPLL) from a premature death, 75 years of age is used as a standard life expectancy. In terms of years of life lost before 75 years of age (YPLL-75), unintentional injuries rank third. However, when one considers all injuries, both intentional and unintentional, then injuries are the leading cause of YPLL-75. Leading causes of YPLL-75 and the number of deaths for various causes of death are shown in **Table 13.1**.[4,5]

Deaths are only a small part of the total cost of injuries. Worldwide, 10.9% of the human burden of disease can be attributed to injuries.[6] Here in the United States, each year,

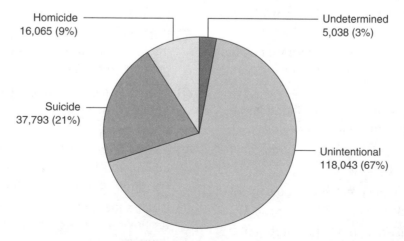

Figure 13.1 Injury deaths: United States, 2010.

Homicide
16,065 (9%)

Undetermined
5,038 (3%)

Suicide
37,793 (21%)

Unintentional
118,043 (67%)

Data from Murphy, S. L., J. Xu, and K. D. Kochanek (2012). "Deaths: Preliminary Data for 2010." *National Vital Statistics Reports*, 60(4): 1–68. Available at http://www.cdc.gov/nchs/data/nvsr/nvsr60/nvsr60_04.pdf.

Table 13.1 Leading Causes of Years of Potential Life Lost (YPLL) and Number of Deaths for Leading Causes of Death: United States, 2008

Disease or Condition	Age-Adjusted YPLL Before Age 75 (per 100,000 population)	Number of Deaths
Injury	1,718	176,695
Cancer	1,438	565,469
Heart disease	1,029	616,828
Stroke	185	134,148
Diabetes mellitus	165	70,553
Chronic lower respiratory diseases	182	141,090
Chronic liver disease and cirrhosis	159	29,963
Human immunodeficiency virus disease	100	10,285
Influenza and pneumonia	81	56,284

Sources: Data from National Center for Health Statistics (2012). *Health, United States, 2011 with Special Feature on Socioeconomic Status and Health*. Hyattsville, MD: National Center for Health Statistics. Available at http://www.cdc.gov/nchs/hus.htm; and Miniño, A. M., S. L. Murphy, J. Xu, and J. D. Kochanek (2011). "Deaths: Final Data for 2008." *National Vital Statistics Reports*, 59(10): 1–152. Available at http://www.cdc.gov/nchs/data/nvsr/nvsr59/nvsr59_10.pdf.

there are approximately 35 million medically consulted injury or poisoning episodes, a rate of 115 episodes per 1,000 population per year. Persons in poor health had higher rates of medically consulted injury or poisoning episodes than those in excellent, very good, good, or fair health.[7]

Injuries place a special burden on our emergency departments (EDs) because they are the leading cause of ED visits, making up more than one-third of the total visits. There were an estimated 39.4 million injury-related ED visits during 2007, or 13.3 visits per 100 persons per year. This made up one-third of all ED visits in 2007. Included in this total were visits for injury, poisoning, or adverse effects of medical treatment.[8]

In addition to the physical and emotional harm caused by these injuries and poisonings, there are significant associated economic costs. For example, in 2010 these costs were estimated at more than $730 billion, including $374 billion in wage and productivity losses, $167 billion in medical expenses, $117 billion in administrative costs, $40 billion in motor vehicle damage, $20 billion in employer uninsured costs, and $11 billion in fire losses.[9] This amounted to about $2,400 per person in the United States.[9] The true economic burden of injuries is much greater than this estimate because it does not include value of life lost to premature mortality, loss of patient and caregiver time, and nonmedical expenditures such as insurance costs, property damage, litigation, decreased quality of life, and disability.

Unintentional Injuries

Unintentional injuries are the cause of nearly two-thirds of all injury-related deaths in the United States; they rank fifth as a leading cause of death and third as a leading cause of YPLL-75. There were 118,043 unintentional injury deaths in 2010.[3] Accounting for those deaths were motor vehicle crashes (30%), followed by unintentional poisonings (26%) and falls (22%), along with other causes.[3] In addition to the human death toll were the economic costs, mentioned earlier. Clearly, unintentional injuries constitute one of the United States' major community health problems. One of the *Healthy People 2020* objectives is to reduce the rate of unintentional injury deaths from 40.0 per 100,000 to 36.0 per 100,000 population; another is to reduce the rate of nonfatal injuries that result in emergency department visits from 9,219.3 per 100,000 to 8,297.4 per 100,000 population.[10,11]

There are four significant characteristics of unintentional injuries: (1) they are unplanned events, (2) they usually are preceded by an unsafe act or condition (hazard), (3) they often are accompanied by economic loss, and (4) they interrupt the efficient completion of tasks.

An **unsafe act** is any behavior that would increase the probability of an unintentional injury; for example, driving an automobile while being impaired by alcohol or operating

unsafe act any behavior that would increase the probability of an injury occurring

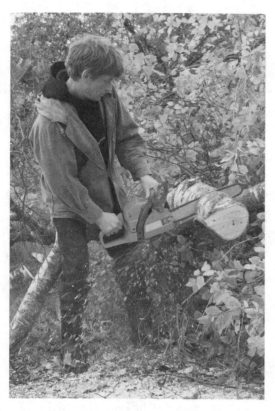

Figure 13.2 An unsafe act is a behavior that increases the probability of any injury. Should this person be wearing eye protection?
© Gala_Kan/ShutterStock, Inc.

a chain saw without eye protection is an unsafe act (see Figure 13.2). An **unsafe condition** is any environmental factor (physical or social) that would increase the probability of an unintentional injury. Icy streets are an example of an unsafe condition. Unsafe acts and unsafe conditions are **hazards**. Whereas hazards do not actually cause unintentional injuries (an alcohol-impaired person may reach home uninjured, even over icy streets), they do increase the probability that an unintentional injury will occur.

Types of Unintentional Injuries

There are many types of unintentional injuries. The majority occur as a result of motor vehicle crashes, poisonings, falls, drowning, suffocation, fires and burns, and firearms. These are discussed briefly here.

hazard an unsafe act or condition

unsafe condition any environmental factor or set of factors (physical or social) that would increase the probability of an injury occurring

Motor Vehicle Crashes

In the United States, motor vehicle crashes are the leading cause of unintentional injury deaths most years. In 2010, 35,080 people were killed[3] and an estimated 2.24 million people were injured in a motor vehicle crash.[12]

Poisonings

Poisonings were the second leading cause of unintentional deaths in the United States in 2010, when unintentional poisoning deaths numbered 30,781.[3] These deaths resulted from unintentional ingestion of fatal doses of medicines and drugs, consumption of toxic foods such as mushrooms and shellfish, and exposure to toxic substances in the workplace or elsewhere.

Falls

Falls, the third leading cause of unintentional fatal injuries, resulted in 25,903 deaths in 2010.[3] The overall rate of non-fatal fall injuries for which a healthcare professional was consulted in 2010 was 43 per 100,000 population; the rate for persons 75 years of age or older was 115 per 100,000.[13]

Other Types of Unintentional Injuries

Other leading causes of unintentional injury deaths in 2010 were drowning (3,696 deaths), all other transport (2,815 deaths), fires and burns (2,737 deaths), and firearms (600 deaths). All other types of unintentional injury deaths numbered about 9,754 in 2010.[3]

Epidemiology of Unintentional Injuries

Unintentional injuries are a major community health concern because they account for a disproportionately large number of early deaths in our society. However, deaths are only a part of the human toll; incapacitation is another significant aspect of the problem. One in six hospital days can be attributed to unintentional injuries. As mentioned earlier, medical costs from unintentional injuries run into the billions of dollars annually. Many of these injuries, such as head and spinal cord injuries, result in long-term or permanent disabilities that can affect individuals and their families for years.

In the following section, we discuss the epidemiology of unintentional injuries. In addition to describing the occurrence of injuries by person (who), place (where), and time (when), we discuss factors that increase one's risk for experiencing an unintentional injury, such as alcohol and other drug use and distracted driving.

Person: Who Experiences Injuries?

Unintentional injuries resulting in death and disability occur in all age groups, genders, races, and socioeconomic groupings. However, certain groups are at greater risk for injury than others.

Age

Unintentional injuries are the leading cause of death of those between 1 and 44 years. They are the fifth leading cause of death in newborns and infants,[14] and the third leading cause of death in the 45- to 54-year age group.[15] In 2008, unintentional injuries accounted for 32.9% of deaths in the 5- to 14-year age group and 43.8% of deaths in the 15- to 24-year age group.[5]

Children and teenagers are at a higher than average risk of dying as a result of unintentional firearm injury. Unintentional nonfatal firearm-related injury rates are highest among persons ages 15 to 24 years; nearly 1 in 4 unintentional firearm deaths occurs in this age group.[16] Nearly 10% of high school males reported carrying a gun at least 1 day in the past 30 days.[17]

For all age groups between 1 and 74 years of age, motor vehicle crashes are the leading cause of unintentional injury deaths.[3] However, rates of involvement in crashes resulting in fatal injuries in 2008 were the highest for drivers ages 16 to 20 (39.1 per 100,000 licensed drivers). This was almost twice the fatal injury involvement rate for all drivers (22.6 per 100,000 licensed drivers).[18]

Among elders (those 65 years or older), injuries are the ninth leading cause of death.[15] Injury deaths would rank higher, but many elders die of other causes resulting from the aging process, such as heart disease, cancer, and stroke. An examination of the rates of death per 100,000 among elders reveals that elders have the highest unintentional injury death rate of any age group (100 per 100,000). For those 85 years or older, the injury death rate climbs to 298 per 100,000.[19]

Falls disproportionately affect elders, who are at nearly three times the average risk of experiencing a medically attended fall injury episode (see **Figure 13.3**).[7,20] Each year in the United States, falls affect approximately 30% of elders (adults 65 years of age or older).[21] Falls are the leading

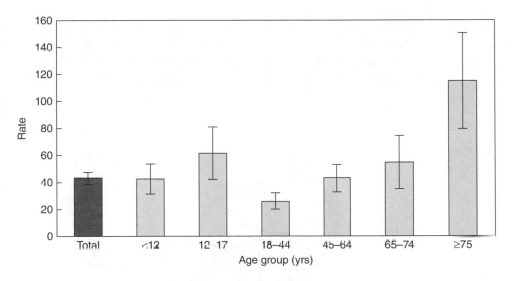

Figure 13.3 Falls disproportionately affect elders, who are at nearly three times the risk of experiencing a medically attended fall injury episode. This figure shows the rate[a] of nonfatal, medically consulted fall injury episodes,[b] by age group.[c]

[a]Per 1,000 population. [b]Annualized rates of injury episodes for which a healthcare professional was contacted either in person or by telephone for advice or treatment. An injury episode refers to a traumatic event in which the person experiences one or more injuries from an external cause. Estimates are based on household interviews of a sample of the civilian, noninstitutionalized population. [c]Estimates are based on household interviews of a sample of the civilian, noninstitutionalized population.

Reproduced from Centers for Disease Control and Prevention. "QuickStats: Rate of Nonfatal, Medically Consulted Fall Injury Episodes, by Age Group." *Morbidity and Mortality Weekly Report*, 61(4): 81; data from Adams, P. F., M. E. Martinez, J. L. Vickerie, and W. K. Kirzinger (2011). "Summary Health Statistics for the U.S. Population: National Health Interview Survey, 2010." *Vital Health Statistics*,10(251).

cause of both nonfatal and fatal injury among elders. They account for 65% of all nonfatal-injury ED visits by elders and more than 50% of the unintentional injury–related deaths of this age group.[9]

Elders are at age-increased risk of dying in car crashes, too. A report published by the American Automobile Association (AAA) Foundation revealed that drivers 65 years of age or over are almost twice as likely to die in car crashes as drivers ages 55 to 64. Drivers 75 or older were two and one-half times as likely to die, and drivers 85 or older were almost four times as likely to die in car crashes compared with drivers ages 55 to 64.[22] Since this article appeared, more attention has been paid to the topic of safe mobility of elders.

Elders also experience high rates of nonfatal injuries. In 2009, elders made 3.4 million injury-related visits to emergency departments.[9] Elders are twice as likely to be hospitalized following an injury as those younger than 65, and to experience longer hospital stays.[7]

Gender

Statistics indicate that, at every age level, males are much more likely to sustain a fatal unintentional injury than are females. Overall, the ratio of male deaths to female deaths is nearly 2:1. In the 15- to 24-year and 25- to 64-year age groups, males die from unintentional injuries at greater than three times the rate of their female counterparts. Although differences in unintentional injury death rates between the sexes decline with age, men retain a marginally

higher rate even in the over-75-year age group. One type of unintentional fatality with a wide disparity in rates per 100,000 is motor vehicle crashes (18.9 in males vs. 7.5 in females in 2008); the type with the narrowest is falls (8.2 in males vs. 7.6 in females).[9]

Minority Status

In 2009, unintentional injuries and adverse effects were the leading cause of death for all age groups 1–44 years for most racial and ethnic groups. However, for black Americans, homicide and unintentional injuries were the leading causes of injury deaths for the 15- to 24-year and 25- to 34-year age groups.[12] Age-adjusted death rates for unintentional injuries in 2008 were highest for the American Indian/Alaska Native population (53.5 per 100,000) and lowest for the Asian/Pacific Islander population (15.4 per 100,000). The white, non-Hispanic population had a rate of 40.2, and the Hispanic population had a lower rate of 27.9 per 100,000 population.[5]

Place: Where Do Injuries Occur?

Unintentional injuries occur wherever people are—at home, on the road, at work, at school, and at play.

Home

People spend more time at home than any other place, so it is not surprising that about half of all episodes of unintentional injuries and poisonings occurred in the home (see **Figure 13.4**).[7] Four-fifths of poisonings occurred in homes,

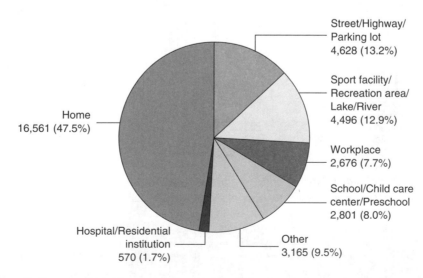

Figure 13.4 Number (in thousands) and percentage of injury episodes by place of occurrence: United States, 2010.

Data from Adams, P. F., M. E. Martinez, J. L. Vickerie, and W. K. Kirsinger (2011). "Summary Health Statistics for the U.S. Population: National Health Interview Survey, 2010." *Vital Health Statistics*, 10(251): 1–117. Available at http://www.cdc.gov/nchs/data/series/sr_10/sr10_251.pdf.

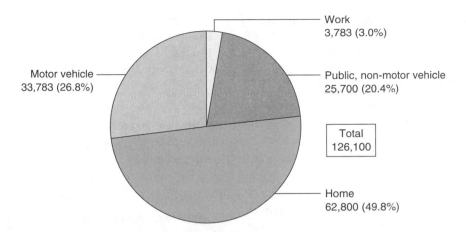

Total
126,100

Work
3,783 (3.0%)

Public, non-motor vehicle
25,700 (20.4%)

Motor vehicle
33,783 (26.8%)

Home
62,800 (49.8%)

Figure 13.5 Unintentional Injury deaths by class: United States, 2010.

Note: Deaths for sections of chart add to more than the total because some deaths are included in more than one section.

Reprinted with permission of the National Safety Council (2012). *Injury Facts 2012 Edition.* Itasca, IL: Author.

where poisonings are the leading cause of injury deaths. For this reason, homes have surpassed highways as the leading site of unintentional injury deaths (see Figure 13.5).[9] Unintentional injuries in the home result from falls, burns, poisonings, accidental shootings and stabbings, and suffocation. Within the home, some areas are more dangerous than others. The presence of appliances (including stoves, toasters, mixers, and so on) and sharp knives in the kitchen makes this room one of the more dangerous in the house.

Another location where many unintentional injuries occur, particularly to the very young and old, is on stairways. Falls can occur from one surface level to another—stairs or ladders, for example—or on the same level. Of the 20,823 deaths resulting from falls in 2010, 18,300 occurred at home, where falls account for 29% of all deaths from unintentional injuries and poisonings.[9] For children, the bathroom, garage, and basement are hazardous areas because of the drugs, cleaning agents, and other poisonous materials that are often stored in these areas.

Highway

According to the 2008 National Health Interview Survey of the U.S. population, 13% of all injuries were sustained on streets, on highways, and in parking lots.[7] However, with regard to all fatal injuries, 26% were sustained at these venues. Fatal injury rates per 100 million vehicle miles traveled (VMT), which has declined almost every year since 1995, reached a record low of 1.14 in 2009. A majority of those killed were drivers (64%), followed by passengers (27%), motorcycle riders (4%), pedestrians (3%), and pedalcyclists (2%).[18] Two of the nation's

Healthy People 2020 objectives were to reduce the number of motor vehicle deaths per 100,000 population from the 2007 baseline of 13.8 to 12.4, and to reduce the number of motor vehicle deaths per 100 million vehicle miles traveled from the 2008 baseline of 1.3 to 1.2 by 2020.[10] By 2009, both these objectives had been met or surpassed.[18]

Streets, highways, and parking lots are no longer the leading venues for fatal injuries. More injury deaths now occur in or around the home. Two reasons explain this change: First, significant progress has been made in reducing motor vehicle–related deaths. Motor vehicle–related deaths have been reduced from a rate of 22.5 per 100,000 people in 1980 to 11.01 per 100,000 people in 2008.[18] This has been achieved through effective interventions, including increasing public awareness, education, legal proscriptions (such as child safety seats and safety belts), innovative vehicle and equipment designs, improved roadways, and enhanced medical systems. The second reason why more deaths now occur at home is because of the recent increase in unintentional poisoning deaths, most of which occur in homes.[5]

One remaining area of concern is the number of unlicensed or improperly licensed drivers on the highways, who may be involved in one in five fatal crashes. These are drivers with a license that is suspended, revoked, expired, cancelled, or denied. Nearly 4% of drivers involved in fatal crashes have no known license at all.[23]

Recreation/Sports Area

The third most likely place to sustain an injury that results in a visit to an ED is a recreation or sports area, such as a soccer field, baseball diamond, or basketball court. Approximately 12.9% of injuries reported in the 2010 National Health Interview Survey occurred in these settings.[7]

School, Preschool, and Child Care Settings

The fourth most common place for injuries to occur is in school, preschool, or child care settings. These settings are not unusually hazardous, but outside the home, these are places where much of our children's time is spent.

Workplace

The workplace ranks fifth as a location where unintentional injuries frequently occur; about 7.7% of reported injuries occurred in the workplace.[7] The number of civilian Americans employed in the labor force is approximately 154.4 million.[24] After home, Americans spend the next largest portion of their time at work; thus, safe and healthy workplaces are essential if the United States is to reach its future health objectives.

An **occupational injury** is any injury that results from a work-related event or from a single, instantaneous exposure in the work environment.[25] The injury can be minor, such as a bruise, cut, abrasion, or minor burn, or major, such as an amputation, fracture, severe laceration, eye loss, acute poisoning, or severe burn. An injury that causes any restriction of normal activity beyond the day of the injury's occurrence is considered a **disabling injury**.

A total of 3.1 million nonfatal injuries were reported in private industry workplaces during 2010, resulting in a rate of 3.5 cases per 100 equivalent full-time workers. About half of the 3.1 million nonfatal injury and illness cases reported in 2010 were classified as a disabling; that is, they required recuperation away from work beyond the day of the incident. The vast majority of these case reports were classified as injuries; about 5% were classified as illnesses.[26]

disabling injury an injury causing any restriction of normal activity beyond the day of the injury's occurrence

occupational injury any injury that results from a work-related event or from a single, instantaneous exposure in the work environment

In extreme cases, occupational injuries can be fatal. In 2010, there were 4,690 fatal work-related injuries, or about 12.8 per day. The fatal work injury rate for 2010 was 3.6 per 100,000 full-time equivalent workers.[27,28] The leading type of workplace fatal injuries were motor-vehicle crashes, with 1,044 deaths (22% of the total); followed by assaults and violent acts, with 832 deaths (18%); other transportation deaths, with

813 deaths (17%); being struck by an object, with 738 deaths (16%); falls, with 646 deaths (14%); exposure to harmful substances or environments, with 414 deaths (9%); and other, with 203 deaths (4%).[28]

The industries with the highest rates of fatal occupational injuries per 100,000 employees in 2010 were agriculture, forestry, fishing, and hunting (27.9); mining (19.8); transportation and warehousing (13.7); and construction (9.8). Industries with the lowest fatality rates per 100,000 employees were educational and health services (0.9), financial activities (1.3), and information (1.5) (see **Figure 13.6**).[27]

Occupational injuries are an economic issue, too. It has been estimated that workplace injuries and deaths cost $176.9 billion in 2010, including $86.8 billion in lost wages and productivity, $43.2 billion in medical expenses, and $32.0 billion in administrative costs and other costs. Thus, each worker in the United States must produce $1,300 in goods or services just to offset the cost of work-related injuries.[9]

Time: When Do Injuries Occur?

The incidence of injuries varies by year, season, and time of day. During the twentieth century, and into the twenty-first, the incidence rates for some types of unintentional injuries declined while others increased. For example, the number of motor vehicle deaths fell from 51,091 to 33,808 during 1980–2010, and the fatality rate per 100 million vehicle miles traveled (VMT) declined from 3.35 to 1.14 during that 30-year period.[18] This remarkable achievement occurred despite the fact that Americans drove twice as many miles in 2010 as they did in 1980.

Since 1975, unintentional deaths from drowning, fires, and burns have declined by more than half, and from firearms by two-thirds. However, deaths from falls, which declined significantly from 1975 to 1986, have begun to increase in the past few years, as the U.S. population ages. Deaths from poisonings have also increased and, in 2010, were the second leading cause of unintentional injury deaths.[5]

Although even one worker death is one too many, it is instructive to note that the work-related fatality rates in the United States have declined significantly over the past 100 years. In 1929, an estimated 20,000 work-related unintentional injury deaths occurred, a death rate of about 16 per 100,000 workers.[9] As mentioned earlier, the death rate per 100,000 workers is now close to 3 per 100,000. Several factors have contributed to this decline: (1) a better educated workforce; (2) regulations, such as the Occupational Safety and Health Act of 1970, requiring safer workplaces;

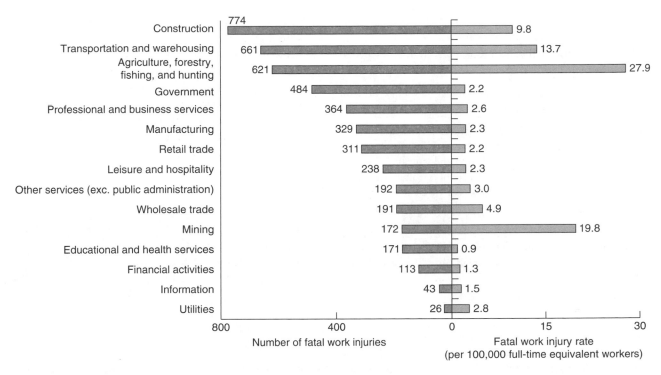

Figure 13.6 Number and rate of fatal occupational injuries, by industry sector, 2010.

Reproduced from U.S. Department of Labor, Bureau of Labor Statistics (2011). "Injuries, Illnesses, and Fatalities: Fatal Occupational Injuries and Workers' Memorial Day." Available at http://www.bls.gov/iif/oshwc/cfoi/worker_memorial.htm.

(3) automation; and (4) the transformation of the United States from a primarily manufacturing and farming economy to more of a service- or information-based economy.

Seasonal variations also occur in the incidence of some types of unintentional injuries. For example, 58% of all drowning occurs in 4 months—May, June, July, and August—when more people take part in water sports. Also, workplace injuries involving outdoor machinery, falling objects, electric current, and explosions are highest in the summer, when farming and construction work increase. Conversely, 62% of all deaths due to fires and burns are recorded during the 6 months from November through April, when furnaces, fireplaces, wood-burning stoves, and electric and kerosene space heaters are most often in use.[9]

Motor vehicle crash rates per 100 million VMT in 2009 were highest during October through February. Motor vehicle–related deaths increase markedly at night. Fatalities also occur at a higher rate on weekends (Friday through Sunday). Although more fatal crashes occur on Saturdays, more crashes of all types occur on Fridays. The hours between midnight and 3 a.m. on Saturdays and Sundays are the most dangerous 3-hour periods to travel by car.[18]

Conversely, workplace fatalities decline on weekends, when fewer people are working.

Much publicity surrounds the number of motor vehicle deaths that occur during the following six major holiday periods: Memorial Day, Fourth of July, Labor Day, Thanksgiving, Christmas, and New Year. However, it has been shown that the number of crash-related deaths for these periods is not significantly greater than that for non holiday periods. However, the proportion of fatal crashes in which the driver is alcohol impaired during holiday periods—40% for New Year's Day, 42% for Memorial Day, 40% for the Fourth of July, 38% for Labor Day, 34% for Thanksgiving, and 37% for Christmas) is higher than during nonholiday periods (32%).[18]

Alcohol and Other Drugs as Risk Factors

Alcohol may be the single most important factor associated with intentional and unintentional injuries. This is certainly the case with fatal motor vehicle crashes, in which 38% of persons killed in traffic crashes in 2009 died in alcohol-related crashes. Although 38% represents a significant decline from the 55% reported in 1982, it is still too high. There has also been a decline in the percentage of those killed in crashes who were intoxicated—that is, who had blood alcohol concentrations (BACs) that exceeded 0.08%—from 48% in 1982 to 32% in 2009.[18]

In 2010, 4 million adults reported an estimated 112,116,000 episodes of alcohol-impaired driving in the United States.

> Sixty percent of those who reported driving while impaired indicated one episode in the past 30 days; however, some respondents reported that they drove while impaired daily. Men accounted for 81% of 2010 alcohol impaired driving episodes. Young men aged 21–34 years, who represented 11% of U.S. adult population, reported 32% of all episodes.[29]

Binge drinking was a factor in episodes of impaired driving, because 85% of all alcohol-impaired episodes were reported by those who also reported binge drinking. Also, the 4.5% of adults who reported binge drinking four or more times per month accounted for 55% of all alcohol-impaired driving episodes.[29]

The percentage of drivers and motorcycle riders in single-vehicle fatal crashes whose BAC exceeded the legal limit (0.08%) was 22% in 2009, but this percentage was nearly four times higher during weekend nighttimes than during daytime on weekdays. Alcohol was involved in 72% of the single-car crashes that occurred on a weekend night in which a 21-year-old or older driver or motorcycle operator was killed (see **Figure 13.7**). Male and female drivers or motorcycle operators are about equally likely to be injured in a vehicle crash, but about three-fourths of all drivers or motorcycle operators who are killed in a vehicle crash are males.[18] Forty percent of drivers or motorcycle operators involved in fatal crashes had a previous record of crashes, license suspension or revocation, driving while intoxicated (DWI) conviction, speeding conviction, or other harmful moving violation conviction.[18]

Unfortunately, drivers are not the only persons killed in alcohol-related motor vehicle crashes. Motor vehicle crashes are the leading cause of death among children age 1 year or older in the United States, and one in four deaths of child passengers age 14 years or older involves alcohol use. Of the 2,355 children who died in alcohol-related crashes during the period 1997 to 2002, 1,588 (68%) were riding with drinking drivers.[30]

Alcohol use often contributes to motor vehicle injuries and deaths in another way. Safety belt use by drinking drivers is lower than for their nondrinking counterparts, thus

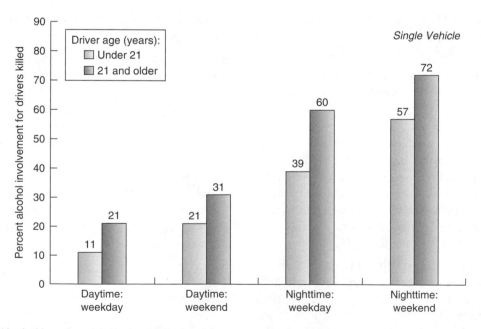

Figure 13.7 Alcohol impairment (BAC ≥ 0.08) for drivers or motorcycle operators killed in single-vehicle crashes, by driver age, time of day, and day of week.

Reproduced from U.S. Department of Transportation, National Highway Traffic Safety Administration (2011). *Traffic Safety Facts 2009: A Compilation of Motor Vehicle Crash Data from the Fatality Analysis Reporting System and the General Estimates System* (DOT HS 811 402). Washington, DC: Author. Available at http://www-nrd.nhtsa.dot.gov/Pubs/811402.pdf.

increasing the likelihood of a fatal outcome if there is a crash. In 1999, safety belts were used by only 19% of fatally injured intoxicated drivers, compared with 30% of fatally injured alcohol-impaired drivers (with BAC levels between 0.01% and 0.09%) and 48% of fatally injured sober drivers. Child passenger restraint use also decreases as the BAC of the driver increases.[30] Of 1,409 child passengers with known restraint information who died while riding with drinking drivers (1997–2002), only 466 (32%) were restrained at the time of the crash. Passage of primary enforcement safety belt laws (laws that allow police to stop and ticket a driver solely because an occupant is unbelted) and stricter enforcement of these laws in all states could reduce child passenger deaths. Excessive drinking can also increase a pedestrian's chances of being killed by a motor vehicle. In 2009, 14% of pedestrians killed by motor vehicles were intoxicated.[18] Alcohol has also been shown to be a risk factor for bicyclists; nearly 11% of those killed in traffic crashes were under the influence of alcohol or other drugs.[18]

Alcohol contributes to water-related deaths as well. Nearly half of those who drown have evidence of alcohol in their blood. Alcohol was the leading contributing factor in 16% of boating fatalities in 2011.[31] A U.S. Coast Guard study estimates that boat operators with a BAC above 0.10% are more than 10 times as likely to be killed in a boating accident than are boat operators with zero BACs.[32] In another study, it was found that nearly half of all boating fatalities occurred when vessels were not underway. This implies that although it is dangerous when the person who is operating the boat is drinking, it is also dangerous when passengers have been drinking (see Figure 13.8). Finally, alcohol

consumption lowers a person's chance of survival should that person end up in the water. In a study conducted in Louisiana, alcohol and/or metabolites of an illicit drug were found in 60% of drowning victims age 13 years or older.[33] Clearly, alcohol consumption and aquatic recreation are a dangerous combination.

Prevention Through Epidemiology

Two *Healthy People 2020* objectives focus on reducing the rate of fatal and nonfatal injuries in the United States. One objective is to reduce the rate of fatal injuries from 59.2 to 53.3 per 100,000; another is to reduce the rate of hospitalization for nonfatal injuries from 617.6 to 555.8 per 100,000 (see Box 13.1).

Unfortunately, sometimes it has been society's nature to wait until after the occurrence of a tragedy to correct an existing hazard or dangerous situation. When properly implemented

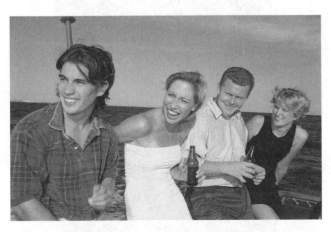

Figure 13.8 Alcohol consumption while boating lowers your chances of survival should you end up in the water.
© Ingram Publishing/Index Stock Imagery, Inc.

Box 13.1 *Healthy People 2020*: Objectives

Objective IVP-1 Reduce fatal and nonfatal injuries
Target setting method: 10% improvement
Data Sources: National Vital Statistics System-Mortality (NVSS-M), CDC, NCHS, National Hospital Discharge Survey (NHDS), CDC, NCHS
Target and baseline:

Objective	2007 Baseline	2020 Target
IVP-1.1 Reduce deaths per 100,000 population	59.2	53.3
IVP-1.2 Reduce hospitalizations for nonfatal injuries per 100,000 population	617.6	555.8

For Further Thought

Injuries are a leading cause of death and years of potential life lost (YPLL-75) in the United States. Millions more are hospitalized because of injuries each year. During the last decade, significant progress was made in reducing fatal and nonfatal injuries on our highways and in our workplaces, in large part through regulation. During the same period, fatal and nonfatal injuries from falls and poisonings have increased. What role do you think well-conceived regulations can play in reducing fatal and nonfatal injuries from poisonings and falls?

Source: Reproduced from U.S. Department of Health and Human Services, Office of Disease Prevention and Health Promotion (2010). *Healthy People 2020.* Available at http://www.healthypeople.gov/2020 /topicsobjectives2020/pdfs/HP2020objectives.pdf.

in a timely manner, however, **injury prevention/injury control** efforts can reduce the number and seriousness of injuries and minimize the number of injury deaths.

A Model for Unintentional Injuries

An understanding of the public health model of communicable diseases (host, agent, and environment) can help conceptualize disease control. A similar **model for unintentional injuries** has been proposed. In this model, the injury-producing agent is energy (see **Figure 13.9**).

Examples of injury-producing energy are plentiful. A moving car, a falling object (or person), and a speeding bullet all have kinetic energy. When one of these moving objects strikes another object, energy is released, often resulting in injury or trauma. Similarly, a hot stove or pan contains energy in the form of heat. Contact with one of these objects results in the rapid transfer of heat. If the skin is unprotected, tissue damage (a burn) occurs. Electrical energy is all around us and represents a potential source of unintentional injuries. Even accidental poisonings fit nicely into the model that incorporates energy as the causative agent of injury. Cleansers, drugs, and medicines represent stored chemical energy that, when released inappropriately, can cause serious injury or death.

Prevention and Control Tactics Based on the Model

Based on the epidemiological model just described, in which energy is considered the agent of injury, four types of injury prevention/injury control actions can be taken. These four tactics are modified from those of William Haddon, Jr.[34] The first is to prevent the accumulation of the injury-producing agent, energy. Examples of implementing this principle include reducing speed limits to decrease motor vehicle injuries, lowering the height of children's high chairs and of diving boards to reduce fall injuries, and lowering the settings on hot water heaters to reduce the number and seriousness of burns. In our electrical example, circuit breakers in the home prevent the accumulation of excess electrical energy.

The second type of action is to prevent the inappropriate release of excess energy or to modify its release in some way. Flame-retardant fabric that will not ignite is an example of such prevention. Currently, there is a law that requires that such a fabric be used in the manufacture of children's pajamas. The use of automobile safety belts is another example. In this case, excess energy (movement of a human body) is released into the safety belt instead of into the car's windshield (see **Figure 13.10**). In the prevention of fall injuries, hand rails, walkers, and nonslip surfaces in bathtubs prevent the inappropriate release of kinetic energy resulting from falls.

The third tactic involves placing a barrier between the host and agent. The insulation around electrical wires and the

injury prevention/ injury control an organized effort to reduce the number and seriousness of injuries and minimize the number of injury deaths

model for unintentional injuries the public health triangle (host, agent, and environment) modified to indicate energy as the causative agent of injuries

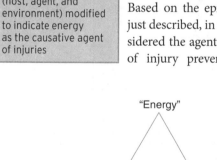

Figure 13.9 The public health model for unintentional injuries.

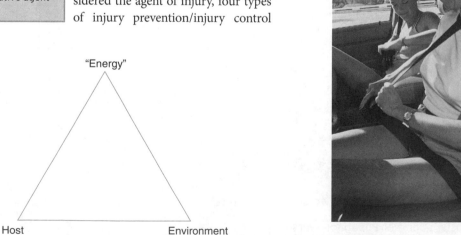

Figure 13.10 Safety belts reduce injuries caused by motor vehicle crashes and save lives.
© Yuri Arcurs/ShutterStock, Inc.

use of potholders and non–heat-transferring handles on cookware are examples of this preventive strategy. The use of sunscreen lotion and the wearing of a hat in the summer place a barrier between the sun's energy and a person's skin. Another example is the cable barriers being installed between opposing traffic lanes on many interstate highways. These cable barriers not only serve as a barrier to protect oncoming traffic, but also modify the release of energy and provide drivers and occupants with a relatively soft landing.

Finally, it is sometimes necessary or useful to completely separate the host from potentially dangerous sources of energy. Examples include the locked gates and high fences around electrical substations and swimming pools. At home, locking up guns and poisons provides protection against the likelihood of unintentional injury of young children.

Other Tactics

By viewing energy as the cause of unintentional injuries and deaths, it is possible to take positive steps in their prevention and control. There are still other actions that a community can take. First, injury-control education in the schools and in other public forums can be helpful. Second, improvements in the community's ability to respond to emergencies, such as encouraging the public to enroll in first aid and cardiopulmonary resuscitation (CPR) classes and expanding 911 telephone services, can limit disability and save lives. Third, communities can ensure that they have superior emergency and paramedic personnel by instituting the best possible training programs. The result will be improved emergency medical care and rehabilitation for the injured. Finally, communities can strengthen ordinances against high-risk behaviors, such as driving while impaired by alcohol, and then support their enforcement.

Community Approaches to the Prevention of Unintentional Injuries

There are four broad approaches to the prevention of unintentional injuries—education, regulation, automatic protection, and litigation.

Education

Injury prevention education is the process of changing people's health-directed behavior in such a way as to reduce unintentional injuries. Many of us remember the school fire drill, lessons on bicycle safety, and the school crossing guard. Education certainly has a place in injury prevention. Undoubtedly, millions of injuries were prevented in these ways. However, injury prevention education has its limitations, because people do not always heed the lessons they learned.

Regulation

Regulation, the enactment and enforcement of laws to control conduct, is a powerful way for societies to reduce the number and seriousness of unintentional injuries. Examples of the success of this approach are evident in our motor vehicle–related, workplace-related, and residential-based injury statistics.

State laws requiring child safety seats and safety belt use are another example of regulation to reduce injuries. Beginning in the 1980s, automobile child restraint and safety belt legislation spread across the United States. Beginning with the 1990 models, auto makers were required to equip all passenger cars with safety belts or air bags. All states now have child passenger safety seat or restraint requirements for children, and all states except for New Hampshire have occupant restraint (safety belt) use laws for adults (18 years of age or older).[18] Enforcement laws and fine levels vary from state to state, as well as seats of the vehicle covered (front seat or all seats), and type of vehicle covered. To check state seat belt laws, visit this text's website. Passage and vigorous enforcement of safety belt regulations are one reason why motor vehicle fatalities have declined in recent years.

Another regulatory change that has helped reduce motor vehicle–related injuries is the lowering of the blood alcohol concentration at which a person is legally intoxicated to 0.08%. In 2004, Delaware became the final state to adopt this standard, which has now been adopted by all 50 states, Puerto Rico, and the District of Columbia. A systematic review of the effectiveness of such laws has revealed that they decrease fatal alcohol-related motor vehicle crashes an average of 7%. This should save 400 to 600 lives per year nationally and significantly decrease the number and seriousness of injuries.[35]

It will be interesting to see how well the regulatory approach will resolve another serious hazard, distracted drivers. A recent survey indicates that distracted driving is becoming increasingly recognized as a roadway hazard for everyone. Thirty-four percent of interviewees indicated they felt less safe on the road today than before, and 31% indicated that distracted driving was the single most common reason for this feeling.[36] Since the first workshop on distracted

injury prevention education the process of changing people's health-directed behavior so as to reduce unintentional injuries

regulation the enactment and enforcement of laws to control conduct

driving research was held by the National Highway Traffic Safety Administration (NHTSA) in 2000, the number of personal electronic devices in use has increased dramatically. Examples are cell phones (including iPhones), Blackberries, personal digital assistants (PDAs), laptops, electronic notebooks, and global positioning devices. In addition, availability of in-car entertainment devices, such as DVD players and gaming devices, is more widespread than in the past. "Drivers using handheld cell phones at any given moment has increased from 4% in 2002 to 6% in 2008," according to the NHTSA.[37]

Use of electronic devices is only part of the problem. Drivers also become distracted when eating or drinking, putting on makeup, tending to children, talking to a passenger, looking for something in the car or in a purse, fidgeting with controls, singing along with music, and reading a map. But add to these all of the technological devices now in widespread use, and the impact of distracted driving on highway safety becomes significant. In 2008, 5,870 of the 37,261 traffic fatalities (16%) were recorded as distracted-related traffic fatalities.[37] Drivers younger than 20 years of age had the highest proportion of fatal crashes in which the driver was reported as being distracted at the time of the crash (16%).

Twenty-seven states, Guam, and the District of Columbia have indicated that distracted driving has become a priority in their Strategic Highway Safety Plans. Eight states have indicated that the governor or legislature has set up a task force or summit on distracted driving. In 2010, 43 states collected data on crashes in which distraction was a factor. Collecting such data may soon become a federal requirement.[37]

No state bans all cell phone use for all drivers, but 10 states; Washington, D.C.; Guam; and the Virgin Islands prohibit all drivers from using handheld cell phones while driving. Thirty-one states ban cell phone use for novice drivers, and 19 states prohibit school bus drivers from cell phone use when passengers are present.[38]

Texting and e-mailing while driving are the latest distracted driving issues. The American Automobile Association's Foundation for Traffic Safety reports that 21% of drivers admit to having read or sent a text message or e-mail while driving in the past 30 days. This figure increases to 40% of drivers younger than 35 and 51%

of drivers 16–19 years of age.[37] States are taking a comprehensive approach to reducing text messaging and e-mailing while driving, including education, legislation, and enforcement. Forty-one states indicate that they have initiated public education/information campaigns on this topic using either traditional methods or new media/social networking, and eight states indicate that they have begun efforts to educate judges on the issue of distracted driving. Text messaging has been banned for all drivers in 38 states and Guam and for novice drivers in an additional 5 states.[38] Efforts to regulate cell phone usage and texting are ongoing; to see the laws in a particular state, visit the Governors' Highway Safety Association website at www.ghsa.org.

Regulation of distracted driving highlights the difficulties involved in relying entirely on regulation as an approach to controlling personal behavior. The recent history of motorcycle helmet legislation provides another example of the problem of achieving a balance between personal freedoms and society's legitimate health interests. Studies show that helmet laws are associated with a 29% to 33% decrease in annual per capita motorcycle fatalities.[39] In 1975, all but two states required motorcyclists to use helmets. Beginning in 1976, states began to repeal these laws. By the end of 2008, only 20 states, Puerto Rico, and the District of Columbia required a helmet for all motorcyclists.[18] To check the motorcycle helmet laws in a particular state, visit this text's website.

One place in which legislation has played a significant role in reducing the number and seriousness of injuries is in the workplace. Some of the earliest laws, passed during the nineteenth century, were aimed at protecting children in the workplace (see **Figure 13.11**). In 1908, following the lead in several states, the federal government passed the first federal **workers' compensation laws**. This set of laws was designed to compensate those workers and their families who suffer injuries, disease, or death from workplace exposure. Although the first laws covered only federal workers, laws in individual states now cover all workers.

By far, the most important federal regulation that protects workers is the **Occupational Safety and Health Act of 1970 (OSH Act)**. The enactment of this legislation validated and reinforced the view that the federal government has a direct interest in the safety and health of U.S. workers. At the time the act was passed, 14,000 workers died each year on the job. The act helped to raise the consciousness of both management and labor regarding the problems of health and safety in the workplace. Today, only about 5,000 workers die each year in the United States, even though the workforce has increased substantially over the past 40-plus years.

Occupational Safety and Health Act of 1970 (OSH Act) comprehensive federal legislation aimed at ensuring safe and healthful working conditions for working men and women

workers' compensation laws a set of federal laws designed to compensate those workers and their families who suffer injuries, disease, or death from workplace exposure

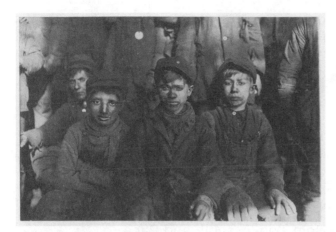

Figure 13.11 Before child labor laws were passed, many children worked long hours at dangerous jobs such as mining.

The purpose of the Occupational Safety and Health Act of 1970 is to ensure that employers in the private sector furnish each employee "employment and a place of employment which are free from recognized hazards that are causing or likely to cause death or serious physical harm."[40] Furthermore, employers were required to comply with all occupational safety and health standards promulgated and enforced under the act by the **Occupational Safety and Health Administration (OSHA)**, which was established by the act.

Also established by the OSH Act was the **National Institute for Occupational Safety and Health (NIOSH)**, a research body now located in the Centers for Disease Control and Prevention of the Department of Health and Human Services. NIOSH is responsible for recommending occupational safety and health standards to OSHA, which is located in the Department of Labor.

The OSH Act contains several noteworthy provisions that, taken together, have made workplaces safer than in the past. Perhaps the most important is the employee's right to request an OSHA inspection. Under this right, any employee or any employee representative may notify OSHA of violations of standards or of the general duty obligation (to provide a safe and healthy workplace) by the employer. Under the act, the employee's name must be withheld if desired, and the employee or a representative may accompany the OSHA inspectors in their inspection. By another provision of the OSH Act, individual states can regain local authority over occupational health and safety by submitting state laws that are and will continue to be as effective as the federal programs.[40]

Some of the injury prevention actions required in the workplace have found their way into residential settings, where they have reduced the number and seriousness of injuries. Electrical, heating, and other codes have improved the safety of homes. Equipment and tools that meet workplace standards (such as stepladders and power hand tools) are available for general purchase.

Automatic Protection

When engineered changes are combined with regulatory efforts, remarkable results can sometimes be achieved. The technique of improving product or environmental design to reduce unintentional injuries is termed **automatic (passive) protection**.[34] A good example is child-proof safety caps (see **Figure 13.12**). Child-proof safety caps on aspirin and other medicine were

> **automatic (passive) protection** the modification of a product or an environment to reduce unintentional injuries
>
> **National Institute for Occupational Safety and Health (NIOSH)** a research body within the U.S. Department of Health and Human Services that is responsible for developing and recommending occupational safety and health standards
>
> **Occupational Safety and Health Administration (OSHA)** the federal agency located within the U.S. Department of Labor and created by the OSH Act that is charged with the responsibility of administering the provisions of the OSH Act

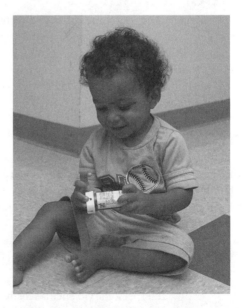

Figure 13.12 Child safety caps are an example of automatic or passive protection.

introduced in 1972. By 1977, deaths attributed to ingestion of analgesics and antipyretics had decreased by 41%.[41] We are all familiar with automatic protection devices. Common examples include automatic shut-off mechanisms on power tools (such as lawn mowers), safety caps on toxic products, and the warning lights and sounds that remind us to buckle our safety belts in motor vehicles.

Litigation

When other methods fail, behavioral changes can sometimes come about through the courts. **Litigation**—lawsuits filed by injured victims or their families—has been successful in removing dangerous products from store shelves or otherwise influencing changes in dangerous behavior. Litigation against a manufacturer of unsafe automobile tires, for example, might result in safer tires. Lawsuits against bartenders and bar owners for serving alcohol to drunken customers, who have later injured other people, have produced more responsible server behavior at public bars. Alcohol-related deaths and injuries on college campuses have caused insurance companies to re-examine their liability insurance policies with fraternities and sororities. This has forced some of these organizations and the universities themselves to restrict the way alcohol is used. The outcome may be a drop in unintentional injuries on these campuses.

Intentional Injuries

Intentional injuries, the outcome of self-directed and interpersonal violence, are a staggering community health problem that result in more than 50,000 deaths and countless nonfatal injuries each year in the United States.[3] In 2010, an estimated 2 million persons were treated for nonfatal physical assault–related injuries in EDs.[8]

Types of Intentional Injuries

The spectrum of violence includes assaults, rapes, suicides, and homicides. These acts of violence can be perpetrated against family members (children, elders, and intimate partners), community members, or complete strangers. In 2008, residents of the United States 12 years of age or older reported being victims of an estimated 3.8 million violent crimes. Violent and property crimes were at or near their lowest levels in more than three decades.[42]

litigation the process of seeking justice for injury through the courts

Interpersonal violence is a costly community health problem, not only because of the loss of life and productivity, but also because of its economic costs to the community, including the costs of extra police, prosecutors, judges, jails, prisons, emergency healthcare services, medical services, social workers, and probation officers. Clearly, this is a problem for which prevention is the most economic approach.

Epidemiology of Intentional Injuries

To better understand the problem of intentional injuries, it is instructive to look more closely at both the victims and the perpetrators of violence. Victims can be classified by gender, age, and racial characteristics. The nature and seriousness of crimes can also be categorized.

Homicide, Assault, and Rape

Males and blacks as well as the poor are more vulnerable to violence. Except for rape and sexual assault, for which females were victims four times more often than males, the violent crime victimization rate is higher for males than for females. In 2010, victimization rates were higher for blacks, American Indian and Alaskan Natives, and persons of mixed race than for whites, Hispanics, or Asian or Pacific Islanders. Persons age 25 or older generally experienced lower violent victimization rates when compared with younger persons.[42]

Violent crimes often result in injuries. Although the overall rate of violent victimizations has declined, the injury rate for victims of violent crimes has risen to 29%. Although injuries are more frequent in males, the rate of emergency department visits for sexual assault–related injuries can be five times higher for females. The highest injury rates for both males and females were for the 15- to 24-year age group.[8]

More violent acts, whether self-directed or directed at others, are committed by males. Firearms are increasingly involved in violent acts, with increasingly fatal consequences. Abuse of drugs, especially alcohol, also contributes to the number of intentional injuries. Additionally, perpetrators of violent acts are more likely to have been abused or neglected as children or exposed to violence and aggression earlier in their lives.

In 2010, 12,996 murders were reported to the Federal Bureau of Investigation (FBI).[43] Although the U.S. homicide rate has declined in recent years and has leveled off at about 6 per 100,000 people, it remains higher than the rates of most other industrialized nations. Homicide and legal intervention fell from the list of the 15 leading causes of death in the United States in 2010. For the 15- to 24-year age group, however, homicide still ranked as the second leading cause of death in 2009.[15] Two-thirds of the homicides in the United States are committed with firearms, which are abundant and easy to acquire. Males accounted for 77.4% of the murder victims, and 90.3% of the offenders.[43]

Overall, it is estimated that about half of all violent crimes were reported to police in 2010. Although the statistics on rape and attempted rape are somewhat incomplete, the data suggest that 78% of all rapes and sexual assaults against females are committed by someone acquainted with, known to, or related to the victim.[42]

Suicide and Attempted Suicide

As previously indicated, more than 30,000 suicides are reported each year in the United States, accounting for one-fifth of all injury mortality. In 2010, 37,793 suicide deaths were reported.[3] The suicide rate for men was nearly four times that for women in 2008.[5] The suicide rate in young people (15 to 24 years of age) in 2008 was 10.1 per 100,000.[5] Senior men (65 years old or older) are much more likely to commit suicide than are senior women.

Firearm Injuries and Injury Deaths

Statistics on fatal and nonfatal firearm injuries include data covering both intentional and unintentional incidents. When one considers all firearm deaths—those that result from both intentional and unintentional acts—firearms were the third leading cause of injury deaths after poisoning and motor vehicle crashes in 2006 (see **Figure 13.13**).[44]

In 2010, there were 30,978 firearm injury deaths. Of these, 19,308 (62%) were classified as suicides, 11,015 (35%) as homicides, 409 (1%) as resulting from legal intervention, and 246 (< 1%) as of undetermined intent. Only 600 (2%) were classified as unintentional deaths. In 2010, firearms were used in 69% of all homicides, 51% of all suicides, and less than 1% of all unintentional injury deaths.[3] Males were six times more likely to die or be treated in an emergency department for a gunshot wound than were females.

At highest risk for homicide and suicide involving firearms are teenage boys and young men, ages 15 to 24 years. A national survey found that in 2009, nearly 10% of high school males had carried a handgun on at least one occasion in the past 30 days.[18] The gun-toting behavior continues even in college. In a random sample of 10,000 undergraduate students, 4.3% reported that they had a working firearm at college, and 1.6% said they had been threatened with a gun while at college.[45] The banning of firearms on college and university campuses was successfully challenged in Utah where, in 2006, the Utah Supreme Court ruled that the University of Utah cannot bar guns from campus.[46] This decision has raised concern among educators and administrators in institutions of higher education, where campus safety is an ever-present concern. Although there have been heinous and well-publicized violent crimes on campuses, statistics reveal that college and university campuses are much safer than other busy venues. The average homicide rate on U.S. campuses is one homicide

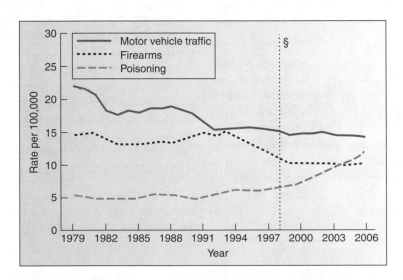

Figure 13.13 Firearms were the third leading cause of injury deaths after motor vehicle accidents and poisonings in 2006.

Data from Centers for Disease Control and Prevention (2009). "QuickStats: Age-Adjusted Death Rates per 100,000 Population for the Three Leading Causes of Injury Death—United States, 1979–2006." *Morbidity and Mortality Weekly Report*, 58(24): 675; and Miller, M., D. Hemenway, and H. Wechsler (2002). "Guns and Gun Threats at College." *Journal of American College Health*, 51(2): 57–65.

per 1 million students. By comparison, the homicide rate in New York City is 70 times greater.[47]

But the presence of more guns on campus could change this. About 40% of college students binge drink regularly, and 85% of campus arrests involve alcohol.[47] Allowing students to possess/carry guns would virtually guarantee that violence on college campuses would become more deadly. Also, college students are under considerable stress, often citing relationship problems, financial matters, or academic or career concerns. The reported suicide ideation rate among college students is estimated at about 10%. Because about 50% of suicides involve firearms, one can assume that increasing the number of firearms on campus would increase the suicide completion rate among college students.

Violence in Our Society and Resources for Prevention

A sixth-grade student brings a gun to school and kills a teacher and three students; a man is killed for "cutting" in line; and a child dies from punishment for breaking a rule at home. These are signs of the violent society in which Americans now find themselves living. Violence seems like the natural and easy way to resolve differences among those who lack verbal negotiation skills or interest in compromise. Violent confrontations can affect the social environment of the community and the health of its members. Violent conflicts take place in our homes, neighborhoods, schools, and places of work.

child abuse the intentional physical, emotional, verbal, or sexual mistreatment of a minor

child maltreatment an act or failure to act by a parent, caretaker, or other person as defined under state law that results in physical abuse, neglect, medical neglect, sexual abuse, or emotional abuse, or an act or failure to act that presents an imminent risk of serious harm to a child

child neglect the failure of a parent or guardian to care for or otherwise provide the necessary subsistence for a child

family violence the use of physical force by one family member against another, with the intent to hurt, injure, or cause death

The availability and proliferation of firearms make this approach particularly deadly. In 2009, homicide and legal intervention were the number-one cause of death for black American males in the 15- to 24-year and 25- to 34-year age groups.[15] Unfortunately, violent confrontations often result in injuries and deaths not only for the victim, but also for others not directly involved in the confrontation.

Violence in Our Homes

One in every six homicides is the result of family violence. **Family violence** includes the maltreatment of children, intimate partner violence, sibling violence, and violence directed toward elder family members. Because children are our most important resources, and because being abused or neglected as a child increases one's risk for violent behavior as an adult, it is of paramount importance that communities prevent domestic violence wherever possible and intervene in cases where prevention has failed. In recent years, family violence, including violence against children and intimate partners, has drawn increased attention.

Child Maltreatment

Child maltreatment is an act or failure to act by a parent, caretaker, or other person as defined under state law that results in physical abuse, neglect, medical neglect, sexual abuse, emotional abuse, or an act or failure to act that presents an imminent risk of serious harm to a child. Also included are other forms of child maltreatment, such as child abandonment and congenital drug addiction. **Child abuse** can be physical, emotional, verbal, or sexual. Physical abuse is the intentional (nonaccidental) inflicting of injury on another person by shaking, throwing, beating, burning, or other means. Emotional abuse can take many forms, including showing no emotion and the failure to provide warmth, attention, supervision, or normal living experiences. Verbal abuse is the demeaning or teasing of another verbally. Sexual abuse includes the physical acts of fondling or intercourse, nonphysical acts such as indecent exposure or obscene phone calls, or violent physical acts such as rape and battery. **Child neglect** is a type of maltreatment that refers to the failure by the parent or legal caretaker to provide necessary, age-appropriate care when financially able to do so, or when offered financial or other means to do so. Neglect may be physical, such as the failure to provide food, clothing, medical care, shelter, or cleanliness. It also may be emotional, such as the failure to provide attention, supervision, or other support necessary for a child's well-being. Or, it may be educational, such as the failure to ensure that a child attends school regularly. Educational neglect is one of the most common categories of neglect, followed by physical, and then emotional neglect.

In 2010, 753,655 children under the age of 18 years were victims of abuse or neglect nationwide at a rate of 10 per 1,000 children.[48] This rate of reported child victimization has declined from 14.7 per 1,000 children in 1996 (see **Figure 13.14**). Of the 753,655 children who were maltreated in 2010, more than 75% suffered neglect, more than 15% suffered physical abuse, and nearly 10% were sexually abused.[48] The highest victimization rates were for infants (20.6 maltreatments per 1,000 children under 1 year of age);

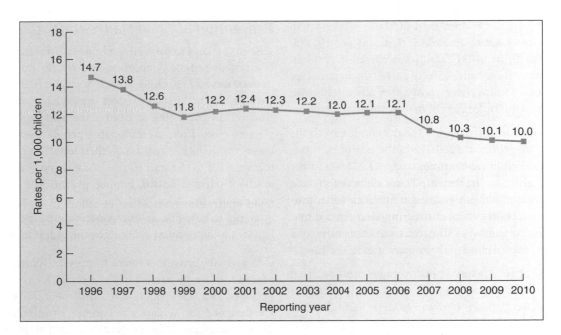

Figure 13.14 There has been a fairly steady decline in child maltreatment rates since 1996, when the rate was 14.7 victims per 1,000 children.

Data from U.S. Department of Health and Human Services, Administration on Children, Youth and Families (2011). *Child Maltreatment 2010*. Available at http://archive.acf.hhs.gov/programs/cb/pubs/cm10/cm10.pdf.

rates then decline with age (see Figure 13.15). Rates of many types of maltreatment are the same for males and females, but the sexual abuse rate for female children was higher than the rate for male children. Victimization rates vary by race and ethnicity. In 2008, the lowest rates were for Asian children (1.9 children per 1,000) and the highest

rates were for African American children (14.6 children per 1,000), children of multiple races (12.7 per 100,000), and American Indian and Alaskan Native children (11.0 children per 1,000).[40] There were 510,824 unique perpetrators (excluding repeated episodes). Eighty-two percent of the perpetrators were parents of the child victim.

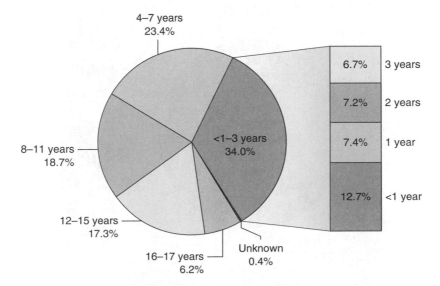

Figure 13.15 The highest rates of child maltreatment occur in the youngest children.

Reproduced from U.S. Department of Health and Human Services, Administration on Children, Youth and Families (2011). *Child Maltreatment 2010*. Available at http://archive.acf.hhs.gov/programs/cb/pubs/cm10/cm10.pdf.

An estimated 1,537 children died of abuse or neglect in 2010, at a rate of approximately 2.07 deaths per 100,000 children. Four-fifths of the fatalities occurred in children under 4 years of age, and 45% occurred in infants (see **Figure 13.16**). Deaths were most often associated with neglect or with multiple types of maltreatment.[48]

Beyond the human suffering lies the economic cost to the community, an estimated $210,012 in the case of each victim of nonfatal child maltreatment, and $1,272,900 in the case of fatal child maltreatment. These estimates include the cost of childhood health care, adult medical costs, productivity losses, child welfare costs, criminal costs, and special education costs. It was estimated for 2008 that the total cost for new cases of child maltreatment was $124 billion.[49]

Children who physically survive maltreatment may be scarred emotionally. Researchers followed 1,575 child victims of abuse and neglect between 1967 and 1971. By the mid-1990s, 49% of the victims had been arrested for some type of non-traffic offense, compared with 38% of the control group (who shared other risk factors such as poverty). Eighteen percent had been arrested for a violent crime, compared with 14% in the control group. These differences were regarded as significant by the researchers. A key finding of the study was that neglected children's rates of arrest for violence were almost as high as physically abused children's. Another key finding was that black individuals who had been abused or neglected as children were being arrested at much higher rates than white individuals with the same background.[50]

Prevention of Child Maltreatment

One of the keys to protecting children from maltreatment is a system of timely reporting and referral to one of the many state and local child protective service (CPS) agencies. Anyone may make such a report (e.g., relative, neighbor, or teacher). In 2010, 60% of child abuse and neglect reports were received from professionals—people who came into contact with the victim through their jobs.[48] Signs of neglect are apparent to the trained professional, such as a teacher, a school nurse, a doctor, a nurse practitioner, or another community health professional. Signs of neglect include extremes in behavior, an uncared-for appearance, evidence of a lack of supervision at home, or the lack of medical care.

CPS agencies provide services to prevent future instances of child abuse or neglect and to remedy harm that has occurred as a result of child maltreatment. These services are designed to increase the parents' child-rearing competence and knowledge of developmental stages of childhood. There may be an assessment of the family's strengths and weaknesses, the development of a plan based on the family's needs, and post-investigative follow-up services. Services might include respite care, parenting education, housing assistance, substance abuse treatment, day care, home visits, counseling, and other services. The goal is to ensure the safety of the child or children.[48]

There are many useful sources of information and support for those interested in preventing child abuse and neglect.

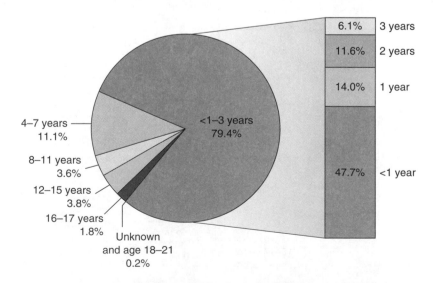

Figure 13.16 Percentage of child fatalities resulting from abuse or neglect by age, 2010.

The Child Welfare Information Gateway, sponsored by the Children's Bureau of the U.S. Department of Health and Human Services' Administration for Children and Families, provides information, products, and technical assistance services to help professionals locate information related to child abuse and neglect and related child welfare issues (available at www.childwelfare.gov). Another source of information is the Committee for Children. Its mission is to promote the safety, well-being, and social development of children (available at www.cfchildren.org). The National Foundation for Abused and Neglected Children (NFANC), created in 1992, is a nonprofit organization dedicated to the prevention of child abuse and neglect (available at www.gangfreekids.org).

Elder Maltreatment

There were more than 40 million elders (persons 65 years of age or older) in the United States in 2010.[51] Although elders experience violent crime and thefts at a lower rate than do people of other age groups (3.1 per 1,000 population vs. 19.3 per 1,000 for the population as a whole in 2008),[42] between 1 million and 2 million of them have been abused, neglected, exploited, or otherwise mistreated.[52] Women over the age of 75 are particularly vulnerable, and elders over 80 are three times more likely to be abused as are younger elders. More than half of the abusers are family members, either adult children or other relatives.[53]

Abuse can be physical, sexual, psychological or emotional, or financial, or may involve abandonment, neglect, or self-neglect. Elders may be kicked, hit, denied food and medical care, or have their Social Security checks or other financial resources stolen or otherwise misappropriated. Most cases of elder abuse are not reported or only become apparent following other legal or medical proceedings; thus, accurate statistics on the incidence of elder abuse are unavailable. As the U.S. population ages, elder maltreatment is likely to become a community health problem of increasing importance.

"Late life domestic violence occurs when a person uses power and control to inflict physical, sexual, emotional, or financial injury or harm upon an older adult with whom they have an ongoing relationship."[54] Domestic violence in later life connotes the abusive use of power and control by a spouse/partner or other person known to the victim. Although domestic violence programs are able to help many older victims of abuse, "the elder abuse network/adult protective services systems have legal responsibility and authority to protect vulnerable elders/adults."[54] More

information about elder abuse is available at the National Center on Elder Abuse website: www.ncea.aoa.gov/ncea-root/Main_Site/index.aspx.

Intimate Partner Violence

Intimate partner violence (IPV) can be defined as rape, physical assault, and stalking perpetrated by current and former dates, spouses, and cohabiting partners (cohabiting means living together at least some of the time as a couple).[55] Each year countless women and men are victimized by their intimate partners. About 552,000 females age 12 or older experienced nonfatal violent victimization (rape/sexual assault, robbery, or aggravated or simple assault) by an intimate partner in 2008.[56] Sometimes intimate partner violence is deadly. In 2008, 1,640 women and 440 men were murdered by an intimate partner.[56] Fifty-seven percent of rapes and sexual assaults against females were committed by an offender whom they knew, 20% by an intimate partner.[56] Injuries to women from intimate partner physical violence are underreported, but more than 500,000 women injured as a result of IPV require medical treatment each year. Women spend more days in bed, miss more work, and suffer more from stress and depression than do men. The healthcare costs of intimate partner rape, physical assault, and stalking exceed $5.8 billion each year.[57]

One in four women residing in the United States has been physically assaulted or raped by an intimate partner; 1 in 14 men has reported such an experience.[56] Women are also more likely than men to be murdered by an intimate partner. In 2007, 45% of all women who were murdered were killed by an intimate partner, whereas only 5% of male murder victims were killed by an intimate partner.[56] Each year, thousands of U.S. children witness IPV within their families. Witnessing such violence is a risk factor for developing long-term physical and mental health problems, including alcohol and substance abuse, becoming a victim of abuse, and perpetrating IPV.[56]

Despite the grim statistics just presented, the rates of victimization by an intimate partner have declined since 1993, when the rates were 9.8 per 1,000 for females and 1.6 per 1,000 for males. In 2008, these rates were 4.3 per 1,000 for females and 0.8 per 1,000 for males.[56]

Risk factors for women who are likely to experience IPV include having a family income below $10,000, being young (19–29 years of age), and living with an intimate partner who uses

intimate partner violence (IPV) rape, physical assault, or stalking perpetrated by current or former dates, spouses, or cohabiting partners

alcohol or other drugs. In a dysfunctional relationship, the male intimate partner may seek to exert power and control over his female intimate partner. The abuser may be possessive or jealous, have rigid role expectations, be controlling or dictatorial, and exhibit low impulse control. Another risk factor is a previous episode of abuse. Repeated episodes result in a cycle in which violence recurs. The typical cycle of violence involves a progression of steps leading up to an attack or episode of violence and the restoration of calm. A violent episode is followed by a crisis state characterized by abuser remorse and forgiveness by the victim. A "honeymoon" period in which calmness prevails ensues. Eventually a prolonged stressful period develops. Stressors may include the loss of a job, a divorce, illness, pregnancy, death of a family member, sexual dysfunction, misbehavior (actual or perceived) of children or an intimate partner, or another factor. The likelihood that a violent and abusive episode will occur is greatly increased if alcohol has been consumed.

Although selected interventions aimed at one factor (for example, the abuser) might mitigate family violence, community efforts to reduce violence should be both comprehensive, involving a variety of approaches, and coordinated among all agencies involved in order to be effective.

Prevention of Intimate Partner Violence

Prevention of IPV involves improvements in identifying and documenting cases of IPV and increasing access to services for victims and perpetrators of IPV and their children. Coordinating community initiatives strengthens the safety networks for high-risk individuals and families. Some communities have established a Violence Coordinating Council that holds monthly meetings to set an agenda and action plans for the community and to determine and clarify the roles and responsibilities of agencies and individuals. It is important for communities to develop and implement a coordinated response with strong advocates from criminal justice, victim services, children's services, and allied professions. One of the important groups of allied professionals are healthcare providers. Educational materials and programs on IPV and sexual assault are available at the National Center for Injury Prevention and Control website (www.cdc.gov/injury/).

Violence in the Workplace

Although only a small number of the incidents of workplace violence that occur each day make the news, some 1.7 million Americans are victims of workplace violence

each year.[58] Many of us have heard about a teacher who was attacked by a student, a female worker who was sexually assaulted in the parking lot, a woman shot in her place of work by an irate boyfriend, or a pizza delivery man killed for a few dollars. In 2008, 526 homicides occurred in the workplace, making homicide the third leading cause of workplace fatalities behind highway incidents and falls, and the second leading cause of workplace deaths among women.[59]

There are many reasons for workplace homicides and violence. Researchers have divided workplace violence into four categories, based on the relationship between the perpetrator and the workplace.[58] These are:

Criminal intent (Type I): The perpetrator has no legitimate relationship to the business or its employees and is usually committing a crime, such as robbery, shoplifting, or trespassing. This category makes up 85% of the work-related homicides.

Customer/client (Type II): The perpetrator has a legitimate relationship with the business and becomes violent while being served. This category includes customers, clients, patients, students, and inmates. This category represents 3% of the work-related homicides.

Worker-on-worker (Type III): The perpetrator is an employee or past employee of the business who attacks or threatens another employee or past employee of the workplace. Worker-on-worker violence accounts for 7% of workplace homicides.

Personal relationship (Type IV): The perpetrator usually does not have a relationship with the business but has a personal relationship with the intended victim. This category, which includes victims of domestic violence assaulted or threatened at work, makes up just 2% of workplace homicides.

Data on nonfatal workplace violence are more difficult to obtain than data on workplace homicides. One estimate is that about 1.7 million people are victims of nonfatal workplace violence each year.[58] Assaults occur almost equally among men and women. Most of these assaults occur in service settings such as hospitals, nursing homes, and social service agencies. Forty-eight percent of nonfatal assaults in the workplace are committed by healthcare patients.[58]

Risk Factors

Risk factors for encountering violence at work are listed in **Box 13.2**. They include working with the public, working around money or valuables, working alone, and working late at night. Additionally, certain industries and occupations put workers at particular risk. For workplace homicides, the taxicab industry has the highest risk at 41.4 per 100,000, nearly 60 times the national average rate of 0.70 per 100,000. Other jobs that carry a higher than average risk for homicide are jobs in liquor stores (7.5), detective and protective services (7.0), gas service stations (4.8), and jewelry stores (4.7). The workplaces that have the highest risk of nonfatal assault (and the highest percentage of all assaults that occurred) are nursing homes (27%), social services (13%), hospitals (11%), grocery stores (6%), and restaurants or bars (5%).[58]

Prevention Strategies for Workplace Violence

Prevention strategies for workplace violence can be grouped into three categories—environmental designs, administrative controls, and behavior strategies. Before these strategies can be implemented, a workplace violence prevention policy should be in place. Such a policy should clearly indicate zero tolerance of violence at work. Just as workplaces have mechanisms for reporting and dealing with sexual harassment, they must also have a policy in place to deal with violence. Such a policy must spell out how such incidents are to be reported, to whom, and how they are to be addressed.

Environmental designs to limit the risk of workplace violence might include implementing safer cash handling procedures, physically separating workers from customers, improving lighting, and installing better security systems at entrances and exits. Administrative controls include staffing policies (having more staff is generally safer than having fewer staff), procedures for opening and closing the workplace, and reviewing employee duties (such as handling money) that may be especially risky. Behavior strategies include training employees in nonviolent response and conflict resolution and educating employees about risks associated with specific duties and about the importance of reporting incidents and adhering to administrative controls. Training should also include instruction on the appropriate use and maintenance of any protective equipment that may be provided.[58]

Violence in Schools

Although schools are one of the safest places for children to spend their time (see **Figure 13.17**), even rare acts of violence strike terror into parents, teachers, and the children themselves. Highly publicized incidents of fatal shootings on school grounds have focused the nation's attention on the question of just how safe (or unsafe) our nation's schools are.

> Our nation's schools should be safe havens for teaching and learning, free of crime and violence. Any instance of crime or violence at school not only affects the individuals involved but also may disrupt the educational process and affect bystanders, the school itself, and the surrounding community.[60]

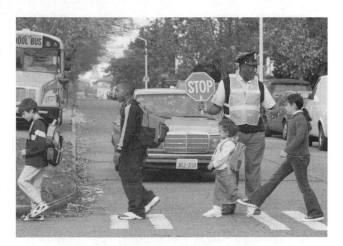

Figure 13.17 Despite several highly publicized tragic events, schools are one of the safest places for students to spend time.

© Blend Images/Alamy Images

The National Center for Educational Statistics (NCES), in the U.S. Department of Education, and the Bureau of Justice Statistics (BJS), in the U.S. Department of Justice, jointly collect and publish data annually on the frequency, seriousness, and incidence of violence in elementary and secondary schools.[61] During the 2009–2010 school year, 33 student, staff, and nonstudent school-associated violent deaths were recorded at school, including 17 homicides and 1 suicide of youths ages 5–18 years. The percentage of homicides of youths at school is just over 1% of all youth homicides, and the percentage of youth suicides has remained less than 1% of all youth suicides occurring nationwide, or about 1 homicide or suicide per 2.1 million students. In 2010, among students ages 12–18 years, there were about 828,000 victims of nonfatal crimes at school, including 470,000 thefts and 359,000 violent crimes (simple assault and serious violent crime). During 2009–2010, 85% of public schools reported that one or more incidents of crime had occurred at their school, and 74% reported one or more violent incidents of violent crime.[61]

Victimization rates have remained steady during the past 3 years at about 4% of students. Theft was reported by 3%, violent victimization by 1%, and serious violent victimization by less than 0.5%. Student victimization rates remained unchanged during 2004–2009. The percentage of teachers who reported being threatened varied by type of school—10% in city schools, 7% in town schools, and 6% in rural schools and suburban schools.[61]

Fighting and weapon carrying are also concerns. In 2009, about 9% of 12- to 18-year-olds reported being the target of hate-related words at school, and 29% reported seeing hate-related graffiti at school. Also, 28% of 12- to 18-year-olds reported being bullied, and 6% reported being cyberbullied in 2009. Thirty-one percent of students in grades 9–12 reported they had been in a fight during the previous year, 11% on school property. Seventeen percent reported having carried a weapon in the past 30 days, 6% on school property. Nearly four times as many males as females (27% vs. 7%) reported carrying a weapon in 2009; 8% of males and 3% of females reported carrying a weapon on school property in 2009.[61]

In 2009–2010, almost all schools utilized some type of security measures, such as requiring visitor sign-ins (94%), controlling access to school buildings during school hours (92%), establishing electronic notification systems for school-wide emergencies (63%), and implementing structured anonymous threats systems (36%). Only 11% of students reported the use of metal detectors in their schools.[61] As zero tolerance and mandatory, predetermined consequences for student offenses have come under fire, school injury prevention and security practices are becoming more widespread. More schools are requiring student, faculty, and staff identification badges (63%), placing telephones in classrooms (74%), and requiring students to wear uniforms (19%).[61]

Safe Schools/Healthy Students Initiative

The Safe Schools/Healthy Students Initiative is a unique federal grant-making program jointly administered by the U.S. Departments of Education, Health and Human Services, and Justice. The program is designed to prevent violence and substance abuse among our nation's youth, schools, and communities. "Since 1999, more than 276 urban, rural, suburban, and tribal school districts—in collaboration with local mental health and juvenile justice providers—have received grants using a single application process."[62] The schools who receive grants develop integrated community-wide plans that must address all of the following elements[62]:

- A safe school environment and violence prevention activities
- Alcohol and other drug prevention activities
- Student behavior, social, and emotional supports
- Mental health services
- Early childhood social and emotional learning programs

Youth Violence After School

Although violence in schools has grabbed the headlines, the real problem area is violence after school. Fewer and fewer children have a parent waiting for them at home after school. Although many youths are able to supervise themselves and their younger siblings responsibly after school or are engaged in sports or other after-school activities, some are not. Statistics show that serious violent crime committed by juveniles peaks in the hours immediately after school. Also, during these after-school hours, juveniles are most likely to become victims of crime, including violent crimes such as robberies and aggravated assaults. This is because at this unsupervised time, youths are more vulnerable to exploitation, injuries, and even death.[63]

For communities that want to become involved in reducing the problem of youth violence, the federal government has a variety of resources. One of these is *Best Practices of Youth Violence Prevention: A Sourcebook for Community Action.*[64] In addition, the federal government has established the Interagency Working Group on Youth Programs (IWGYP), which provides resources for communities that want to develop positive programs for youths.[65] The website provides links to successful after-school programs, ideas for after-school activities, and websites for youths to visit after school. Additional information and resources are available at the National Center for Injury Prevention and Control's website.[66]

Violence in Our Communities

Youth gangs and gang violence contribute to the overall level of violence in the community and are a drain on community resources.

Youth Gang Violence

The **youth gang** is a self-formed association of peers bound together by mutual interests, with identifiable leadership and well-defined lines of authority. Youth gangs act in concert to achieve a specific purpose, and their acts generally include illegal activities and control over a particular territory or enterprise. Types of illegal activities in which gang members participate include larceny/theft, aggravated assault, burglary/breaking and entering, and street drug sales.

A recent survey of a large, representative sample of local law enforcement agencies revealed youth gang activity in 34.5% of the districts under their jurisdiction. This is a significant decline since 1996, when 53% of jurisdictions reported youth gang activity. An estimated 28,100 gangs were active in the United States in 2009. Gang activity is more prevalent in cities with a population of 250,000 or greater. There were more than 731,000 active gang members in 2008.[67]

In some cities, gang homicides account for a substantial proportion of youth homicides. On average, gang homicides claim more young victims, are more likely to involve firearms, and are more likely to occur on streets than do nongang homicides. Gang homicides were found to be less likely be drug related than previously thought, retaliation more often being the motivating factor.[68]

Costs to the Community

Youth gangs and youth-gang–related violence present an enormous drain on the law enforcement resources of a community beyond the injuries and injury deaths that result from their activities. Pressured to "do something," field officers may be pulled from other duties and not replaced. If additional police are hired, it can cost the community $50,000 per year per officer. Next, there is the additional need to strengthen the prosecutor's office if the operation is to be effective. In short, the suppression of gangs by law enforcement is costly for communities,

often depleting resources for other needed community improvements. Another problem is vandalism and the defacing of public and private buildings by gang-related graffiti. This money spent repairing damage and erasing graffiti could be used to hire teachers or to support educational activities.

Community Response

Many communities have responded effectively to the increased violence resulting from gang-related activity. Perhaps the best approach is a multifaceted effort involving law enforcement, education, diversion activities, and social services support. Suppression of gang activity by law enforcement is justified because many gang-related activities—such as selling illicit drugs, carrying and discharging weapons, and defacing property—are illegal. Education of children, teachers, parents, and community leaders is another facet of gang-related violence prevention. Just as there are drug abuse prevention curricula in schools, there are now anti-gang awareness programs in some schools. Diversion activities, including job opportunities and after-school activities such as enrichment programs, sports, and recreation, can reduce the attractiveness of less wholesome uses of free time. Sports and recreational activities have long been touted as a healthy outlet for pent-up physical energy. It seems logical to assume that young persons who participate in such activities would be less likely to become involved in destructive, violent behavior.

State Response

By searching the Internet using the words "injury prevention" or "violence prevention," and "state," one can find many of these state-funded agencies and programs. Most, if not all, states have agencies with programs aimed at preventing or reducing the level of injuries caused by intentional violence; however, these agencies may be located with departments that administer unintentional injury prevention as well as intentional injury prevention. For example, one agency might include programs for child occupant safety, older driver safety, residential fire prevention, domestic violence or violence against women programs, youth violence prevention, suicide prevention, and so on, with links to other injury prevention and control agency websites. Funding sources for these programs vary. Some are

youth gang an association of peers, bound by mutual interests and identifiable lines of authority, whose acts generally include illegal activity and control over a territory or an enterprise

funded as line items on state budgets; other programs are grant driven.

Federal Response

Several federal agencies house programs aimed at preventing or reducing the number and seriousness of intentional and unintentional injuries resulting from violence. The Centers for Disease Control and Prevention, in the Department of Health and Human Services, has a website that provides links to a vast array of programs specifically aimed at preventing injury and violence and promoting safety (www.cdc.gov/InjuryViolenceSafety/).[69] Programs and topics are wide-ranging, from child abuse/maltreatment, to dog bites, to falls among older adults, to youth violence, just to name a few.

The Office of Justice Programs is another federal agency whose mission includes improving public safety by supporting law enforcement and the justice system.[70] The agency monitors crime and victimization, gang-related activity, substance abuse and crime, juvenile justice, and the corrections system. The Office of Justice Programs offers a variety of programs to state and local agencies aimed at reducing intentional violence. Included are programs to empower communities (Community Prosecution, Safe Schools Initiative, Safe Start, Weed and Seed, and Offender Reentry). There are also programs aimed at breaking the cycle of drug abuse and crime (the Drug Free Communities Program, the Drug Prevention Demonstration Program, and Enforcing Underage Drinking).

Injuries, including intentional injuries, are a worldwide problem, but here in the United States, firearm availability is much greater than in most other countries. Legislative attempts aimed at making it more difficult for certain persons to acquire handguns and/or automatic weapons have failed to reduce the level of firearm injuries and deaths.[71] Some local governments have banned guns in their jurisdictions in an effort to reduce the frequency of firearm injuries; however, many of these bans are now in jeopardy. In June 2010, the Supreme Court ruled 5–4 that the Second Amendment applies to states and city governments in regard to gun laws and ended a nearly 30-year handgun ban in the city of Chicago.

In conclusion, intentional injuries resulting from interpersonal violence remain a national as well as a community concern. Significant resources are available at the federal level (from the Departments of Health and Human Services and Justice) to help states and local communities reduce the number and seriousness of violence-related injuries. It is up to each concerned citizen to make sure that his or her own community is taking advantage of these resources.

Chapter Summary

- Injuries are the fifth leading cause of death in the United States.
- Unintentional and intentional injuries represent a major community health problem, not only because of the loss of life, but also because of lost productivity, medical costs, and the increase in the number of disabled Americans.
- Unintentional injuries, injuries that occur with no one intending harm to be done, are unplanned events, usually preceded by an unsafe act or condition, accompanied by economic loss, and interrupt the efficient completion of a task.
- Unintentional injuries occur across all age groups; however, they are the leading cause of death for Americans ages 1–44 years.
- Males and certain minority groups experience proportionately more unintentional injuries.
- More fatal and nonfatal unintentional injuries occur in the home than at any other location.
- Motor vehicle crashes were the leading cause of unintentional injury deaths in 2010, followed by unintentional poisonings, falls, fires and burns, and drowning.
- Fatal injury rates for highways and workplaces have declined over the years.
- Prevention and control of unintentional injuries and fatalities can be instituted based on a model in which energy is the causative agent for injuries.
- Four broad approaches can be used to reduce the numbers and seriousness of unintentional injuries in the community: education, regulation, automatic protection, and litigation.
- Intentional injuries, the outcome of self-directed or interpersonal violence, include those that result from assaults, rapes, robberies, suicides, and homicides.
- Minorities and young adults are at highest risk for injury or death from an intentional violent act.

- Family violence, including child and elder maltreatment and intimate partner violence, is a serious and pervasive community health problem.
- Schools remain a relatively safe place for the nation's youth, despite the occurrence of several widely publicized fatal shootings in schools.
- Youth violence, including youth gang violence, remains a federal, state, and local government concern.

- Significant resources are available at the state and federal levels (from the Departments of Health and Human Services and Justice) to assist local communities in reducing the number and seriousness of violence-related injuries.

Review Questions

1. List the ways in which injuries are costly to society, and quantify these costs.
2. Identify the leading types of unintentional injury deaths and the risk factors associated with each type of death.
3. What is a hazard? Do hazards cause accidents? Explain your answer.
4. What types of injuries are most likely to occur in the home, and in which rooms are they most likely to occur?
5. Characterize trends in rates of injuries from the following activities by time (over the years, seasonally, and by time of day)—motor vehicle driving, swimming, and heating the home.
6. How does alcohol consumption contribute to unintentional injuries?
7. How did William Haddon, Jr. contribute to injury prevention and control?
8. Describe the epidemiological model for injuries and provide three examples of how energy causes injuries.
9. For each of your examples from Question 8, explain how the injury could have been prevented using prevention and control tactics.

10. List four broad strategies for the reduction of unintentional injuries, and give an example of each.
11. Identify the types of violent behavior that result in intentional injuries.
12. Describe the cost of intentional injuries to society.
13. Who are the victims of intentional injury? Who are the perpetrators?
14. Explain the difference between child abuse and child neglect. List some contributing factors to these phenomena.
15. What is intimate partner violence?
16. How safe are our schools? How are schools responding to safety concerns?
17. What are youth gangs? How do their activities affect communities?
18. Describe the best ways for communities to respond to youth gang activity.
19. What resources are available at the state and federal levels to help communities reduce the number and seriousness of injuries?

Activities

1. Obtain a copy of a local newspaper and find three stories dealing with unintentional injuries. Provide a two- or three-sentence summary of each article and then provide your best guess of (a) what the unsafe act or condition that preceded the event was, (b) what the resulting economic loss or injury was, and (c) what task was not completed.

2. Make an appointment and interview the director of safety on your campus. Find out what types of unintentional and intentional injuries occur most frequently on your campus, what strategies have been used to deal with them, and what could be done to eliminate them.

References

1. Baker, S. P. (1989). "Injury Science Comes of Age." *Journal of the American Medical Association*, 262(16): 2284-2285.

2. Miniño, A. M., and R. N. Anderson (2006). "Deaths: Injuries, 2002." *National Vital Statistics Reports*, 54(10): 1-128.

3. Murphy, S. L., J. Xu, and K. D. Kochanek (2012). "Deaths: Preliminary Data for 2010." *National Vital Statistics Reports*, 60(4): 1-68. Available at http://www.cdc.gov/nchs/data/nvsr/nvsr60/nvsr60_04.pdf.

4. National Center for Health Statistics (2012). *Health, United States, 2011 with Special Feature on Socioeconomic Status and Health*. Hyattsville, MD: National Center for Health Statistics. Available at http://www.cdc.gov/nchs/hus.htm.

5. Miniño, A. M., S. L. Murphy, and J. Xu (2011). "Deaths: Final Data for 2008." *National Vital Statistics Reports*, 59(10): 1-152. Available at http://www.cdc.gov/nchs/data/nvsr/nvsr59/nvsr59_10.pdf.

6. Lopez, A.S., C. D. Mathers, M. Ezzati, D. T. Jamison, and C. Murray (2006). *Global Burden of Disease and Risk Factors*. New York: World Bank and Oxford University Press.

7. Adams, P. F., M. E. Martinez, J. L. Vickerie, and W. K. Kirsinger (2011). "Summary Health Statistics for the U.S. Population: National Health Interview Survey, 2010." *Vital Health Statistics*, 10(251): 1-117. Available at http://www.cdc.gov/nchs/data/series/sr_10/sr10_251.pdf.

8. Niska, R., F. Bhuiya, and J. Xu (2010). "National Hospital Ambulatory Medical Care Survey: 2007 Emergency Department Summary." *National Health Statistics Reports*, 26: 1-32. Available at http://www.cdc.gov/nchs/data/nhsr/nhsr026.pdf.

9. National Safety Council (2012). *Injury Facts 2012 Edition*. Itasca, IL: Author.

10. U.S. Department of Health and Human Services, Office of Disease Prevention and Health Promotion (2012). *Healthy People 2020*. Available at http://www.healthypeople.gov/2020/default.aspx.

11. U.S. Department of Health and Human Services (2009). *Data 2010: The Healthy People 2010 Database*. Available at http://wonder.cdc.gov/data2010/focus.htm.

12. U.S. Department of Transportation, National Highway Traffic Safety Administration (2012). "2010 Motor Vehicle Crashes: Overview." *Traffic Safety Facts Research Note* (DOT HS 811 552). Available at http://www-nrd.nhtsa.dot.gov/Pubs/811552.pdf.

13. Centers for Disease Control and Prevention, National Center for Health Statistics (2012). "Rate of Nonfatal, Medically Consulted Fall Injury Episodes, by Age Group—National Health Interview Survey, United States, 2010." *Morbidity and Mortality Weekly Report*, 61(40): 81.

14. Centers for Disease Control and Prevention (2012). "Vital Signs: Unintentional Injury Deaths Among Persons Aged 0-19 Years—United States, 2000-2009." *Morbidity and Mortality Weekly Report*, 61(15): 270-276. Available at http://www.cdc.gov/mmwr/PDF/wk/mm6115.pdf.

15. Centers for Disease Control and Prevention, National Center for Injury Prevention and Control (2012). "WISQARS: Leading Cause of Death Reports, National and Regional, 1999-2009." Available at http://webappa.cdc.gov/sasweb/ncipc/leadcaus10_us.html.

16. Centers for Disease Control and Prevention (2011). "Surveillance for Violent Deaths–National Violent Death Reporting System, 16 States, 2008." *Morbidity and Mortality Weekly Report*, 60(10). Available at http://www.cdc.gov/mmwr/pdf/ss/ss6010.pdf.

17. Centers for Disease Control and Prevention (2010). "Youth Risk Behavior Surveillance–United States, 2009." *Morbidity and Mortality Weekly Report*, 59(SS-5): 1-146. Available at http://www.cdc.gov/mmwr/pdf/ss/ss5905.pdf.

18. U.S. Department of Transportation, National Highway Traffic Safety Administration (2011). *Traffic Safety Facts 2009: A Compilation of Motor Vehicle Crash Data from the Fatality Analysis Reporting System and the General Estimates System* (DOT HS 811 402). Washington, DC: U.S. DOT. Available at http://www-nrd.nhtsa.dot.gov/Pubs/811402.pdf.

19. Bergen, G., L. H. Chen, M. Warner, and L. A. Fingerhut (2008). *Injury in the United States: 2007 Chartbook*. Hyattsville, MD: National Center for Health Statistics. Available at http://www.cdc.gov/nchs/data/misc/injury2007.pdf.

20. Centers for Disease Control and Prevention (2012). "Rate of Nonfatal, Medically Consulted Fall Injury Episodes, By Age Group—National Health Interview Survey, United States, 2010." *Morbidity and Mortality Weekly Report*, 61(4): 81.

21. Centers for Disease Control and Prevention (2006). "Fatalities and Injuries from Falls Among Older Adults–United States, 1993-2003 and 2001-2005." *Morbidity and Mortality Weekly Report*, 55(45): 1221-1224.

22. Griffin III, L. I. (2004). *Older Driver Involvement in Injury Crashes in Texas, 1975-1999*. Washington, DC: AAA Foundation for Traffic Safety. Available at https://www.aaafoundation.org/sites/default/files/OlderDriverInvolvementInInjuryCrashes.pdf.

23. Griffin, L. I., and S. DeLaZerda (2000). *Unlicensed to Kill*. Washington, DC: AAA Foundation for Traffic Safety. Available at https://www.aaafoundation.org/sites/default/files/unlicensed2kill.PDF.

24. U.S. Department of Labor, Bureau of Labor Statistics (2012). "Employment Status of the Civilian Population by Sex and Age." Available at http://www.bls.gov/news.release/empsit.t01.htm.

25. U.S. Department of Labor, Bureau of Labor Statistics (2008). *BLS Information: Glossary*. Available at http://www.bls.gov/bls/glossary.htm.

26. U.S. Department of Labor, Bureau of Labor Statistics (2011). "Economic News Release: Workplace Injury and Illness Summary–2010." Available at http://www.bls.gov/news.release/osh.nr0.htm.

27. U.S. Department of Labor, Bureau of Labor Statistics (2011). "Injuries, Illnesses, and Fatalities: Fatal Occupational Injuries and Workers' Memorial Day." Available at http://www.bls.gov/iif/oshwc/cfoi/worker_memorial.htm.

28. U.S. Department of Labor, Bureau of Labor Statistics (2011). "Revisions to the 2010 Census of Fatal Occupational Injuries (CFOI) Counts." Available at http://www.bls.gov/iif/oshwc/cfoi/cfoi_revised10.pdf.

29. Centers for Disease Control and Prevention (2011). "Vital Signs: Alcohol-Impaired Driving Among Adults–United States, 2010." *Morbidity and Mortality Weekly Report*, 60(39): 1351-1357. Available at http://www.cdc.gov/mmwr/PDF/wk/mm6039.pdf.

30. Centers for Disease Control and Prevention (2004). "Child Passenger Deaths Involving Drinking Drivers–United States, 1997-2002." *Morbidity and Mortality Weekly Report*, 53(4): 77-79.

31. U.S. Department of Homeland Security, U.S. Coast Guard (2012). *Recreational Boating Statistics 2011* (COMDTPUB P16754.25). Available at http://www.uscgboating.org/assets /1/workflow_staging/Publications/557.PDF.

32. U.S. Department of Homeland Security, U.S. Coast Guard (2000). *Boating Statistics–1999* (COMDTPUB P16754.16). Available at http://www.uscgboating.org/assets/1/Publications /Boating_Statistics_1999.pdf.

33. Centers for Disease Control and Prevention (2001). "Drowning–Louisiana, 1998." *Morbidity and Mortality Weekly Report*, 50(20): 413-414.

34. Christoffel, T., and S. S. Gallagher (2006). *Injury Prevention and Public Health: Practical Knowledge, Skills, and Strategies*, 2nd ed. Sudbury, MA: Jones & Bartlett.

35. Centers for Disease Control and Prevention (2010). "Effectiveness of 0.08% Blood Alcohol Concentration (BAC) Laws." Available at http://www.thecommunityguide.org/mvoi /AID/BAC-laws.html.

36. AAA Foundation for Traffic Safety (2009). *2009 Traffic Safety Culture Index*. Washington, DC: Author. Available at https://www.aaafoundation.org/sites/default/files /2009TSCIndexFinalReport.pdf.

37. Vermette, E. (2010). *Curbing Distracted Driving: 2010 Survey of State Safety Programs*. Washington, DC: Governors Highway Safety Association. Available at http://www.ghsa .org/html/publications/pdf/survey/2010_distraction.pdf.

38. Governors Highway Safety Association (2012). "Cell Phone and Texting Laws." Available at http://www.ghsa.org/html /stateinfo/laws/cellphone_laws.html.

39. Waller, P. F. (2002). "Challenges in Motor Vehicle Safety." *Annual Review of Public Health*, 23: 93-113.

40. Ashford, N. A. (1976). *Crisis in the Workplace. Occupational Disease and Injury–A Report to the Ford Foundation*. Cambridge, MA: MIT Press.

41. Centers for Disease Control and Prevention (1982). "Unintentional and Intentional Injuries–United States." *Morbidity and Mortality Weekly Report*, 31(18): 240-248.

42. Truman, J. L. (2011). "Criminal Victimization, 2010." *National Crime Victimization Survey* (NCJ 235508). Washington, DC: U.S. Department of Justice, Bureau of Justice Statistics. Available at http://bjs.ojp.usdoj.gov/content /pub/pdf/cv10.pdf.

43. Federal Bureau of Investigation (2011). "Crime in the United States 2010: Expanded Homicide Data." Available at http://www.fbi.gov/about-us/cjis/ucr/crime-in-the-u.s/2010 /crime-in-the-u.s.-2010/offenses-known-to-law-enforcement /expanded/expandhomicidemain.

44. Centers for Disease Control and Prevention (2009). "QuickStats: Age-Adjusted Death Rates per 100,000 Population for the Three Leading Causes of Injury Death– United States, 1979-2006." *Morbidity and Mortality Weekly Report*, 58(24): 675.

45. Miller, M., D. Hemenway, and H. Wechsler. (2002). "Guns and Gun Threats at College." *Journal of American College Health*, 51(2): 57-65.

46. Jaschik, S. (2006). "Gun Rights vs. College Rights." Available at http://www.insidehighered.com/news/2006/09 /11/guns.

47. Schwartz, V., J. Kay, and P. Appelbaum. (12 May 2010). "Keep Guns off College Campuses." Available at http://www .huffingtonpost.com/victor-schwartz/keep-guns-off-college -cam_b_573634.html.

48. U.S. Department of Health and Human Services, Administration on Children, Youth and Families (2011). *Child Maltreatment 2010*. Available at http://www.acf.hhs.gov /programs/cb/stats_research/index.htm#can.

49. Fang, X., D. S. Brown, C. S. Florence, and J. A. Mercy (2012). "The Economic Burden of Child Maltreatment in the United States and Implications for Prevention." *Child Abuse and Neglect,* 36: 156-165. Available at http://www.sciencedirect .com/science/article/pii/S0145213411003140.

50. National Institute of Justice (1996). *The Cycle of Violence Revisited*. Washington, DC: U.S. Department of Justice.

51. U.S. Census Bureau (2010). "U.S. Population Projections." Available at http://www.census.gov/population/www /projections/2008projections.

52. Bonnie, R. J., and R. B. Wallace (2003). *Elder Mistreatment: Abuse, Neglect, and Exploitation in an Aging America*. Washington, DC: National Academies Press.

53. Teaster, P. B., T. A. Dugar, M. S. Mendiondo, E. L. Abner, and K. A. Cecil (2007). *The 2004 Survey of State Adult Protective Services: Abuse of Adults 60 Years of Age and Older*. Available at http://www.ncea.aoa.gov/ncearoot/Main_Site /pdf/APS_2004NCEASurvey.pdf.

54. U.S. Department of Health and Human Services, Administration on Aging, National Center on Elder Abuse, National Association of State Units on Aging (2006). "Late Life Domestic Violence: What the Aging Network Needs to Know." Available at http://ncea.aoa.gov/ncearoot/main_site /pdf/publication/nceaissuebrief.DVforagingnetwork.pdf.

55. Tjaden, P. and N. Thoennes (2000). *Extent, Nature, and Consequences of Intimate Partner Violence: Findings from the National Violence Against Women Survey* (NCJ 181867). Washington, DC: U.S. Department of Justice, Office of Justice Programs, National Institute of Justice.

56. Catalano, S., E. Smith, H. Snyder, and M. Rand (2009). "Female Victims of Violence" (NCJ 228356). Available at http://bjs.ojp .usdoj.gov/content/pub/pdf/fvv.pdf.

57. Centers for Disease Control and Prevention, National Center for Injury Control and Prevention (2009). *Understanding Intimate Partner Violence*. Available at http://www.cdc.gov /violenceprevention/pdf/IPV_factsheet-a.pdf.

58. Centers for Disease Control and Prevention, National Institute for Occupational Safety and Health (2004). *Violence on the Job* (NIOSH pub. no. 2004-100d). Available at http://www.cdc .gov/niosh/docs/video/violence.html.

59. U.S. Department of Health and Human Services, Centers for Disease Control and Prevention, National Institute for Occupational Safety and Health (2004). *Worker Health Chartbook, 2004* (DHHS [NIOSH] pub. no. 2004-146). Available at http://www.cdc.gov/niosh/docs/2004-146.

60. Henry, S. (2000). "What Is School Violence? An Integrated Definition." *Annals of the American Academy of Political and Social Science*, 567: 16-29. As cited in U.S. Department of Education, National Center for Education Statistics (2007). "Indicators of School Crime and Safety: 2006" (NCES 2007-003/NCJ 214262). Washington, DC: National Center for Education Statistics, Institute of Education Sciences, U.S. Department of Education, and Bureau of Justice Statistics,

Office of Justice Programs, U.S. Department of Justice. Available at http://nces.ed.gov/pubs2007/2007003.pdf

61. Robers, S., J. Zhang, J. Truman, and T. D. Snyder (2012). *Indicators of School Crime and Safety: 2011* (NCES 2012–002/ NCJ 236021). Washington, DC: National Center for Education Statistics, Institute of Education Sciences, U.S. Department of Education, and Bureau of Justice Statistics, Office of Justice Programs, U.S. Department of Justice. Available at http://nces.ed.gov/pubs2012/2012002.pdf.

62. Substance Abuse and Mental Health Services Administration, Department of Health and Human Services (2012). "About the Safe Schools/Healthy Students (SS/HS) Initiative." Available at http://www.sshs.samhsa.gov/initiative /about.aspx.

63. U.S. Department of Justice, Office of Juvenile Justice and Delinquency Prevention (2006). "Statistical Briefing Book, Juveniles as Victims: School Crime Victimization." Available at http://www.ojjdp.gov/ojstatbb/victims/qa02203 .asp?qaDate=2001.

64. Thornton, T. N., C. A. Craft, L. L. Dahlberg, B. S. Lynch, and K. Baer (2002). *Youth Violence: Best Practices of Youth Violence Prevention: A Sourcebook for Community Action*. Atlanta, GA: Centers for Disease Control and Prevention, National Center for Injury Prevention and Control. Available at http://www.cdc.gov/violenceprevention/pub /YV_bestpractices.html.

65. Interagency Working Group on Youth Programs (n.d.). "About the Working Group." Available at http://findyouthinfo.gov /about-us/.

66. Centers for Disease Control and Prevention, National Center for Injury Prevention and Control (2007). "Injury Center: Violence Prevention, Youth Violence." Available at http://www .cdc.gov/ViolencePrevention/youthviolence/.

67. Egley, Jr., A., and J. C. Howell (2011). "Highlights of the 2009 National Youth Gang Survey" (OJJDP Fact Sheet, NCJ 233581). Available at https://www.ncjrs.gov/pdffiles1 /ojjdp/233581.pdf.

68. Centers for Disease Control and Prevention (2012). "Gang Homicides–Five U.S. Cities, 2003-2008." *Morbidity and Mortality Weekly Report*, 61(3): 46-51. Available at http://www .cdc.gov/mmwr/PDF/wk/mm6103.pdf.

69. Centers for Disease Control and Prevention (n.d.). "Injury, Violence and Safety." Available at http://www.cdc.gov /InjuryViolenceSafety/.

70. U.S. Department of Justice, Office of Justice Programs (n.d.). "Mission and Vision." Available at http://www.ojp.usdoj.gov /about/mission.htm.

71. Centers for Disease Control and Prevention (2003). "First Reports Evaluating the Effectiveness of Strategies for Preventing Violence: Firearm Laws: Findings from the Task Force on Community Preventive Services." *Morbidity and Mortality Weekly Report*, 52(RR-14): 11-20.

Glossary

absorption field The element of a septic system in which the liquid portion of waste is distributed.

accreditation The process by which an agency or organization evaluates and recognizes an institution as meeting certain predetermined standards.

acculturated The cultural modification of an individual or a group by adapting to or borrowing traits from another culture.

activities of daily living (ADLs) Eating, toileting, dressing, bathing, walking, getting into and out of a bed or chair, and getting outside.

acute disease A disease in which the peak severity of symptoms occurs and subsides within 3 months of onset, usually within days or weeks.

adolescents and young adults Individuals between the ages of 15 and 24 years.

adult day care programs Daytime care provided to seniors who are unable to be left alone.

advanced practice registered nurse (APRN) A registered nurse who has completed graduate training as a clinical nurse specialist, nurse anesthetist, nurse-midwife, or nurse practitioner.

aftercare The continuing care provided to former drug abusers or drug-dependent persons.

age-adjusted rates Rates used to make comparisons of relative risks across groups and over time when groups differ by age structure.

aged The state of being old.

agent (pathogenic agent) The cause of the disease or health problem; the factor that must be present for the disease to occur.

aging The physiological changes that occur normally in plants and animals as they grow older.

air pollution Contamination of the air that interferes with the comfort, safety, and health of living things or alters climate.

Air Quality Index (AQI) An index (number between 0 and 500) that indicates the level of pollution in the air and its associated health risk.

alcoholism A disease characterized by impaired control over drinking, preoccupation with drinking, and continued use of alcohol despite adverse consequences.

alien A person born in and owing allegiance to a country other than the one in which he or she lives.

allied healthcare professionals Healthcare workers who provide services that assist, facilitate, and complement the work of physicians and other healthcare specialists.

allopathic providers Independent healthcare providers whose remedies for illnesses produce effects different from those of the disease. These people are doctors of medicine (MDs).

American Health Security Act of 1993 The comprehensive healthcare reform introduced by then-President Clinton; this legislation was never enacted.

American Red Cross A nonprofit, humanitarian organization led by volunteers and guided by its Congressional Charter that provides relief to victims of disasters.

amotivational syndrome A pattern of behavior characterized by apathy, loss of effectiveness, and a more passive, introverted personality.

amphetamines A group of synthetic drugs that act as stimulants.

anabolic/androgenic drugs Compounds, structurally similar to the male hormone testosterone, that increase protein synthesis.

analytic study A type of epidemiological study aimed at testing hypotheses (e.g., observational, experimental).

anthroponosis   A disease that infects only humans.

aquifers   Porous, water-saturated layers of underground bedrock, sand, and gravel that can yield economically significant amounts of water.

asbestos   A naturally occurring mineral fiber that has been identified as a class A carcinogen by the Environmental Protection Agency.

asbestosis   Acute or chronic lung disease caused by the deposit of asbestos fibers on lungs.

assisted-living facility   "A special combination of housing, personalized supportive services, and health care designed to meet the needs—both scheduled and unscheduled—of those who need help with activities of daily living."[1]

attack rate   A special incidence rate calculated for a particular population for a single disease outbreak and expressed as a percentage.

automatic (passive) protection   The modification of a product or the environment in such a way as to reduce unintentional injuries.

bacteriological period   The period in public health history from 1875 to 1900 during which the causes of many bacterial diseases were discovered.

barbiturates   Depressant drugs based on the structure of barbituric acid; for example, phenobarbital.

benzodiazapines   Nonbarbiturate depressant drugs; examples include Librium and Valium.

best experience   Intervention strategies used in prior or existing programs that have not gone through critical research and evaluation studies and thus fall short of best practice criteria.

best practices   "Recommendations for interventions based on critical review of multiple research and evaluation studies that substantiate the efficacy of the intervention."[2]

best processes   Original intervention strategies that the planners create based on their knowledge and skills of good planning processes, including the involvement of those in the priority population and the use of theories and models.

binge drinking   Consuming five or more alcoholic drinks in a row for males, four or more for females.

biogenic pollutants   Airborne biological organisms or their particles or gases or other toxic materials that can produce illness.

bioterrorism   The threatened or intentional release of biological agents for the purpose of influencing the conduct of government or intimidating or coercing a civilian population to further political or social objectives.

bipolar disorder   An affective disorder characterized by distinct periods of elevated mood alternating with periods of depression.

blood alcohol concentration (BAC)   The percentage of concentration of alcohol in the blood; a BAC of 0.08% or greater is regarded as the legal level of intoxication in all states.

Bloodborne Pathogen Standard   A set of regulations promulgated by the Occupational Safety and Health Administration (OSHA) that sets forth the responsibilities of employers and employees with regard to precautions to be taken concerning bloodborne pathogens in the workplace.

bloodborne pathogens   Disease agents, such as human immunodeficiency virus (HIV), that are transmissible in blood and other body fluids.

body mass index (BMI)   The ratio of weight (in kilograms) to height (in meters, squared). To calculate in pounds and inches, divide ([weight in pounds]/2.2) by ([height in inches]/32.27)^2.

brownfields   Property where reuse is complicated by the presence of hazardous substances from prior use.

Bureau of Alcohol, Tobacco, Firearms, and Explosives (ATF)   The federal agency in the U.S. Department of Justice that regulates alcohol, tobacco, firearms, and explosives.

byssinosis   Acute or chronic lung disease caused by the inhalation of cotton, flax, or hemp dusts; those affected include workers in cotton textile plants (sometimes called brown lung disease).

capitation   A method of paying for covered healthcare services on a per-person premium basis for a specific time period prior to the service being rendered

carcinogens   Agents, usually chemicals, that cause cancer.

care manager   One who helps identify the healthcare needs of an individual but does not actually provide the healthcare services.

care provider   One who helps identify the healthcare needs of an individual and also personally performs the caregiving service.

carrier   A person or animal that harbors a specific communicable disease agent in the absence of discernible clinical disease and serves as a potential source of infection to others.

carrying capacity   The maximum population of a particular species that a given habitat can support over a given period of time.

case fatality rate (CFR)   The percentage of cases of a particular disease that result in death.

case/control study   An epidemiological study that seeks to compare those diagnosed with a disease (cases) with those who do not have the disease (controls) for prior exposure to specific risk factors.

cases   People afflicted with a disease.

categorical programs   Those programs available only to people who can be categorized into a specific group based on disease, age, family means, geography, or other variables.

cause-specific mortality rate (CSMR)   An expression of the death rate due to a particular disease; the CSMR is calculated by dividing the number of deaths due to a particular disease by the total population and multiplying by 100,000.

cerebrovascular disease (stroke)   A disease in which the blood supply to the brain is interrupted.

chain of infection   A model to conceptualize the transmission of a communicable disease from its source to a susceptible host.

chemical straitjacket   A drug that subdues a mental patient's behavior.

child abuse   The intentional physical, emotional, verbal, or sexual mistreatment of a minor.

child maltreatment   An act or failure to act by a parent, caretaker, or other person as defined under state law that results in physical abuse, neglect, medical neglect, sexual abuse, or emotional abuse, or an act or failure to act that presents an imminent risk of serious harm to the child.

child neglect   The failure of a parent or guardian to care for or otherwise provide the necessary subsistence for a child.

Children's Health Insurance Program (CHIP)   A title insurance program under the Social Security Act that provides health insurance to uninsured children.

chiropractor   A nonallopathic, independent healthcare provider who treats health problems by adjusting the spinal column.

chlorpromazine   The first and most famous antipsychotic drug, introduced in 1954 under the brand name Thorazine.

chronic disease   A disease or health condition that lasts longer than 3 months, sometimes for the remainder of one's life.

Clean Air Act (CAA)   The federal law that provides the government with authority to address interstate air pollution.

Clean Water Act (CWA)   The federal law aimed at ensuring that all rivers are swimmable and fishable and that limits the discharge of pollutants in U.S. waters to zero.

club drugs   A general term for those illicit drugs, primarily synthetic, that are most commonly encountered at night clubs and "raves." Examples include MDMA, LSD, GHB, GBL, PCP, ketamine, Rohypnol, and methamphetamines.

coal workers' pneumoconiosis (CWP)   Acute and chronic lung disease caused by the inhalation of coal dust (sometimes called black lung disease).

coalition   "A formal alliance of organizations that come together to work for a common goal."[3]

cocaine   The psychoactive ingredient in the leaves of the coca plant, *Erythroxylon coca*.

cognitive-behavioral therapy   Treatment based on learning new thought patterns and adaptive skills, with regular practice between therapy sessions.

cohort   A group of people who share some important demographic characteristic—year of birth, for example.

cohort study   An epidemiological study in which a cohort is selected, classified on the basis of exposure to one or more specific risk factors, and observed to determine the rates at which disease develops in each class.

co-insurance   Portion of an insurance company's approved amounts for covered services that the beneficiary is responsible for paying.

combustion (incineration)   The burning of solid wastes.

combustion by-products   Gases and other particles generated by burning.

communicable disease (infectious disease)   An illness due to a specific communicable agent or its toxic products, which arises through transmission of that agent or its products from an infected person, animal, or inanimate reservoir to a susceptible host.

communicable disease model   A visual representation of the interrelationships of agent, host, and environment—the three entities necessary for communicable disease transmission.

community   "A collective body of individuals identified by common characteristics such as geography, interests, experiences, concerns, or values."[4]

community analysis   A process by which community needs are identified.

community building   "[A] 'strategic framework' as an orientation to community through which people who identify as members engage together in building community capacity rather than 'fixing problems' through the application of specific and externally driven strategies."[5]

community capacity   "The characteristics of communities that affect their ability to identify, mobilize, and address social and public health problems."[6]

community diagnosis   See *community analysis*.

community health   The health status of a defined group of people and the actions and conditions to promote, protect, and preserve their health.

community mental health center (CMHC)   A fully staffed center originally funded by the federal government that provides comprehensive mental health services to local populations.

community organizing   "The process by which community groups are helped to identify common problems or change targets, mobilize resources, and develop and implement strategies to reach their collective goals."[7]

complementary/alternative medicine (CAM)   "A group of diverse medical and health care systems, practices, and products that are not presently considered to be a part of conventional medicine."[8]

composting   The natural, aerobic biodegradation of organic plant and animal matter to compost.

Comprehensive Environmental Response, Compensation, and Liability Act (CERCLA)   The federal law (known as the Superfund) created to clean up abandoned hazardous waste sites.

congregate meal programs   Community-sponsored nutrition programs that provide meals at a central site, such as a senior center.

consumer-directed health plans (CDHPs)   Health plan options that combine more consumer responsibility for decisions with a tax-sheltered account to pay for out-of-pocket costs for health care and a high-deductible health insurance policy.

continuing-care retirement communities (CCRCs)   Planned communities for elders that guarantee a lifelong residence and health care.

controlled substances   Drugs regulated by the Comprehensive Drug Abuse Control Act of 1970, including all illegal drugs and many legal drugs that can produce dependence.

Controlled Substances Act of 1970 (Comprehensive Drug Abuse Control Act of 1970)   The central piece of federal drug legislation that regulates illegal drugs and legal drugs that have a high potential for abuse.

coordinated school health program (CSHP)   "[A]n organized set of policies, procedures, and activities designed to protect, promote, and improve the health and well-being of pre-K through grade 12 students and staff, thus improving a student's ability to learn. It includes, but is not limited to comprehensive school health education; school health services; a healthy school environment; school counseling; psychological and social services; physical education; school nutrition services; family and community involvement in school health; and school-site health promotion for staff."[9]

copayment A negotiated set amount the insured will pay for a certain service after paying the deductible.

core functions of public health Health assessment, policy development, and health assurance.

coronary heart disease (CHD) A noncommunicable disease characterized by damage to the coronary arteries, which supply blood to the heart.

criteria of causation Criteria or factors that should be considered when deciding whether an association between a disease and a possible risk factor might be one of causation.

criteria pollutants The most pervasive air pollutants in the United States.

crude birth rate (CBR) An expression of the number of live births per unit of population in a given period of time. For example, the crude birth rate in the United States in 2010 was 13.0 births per 1,000 population.

crude death rate (CDR) An expression of the total number of deaths (from all causes) per unit of population in a given period of time. For example, the crude death rate in the United States in 2010 was 798.7 per 100,000 population.

crude rate A rate in which the denominator includes the total population.

cultural competence A service provider's degree of compatibility with the specific culture of the population served, for example, proficiency in language(s) other than English, familiarity with cultural idioms of distress or body language, folk beliefs, and expectations regarding treatment procedures (such as medication or psychotherapy) and likely outcomes.

cultural and linguistic competence A set of congruent behaviors, attitudes, and policies that come together in a system, in an agency, or among professionals that enables effective work in cross-cultural situations.

curriculum Written plan for instruction.

deductible The amount of expense that the beneficiary must incur before the insurance company begins to pay for covered services.

deinstitutionalization The process of discharging, on a large scale, patients from state mental hospitals to less restrictive community settings.

demography The study of a population and those variables bringing about change in that population.

dependency ratio A ratio that compares the number of individuals whom society considers economically productive (the working population) to the number of those it considers economically unproductive (the nonworking or dependent population).

depressant A psychoactive drug that slows down the central nervous system.

descriptive study An epidemiological study that describes an epidemic with respect to person, place, and time.

diagnosis-related groups (DRGs) A procedure used to classify the health problems of all Medicare patients when they are admitted to a hospital.

direct contract HMO Contracts with individual physicians as opposed to group practices.

direct transmission The immediate transfer of an infectious agent by direct contact between infected and susceptible individuals.

disability-adjusted life years (DALYs) A measure for the burden of disease that takes into account premature death and years lived with disability of specified severity and duration. One DALY is one lost year of healthy life.

disabling injury An injury causing any restriction of normal activity beyond the day of the injury's occurrence.

diseases of adaptation Diseases that result from chronic exposure to excess levels of stressors that elicit the General Adaptation Syndrome.

disinfection The killing of communicable disease agents outside the host, on countertops, for example.

dose The number of program units as part of the intervention.

drug A substance other than food or vitamins that, upon entering the body in small amounts, alters one's physical, mental, or emotional state.

drug abuse Use of a drug despite the knowledge that continued use is detrimental to one's health or well-being.

drug abuse education Providing information about the dangers of drug abuse, changing attitudes and beliefs about drugs, providing skills necessary to abstain from drugs, and ultimately changing drug abuse behavior.

drug (chemical) dependence A psychological and sometimes physical state characterized by a craving for a drug.

Drug Enforcement Administration (DEA) The federal government's lead agency with the primary responsibility for enforcing the nation's drug laws, including the Controlled Substances Act of 1970.

drug misuse Inappropriate use of prescription or nonprescription drugs.

drug use A nonevaluative term referring to drug-taking behavior in general; any drug-taking behavior.

elderly (or elder) Individuals older than 65 years of age.

electroconvulsive therapy (ECT) A method of treatment for mental disorders involving the administration of electric current to induce convulsions and unconsciousness.

employee assistance programs (EAPs) Worksite-based, employer-sponsored programs that assist employees whose work performance suffers because of substance abuse or domestic, psychological, or social problems.

encore careers When individuals transition out of their work careers and into jobs and volunteer opportunities in nonprofit and public sectors.

endocrine-disrupting chemical (EDC) A chemical that interferes in some way with the body's endocrine (hormone) system.

end-of-life practice Healthcare services provided to individuals shortly before death.

endemic disease A disease that occurs regularly in a population as a matter of course.

environmental hazards Factors or conditions in the environment that increase the risk of human injury, disease, or death.

environmental health The study and management of environmental conditions that affect the health and well-being of humans.

Environmental Protection Agency (EPA) The federal agency primarily responsible for setting, maintaining, and enforcing environmental standards.

environmental tobacco smoke (ETS) Tobacco smoke in the environment that can be inhaled.

epidemic An unexpectedly large number of cases of an illness, specific health-related behavior, or other health-related event.

epidemic curve A graphic display of the cases of disease according to the time or date of onset of symptoms.

epidemiologist An investigator who studies the occurrence of disease or other health-related conditions or events in defined populations.

epidemiology The study of the distribution and determinants of health-related states or events in specific populations, and the application of this study to control health problems.

eradication The complete elimination or uprooting of a disease (e.g., smallpox eradication).

etiology The cause of a disease (e.g., the etiology of mumps is the mumps virus).

evaluation Determining the value or worth of the objective of interest.

evidence-based practices Ways of delivering services to people using scientific evidence that shows that the services actually work.

exclusion A condition that is written into a health insurance policy indicating what is not covered by the policy.

experimental study An analytic, epidemiological study in which investigators allocate exposure to the risk factor(s) and follow the subjects to observe disease development.

Family and Medical Leave Act (FMLA) Federal legislation that provides up to a 12-week unpaid leave to men and women after the birth of a child, an adoption, or an event of illness in the immediate family.

family planning The process of determining the preferred number and spacing of children in one's family and choosing the appropriate means to achieve this preference.

family violence The use of physical force by one family member against another, with the intent to hurt, injure, or cause death.

fatal injury An injury that results in one or more deaths.

fatality rate See *mortality (fatality) rate*.

Federal Emergency Management Agency (FEMA) The nation's official emergency response agency.

fee-for-service A method of paying for health care in which a bill (fee) is paid after the care (service) is rendered.

fetal alcohol syndrome (FAS) A group of abnormalities that may include growth retardation, abnormal appearance of face and head, and deficits of central nervous system function including mental retardation in babies born to mothers who have consumed heavy amounts of alcohol during their pregnancies.

fight or flight reaction An alarm reaction that prepares one physiologically for sudden action.

fixed indemnity The maximum amount an insurer will pay for a certain service.

Food and Drug Administration (FDA) An operating division of the Centers for Disease Control and Prevention, U.S. Department of Health and Human Services, that regulates most food, over-the-counter and prescription drugs, tobacco products, medical devices, and cosmetics.

foodborne disease outbreak (FBDO) The occurrence of two or more cases of a similar illness resulting from the ingestion of food.

formaldehyde (CH_2O) A water-soluble gas used in aqueous solutions in hundreds of consumer products.

formative evaluation The evaluation that is conducted during the planning and implementing processes to improve or refine a program.

full-service hospitals Hospitals that offer services in all or most of the levels of care defined by the spectrum of health care.

functional limitations Difficulty in performing personal care and home management tasks.

gag rule Regulations that bar physicians and nurses in clinics receiving federal funds from counseling clients about abortions.

gatekeepers Those who control, both formally and informally, the political climate of the community.

General Adaptation Syndrome (GAS) The complex physiological responses resulting from exposure to stressors.

geriatrician "A physician specializing in the care of patients with multiple chronic diseases who may not be able to be cured but whose care can be managed."[10]

geriatrics "The branch of medicine concerned with medical problems and care of the elderly."[10]

gerontology "The multidisciplinary study of the biological, psychological, and social processes of aging and the elderly."[10]

global health "[H]ealth problems, issues, and concerns that transcend national boundaries, may be influenced by circumstances or experiences in other countries, and are best addressed by cooperative actions and solutions."[11]

government hospital A hospital that is supported and managed by governmental jurisdictions.

governmental health agency Health agencies that are part of the governmental structure (federal, state, or local) and that are funded primarily by tax dollars.

grass-roots community organizing A process that begins with those affected by the problem/concern.

greenhouse gases Atmospheric gases, principally carbon dioxide, chlorofluorocarbons, ozone, methane, water vapor, and nitrous oxide, that are transparent to visible light but absorb infrared radiation.

groundwater   Water located under the surface of the ground.

group model HMO   A health maintenance organization (HMO) that contracts with a multispecialty group practice.

hallucinogens   Drugs that produce profound distortions of the senses.

hazard   An unsafe act or condition.

hazardous waste   A solid waste or combination of solid wastes that is dangerous to human health or the environment.

health   A dynamic state or condition of the human organism that is multidimensional in nature, a resource for living, and results from a person's interactions with and adaptations to his or her environment; therefore, it can exist in varying degrees and is specific to each individual and his or her situation.

health disparities   The difference in health between different populations.

health education   "Any combination of planned learning experiences using evidence based practices and/or sound theories that provide the opportunity to acquire knowledge, attitudes, and skills needed to adopt and maintain health behaviors."[9]

health maintenance organizations (HMOs)   Groups that supply prepaid comprehensive health care with an emphasis on prevention.

health promotion   "Any planned combination of educational, political, environmental, regulatory, or organizational mechanisms that support actions and conditions of living conducive to the health of individuals, groups, and communities."[9]

health resources development period   The period in public health history from 1900 to 1960; a time of great growth in healthcare facilities.

health-adjusted life expectancy (HALE)   The number of years of healthy life expected, on average, in a given population.

healthy school environment   "The promotion, maintenance, and utilization of safe and wholesome surroundings, organization of day-by-day experiences and planned learning procedures to influence favorable emotional, physical and social health."[12]

herd immunity   The resistance of a population to the spread of an infectious agent based on the immunity of a large portion of individuals.

home health care   Care that is provided in the patient's residence for the purpose of promoting, maintaining, or restoring health.

home healthcare services   Healthcare services provided in the patient's place of residence (home or apartment).

homebound   A person unable to leave home for normal activities such as shopping, meals, or other activities.

hospice care   "[A] cluster of special services for the dying, which blends medical, spiritual, legal, financial, and family-support services."[13]

Hospital Survey and Construction Act of 1946 (Hill-Burton Act)   Federal legislation that provided substantial funds for hospital construction.

host   A person or other living animal that affords subsistence or lodgment to a communicable agent under natural conditions.

hypercholesterolemia   High levels of cholesterol in the blood.

hypertension   Systolic pressure equal to or greater than 140 mm of mercury (Hg) and/or diastolic pressure equal to or greater than 90 mm Hg for extended periods of time.

illegal alien   An individual who entered this country without permission.

illicit (illegal) drugs   Drugs that cannot be legally manufactured, distributed, bought, or sold and that lack recognized medical value.

immigrants   Individuals who migrate to this country from another country for the purpose of seeking permanent residence.

impact evaluation   Focuses on the immediate observable effects of a program.

impairments   Defects in the functioning of one's sense organs or limitations in one's mobility or range of motion.

implementation   Putting a planned program into action.

incidence rate   The number of new health-related events or cases of a disease in a population exposed to that risk during a particular period of time, divided by the total number in that same population.

incubation period   The period of time between exposure to an infectious agent and the onset of symptoms.

independent practice associations (IPAs)   Legal entities separate from the health maintenance organization (HMO) that are physician organizations composed of community-based independent physicians in solo or group practices that provide services to HMO members.

independent providers   Healthcare professionals with the education and legal authority to treat any health problem.

indirect transmission   Communicable disease transmission involving an intermediate step; for example, airborne, vehicleborne, or vectorborne transmission.

industrial hygienist   A health professional concerned with health hazards in the workplace, including such things as problems with ventilation, noise, and lighting; also responsible for measuring air quality and recommending plans for improving the healthiness of work environments.

industrial smog   Smog formed primarily by sulfur dioxide and suspended particles from the burning of coal (also known as gray smog).

infectivity   The ability of a pathogen to lodge and grow in a host.

informal caregiver   One who provides unpaid care or assistance to someone who has some physical, mental, emotional, or financial need that limits his or her independence.

inhalants   Breathable substances that produce mind-altering effects; for example, glue.

injury   Physical harm or damage to the body resulting from an exchange, usually acute, of mechanical, chemical, thermal, or other environmental energy that exceeds the body's tolerance.

injury prevention education The process of changing people's health-directed behavior in such a way as to reduce unintentional injuries.

injury prevention/injury control An organized effort to reduce the number and seriousness of injuries and to minimize the number of injury deaths.

instrumental activities of daily living (IADLs) Measure of more complex tasks such as handling personal finances, preparing meals, shopping, doing housework, traveling, using the telephone, and taking medications.

intentional injury An injury that is judged to have been purposely inflicted, either by the victim or another person.

intervention An activity or activities designed to create change in people.

intimate partner violence (IPV) Rape, physical assault, or stalking perpetrated by current or former dates, spouses, or cohabiting partners (cohabiting means living together at least some of the time as a couple).

ionizing radiation High-energy radiation (ultraviolet radiation, gamma rays, X-rays, alpha and beta particles) that can knock an electron out of orbit, creating an ion, and can thereby damage living cells and tissues.

isolation The separation of infected persons from those who are susceptible.

Joint Commission The predominant organization responsible for accrediting healthcare facilities.

labor-force ratio A ratio of the total number of those individuals who are not working (regardless of age) to the number of those who are.

law enforcement The application of federal, state, and local laws to arrest, jail, bring to trial, and sentence those who break drug laws or break laws because of drug use.

leachates Liquids created when water mixes with wastes and removes soluble constituents from them by percolation.

lead A naturally occurring mineral element found throughout the environment and used in large quantities for industrial products, including batteries, pipes, solder, paints, and pigments.

licensed practical nurse (LPN) Those prepared in 1- to 2-year programs to provide nontechnical bedside nursing care under the supervision of physicians or registered nurses.

life expectancy The average number of years a person from a specific cohort is projected to live from a given point in time.

limited (restricted) care providers Healthcare providers who provide care for a specific part of the body; for example, dentists.

limited-service hospitals Hospitals that offer only the specific services needed by the population served.

litigation The process of seeking justice for injury through courts.

lobotomy Surgical severance of nerve fibers of the brain by incision.

long-term care Different kinds of help that people with chronic illnesses, disabilities, or other conditions need to deal with the circumstances that limit them physically or mentally.

low-birth-weight infant An infant who weighs less than 2,500 grams, or 5.5 pounds, at birth.

mainstream smoke Tobacco smoke inhaled and exhaled by the smoker.

major depression An affective disorder characterized by a dysphoric mood, usually depression, or loss of interest or pleasure in almost all usual activities or pastimes.

majority Those with characteristics that are found in more than 50% of a population.

malignant neoplasm Uncontrolled new tissue growth resulting from cells that have lost control over their growth and division.

managed care "[A]rrangements that link health care financing and service delivery and allows payers to exercise significant economic control over how and what services are delivered."[14]

marijuana Dried plant parts of *Cannabis sativa*.

maternal, infant, and child health The health of women of childbearing age from pre-pregnancy through pregnancy, labor and delivery, and the postpartum period, and the health of the child prior to birth through adolescence.

Meals on Wheels program A community-supported nutrition program in which prepared meals are delivered to elders in their homes, usually by volunteers.

median age The age at which half of the population is older and half is younger.

Medicaid A national federal–state health insurance program for low-income Americans.

medical preparedness "The ability of the health care system to prevent, protect against, quickly respond to, and recover from health emergencies, particularly those whose scale, timing, or unpredictability threatens to overwhelm routine capabilities."[15]

medically indigent Those lacking the financial ability to pay for their own medical care.

Medicare A national health insurance program for people 65 years of age or older, certain younger disabled people, and people with permanent kidney failure.

Medigap Private health insurance to supplement Medicare benefits—that is, to fill in the gaps of Medicare.

mental disorders Health conditions characterized by alterations in thinking, mood, or behavior (or some combination thereof) associated with distress and/or impaired functioning.

mental health Emotional and social well-being, including one's psychological resources for dealing with the day-to-day problems of life.

mental illness A collective term for all mental disorders.

Mental Retardation Facilities and Community Mental Health Centers (CMHC) Act A law that made the federal government responsible for assisting in the funding of mental health facilities and services.

metastasis The spread of a disease, such as cancer, by the transfer of cells by means of the blood or lymphatics.

methamphetamine The amphetamine drug most widely abused.

methaqualone An illicit depressant drug.

migration   Movement of people from one country to another.

minority groups   Subgroups of the population that consist of less than 50% of the population.

minority health   The morbidity and mortality of American Indians/Alaska Natives, Asian Americans and Pacific Islanders, black Americans, and Americans of Hispanic origin in the United States.

mixed model HMO   A hybrid form of a health maintenance organization.

model for unintentional injuries   The public health triangle (host, agent, and environment) modified to indicate energy as the causative agent of injuries.

modern era of public health   The era of U.S. public health that began in 1850 and continues today.

modifiable risk factors   Factors contributing to the development of a noncommunicable disease that can be altered by modifying one's behavior or environment; for example, cigarette smoking is a modifiable risk factor for coronary heart disease.

moral treatment   A nineteenth century treatment in which people with mental illness were removed from the everyday life stressors of their home environments and given "asylum" in a rural setting, including rest, exercise, fresh air, and amusements.

morbidity rate   The rate of illness in a population.

mortality (fatality) rate   The rate of deaths in a population.

multicausation disease model   A visual representation of the host, together with various internal and external factors that promote and protect against disease.

multiplicity   The number of activities that make up an intervention.

municipal solid waste (MSW)   Waste generated by individual households, businesses, and institutions located within municipalities.

narcotics   Drugs similar to morphine that reduce pain and induce a stuporous state.

natality (birth) rate   The rate of births in a population.

National Alliance on Mental Illness (NAMI)   A national grassroots mental health organization dedicated to support, education, advocacy, and research for people living with mental illness.

National Ambient Air Quality Standards (NAAQSs)   Standards created by the EPA for allowable concentration levels of outdoor air pollutants.

National Electronic Telecommunications System (NETS)   The electronic reporting system by which state health departments send health records to the Centers for Disease Control and Prevention (CDC).

National Institute for Occupational Safety and Health (NIOSH)   A research body within the Centers for Disease Control and Prevention, Department of Health and Human Services, that is responsible for developing and recommending occupational safety and health standards.

National Institute of Mental Health (NIMH)   The nation's leading mental health research agency; housed in the National Institutes of Health.

National Institute on Drug Abuse (NIDA)   The federal government's lead agency for drug abuse research; part of the National Institutes of Health.

natural disaster   A natural hazard that results in substantial loss of life or property.

natural hazards   Naturally occurring phenomena or events that produce or release energy in amounts that exceed human endurance, causing injury, disease, or death (such as radiation, earthquakes, tsunamis, volcanic eruptions, hurricanes, tornados, and floods).

needs assessment   The process of collecting and analyzing information to develop an understanding of the issues, resources, and constraints of the priority population, as related to the development of health promotion programs.

net migration   The population gain or loss resulting from migration.

network model HMO   A type of health maintenance organization that contracts with more than one medical group practice.

neuroleptic drugs   Drugs that reduce nervous activity; another term for antipsychotic drug.

nonallopathic providers   Independent providers who provide nontraditional forms of health care.

noncommunicable disease (noninfectious disease)   A disease not caused by a communicable agent, and that thus cannot be transmitted from infected host to susceptible host.

nonphysician practitioners (NPPs)   "[C]linical professionals who practice in many of the areas similar to those in which physicians practice, but who do not have an MD or DO degree."[13]

nonpoint source pollution   All pollution that occurs through the runoff, seepage, or falling of pollutants into the water.

notifiable diseases   Infectious diseases for which health officials request or require reporting for public health reasons.

observational study   An analytic, epidemiological study in which an investigator or investigators observe the natural course of events, noting exposed and unexposed subjects and disease development.

occupational injury   An injury that results from exposure to a single incident in the work environment (e.g., cut, fracture, sprain, amputation).

Occupational Safety and Health Act of 1970 (OSH Act)   Comprehensive federal legislation aimed at ensuring safe and healthy working conditions for working men and women.

Occupational Safety and Health Administration (OSHA)   The federal agency located within the Department of Labor and created by the Occupational Safety and Health Act of 1970 (OSH Act) that is charged with the responsibility of administering the provisions of the OSH Act.

odds ratio   A probability statement about the association between a particular disease and a specific risk factor, often the outcome of a case/control epidemiologic study.

Office of National Drug Control Policy (ONDCP)   The headquarters of the United States' drug control effort, located in the executive branch of the federal government and headed by a director appointed by the president.

Older Americans Act of 1965 (OAA)   Federal legislation to improve the lives of elders.

operationalize (operational definition)   To provide working definitions.

osteopathic providers   Independent healthcare providers whose remedies emphasize the interrelationships of the body's systems in prevention, diagnosis, and treatment.

outcome evaluation   Focuses on the end result of the program.

outpatient care facilities   Any facility in which the patient receives care and does not stay overnight.

ozone (O_3)   An inorganic molecule considered to be a pollutant in the atmosphere because it harms human tissue but considered beneficial in the stratosphere because it screens out ultraviolet radiation.

packaged pricing   Several related health services are included in one price.

pandemic   An outbreak of disease over a wide geographic area, such as a continent.

passive smoking   The inhalation of environmental tobacco smoke by nonsmokers.

pathogenicity   The capability of a communicable agent to cause disease in a susceptible host.

peer counseling programs   School-based drug education programs in which students discuss alcohol and other drug-related problems with other students.

pesticides   Synthetic chemicals developed and manufactured for the purpose of killing pests.

pharmaceuticals and personal care products (PPCPs)   Synthetic chemicals found in everyday consumer healthcare products and cosmetics.

phasing in   Implementation of an intervention with small groups prior to its implementation with the entire priority population.

philanthropic foundation   An endowed institution that donates money for the good of humankind.

photochemical smog   The visible, photochemical smog formed when air pollutants interact with sunlight.

physical dependence   Drug dependence in which discontinued use results in the onset of physical illness.

pilot test   Presentation of an intervention to just a few individuals, who are either from the intended priority population or from a very similar population.

placebo   A blank treatment (e.g., a sugar pill).

pneumoconiosis   Fibrotic lung disease caused by the inhalation of dusts, especially mineral dusts.

point-of-service (POS) option   An option of a health maintenance organization plan that allows enrollees to be at least partially reimbursed for selecting a healthcare provider outside the plan.

point source epidemic curve   An epidemic curve depicting a distribution of cases that can all be traced to a single source of exposure.

point source pollution   Pollution that can be traced to a single identifiable source.

polydrug use   Concurrent use of multiple drugs.

population at risk   Those in the population who are susceptible to a particular disease or condition.

population-based public health practice   Incorporates interventions aimed at disease prevention and health promotion, specific protection, and case findings.

population health   The health status of people who are not organized and have no identity as a group or locality and the actions and conditions to promote, protect, and preserve their health.

preconception health care (pre- or interconception health)   Health care that begins before pregnancy, or in between pregnancies, when a woman is considering becoming pregnant.

pre-existing condition   A medical condition that was diagnosed or treated usually within 6 months before the date a health insurance policy goes into effect.

preferred provider organization (PPO)   An organization that buys fixed-rate (discount) health services from providers and sells them (via premiums) to consumers.

prenatal health care (prenatal care)   One of the fundamentals of a healthy pregnancy program that includes three major components: risk assessment, treatment for medical conditions or risk reduction, and education. Prenatal health care should begin *preconceptionally* (before pregnancy), when a woman is considering becoming pregnant, and should continue throughout pregnancy.

prescription drugs   Drugs that can be purchased only with written instructions from a physician, dentist, or other licensed independent healthcare provider (a prescription).

prevalence rate   The number of new and old cases of a disease in a population in a given period of time, divided by the total number of that population.

prevention   The planning for and taking of action to forestall the onset of a disease or other health problem before the occurrence of undesirable health events.

primary care   "[C]linical preventive services, first-contact treatment services, and ongoing care for commonly encountered medical conditions."[16]

primary pollutants   Air pollutants emanating directly from transportation, power and industrial plants, and refineries.

primary prevention   Preventive measures that forestall the onset of illness or injury during the prepathogenesis period.

priority population (audience)   Those whom a program is intended to serve.

pro-choice   A medical/ethical position that holds that women have a right to reproductive freedom.

pro-life   A medical/ethical position that holds that performing an abortion is an act of murder.

problem drinker   One for whom alcohol consumption results in personal, economic, medical, social, or any other type of problem.

professional nurse   A registered nurse holding a bachelor of science degree in nursing (BSN).

program planning   A process by which an intervention is planned to help meet the needs of a priority population.

propagated epidemic curve   An epidemic curve depicting a distribution of cases traceable to multiple sources of exposure over time.

proportionate mortality ratio (PMR)   The percentage of overall mortality in a population that can be assigned to a particular cause or disease.

prospective reimbursement   "[U]ses certain established criteria to determine the amount of reimbursement in advance, before services are delivered."[13]

providers   Healthcare facilities or health professionals that provide healthcare services.

psychiatric rehabilitation   Intensive, individualized services encompassing treatment, rehabilitation, and support delivered by a team of providers over an indefinite period to individuals with severe mental disorder to help them maintain stable lives in the community.

psychoactive drugs   Mind-altering drugs; drugs that affect the central nervous system.

psychological dependence   A psychological state characterized by an overwhelming desire to continue use of a drug.

psychopharmacological therapy   Treatment for mental illness that involves medications.

psychotherapy   A treatment that involves verbal communication between the patient and a trained clinician.

public health   "[W]hat we as a society do collectively to assure the conditions in which people can be healthy."[15]

public health preparedness   "The ability of the public health system, community, and individuals to prevent, protect against, quickly respond to, and recover from health emergencies, particularly those in which scale, timing, or unpredictability threatens to overwhelm routine capabilities."[16]

public health system   "[A]ctivities undertaken within the formal structure of government and the associated efforts of private and voluntary organizations and individuals."[15]

public hospitals   Hospitals that are supported and managed by governmental jurisdictions.

public policy   The guiding principles and courses of action pursued by governments to solve practical problems affecting society.

quality management and utilization review   The analysis of provided health care for its appropriateness by someone other than the patient and provider.

quarantine   Limitation of freedom of movement of those who have been exposed to a disease and may be incubating it.

quasi-governmental health organizations   Organizations that have some responsibilities assigned by the government but operate more like voluntary agencies; for example, the American Red Cross.

radiation   A process in which energy is emitted as particles or waves.

radon   A naturally occurring, colorless, tasteless, odorless, radioactive gas formed during the radioactive decay of uranium-238.

rate   The number of events (cases of disease) that occur in a given period of time.

recovery   Outcome sought by most people with mental illness; includes increased independence, effective coping, supportive relationships, community participation, and sometimes gainful employment.

recycling   The collecting, sorting, and processing of materials that would otherwise be considered waste into raw materials for manufacturing new products, and the subsequent use of those new products.

reform phase of public health   The period of public health from 1900 to 1920, characterized by social movements to improve health conditions in cities and in the workplace.

refugee   A person who flees one area or country to seek shelter or protection from danger in another.

registered environmental health specialists (REHSs) (sanitarians)   Environmental workers responsible for the inspection of restaurants, retail food outlets, public housing, and other sites to ensure compliance with public health codes.

registered nurse (RN)   One who has successfully completed an accredited academic program and a state licensing examination.

regulation   The enactment and enforcement of laws to control conduct.

rehabilitation center   A facility in which restorative care is provided following injury, disease, or surgery.

reimbursement   Payments made by the third-party payers to providers.

relative risk   A statement of the relationship between the risk of acquiring a disease when a specific risk factor is present and the risk of acquiring that same disease when the risk factor is not present.

resident   A physician who is training in a specialty.

resource-based relative value scale   Reimbursement to physicians according to the relative value of the service provided.

Resource Conservation and Recovery Act of 1976 (RCRA)   The federal law that sets forth guidelines for the proper handling and disposal of solid and hazardous wastes.

respite care   Planned short-term care, usually for the purpose of relieving a full-time informal caregiver.

restorative care   Care provided to patients after a successful treatment or when the progress of an incurable disease has been arrested.

retirement communities   Residential communities that have been specifically developed for those in their retirement years.

risk factors   Factors that increase the probability of disease, injury, or death.

Roe v. Wade   A 1973 Supreme Court decision that made it unconstitutional for state laws to prohibit abortions.

Rohypnol (flunitrazepam)   A depressant in the benzodiazepine group that has achieved notoriety as a date rape drug.

runoff   Water that flows over land surfaces (including paved surfaces), typically from precipitation.

Safe Drinking Water Act (SDWA)   The federal law that regulates the safety of public drinking water.

sanitary landfills   Waste disposal sites on land suited for this purpose and on which waste is spread in thin layers, compacted, and covered with a fresh layer of clay or plastic foam each day.

sanitation   The practice of establishing and maintaining healthy or hygienic conditions in the environment.

school health advisory committee "[S]chool, health, and community representatives who act collectively to advise the school district or school on aspects of Coordinated School Health sometimes referred to as a school wellness council."[9]

school health coordinator A professional at the district (or school) level responsible for management and coordination of all school health policies, activities, and resources.

school health education The development, delivery, and evaluation of a planned curriculum, kindergarten through grade 12.

school health policies Written statements that describe the nature and procedures of a school health program.

school health services Health services provided by school health workers to appraise, protect, and promote the health of students and school personnel.

scope Part of the curriculum that outlines what will be taught.

secondary medical care Specialized attention and ongoing management for common and less frequently encountered medical conditions, including support services for people with special challenges due to chronic or long-term conditions.

secondary pollutants Air pollutants formed when primary air pollutants react with sunlight and other atmospheric components to form new harmful compounds.

secondary prevention Preventive measures that lead to early diagnosis and prompt treatment of a disease or injury to limit disability and prevent more severe pathogenesis.

secondhand smoke See *environmental tobacco smoke*.

self-funded insurance program A program that pays the healthcare costs of its employees with the premiums collected from the employees and the contributions made by the employer.

self-help groups Groups of concerned members of the community who are united by a shared interest, concern, or deficit not shared by other members of the community (Alcoholics Anonymous, for example).

septic tank A watertight concrete or fiberglass tank that holds sewage; one of two main parts of a septic system.

sequence Part of the curriculum that states in what order the content will be taught.

sick building syndrome A situation in which the air quality in a building produces generalized signs and symptoms of ill health in the building's occupants.

sidestream tobacco smoke The smoke that comes off the end of burning tobacco products.

silicosis Acute or chronic lung disease caused by the inhalation of free crystalline silica; those affected include workers in mines, stone quarries, sand and gravel operations, and abrasive blasting operations.

sliding scale fee A fee based on ability to pay.

social capital "Relationships and structures within a community that promote cooperation for mutual benefit."[7]

socioeconomic status A demographic term that takes into consideration the combination of social and economic factors.

solid waste Solid refuse from households, agriculture, and businesses.

solid waste management (integrated waste management) The collection, transportation, and disposal of solid waste.

source reduction A waste management approach involving the reduction or elimination of use of materials that produce an accumulation of solid waste.

Special Supplemental Food Program for Women, Infants, and Children See *WIC*.

specific rate A rate of a specific disease in a population or the rate of events in a specific population (e.g., cause-specific death rate, age-specific death rate).

spectrum of healthcare delivery The array of types of care—from preventive to continuing, or long-term, care. It comprises four levels of care.

staff model HMO A health maintenance organization that hires its own staff of health care providers.

standard of acceptability A comparative mandate, value, norm, or group.

Statistical Abstract of the United States The standard summary of statistics on the social, political, and economic organization of the United States published by the U.S. Census Bureau.

stimulant A drug that increases the activity of the central nervous system; for example, methamphetamine.

student assistance programs (SAPs) School-based drug education programs to assist students who have alcohol or other drug problems.

Substance Abuse and Mental Health Services Administration (SAMHSA) An operating division of the U.S. Department of Health and Human Services whose stated mission is the reduction of the incidence and prevalence of alcohol and other drug abuse and mental disorders, the improvement of treatment outcomes, and the curtailment of the consequences of mental health problems for families and communities.

sudden infant death syndrome (SIDS) Sudden unanticipated death of an infant in whom, after examination, there is no recognized cause of death.

sudden unexpected infant death (SUID) "[D]eaths in infants less than 1 year of age that occur suddenly and unexpectedly, and whose cause of death are not immediately obvious prior to investigation."[17]

summative evaluation The evaluation that determines the impact of a program on the priority population.

Superfund legislation See *Comprehensive Environmental Response, Compensation, and Liability Act (CERCLA)*.

Supplemental Security Program of the Social Security Administration that provides cash benefits to elderly, blind, and disabled Americans with minimal resources.

surface water Precipitation that does not infiltrate the ground or return to the atmosphere by evaporation; the water in streams, rivers, and lakes.

Synar Amendment A federal law that requires states to set the minimum legal age for purchasing tobacco products at 18 years and that requires states to enforce this law.

synesthesia Impairment of the mind (by hallucinogens) characterized by a sensation that senses are mixed (e.g., seeing sounds, hearing images).

tardive dyskinesia An irreversible condition of involuntary and abnormal movements of the tongue, mouth, arms, and legs, which can result from long-term use of certain antipsychotic drugs (such as chlorpromazine).

task force "A self-contained group of 'doers' that is not ongoing, but rather brought together due to a strong interest in an issue and for a specific purpose."[3]

terrorism Calculated use of violence (or threat of violence) against civilians to attain goals that are political, religious, or ideological in nature.

tertiary medical care Specialized and technologically sophisticated medical and surgical care for those with unusual or complex conditions (generally no more than a few percent of the need in any service category).

tertiary prevention Measures aimed at rehabilitation following significant pathogenesis.

thermal inversion Condition that occurs when warm air traps cooler air at the surface of the earth.

third-party payment system A health insurance term indicating that bills will be paid by the insurer (the government or private insurance company) and not the patient (the first party) or the healthcare provider (the second party).

Thorazine See *chlorpromazine*.

Title X A portion of the Public Health Service Act of 1970 that provides funds for family planning services for low-income people.

tolerance Physiological and enzymatic adjustments that occur in response to the chronic presence of drugs, reflected in the need for ever-increasing doses to achieve a previous level of effect.

top-down funding A method of funding in which funds are transmitted from the federal or state government to the local level.

total dependency ratio The dependency ratio that includes both youth and elders.

transinstitutionalization Transferring patients from one type of public institution to another, usually as a result of policy change.

treatment (for drug abuse and dependence) Care that removes the physical, emotional, and environmental conditions that have contributed to drug abuse and/or dependence.

ultraviolet (UV) radiation Radiation energy with wavelengths 0 to 400 nanometers.

unintentional injury An injury judged to have occurred without anyone intending that harm be done.

unmodifiable risk factors Factors contributing to the development of a noncommunicable disease that cannot be altered by modifying one's behavior or environment.

unsafe act Any behavior that would increase the probability of an injury occurring.

unsafe condition Any environmental factor or set of factors (physical or social) that would increase the probability of an injury occurring.

U.S. Census The enumeration of the population of the United States that is conducted every 10 years; begun in 1790.

vector A living organism, usually an arthropod, that can transmit a communicable disease agent to a susceptible host (e.g., mosquitoes, ticks, lice, fleas).

vectorborne disease outbreak (VBDO) An occurrence of an unexpectedly large number of cases of disease caused by an agent transmitted by insects or other arthropods.

vehicle An inanimate material or object, such as clothes, bedding, toys, or hypodermic needles, or nonliving biological materials, such as food, milk, water, blood, serum or plasma, tissues, or organs, that can serve as a source of infection.

vehicleborne disease A communicable disease transmitted by nonliving objects; for example, typhoid fever can be transmitted by water.

visitor services A community social service involving one individual taking time to visit with another who is unable to leave his or her residence.

vital statistics Statistical summaries of vital records—records of major life events, such as births, deaths, marriages, divorces, and infant deaths.

volatile organic compounds (VOCs) Compounds that exist as vapors over the normal range of air pressures and temperatures.

voluntary health agency A nonprofit organization created by concerned citizens to deal with health needs not met by governmental health agencies.

voluntary hospital A nonprofit hospital administered by a religious, fraternal, or other charitable community organization.

wastewater The aqueous mixture that remains after water has been used or contaminated by humans.

wastewater treatment The process of improving the quality of wastewater (sewage) to the point that it can be released into a body of water without seriously disrupting the aquatic environment, causing health problems in humans, or causing nuisance conditions.

water pollution Any physical or chemical change in water that can harm living organisms or make the water unfit for other uses.

waterborne disease outbreak (WBDO) A disease in which at least two persons experience a similar illness after the ingestion of drinking water or after exposure to water used for recreational purposes and epidemiological evidence implicates water as the probable source of the illness.

watershed The area of land from which all of the water that is under it or drains from it goes into the same place and drains in one point; for example, the Mississippi River watershed drains and collects all the water from the land extending from east of the Rocky Mountains to the Appalachian Mountains and from the upper Midwest all the way south to the Gulf of Mexico.

WIC A federal program sponsored by the U.S. Department of Agriculture designed to provide supplemental foods, nutrition and health education, and referrals for health and social services to improve the health of at-risk, economically disadvantaged women who are pregnant or are caring for infants and children under age 5.

(Also known as the Special Supplemental Food Program for Women, Infants, and Children.)

withdrawal illness (abstinence syndrome) The unpleasant feelings or painful, clinically recognized symptoms that arise when one abstains from a dependence-producing drug after tolerance develops.

workers' compensation laws A set of federal laws designed to compensate those workers and their families who suffer injuries, disease, or death from workplace exposure.

World Health Assembly Body of delegates of the member nations of the World Health Organization.

World Health Organization (WHO) The most widely recognized international governmental health organization today. Created in 1948 by representatives of United Nations countries.

years of potential life lost (YPLL) The number of years lost when death occurs before the age of 65 or 75.

young old Those 65 to 74 years of age.

youth dependency ratio The dependency ratio that includes only youth.

youth gang A self-formed association of peers, bound together by mutual interests, with identifiable leadership and well-defined lines of authority, who act in concert to achieve a specific purpose and whose acts generally include illegal activity and control over a territory or an enterprise.

zoonosis A communicable disease transmissible under natural conditions from vertebrate animals to humans.

References

1. Assisted Living Federation of America (2010). "What Is Assisted Living?" Available at http://www.alfa.org/alfa/Assisted_Living_Information.asp?SnID=1383416766.
2. Green, L. W., and M. W. Kreuter (2005). *Health Program Planning: An Educational and Ecological Approach*, 4th ed. Boston: McGraw-Hill.
3. Butterfoss, F. D. (2007). *Coalitions and Partnerships in Community Health*. San Francisco, CA: Jossey-Bass.
4. Minkler, M., N. Wallerstein, and N. Wilson (2008). "Improving Health Through Community Organizing and Community Building." In K. Glanz, B. K. Rimer, and K. Viswanath, eds., *Health Behavior and Health Education Practice: Theory, Research, and Practice*, 4th ed. San Francisco: Jossey-Bass, 287–312.
5. Minkler, M. (2012). "Introduction to Community Organizing and Community Building." In M. Minkler, ed., *Community Organizing and Community Building for Health and Welfare*, 3rd ed. New Brunswick, NJ: Rutgers University Press, 5–26.
6. Goodman, R. M., M. A. Speers, K. McLeroy, S. Fawcett, M. Kegler, E. Parker, S. R. Smith, T. D. Sterling, and N. Wallerstein (1998). "Identifying and Defining the Dimensions of Community Capacity to Provide a Basis for Measurement." *Health Education and Behavior*, 25(3): 258–278.
7. Minkler, M., and N. Wallerstein (2012). "Improving Health through Community Organizing and Community Building: Perspectives from Health Education and Social Work." In M. Minkler, ed., *Community Organizing and Community Building for Health and Welfare*, 3rd ed. New Brunswick, NJ: Rutgers University Press, 37–58.
8. National Institutes of Health, National Center for Complementary and Alternative Medicine (2011). "What Is Complementary and Alternative Medicine?" Available at http://nccam.nih.gov/health/whatiscam.
9. Joint Committee on Health Education and Promotion Terminology (2012). *Report of the 2011 Joint Committee on Health Education and Promotion Terminology*. Reston, VA: American Association of Health Education.
10. Slee, D. A., V. N. Slee, and H. J. Schmidt (2008). *Slee's Health Care Terms*, 5th ed. Sudbury, MA: Jones & Bartlett.
11. Institute of Medicine (1997). *America's Vital Interest in Global Health: Protecting Our People, Enhancing Our Economy, and Advancing Our International Interests*. Washington, DC: National Academies Press. Available at http://books.nap.edu/openbook.php?record_id=5717&page=R1.
12. Joint Committee on Health Education Terminology (1974). "New Definitions: Report of the 1972–73 Joint Committee on Health Education Terminology." *Journal of School Health*, 44(1): 33–37.
13. Shi, L., and D. A. Singh (2012). *Delivering Health Care in America: A Systems Approach*, 5th ed. Burlington, MA: Jones & Bartlett Learning.
14. Sultz, H. A., and K. M. Young (2011). *Health Care USA: Understanding Its Organization and Delivery*, 7th ed. Burlington, MA: Jones & Bartlett.
15. Institute of Medicine (1988). *The Future of Public Health*. Washington, DC: National Academies Press.
16. Centers for Disease Control and Prevention (2012). *Emergency Preparedness and Response: What CDC Is Doing*. Available at http://www.bt.cdc.gov/cdc.
17. Centers for Disease Control and Prevention (2012). "Sudden Unexpected Infant Death." Available at http://www.cdc.gov/SIDS.

Index